MRI and CT of the Brain

MRI and CT of the Brain

Edited by

James E Gillespie DMRD FRCR
Consultant Neuroradiologist, Manchester Royal Infirmary; Lecturer in Diagnostic Radiology, University of Manchester, Manchester, UK

Alan Jackson PhD MRCP FRCR
Professor of Neuroradiology, Division of Imaging Sciences and Biomedical Engineering, University of Manchester Medical School; Honorary Consultant Neuroradiologist, Manchester Royal Infirmary, Manchester, UK

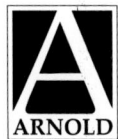

A member of the Hodder Headline Group
LONDON
Co-published in the United States of America by
Oxford University Press Inc., New York

First published in Great Britain in 2000 by
Arnold, a member of the Hodder Headline Group,
338 Euston Road, London NW1 3BH

http://www.arnoldpublishers.com

© 2000 Arnold

All rights reserved. No part of this publication may be reproduced or
transmitted in any form or by any means, electronically or mechanically,
including photocopying, recording or any information storage or retrieval
system, without either prior permission in writing from the publisher or a
licence permitting restricted copying. In the United Kingdom such licences
are issued by the Copyright Licensing Agency: 90 Tottenham Court Road,
London W1P 9HE.

Whilst the advice and information in this book are believed to be true and
accurate at the date of going to press, neither the author[s] nor the publisher
can accept any legal responsibility or liability for any errors or omissions
that may be made. In particular (but without limiting the generality of the
preceding disclaimer) every effort has been made to check drug dosages;
however it is still possible that errors have been missed. Furthermore,
dosage schedules are constantly being revised and new side-effects
recognized. For these reasons the reader is strongly urged to consult the
drug companies' printed instructions before administering any of the drugs
recommended in this book.

British Library Cataloguing in Publication Data
A catalogue record for this book is available from the British Library

Library of Congress Cataloguing-in-Publication Data
A catalog record for this book is available from the Library of Congress

ISBN 0 340 761 21 0

1 2 3 4 5 6 7 8 9 10

Commissioning Editor: Nick Dunton
Production Editor: Anke Ueberberg
Production Controller: Iain McWilliams
Project Manager: Jane Duncan

Typeset by Phoenix Photosetting, Chatham, Kent
Printed and bound in the United Kingdom by
The Bath Press, Bath

What do you think about this book? Or any other Arnold title?
Please send your comments to feedback.arnold@hodder.co.uk

To my wife Denise and children, Jenny, Mark and David
for their never-ending love and support

JEG

To my wife Susan
with love

AJ

Contents

List of Contributors		ix
Preface		xi
Acknowledgement		xii

PART 1 ATLAS OF NORMAL BRAIN ANATOMY 1

PART 2 ATLAS OF BRAIN PATHOLOGY 22

PART 3

1	Congenital abnormalities James E Gillespie	44
2	Trauma Donald M Hadley, Evelyn M Teasdale	73
3	Supratentorial tumours Shawn F S Halpin	98
4	Infratentorial tumours Margaret D Hourihan	140
5	Haemorrhagic vascular disease Paul D Griffiths, Anil Gholkar	162
6	Non-haemorrhagic vascular disease Paul Butler	187
7	Infections and inflammatory diseases Charles A J Romanowski	212
8	Neurodegenerative and white matter diseases Alan Jackson	241
9	Hydrocephalus Roger D Laitt, David G Hughes	266
10	Advanced techniques in neuroradiology Alan Jackson, Steve Williams	280
	Colour plate section	following page 292
	INDEX	293

Contributors

Paul Butler MRCP FRCR
Consultant Neuroradiologist, The Royal London Hospital, London, UK

Anil Gholkar FRCP
Consultant Neuroradiologist, Newcastle General Hospital, Newcastle upon Tyne, UK

James E Gillespie DMRD FRCR
Consultant Neuroradiologist, Manchester Royal Infirmary and Lecturer in Diagnostic Radiology, Universtiy of Manchester, Manchester, UK

Paul D Griffiths PhD FRCR
Professor, Section of Radiology, Royal Hallamshire Hospital, Sheffield, UK

Donald M Hadley PhD FRCR DMRD
Consultant Neuroradiologist, Professor of Radiology, Institute of Neurological Sciences and Senior Radiological Research Fellow, University of Glasgow, Scotland

Shawn F S Halpin MRCP FRCR
Consultant Neuroradiologist, University Hospital of Wales, Cardiff, Wales

Margaret D Hourihan FRCR
Consultant Neuroradiologist, University Hospital of Wales, Cardiff, Wales

David G Hughes MRCP FRCR
Consultant Neuroradiologist, Hope Hospital, Salford, UK

Alan Jackson PhD MRCP FRCR
Professor of Neuroradiology, Division of Imaging Sciences and Biomedical Engineering, University of Manchester Medical School and Honorary Consultant Neuroradiologist, Manchester Royal Infirmary, Manchester, UK

Roger D Laitt MRCP FRCR
Consultant Neuroradiologist, Manchester Royal Infirmary, Manchester, UK

Charles A J Romanowski BSc MRCP FRCR
Consultant Neuroradiologist, Royal Hallamshire Hospital, Sheffield, UK

Evelyn M Teasdale MRCP FRCR
Consultant Neuroradiologist, Institute of Neurological Sciences and Senior Lecturer, University of Glasgow, Scotland

Steve Williams MA DPhil
Professor of Imaging Sciences, University of Manchester, Manchester, UK

Preface

Cross-sectional imaging of the brain has advanced beyond all recognition since the advent of computed tomography (CT) in 1973. Current generation CT scanners produce high quality bone and soft tissue images in seconds and are considered standard equipment in modern general hospitals. Magnetic resonance imaging (MRI) produces anatomical images of even greater quality and is expanding our horizons further with physiological or functional brain imaging.

Although most highly specialized neurological studies and imaging research are performed in specialized neuroscience units, the widespread availability of CT and, increasingly, MR scanners has resulted in many patients having their initial imaging investigations conducted in non-specialist units. Consequently, general radiologists must become adept in the interpretation of brain CT and MRI. This evolving situation was the stimulus for this volume.

The book is divided into three parts. As a basic understanding of cerebral anatomy is the starting point in image interpretation and accurate communication of information to clinical colleagues, Part 1 is a multiplanar anatomical atlas of CT and MR images. The CT images are in the axial plane with 5mm slices through the posterior fossa and 10mm slices to the vertex. The MR images are from a 1.5 T Philips NT system presented in the three orthogonal planes, using an inversion-recovery turbo-spin echo sequence with data reconstruction optimized for grey and white matter differentiation. Also included are drawings of specific areas of anatomical complexity.

The next stage of image interpretation involves an analysis of lesion configuration, density/signal and enhancement characteristics. Combining this with anatomical location should lead to a differential diagnosis. Part 2 of the book is therefore an atlas of differential diagnoses. To keep this part a manageable size the number of illustrated lists we could include was limited and each list contains what we consider the five most common individual lesions or categories of pathology encountered. Nevertheless we hope this section will provide a useful starting point in formulating a differential diagnosis which can be supplemented by reading Part 3.

Part 3 is the largest and most detailed portion of the book and contains ten chapters covering the major categories of brain pathology in both adults and children. Because of their frequency in everyday practice cerebral vascular disease and neoplasms are given two chapters each. The final chapter is an overview of recent technical advances in cerebral imaging including diffusion and perfusion imaging, and spectroscopy.

Though written primarily for general radiologists and radiologists in training, we hope the book will appeal to neurosurgeons, neurologists or others with an interest in neuroimaging.

James E Gillespie
Alan Jackson

The Editors and Publisher
are grateful to acknowledge financial support from
Philips Medical Systems
for the reproduction of colour images in this book

Part 1: Atlas of normal brain anatomy

Sagittal images

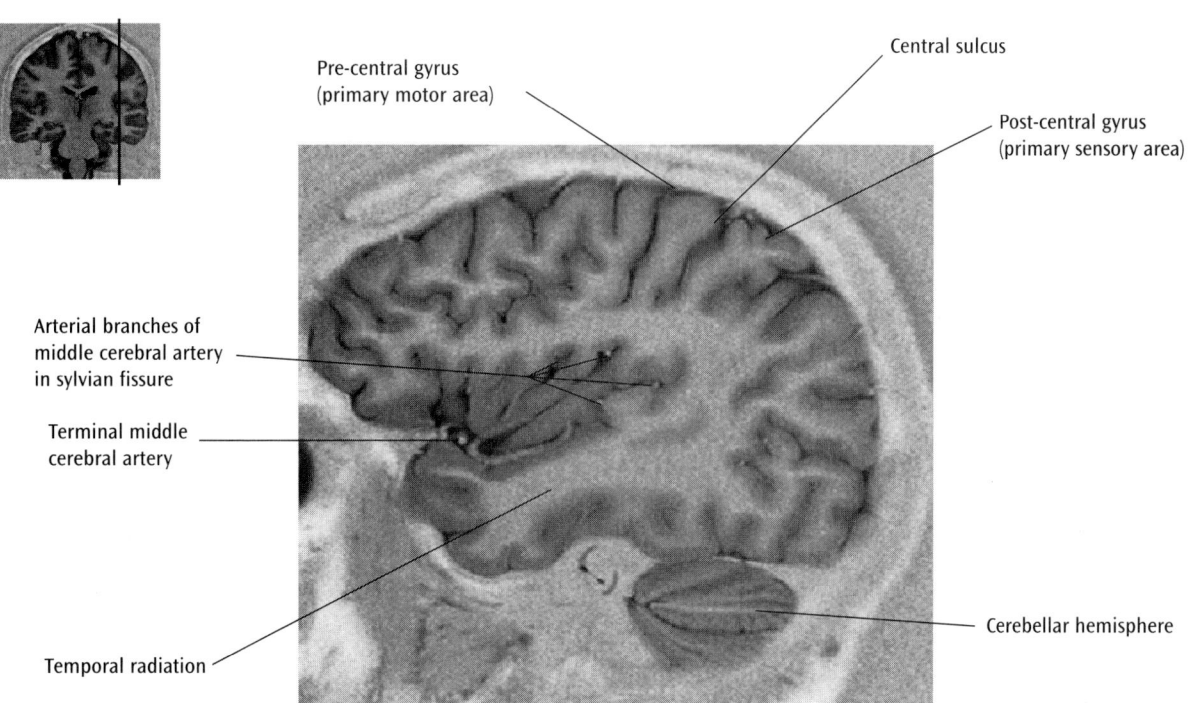

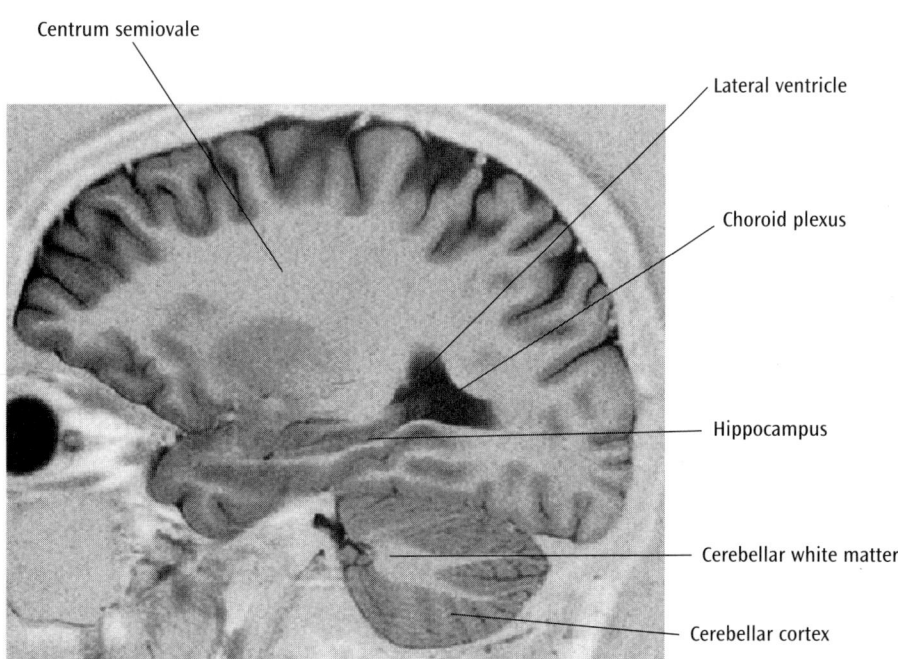

Sagittal images

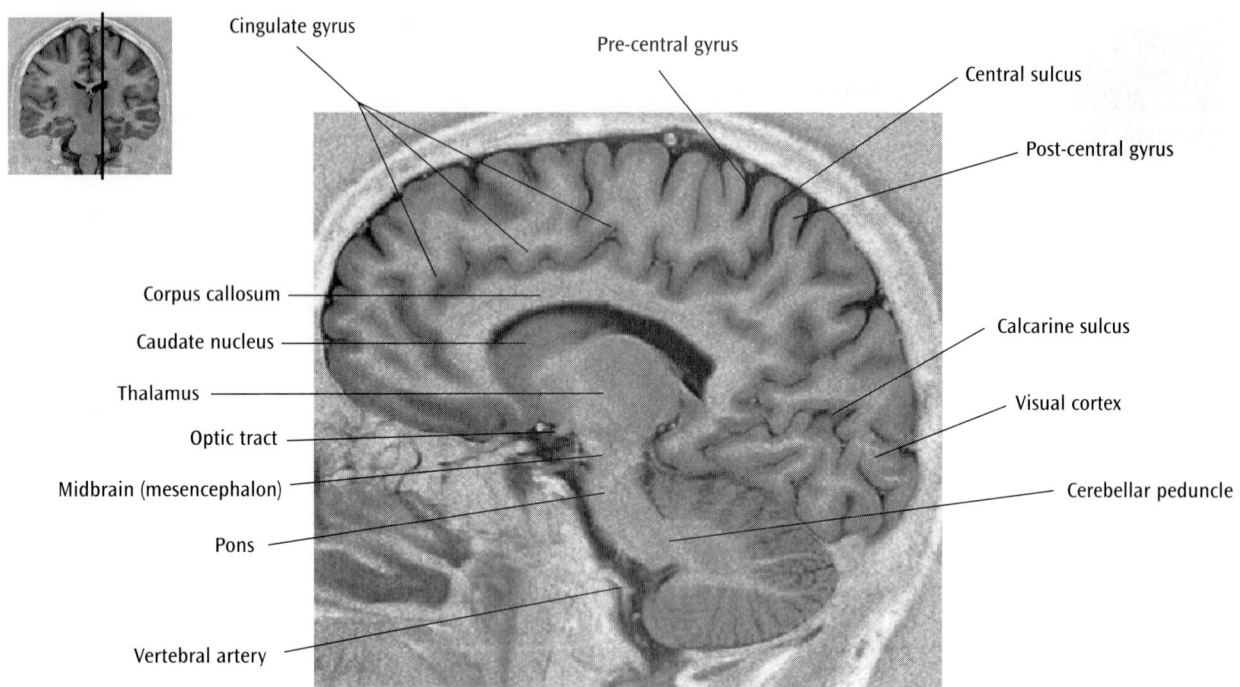

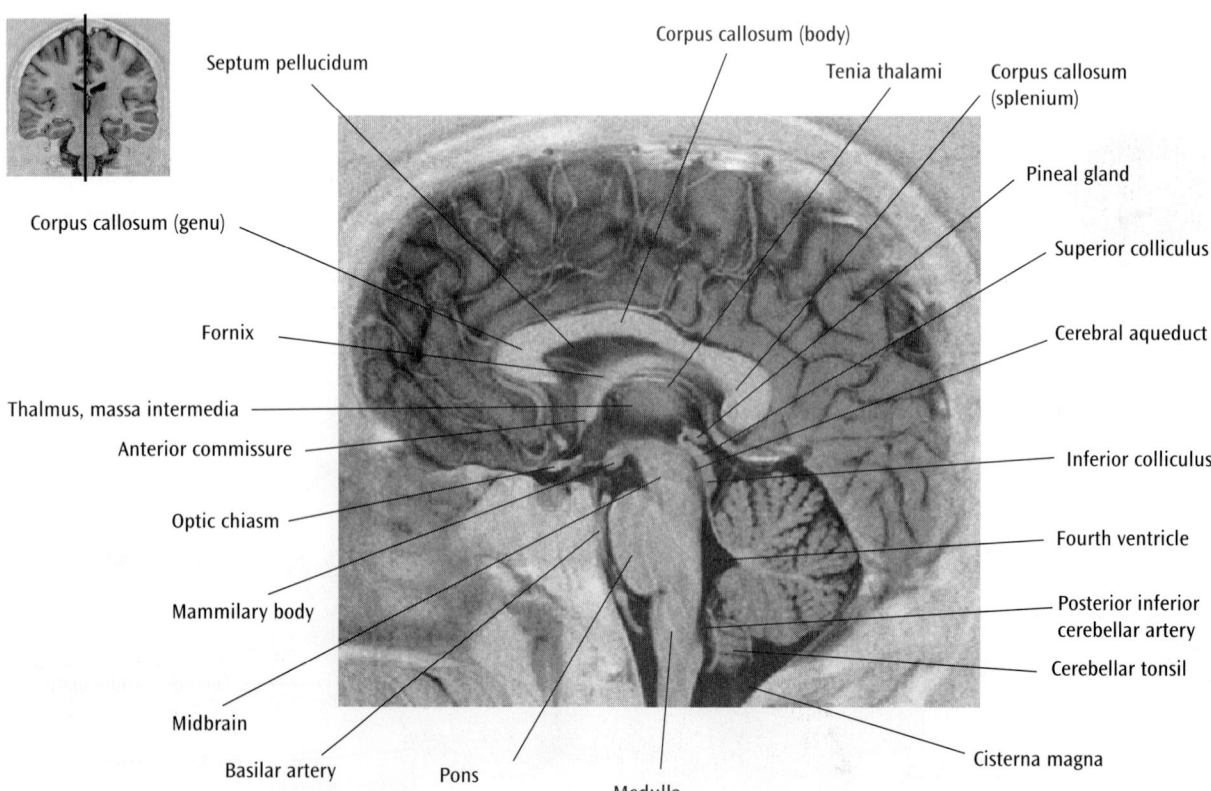

Coronal images

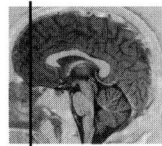
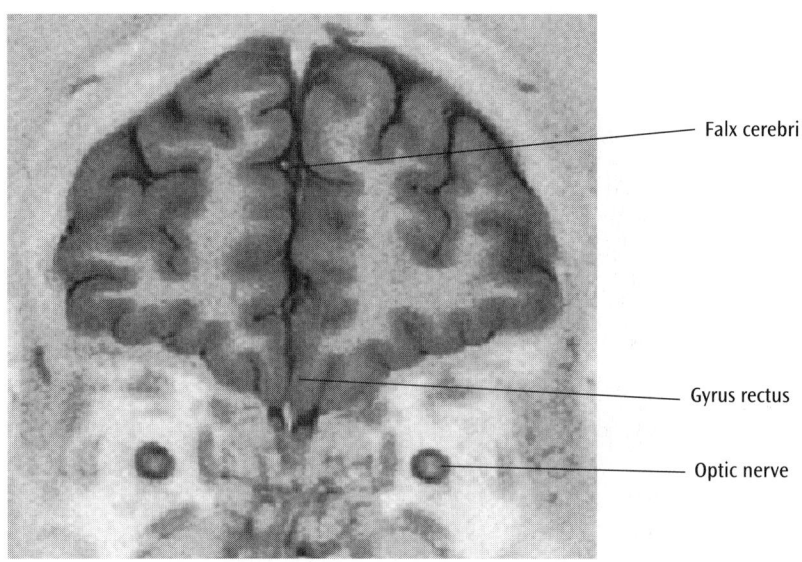

- Falx cerebri
- Gyrus rectus
- Optic nerve

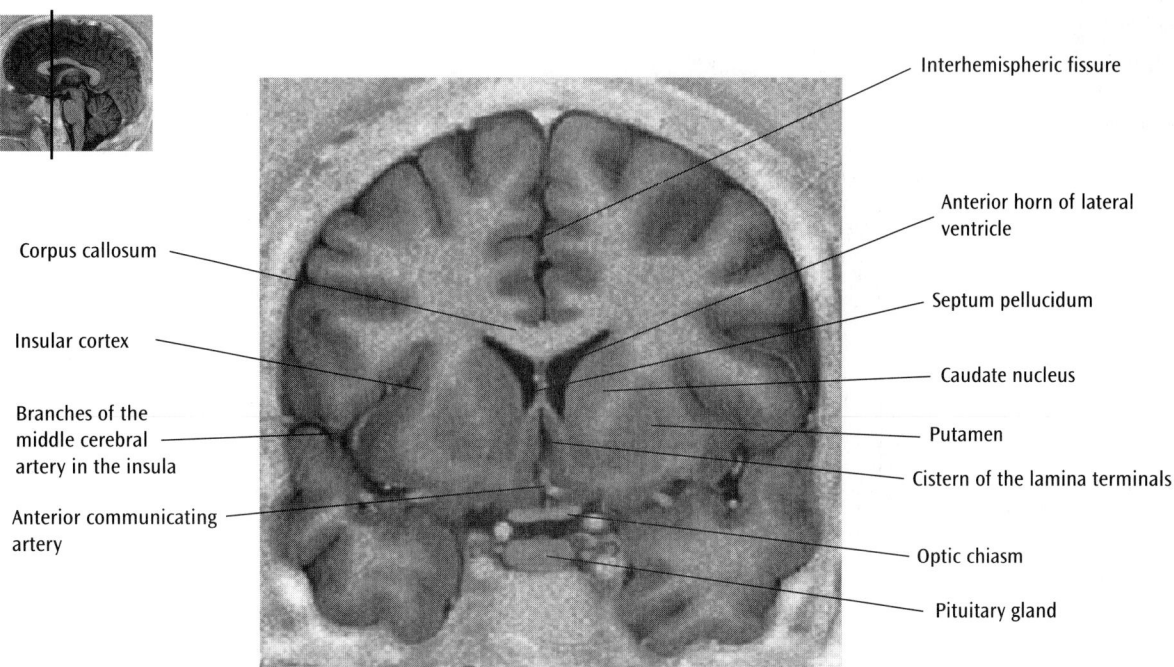

- Interhemispheric fissure
- Anterior horn of lateral ventricle
- Septum pellucidum
- Caudate nucleus
- Putamen
- Cistern of the lamina terminals
- Optic chiasm
- Pituitary gland
- Corpus callosum
- Insular cortex
- Branches of the middle cerebral artery in the insula
- Anterior communicating artery

Coronal images

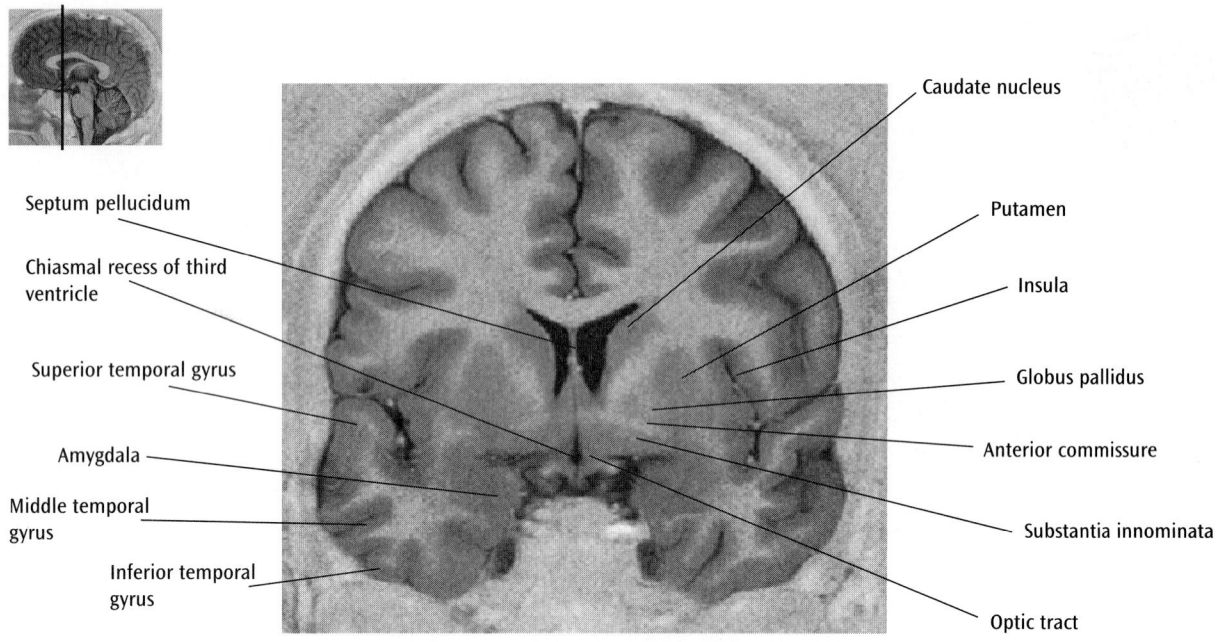

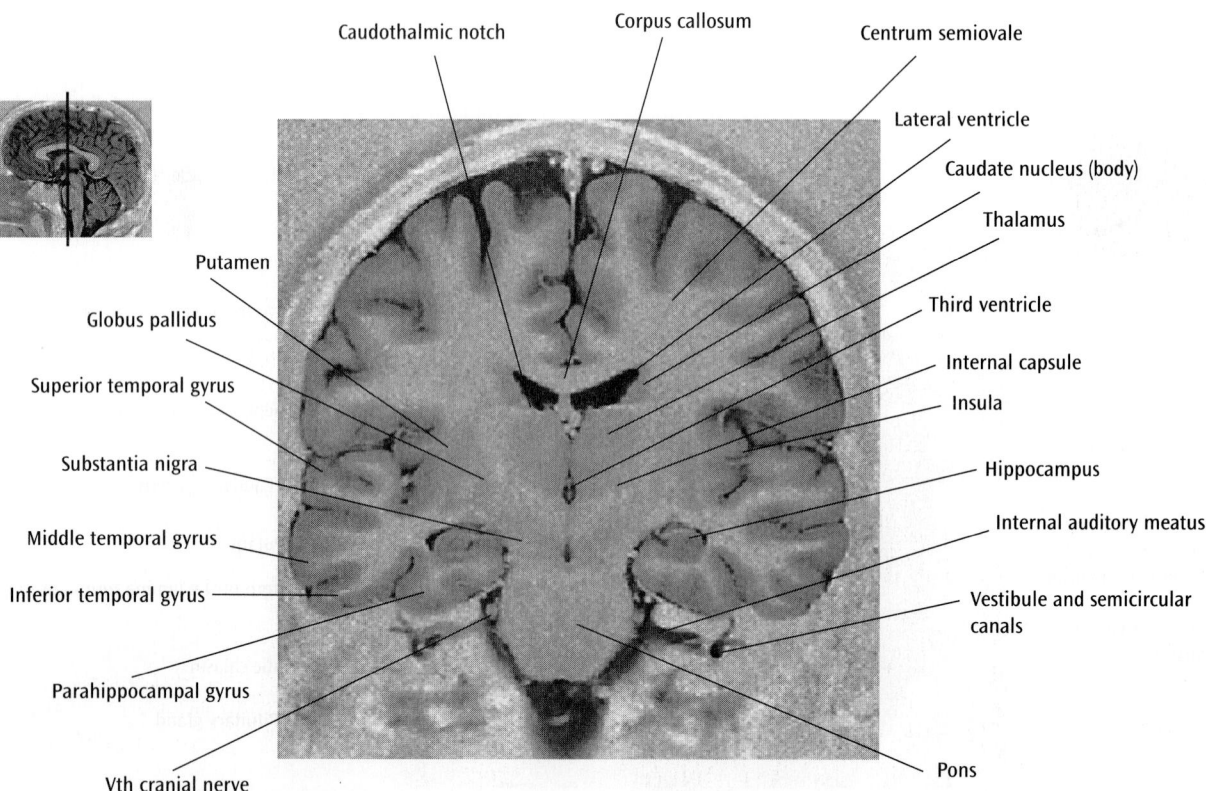

Coronal images

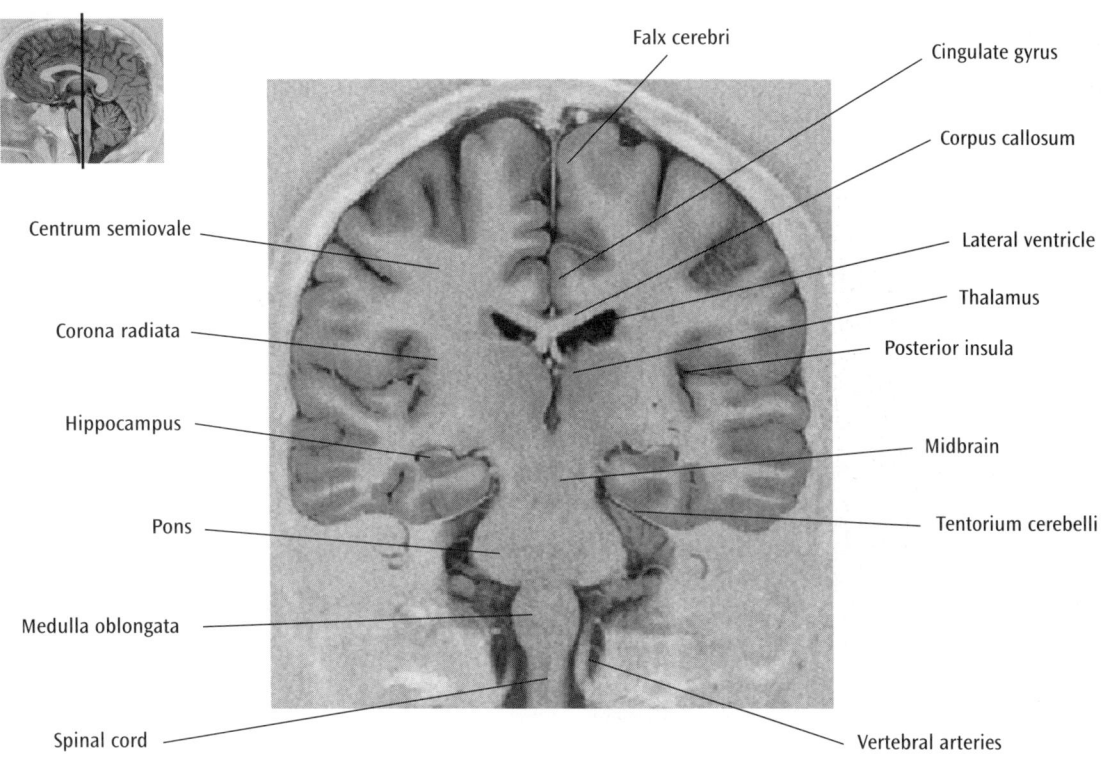

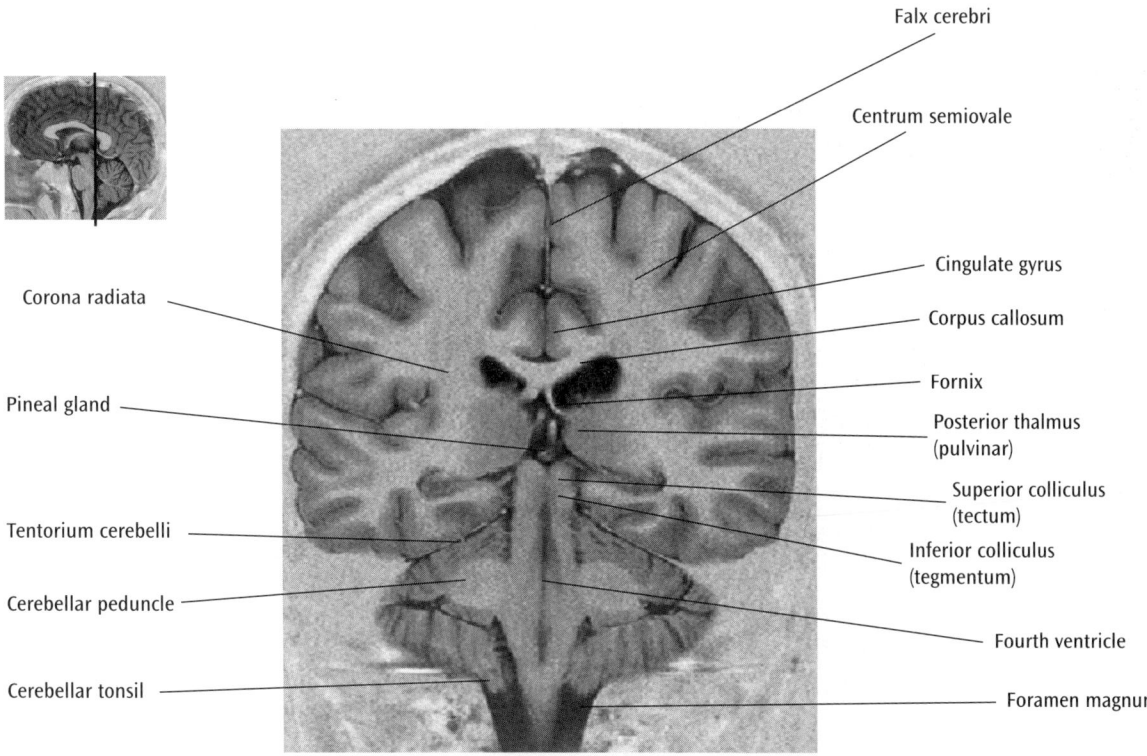

Coronal images

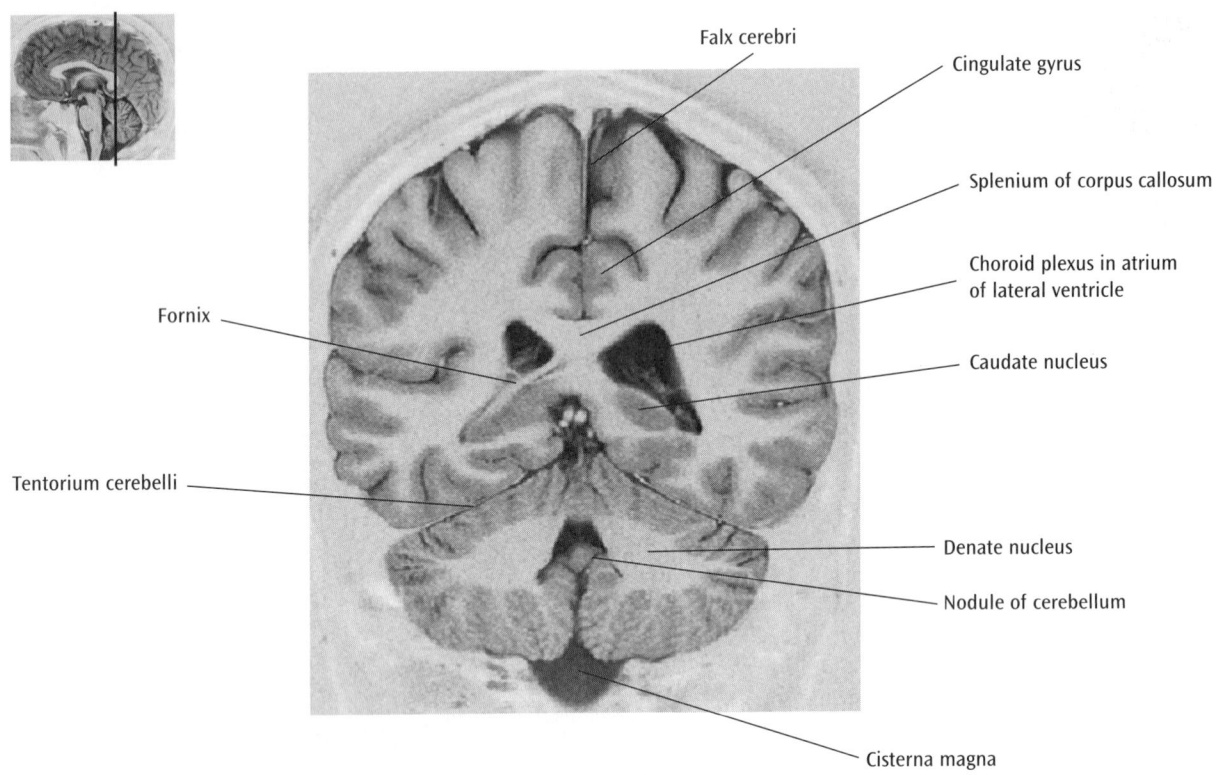

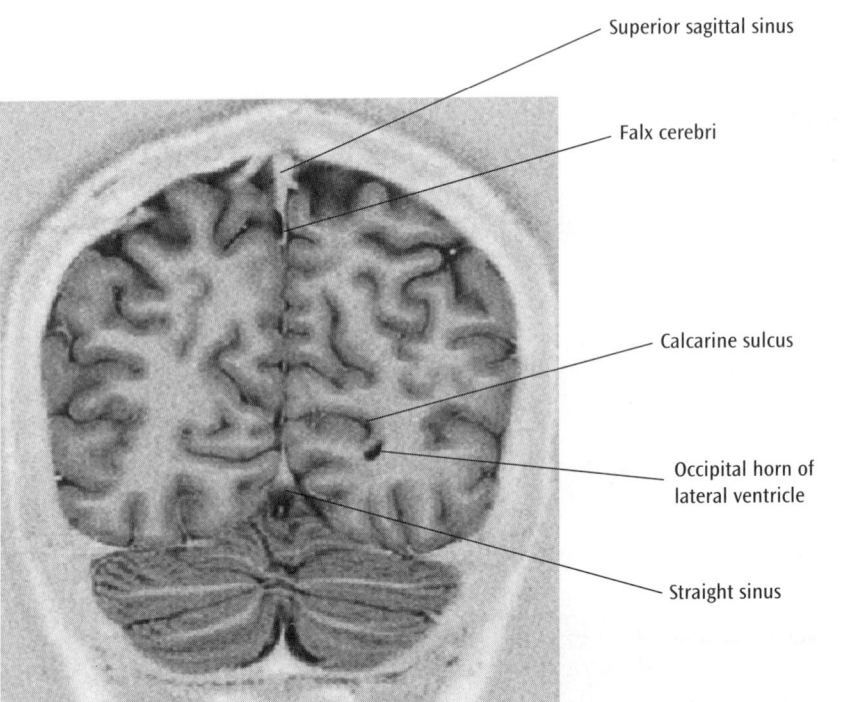

Axial images

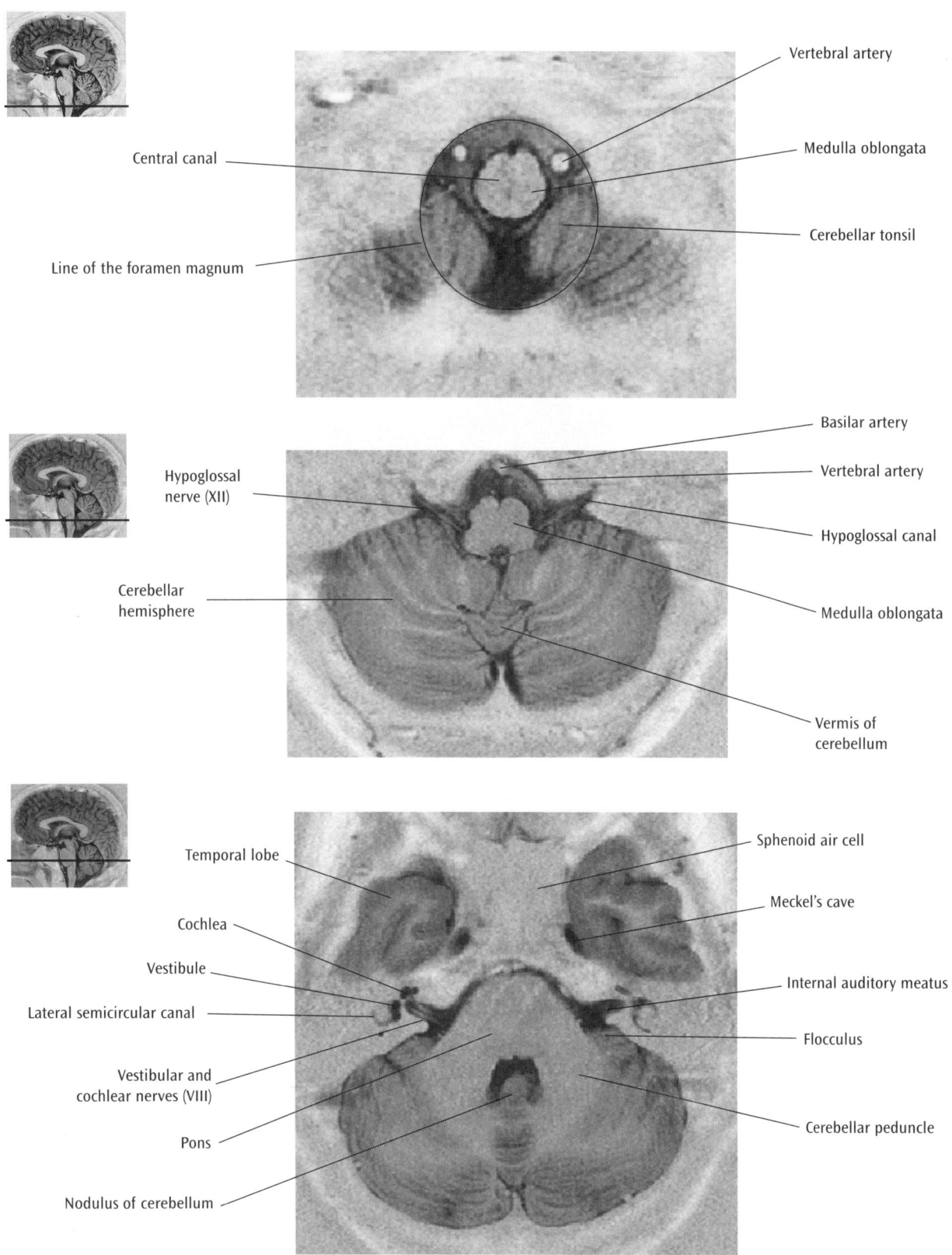

Axial images

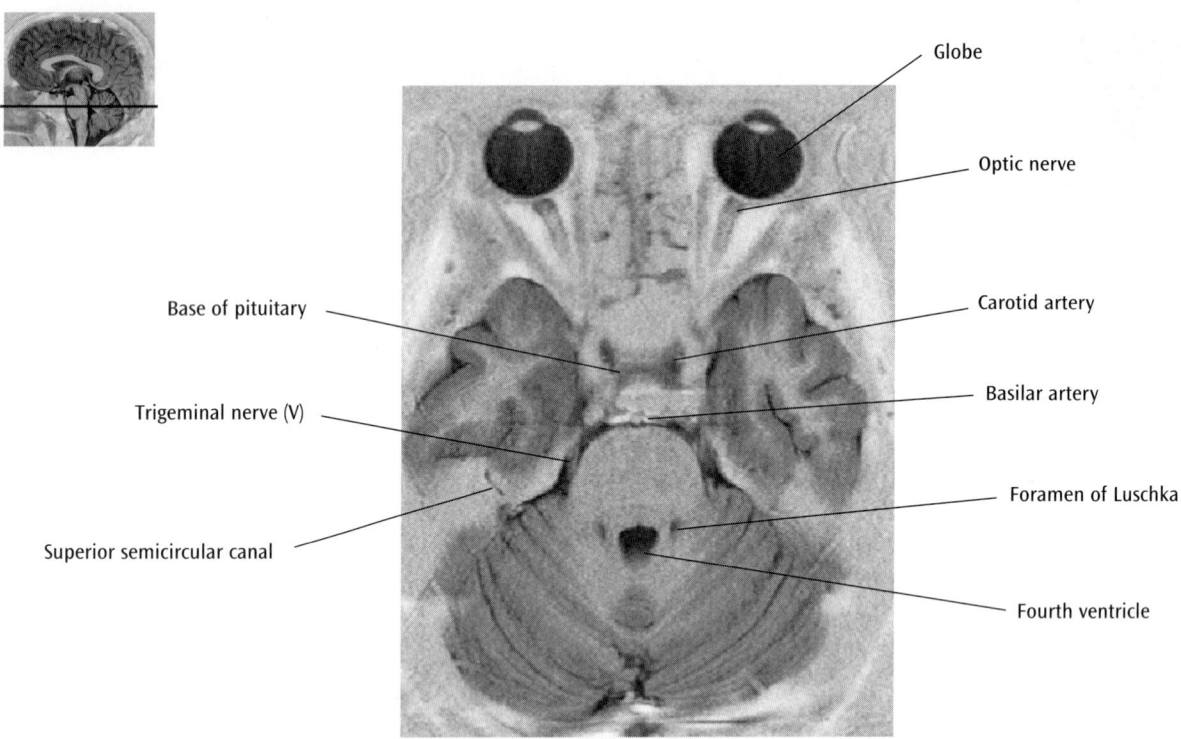

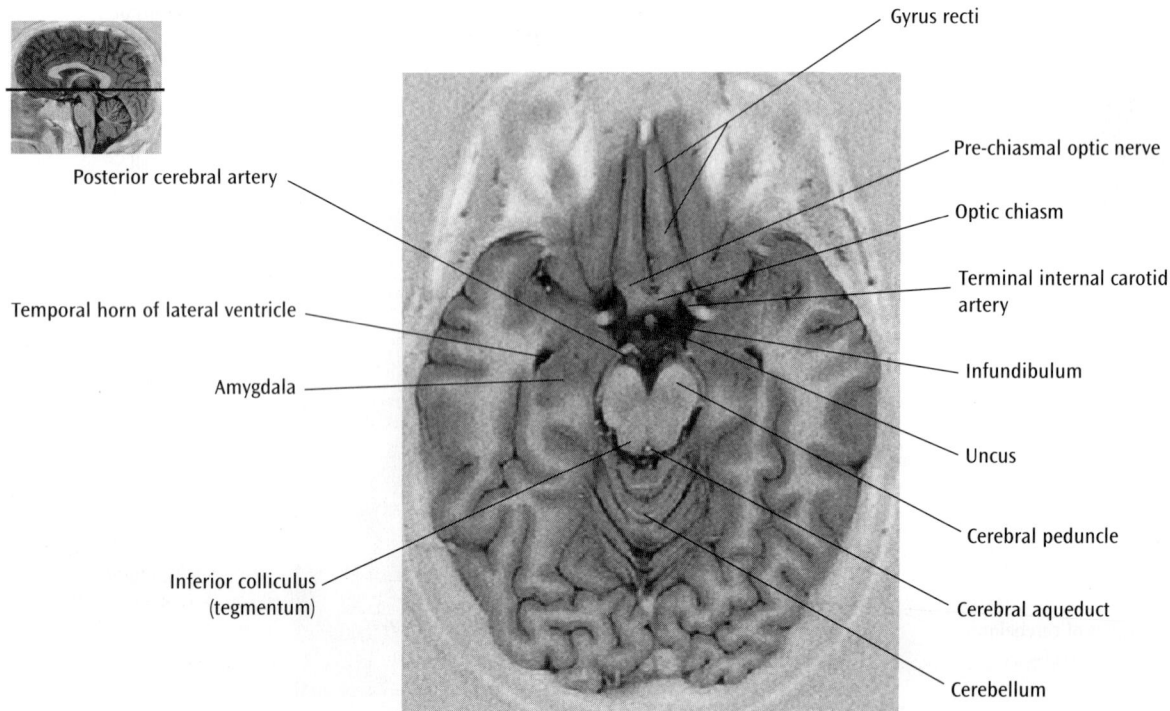

Axial images

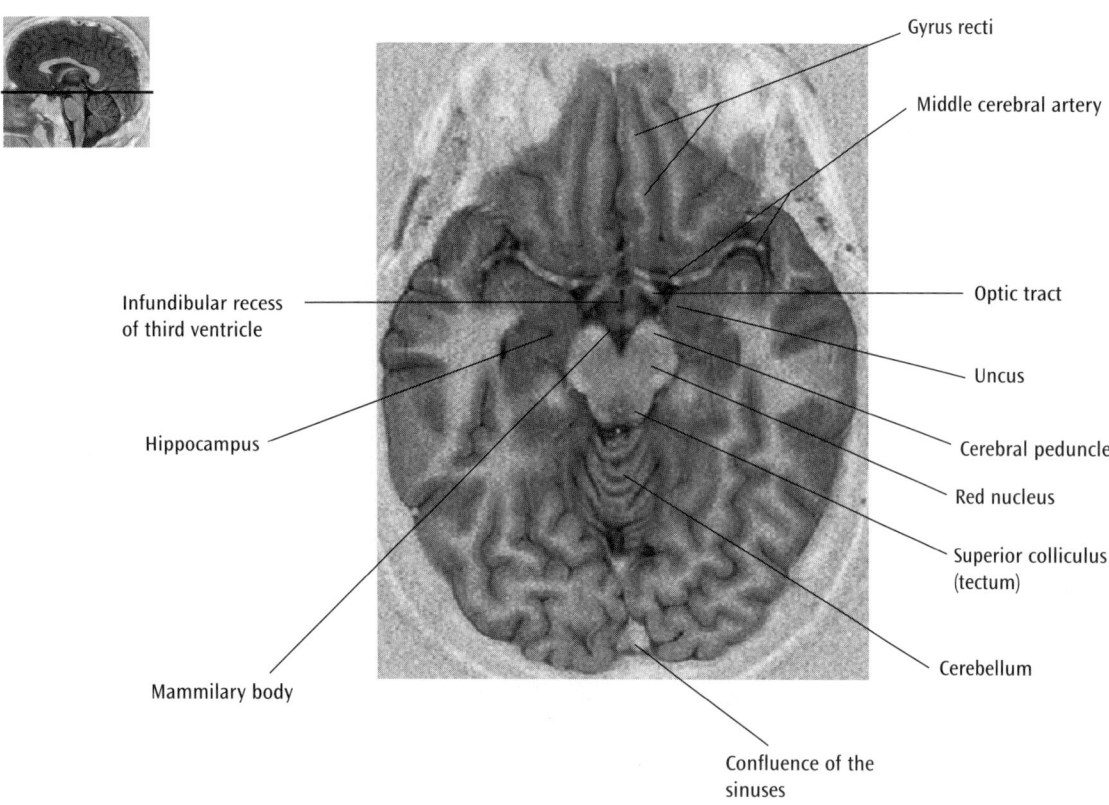

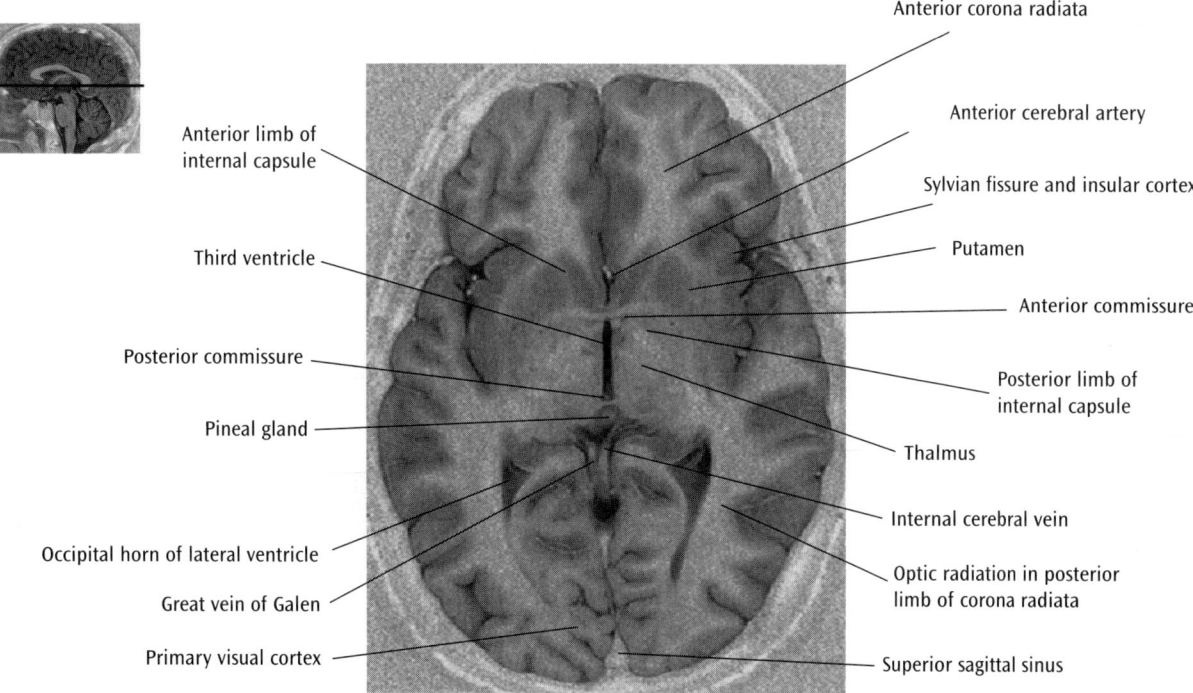

Axial images

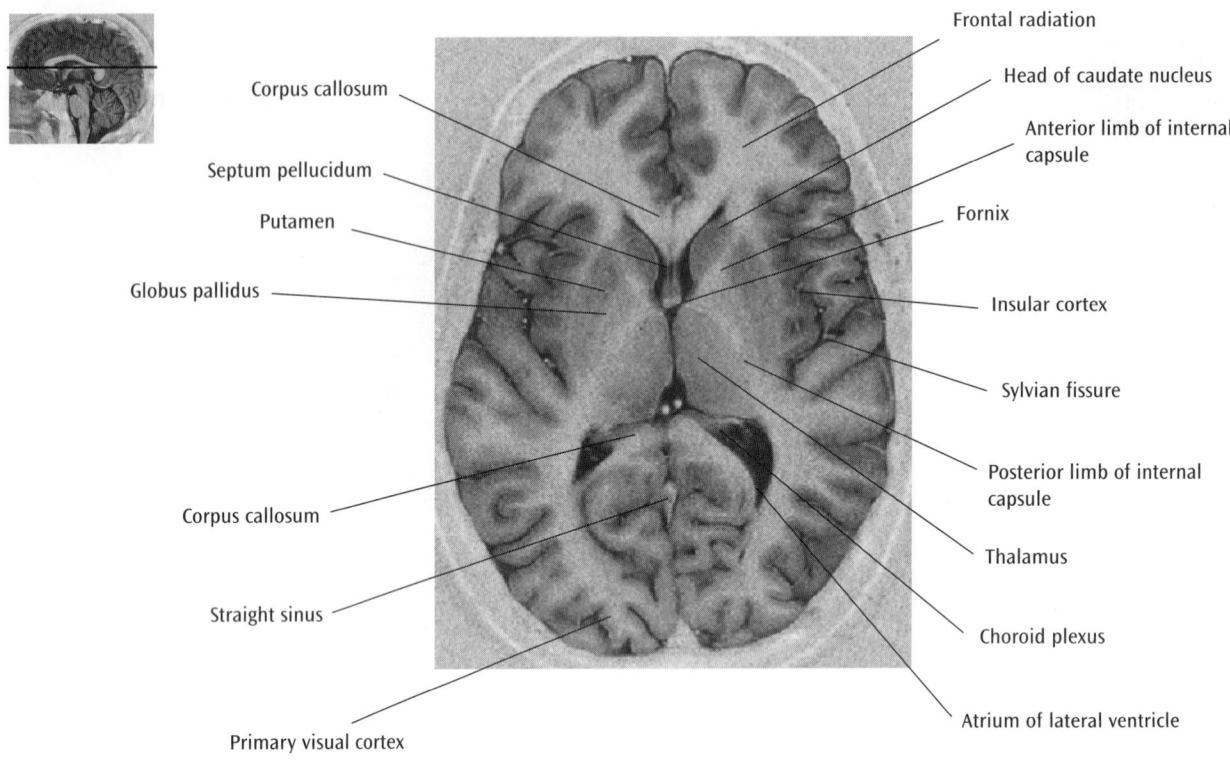

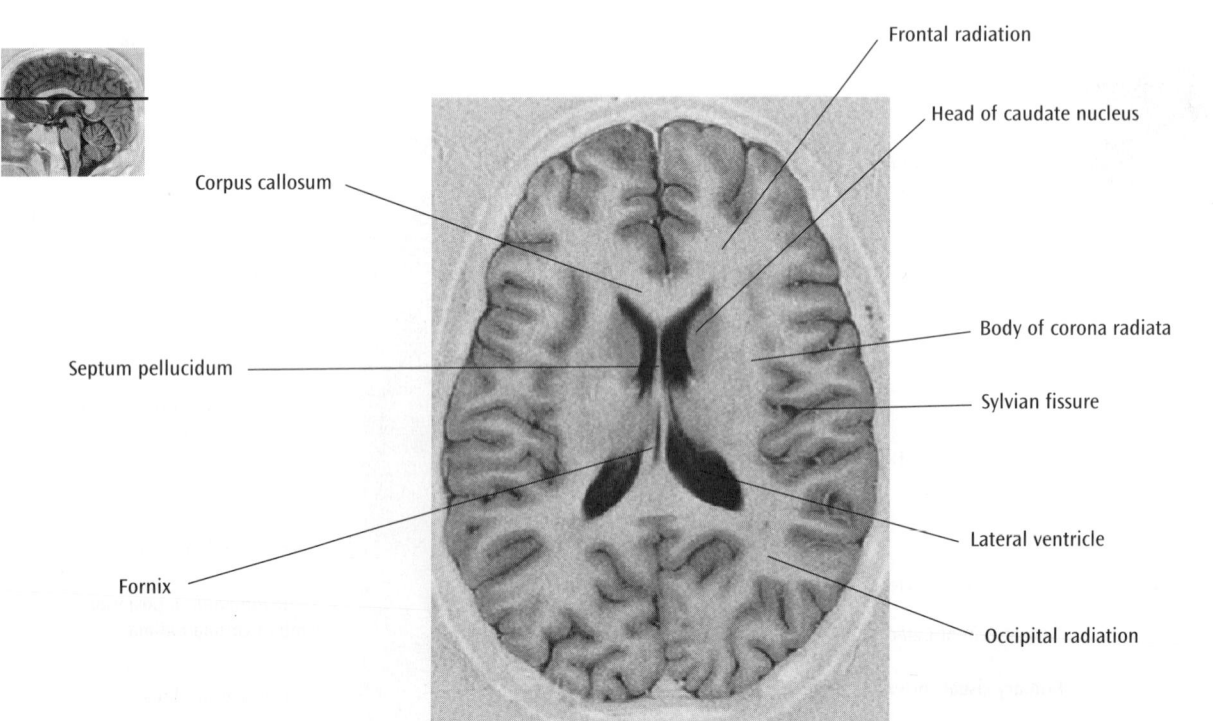

Axial images

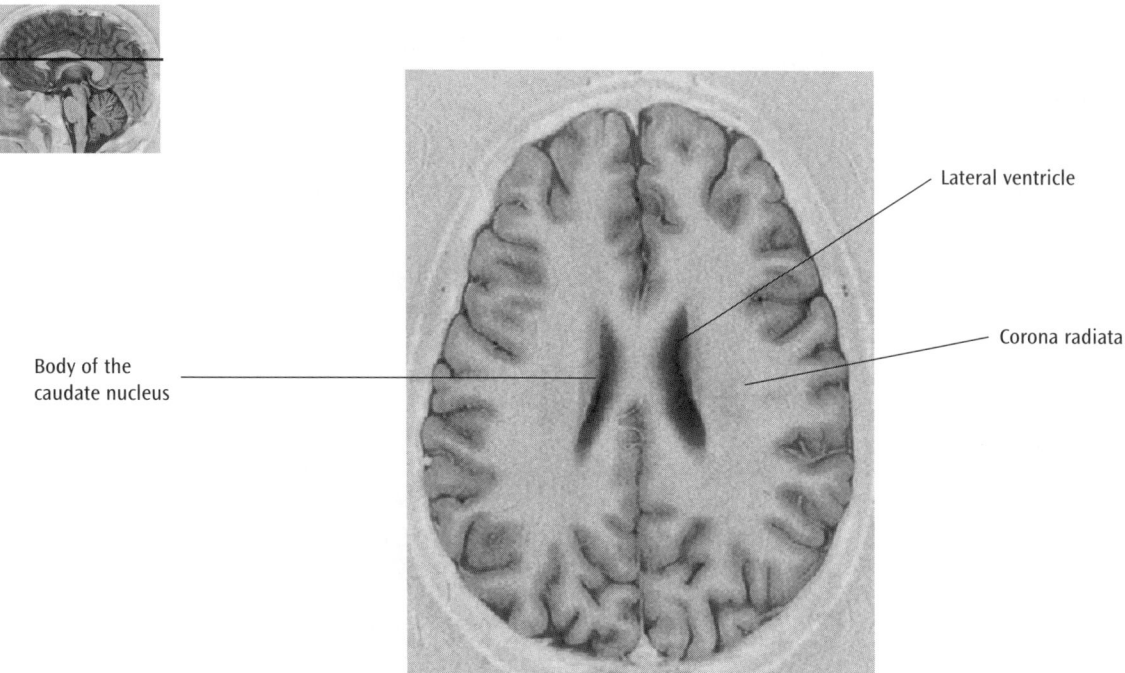

Body of the caudate nucleus

Lateral ventricle

Corona radiata

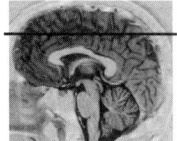

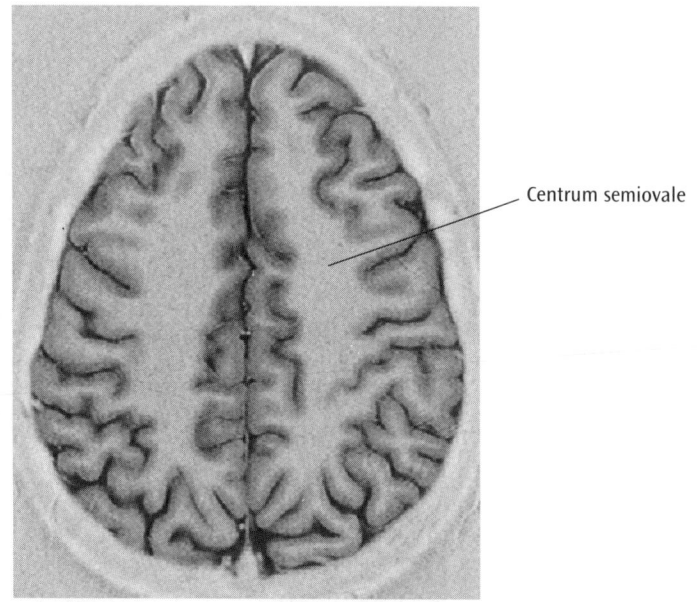

Centrum semiovale

Computed tomography

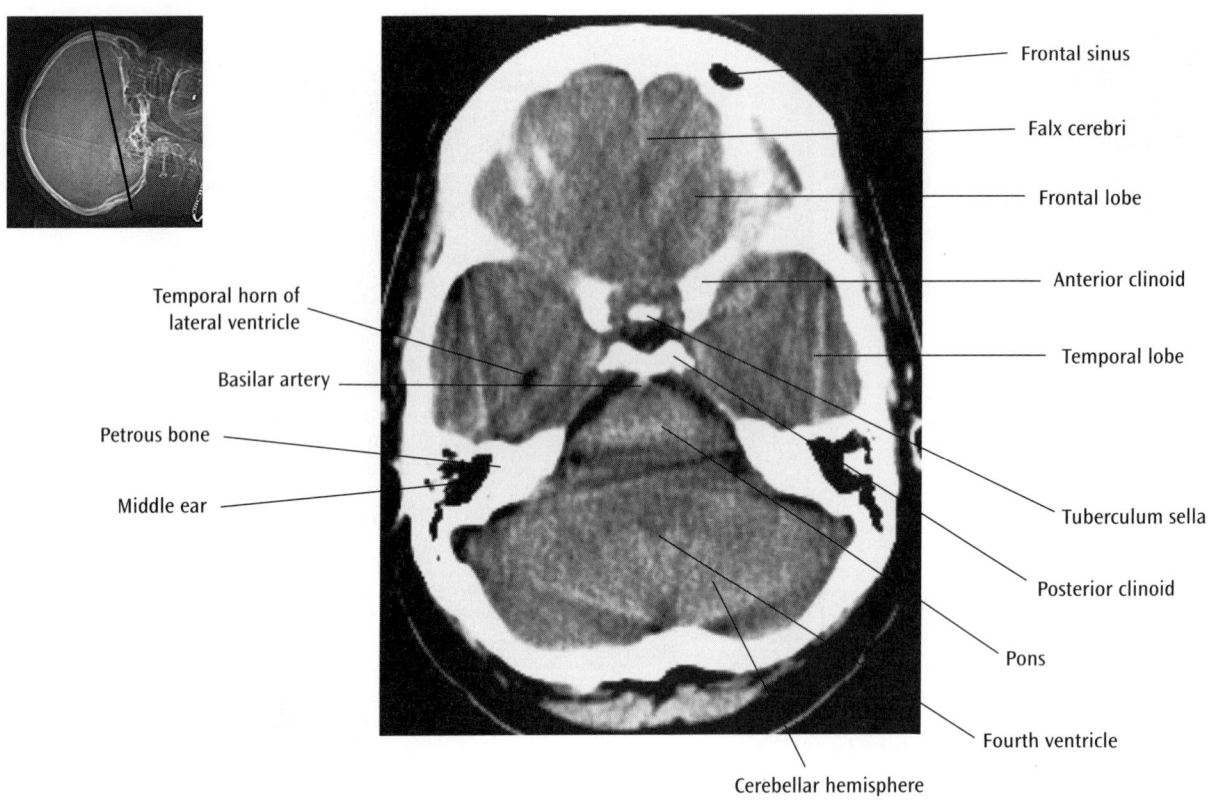

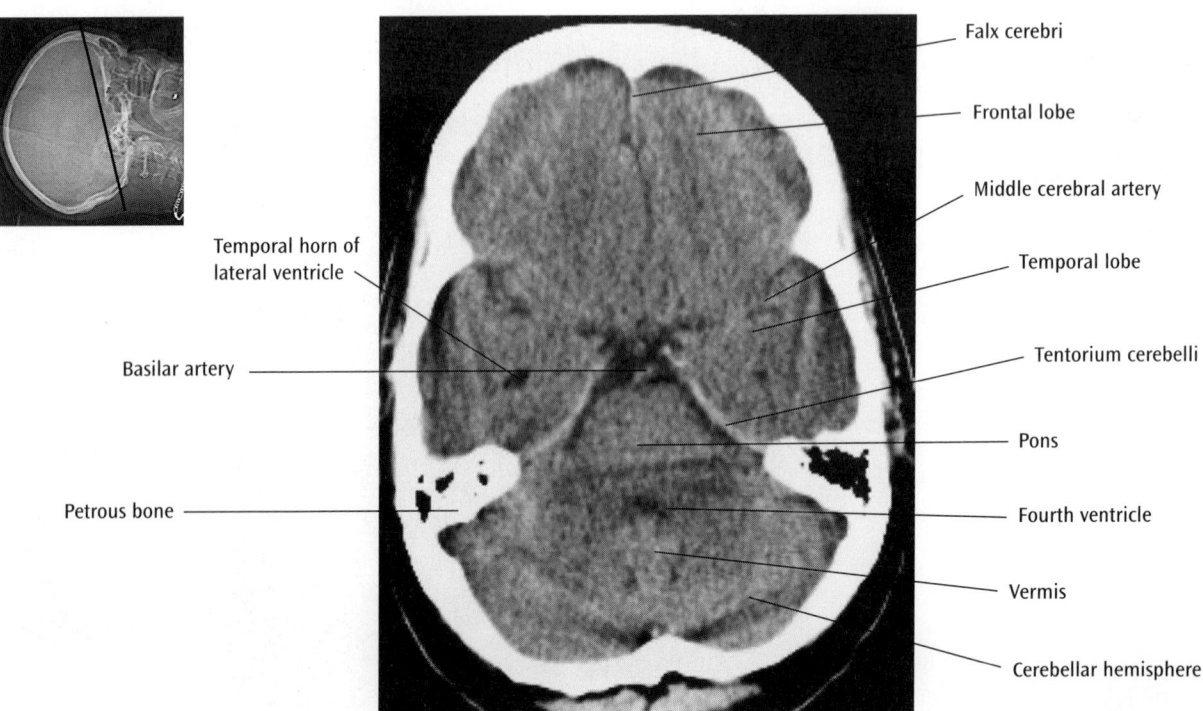

Computed tomography

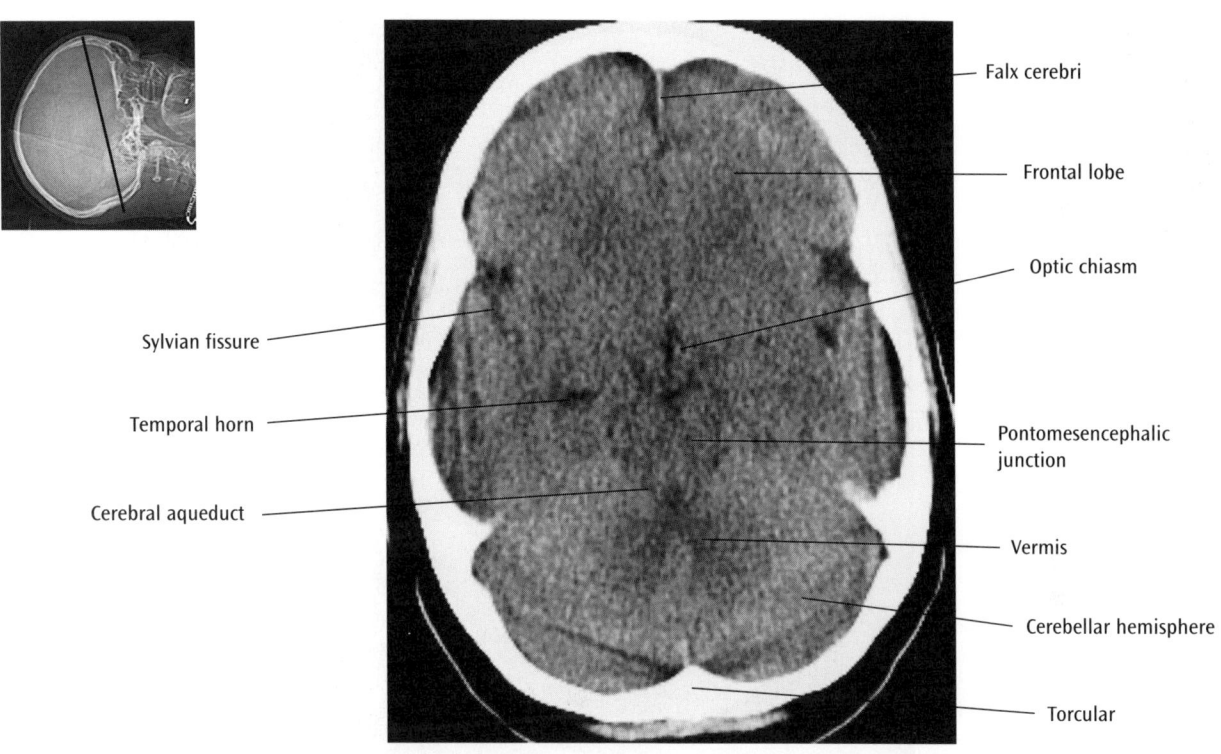

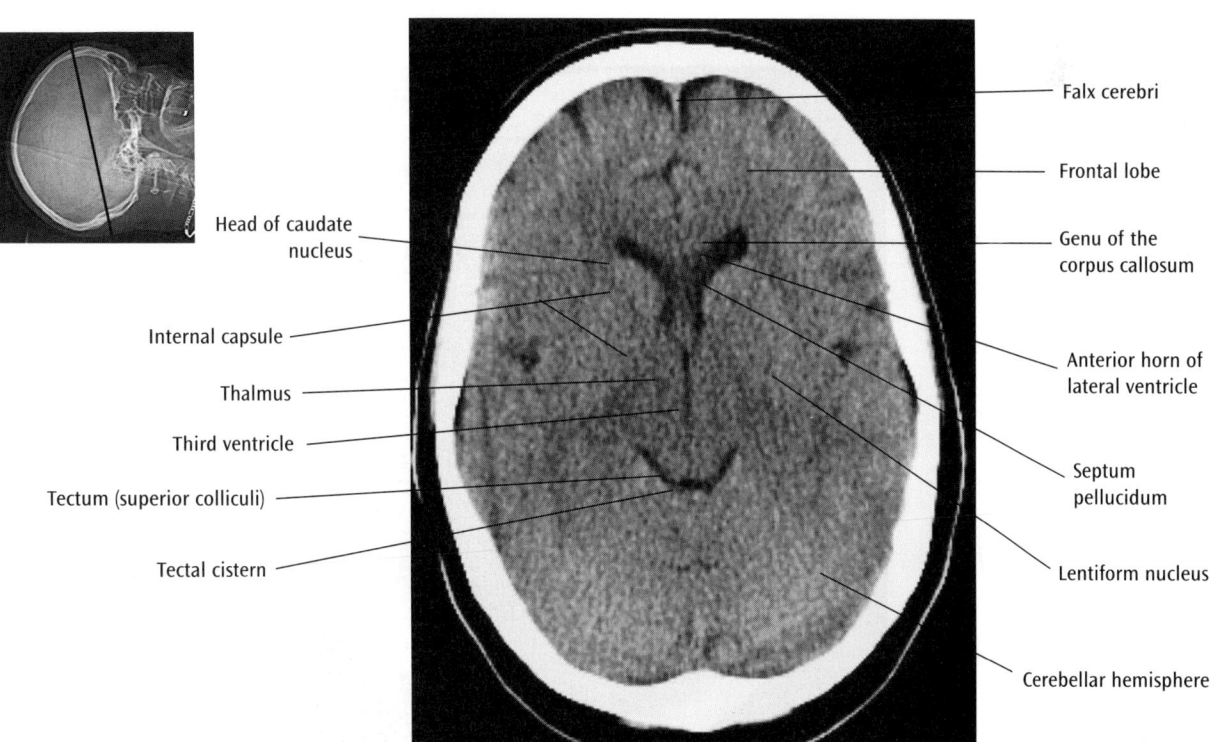

Computed tomography

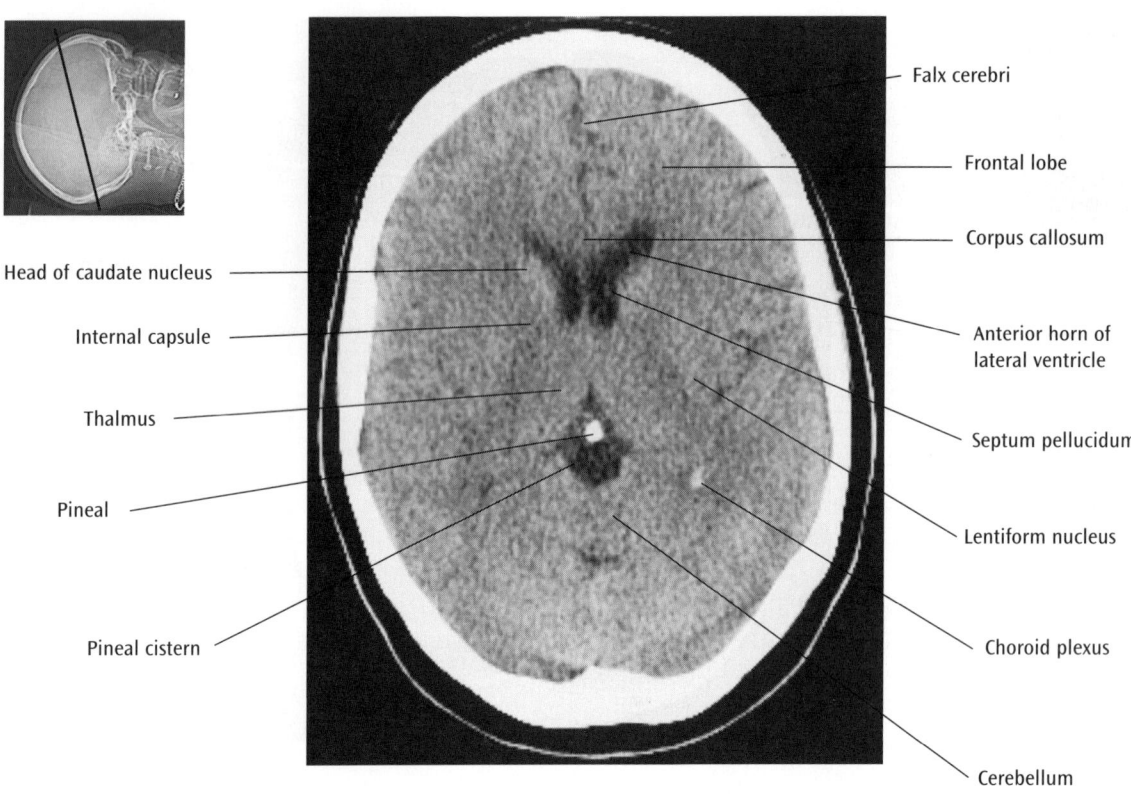

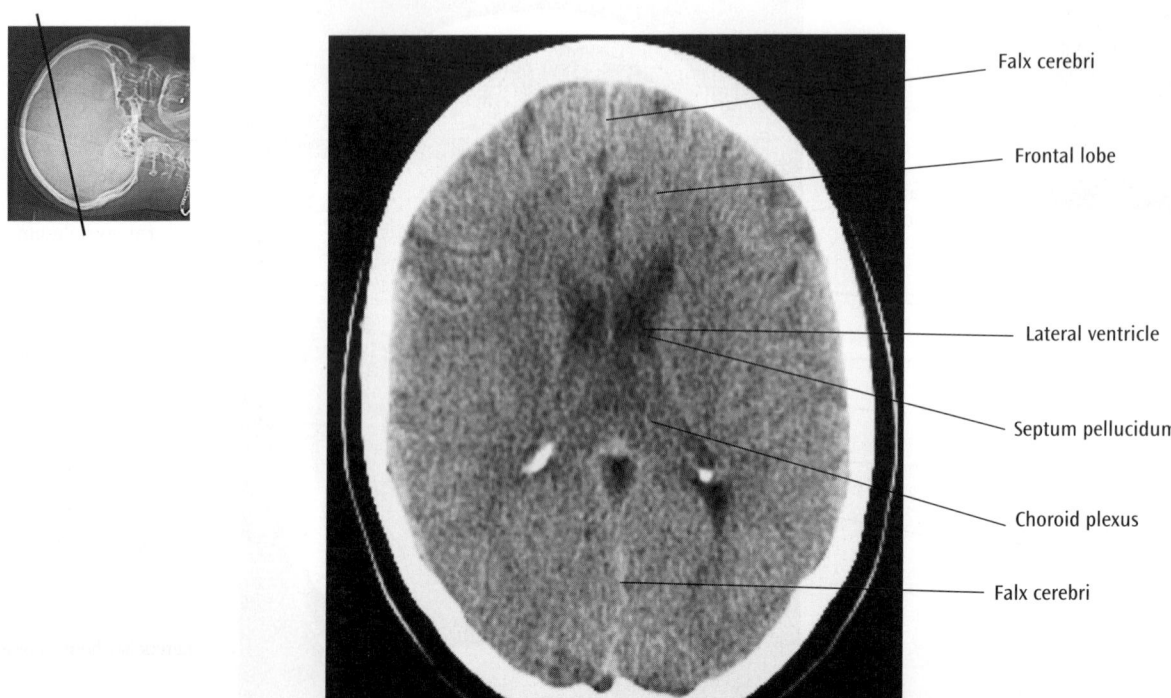

Computed tomography

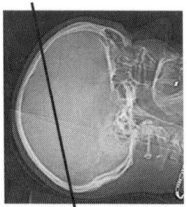

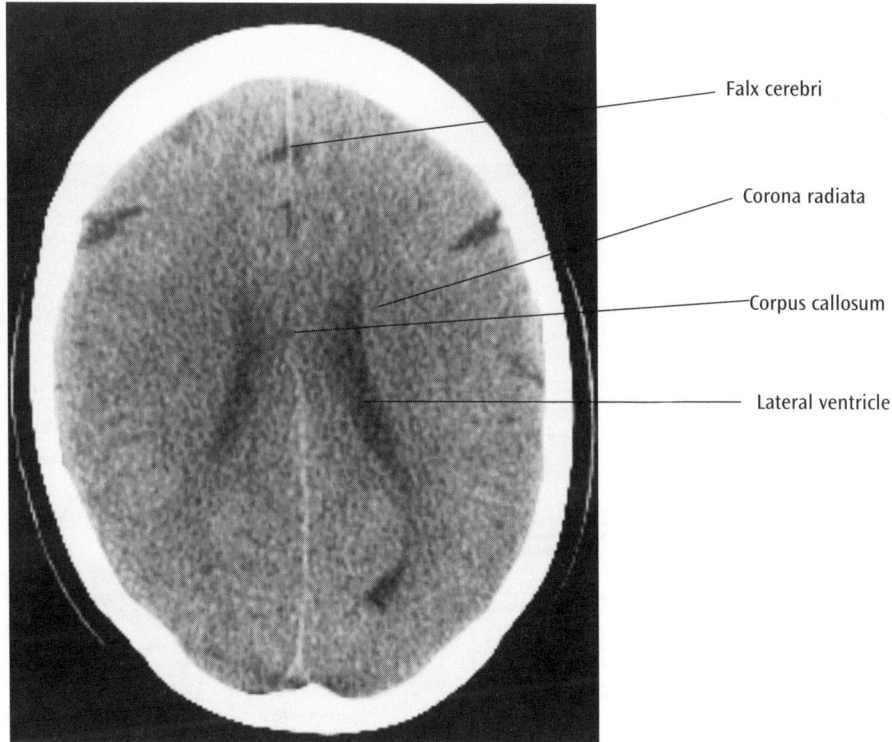

- Falx cerebri
- Corona radiata
- Corpus callosum
- Lateral ventricle

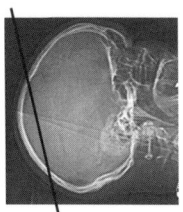

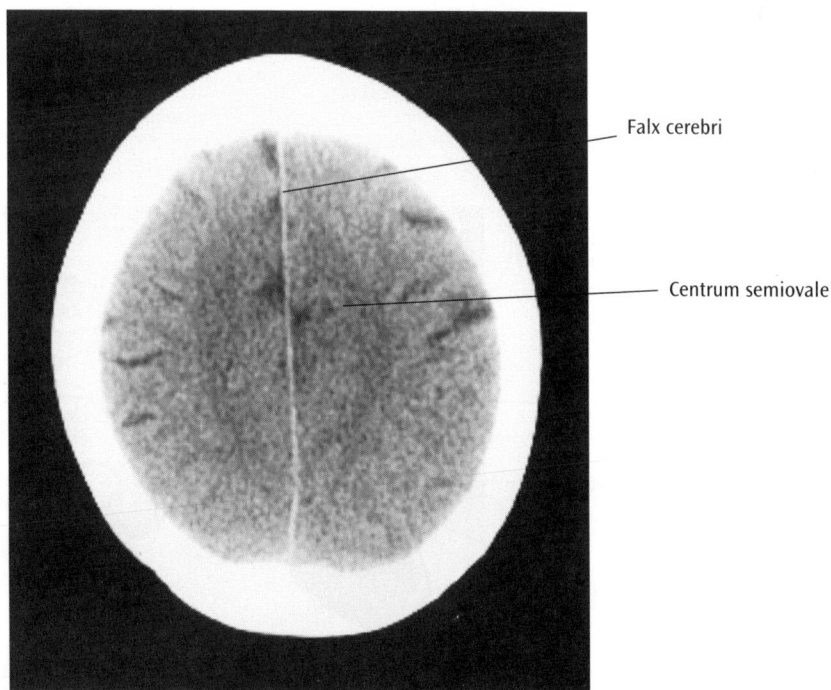

- Falx cerebri
- Centrum semiovale

Suprasellar cistern and parasellar region

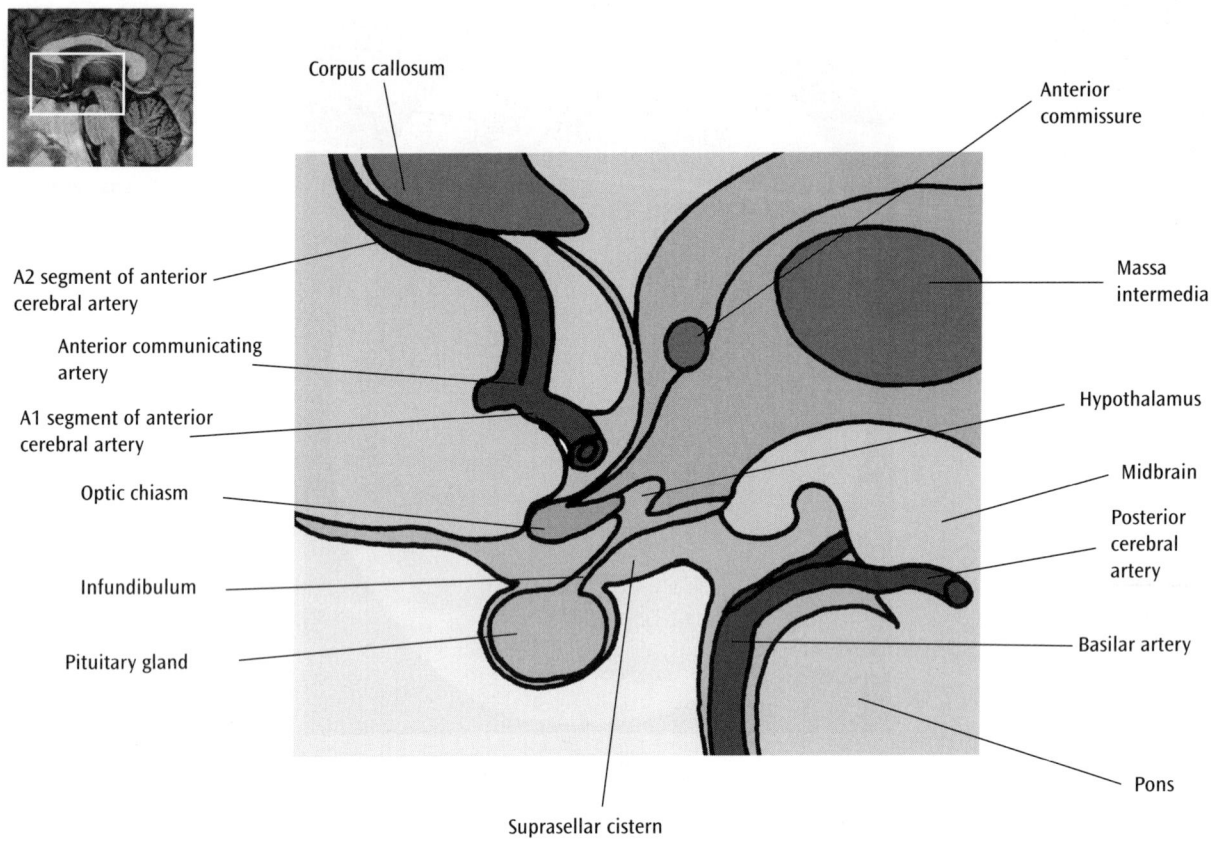

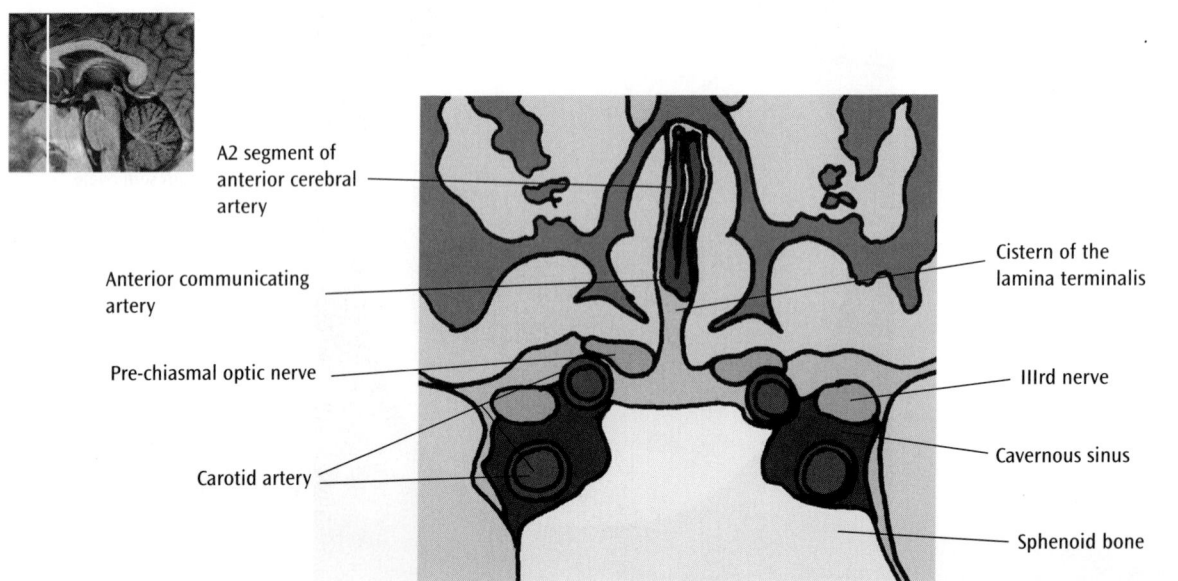

Suprasellar cistern and parasellar region

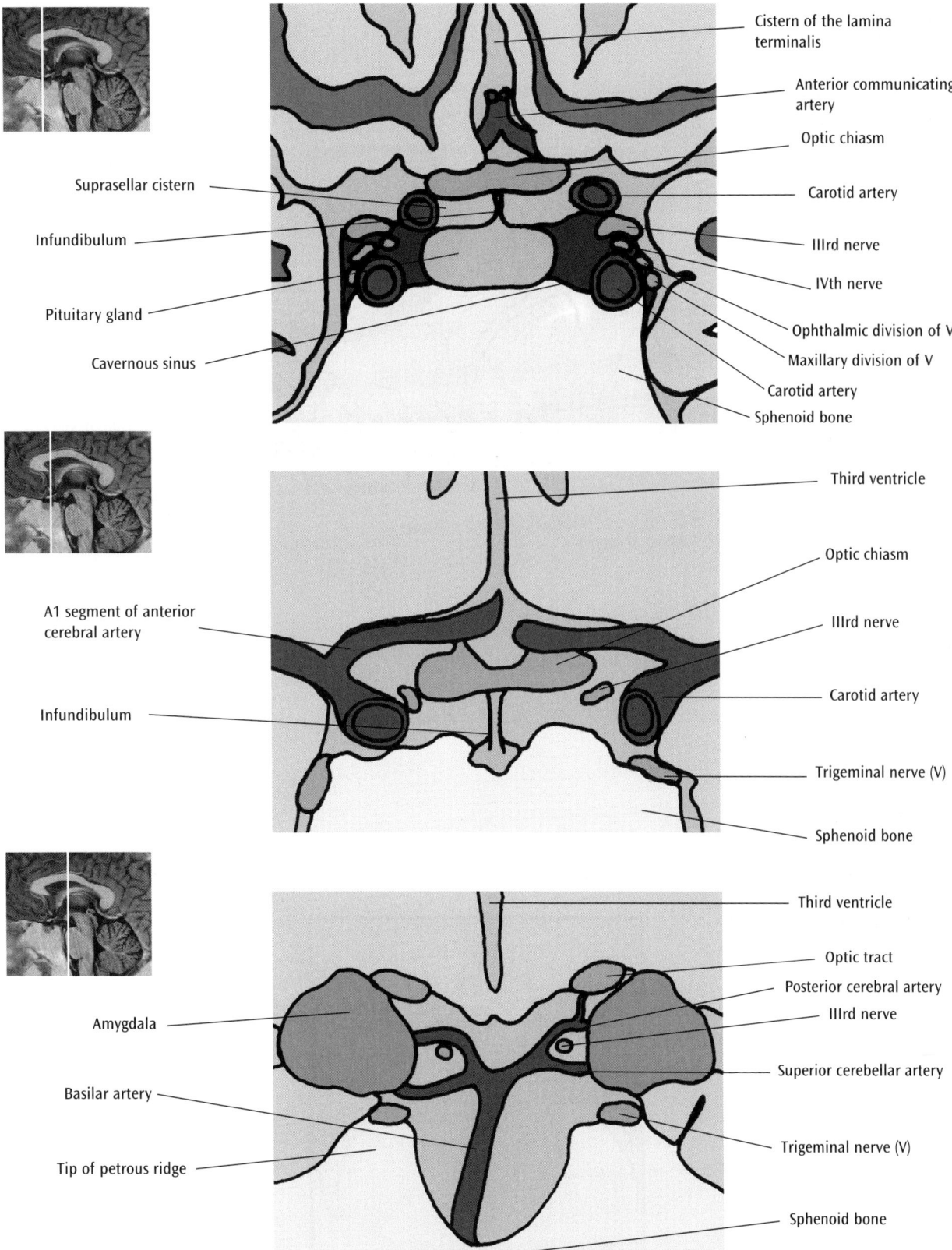

Pineal region

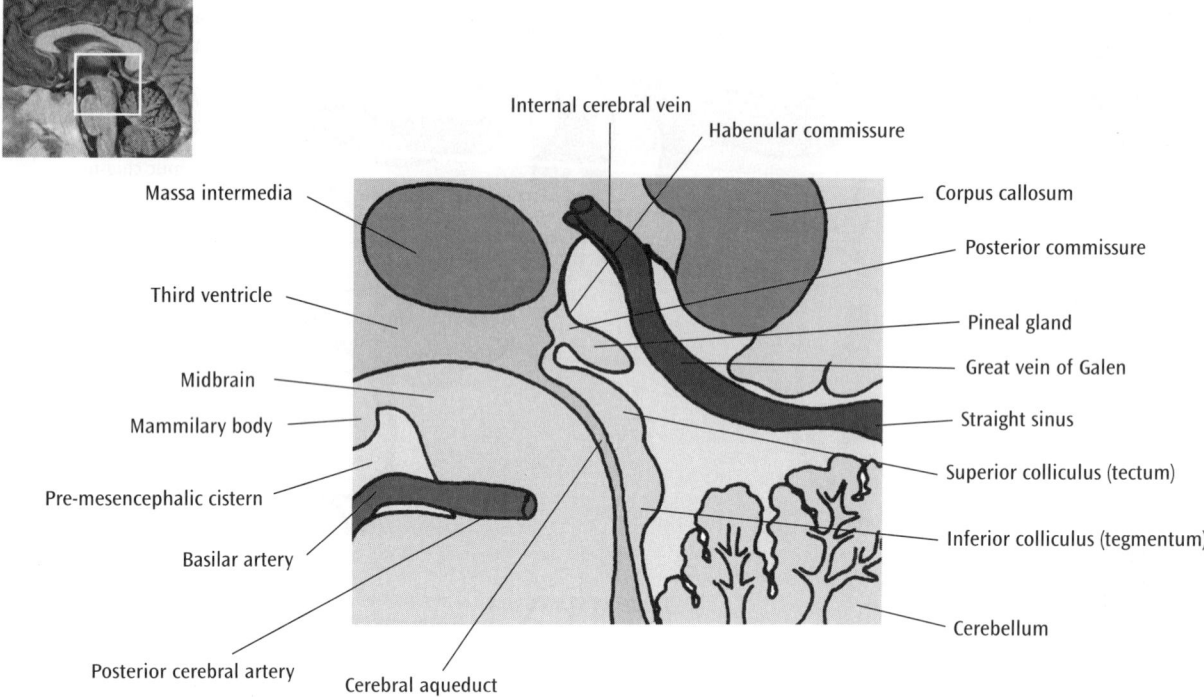

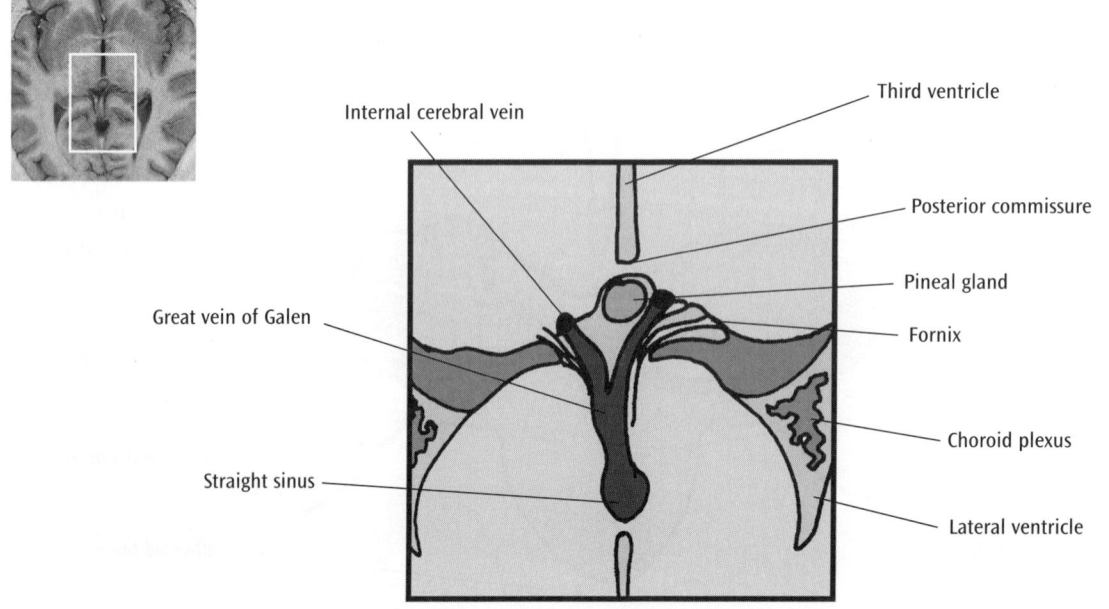

Cerebellopontine angle

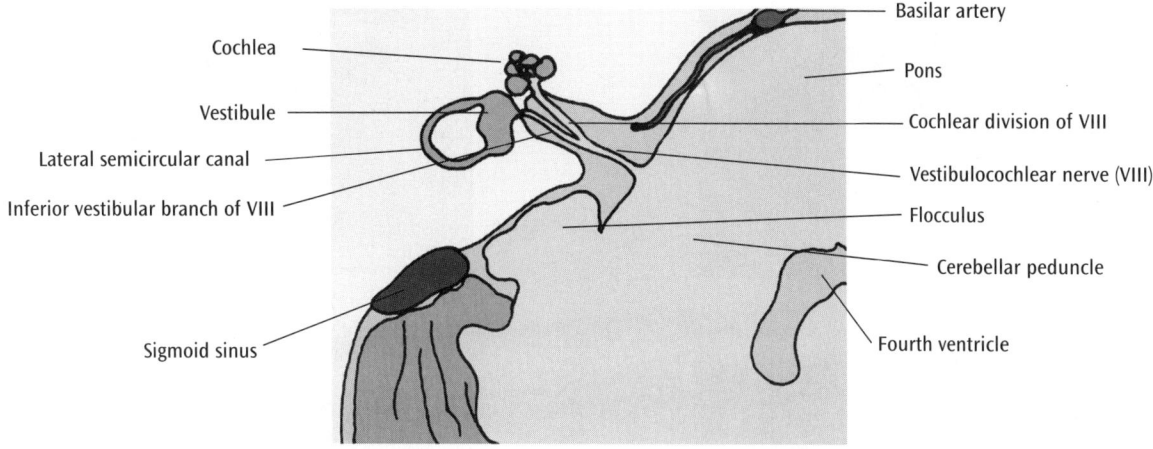

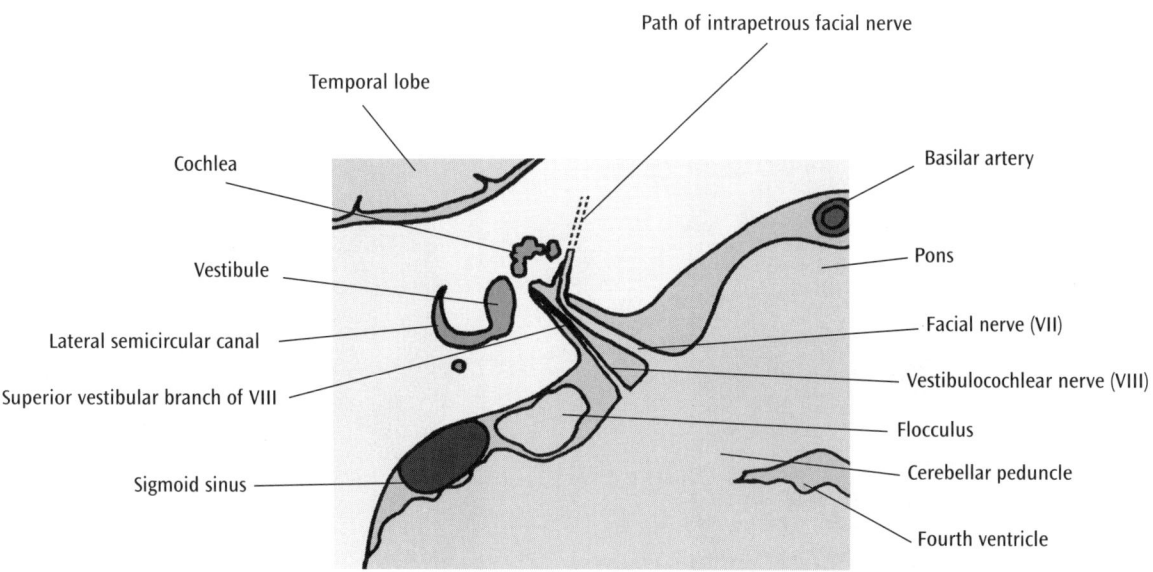

Cerebral artery territories
Cerebral/cerebellar lobes

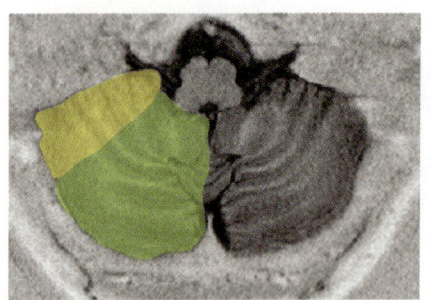
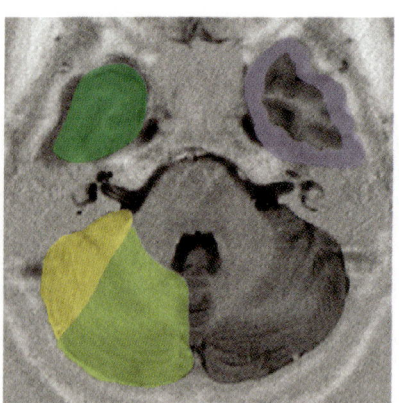
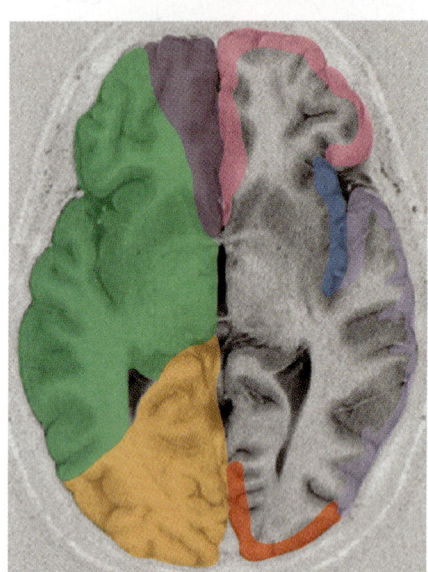
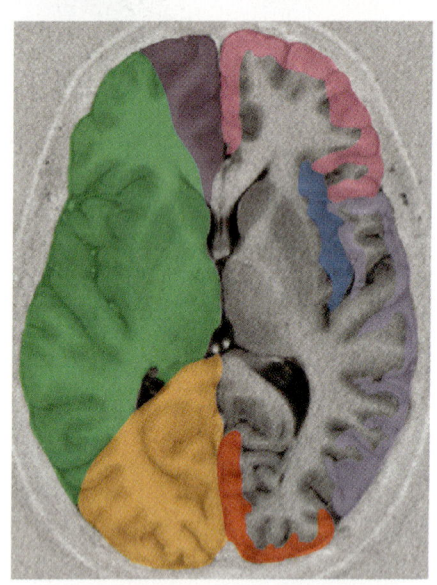
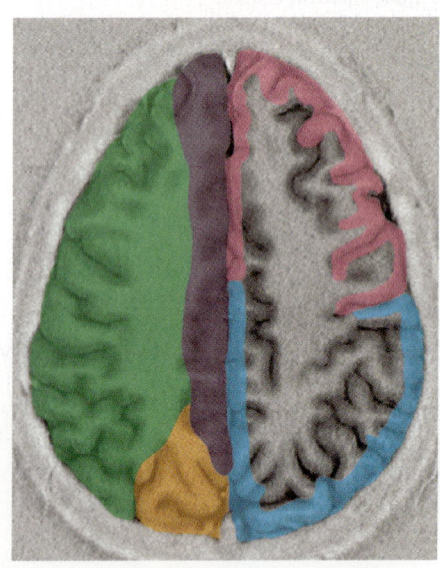
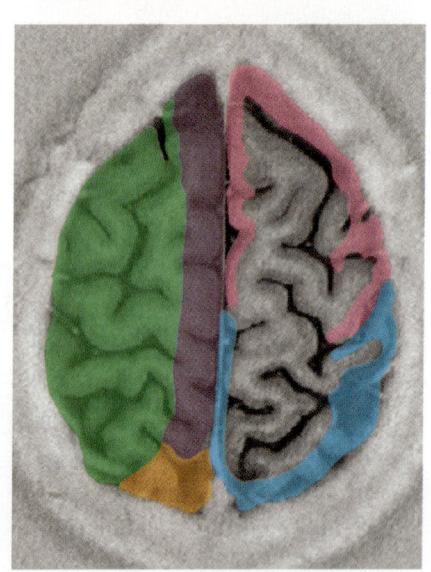

Cerebral artery territories
Cerebral/cerebellar lobes

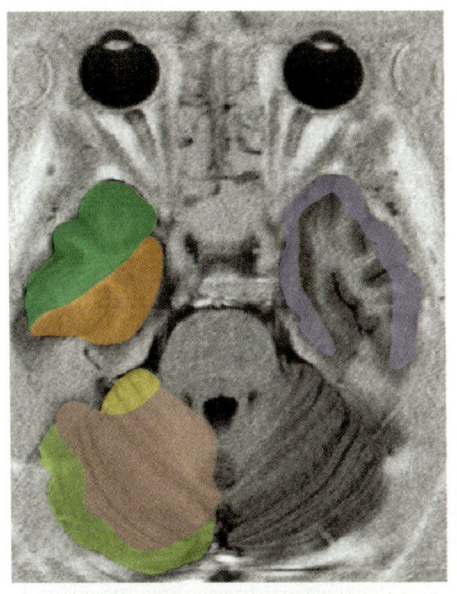

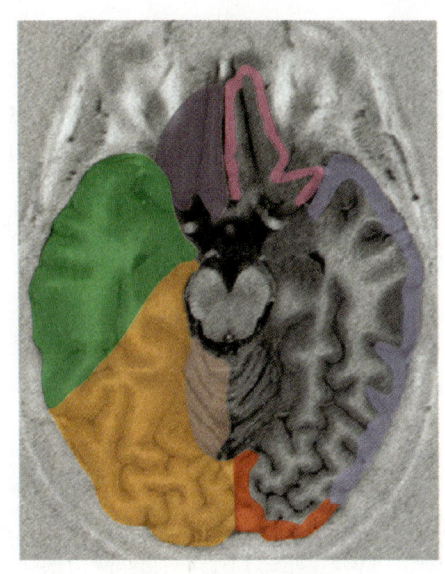

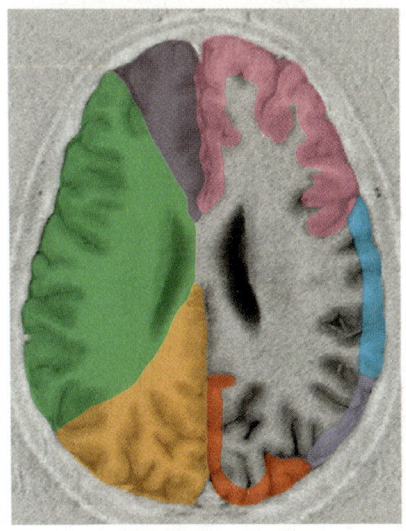

Cerebral artery territories

- Anterior inferior cerebellar artery
- Posterior inferior cerebellar artery
- Superior cerebellar artery
- Posterior cerebral artery
- Middle cerebral artery
- Anterior cerebral artery

Cerebral lobes

- Frontal
- Occipital
- Parietal
- Rolandic (Insular)
- Temporal

Key
Cerebral artery territories (left side of images)
Cerebral and cerebellar lobes (right side of images)

Part 1: Atlas of normal brain anatomy

Part 2: Atlas of brain pathology

Intra-axial mass lesion: Supratentorial

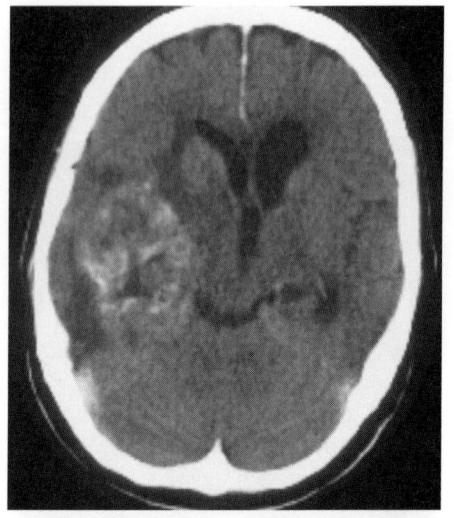

Glioma

High grade glioma

Enhancing solitary mass lesion. Often heterogeneous due to internal necrosis and cyst formation. Edge is often ill-defined with surrounding oedema. Can grow through midline in corpus callosum (butterfly glioma). Occasional internal haemorrhage.

Low grade glioma

Homogeneous solitary mass lesion. Enhancement indicates de-differentiation to higher grade. Calcification common in oligodendrogliomas. Oedema necrosis and cyst formation rare.

◀ **High grade glioma**

Metastases

Commonest intrinsic neoplasm in adults. Presents as enhancing solid or 'target' lesions. Multiple lesions highly suggestive. Commonest at grey/white matter boundary. Oedema is a normal feature. Calcification rare and suggests adenocarcinoma of colon, carcinoid or osteosarcoma. Intratumoural haemorrhage suggests melanoma or, renal cell carcinoma.

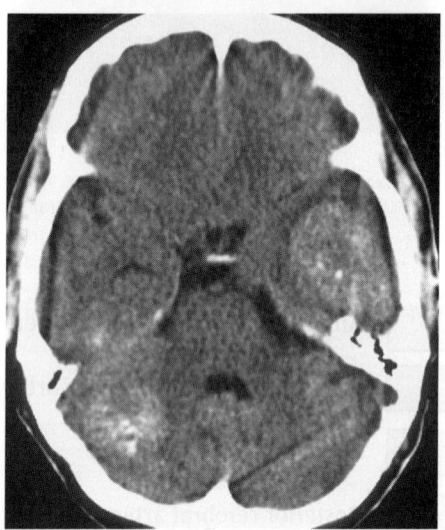

◀ **Enhancing metastases in temporal lobe and cerebellum**

Acute infarction

Arterial

Acute infarct can present as a mass lesion mimicking glioma. Mass effect can persist for several days after onset. Peripheral enhancement in adjacent brain and internal haemorrhage are common. Oedema in adjacent brain can occur. Identification of infarction usually depends on acute onset of clinical features, localization of abnormality to arterial vascular territories and resolution of mass effect on follow-up scan.

Venous

Thrombotic and occlusive venous disease can cause infarction due to obstruction of venous outflow. Swelling, non-arterial in distribution and hemorrhage are suggestive features. Commonest in the anterior part of the hemisphere. Features rarely resolve spontaneously and rapid progression may occur. MRI venography can confirm the diagnosis.

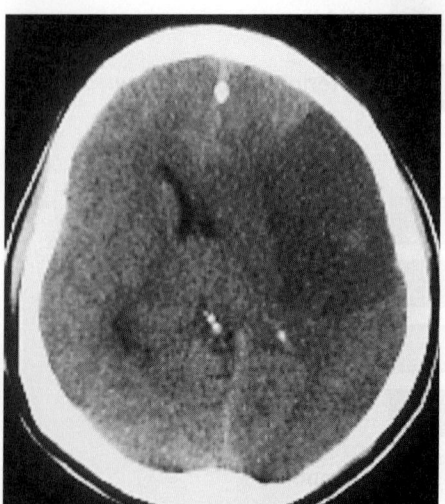

◀ **Acute left parietal infarct**

Intra-axial mass lesion: Supratentorial

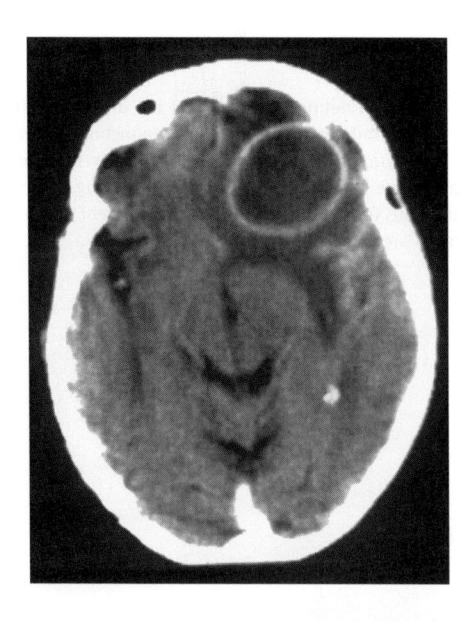

Abscess

Single or multiple (suggests haematogenous spread) ring enhancing mass lesions. Oedema is a prominent feature. The enhancing wall is usually thin and regular. Commonly located near opacified paranasal sinuses or petrous air spaces. Commonly associated with secondary venous thrombosis.

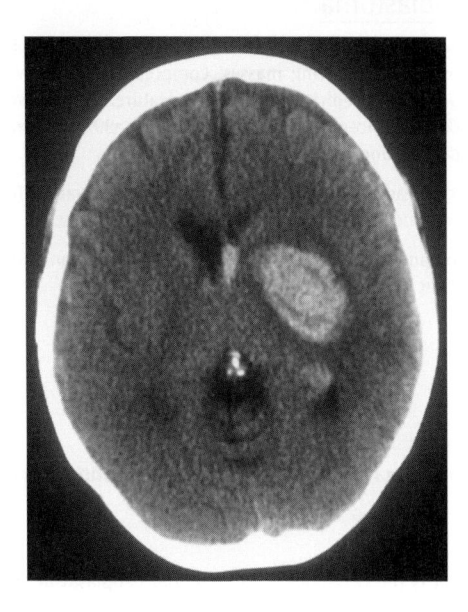

◀ Large ring enhancing abscess

Haematomas

Well defined mass lesion initially homogeneous on CT and MRI. Mass effect and oedema decrease over time. Initially high attenuation on CT gradually decreasing over several weeks. MRI appearances are usually dramatic with extremes (high and low) of signal intensity on T1- and T2-weighted images. MRI appearances undergo specific changes as the haematoma matures. Position and clinical features suggest possible aetiology, i.e. 1) Spontaneous haemorrhage commonest in basal ganglia. 2) Haematomas adjacent to brain surface and circle of Willis suggests aneurysmal bleed.

◀ Left basal ganglia haematoma

Remember

1 In children the differential diagnosis of low grade glioma includes dysembryoplastic neuroepithelial tumours (DNT) and gangliogioma.
2 Acute plaques in multiple sclerosis can present as large enhancing, often cystic, mass lesions.
3 The differential diagnoses in immunocompromised patients differ with increased incidence of less common disorders (i.e. lymphoma).
4 Extra-axial lesions may mimic intra-axial lesions (i.e. meningioma with associated oedema).

Intra-axial mass lesion: Infratentorial

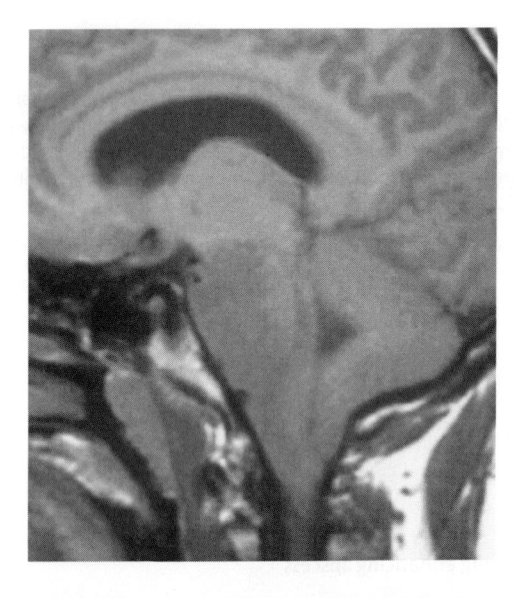

Brainstem glioma

Usually present as ill defined expansion of the brainstem often centered in the pons initially. Cervicomedullary junction is also a common site. Exophytic growth may occur particularly into the fourth ventricle and more commonly in children. Loss of the brainstem cisterns is suspicious of brainstem glioma. Enhancement and secondary hydrocephalus are late features.

◀ **Brainstem glioma (T1)**

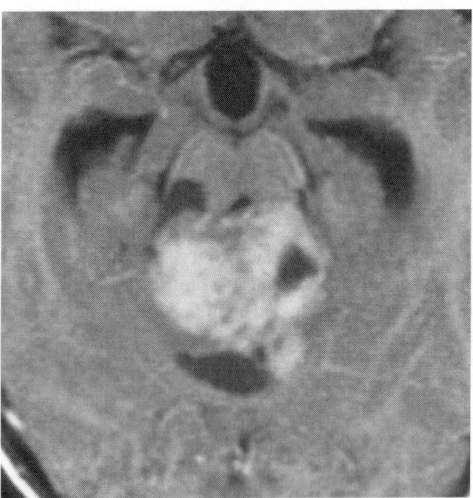

Medulloblastoma

Account for one-third of posterior fossa neoplasms in children. Typically midline enhancing masses. Compress the fourth ventricle from behind. Hydrocephalus is an early feature. Many have cystic areas (50%). Enhancement normally present (>90%) but variable. Tumoral calcification seen in a minority (15%).

Appearance in adults and older children is more variable. Tumours may be eccentric and can occur in cerebellar hemispheres.

Tumour spread by cerebrospinal fluid seeding is common and is present in 50% at diagnosis.

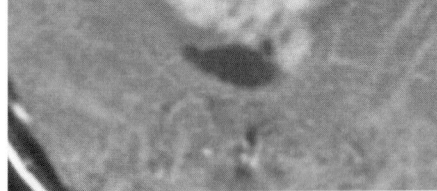

◀ **Medulloblastoma (note intact fourth ventricle anteriorly (T1+C)**

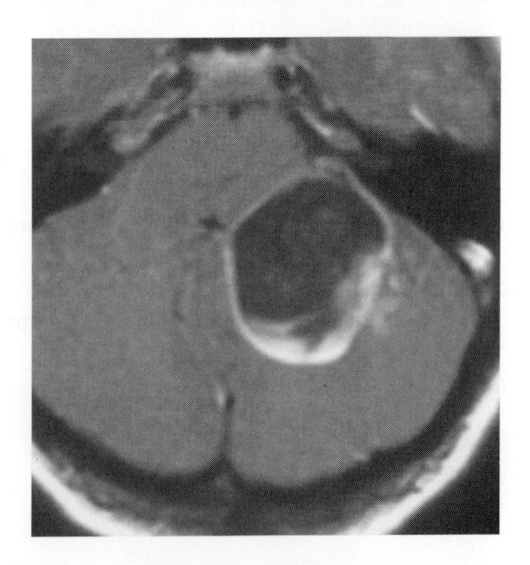

Astrocytoma

Astrocytoma is the commonest infratentorial neoplasm in children. Most are pilocytic and carry a favourable prognosis; 60–80% are cystic. Most cystic lesions have an enhancing tumour nodule in the wall of the cyst (50%). The remainder appear as a solid tumour with a cystic/necrotic centre. Calcification is unusual (10–15%). Most occur in the vermis of the cerebellum or cerebellar hemisphere.

◀ **Cystic astrocytoma (T1+C)**

Intra-axial mass lesion: Infratentorial

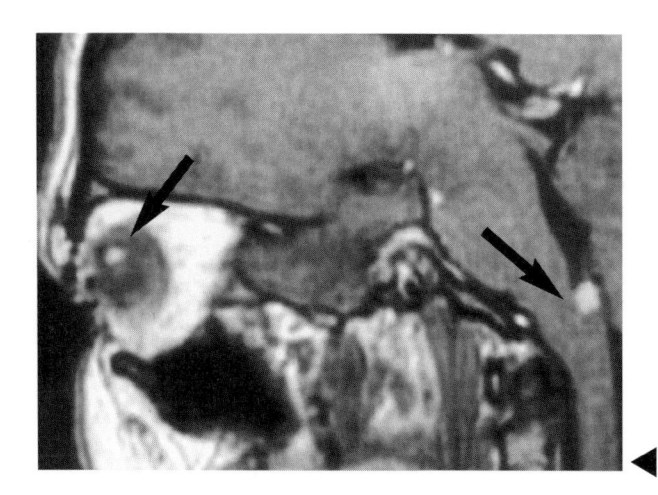

Haemangioblastoma

Represent only 1% of brain tumours but are the commonest primary neoplasm of the posterior fossa in adults. Occur in 40–50% of patients with Von Hippel-Lindau syndrome and are often multiple.

In all, 80% are cerebellar; the remainder occur principally in the spinal cord and brainstem; 40% are solid; 60% are cystic with an enhancing mural nodule. Solid components enhance. Haemorrhage, calcification and necrosis very rare.

◀ Von Hippell–Lindau syndrome with brainstem haemangioblastoma and choroidal haemangioblastoma (arrowed, T1+C)

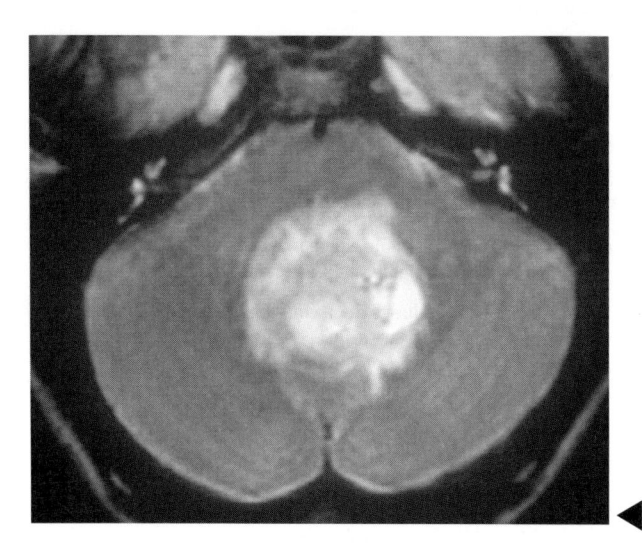

Ependymoma

Although ependymoma usually arises in the ventricle it is included here since it forms the most common differential diagnosis for medulloblastoma and astrocyoma in children, representing 15% of posterior fossa neoplasms.

Most present as a mass in the fourth ventricle. Small cysts and punctate calcification are common. Most enhance. Direct growth into the adjacent cerebrospinal fluid cisterns is common. Dissemination via cerebrospinal fluid seeding occurs but is unusual (10%).

◀ Ependymoma (T2)

Remember

1 Abscesses, metastases and infarcts (see previous page) also occur commonly in the posterior fossa.
2 Intraventricular masses can be difficult to distinguish from intra-axial masses in and around the fourth ventricle. (i.e. ependymoma, choroid plexus papilloma).

Non space-occupying lesions

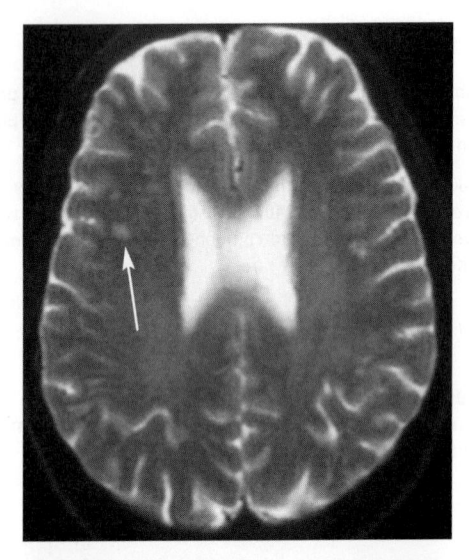

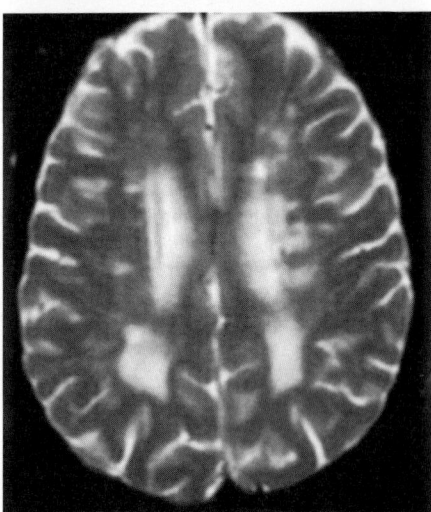

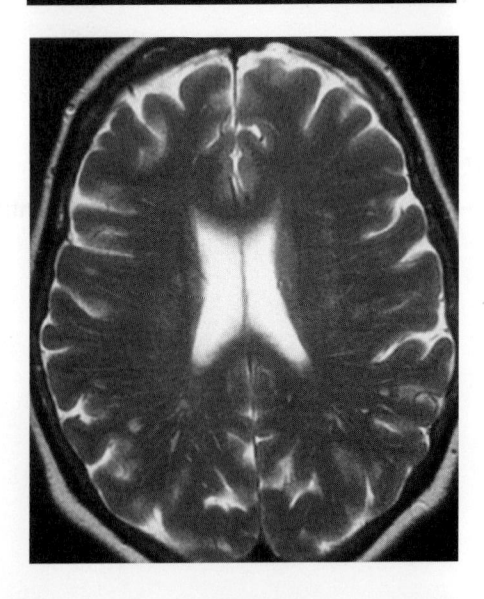

Diffuse white matter hyperintensity (DWMH)

Small areas of high signal on T2-weighted images are common over the age of 50 years. Incidence increases to >40% at age 80. Commonest in corona radiata and centrum semiovale. Lesions have no mass effect and do not enhance. Incidence related to vascular risk factors and lesions are presumed to be vascular in origin.

The main importance of these lesions is that they may be mistaken for clinically significant lesions such as demyelinating plaques in multiple sclerosis.

◄ **Normal brain in a 58-year-old showing areas high signal in the deep white matter (arrowed, T2).**

Periventricular hyperintensity (PVH)

PVH, seen on T2-weighted images, is most commonly due to increased extracellular fluid. PVH can be a normal feature of ageing. Many pathological processes are associated with PVH due to disruption of normal cerebral homeostatic mechanisms. These include tumours, inflammatory disorders and stroke. PVH in these circumstances forms a smooth periventricular halo which may also be evident as decreased signal/density on T1-weighted MRI/CT images.

Less commonly PVH is due to demyelination or gliosis around the ventricle. This is commonly seen in MS where it has a 'lumpy bumpy' appearance.

◄ **Multiple areas of hyperintensity around the body and occipital horns of the lateral ventricles (T2).**

Virchow–Robin spaces (VRS)

These are cerebrospinal fluid spaces extending into the brain around penetrating arteries. They are normally seen around the anterior commisure at the base of the brain and can appear circular or tubular. They are isointense to cerebrospinal fluid on all sequences. They become more prominent with increasing age and may be seen in the mesencephalon and corona radiata.

◄ **Multiple linear areas of hyperintensity on a T2-weighted image due to dilated VRS.**

Non space-occupying lesions

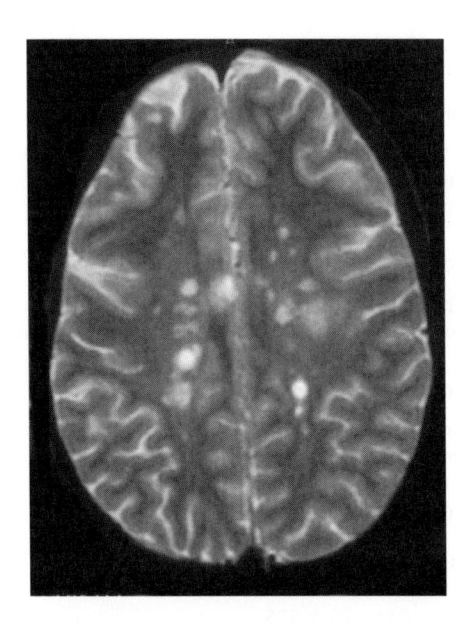

Demyelinating diseases

In multiple sclerosis (MS) demyelinating plaques appear high signal on T2-weighted images. Acute lesions may enhance and chronic lesions may become low signal on T1-weighted images. They are commonly seen in the white matter around the lateral ventricles and in the centrum semiovale and corona radiata. In the brainstem, lesions commonly occur at cerebrospinal fluid surfaces and in the pontine reticular formation and cerebellum. Some lesions are more specific to MS (e.g. callososeptal interface lesions). Distinctive patterns of myelin damage may also be seen in other, rarer, demyelinating and dysmyelinating diseases (e.g. central pontine myelinolysis) and following radiation and chemotherapy.

Multiple areas of hyperintensity in the centrum semiovale on a T2-weighted image due to demyelination in multiple sclerosis (T2).

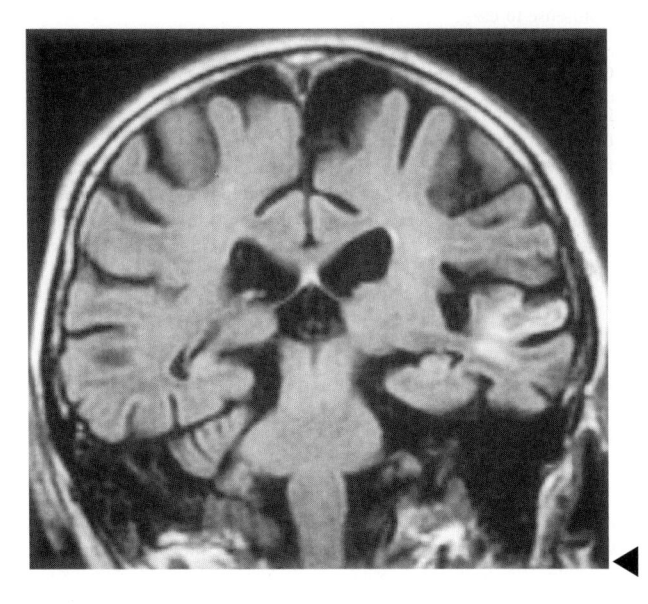

Infarction

Cortical infarcts appear as rounded or wedge shaped lesions characterized by regional atrophy with widening of adjacent sulci. Some infarcts show increased signal intensity on T2-weighted images. Longstanding cortical lesions may be visible only as regions of focal atrophy. CT demonstrates focal atrophy and areas of decreased attenuation in adjacent areas of the brain. Multiple cortical and basal lacunar infarcts may co-exist in patients with vascular disease. Lacunar infarcts are seen as cystic lesions 0.5–1.5 cm in size. They are located in region of the basal ganglia occurring along the path of the penetrating striothalamic arteries.

Chronic left-sided temporal lobe infarct showing regional atrophy and high signal change due to gliosis. The image is a fluid suppressed T2-weighted image (FLAIR).

Remember

1 Many non-space occupying lesions (e.g. infarction and demyelinating plaque) are space occupying in their acute stages.

Intraventricular masses

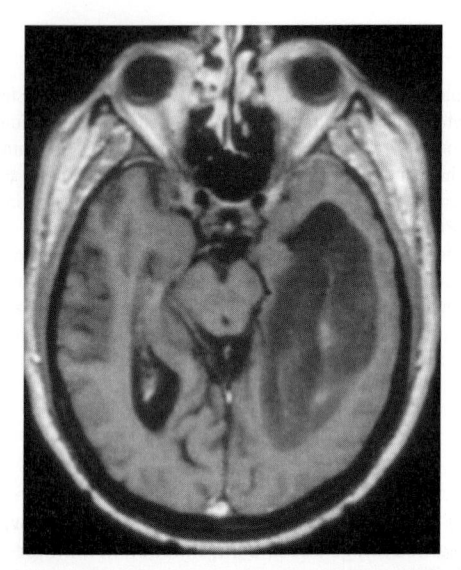

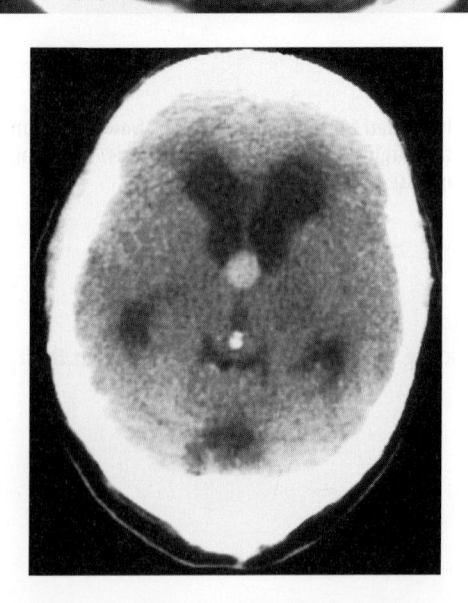

Gliomas and neurocytoma

Astrocytoma

Commonest primary neoplasm arising from septum. Periventricular astrocytomas may show intraventricular extension. Appearances typical of astrocytoma elsewhere.

Oligodendroglioma

Typically presents as a mass in the body of the lateral ventricle. Calcification common, may be extensive. Enhancement variable.

Neurocytomas

Typically at or near the foramen of Munro arising from the septum pellucidum. Sharply demarcated, 50% show areas of calcification. Necrosis and cyst formation common. Difficult to distinguish from oligodendroglioma.

◄ **Large left-sided intraventricular astrocytoma (T1).**

Choroid plexus masses

Non-neoplastic cysts in the glomus of the choroid plexus are a common incidental finding. They are thin walled, frequently bilateral and isointense to CSF.

Choroid plexus papilloma

Commonest in children under 5 years. Typically located in the trigone or atria of the lateral ventricles. In adults they are commonest in the fourth ventricle. Calcification is present in 25%. Imaging appearances are of a heterogeneous, lobulated frond-like mass with intense enhancement. Secondary hydrocephalus is common. CSF seedling may occur especially after malignant transformation which occurs in 10–20%.

◄ **Fourth ventricular choroid plexus papilloma (T1+C).**

Colloid cysts

These benign lesions occur in the anterior part of the third ventricle adjacent to the foramen of Munro. They appear as well defined thin walled cysts which are usually hyperdense on CT. MRI appearances are variable. They do not enhance or calcify. Secondary obstructive hydrocephalus is common and may be intermittent and postural in nature.

◄ **Colloid cyst (CT)**

Intraventricular masses

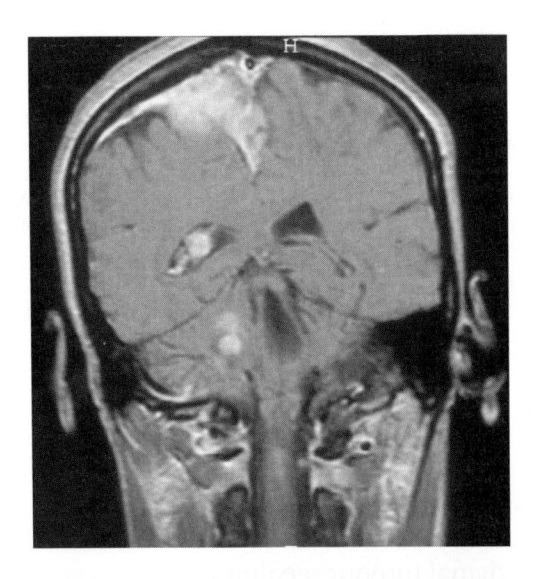

Meningioma

Most commonly seen in the atrium, occipital and temporal horns of the lateral ventricles. Appearances typical of meningiomas elsewhere. Typically well defined, 75% hyperdense on CT, 20–25% calcify, >90% enhance. Intraventricular haemorrhage is a rare but recognized complication.

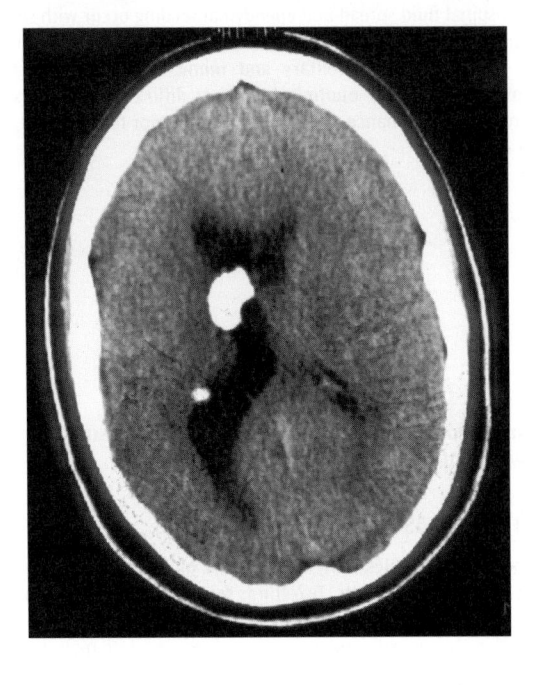

◀ Meningioma in the right occipital horn in a patient with neurofibromatosis. Note also convexity meningioma and high signal in cerebellum due to acoustic neuroma (T1+C).

Giant cell astrocytoma

Subependymal giant cell astrocytomas are usually associated with tuberous sclerosis (TS) and represent proliferation of one of the subependymal hamartomas which are the hallmark of this disease. Other stigma of TS are usually present. Lesions enhance strongly. Calcification and secondary hydrocephalus are common.

Usually present before the age of 20.

◀ Calcified giant cell astrocytoma in tuberous sclerosis. Note also calcified tuber on the right (CT)

Remember

1 Ependymomas are also intraventricular tumours (see previous page).
2 In children medulloblastoma and pilocytic astrocytoma may present as predominantly intraventricular masses.
3 Metastases often present with intraventricular masses particularly in the atrium, occipital and temporal horns of the lateral ventricle.
4 Craniopharyngiomas may grow up from the suprasellar region into the third ventricle to become predominantly intraventricular.
5 Periventricular lesions may present as intraventricular mass lesions (see next page).

Periventricular lesions

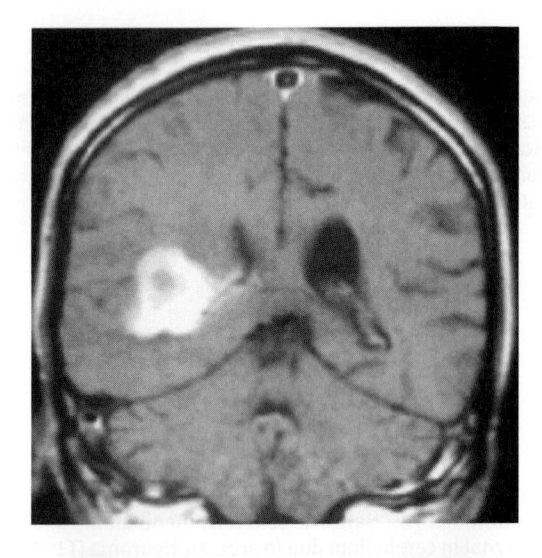

Lymphoma

Periventricular and deep grey matter lesions are the most common imaging features in cerebral lymphoma. Lesions may cause diffuse infiltration or focal abnormalities. Mass effect is minimal, haemorrhage and necrosis are rare. Most lesions are iso to slightly hyperintense on T2-weighted and iso to hypointense on T1-weighted images. Strong homogeneous enhancement is typical, ring enhancement may be seen in immunocompromised individuals.

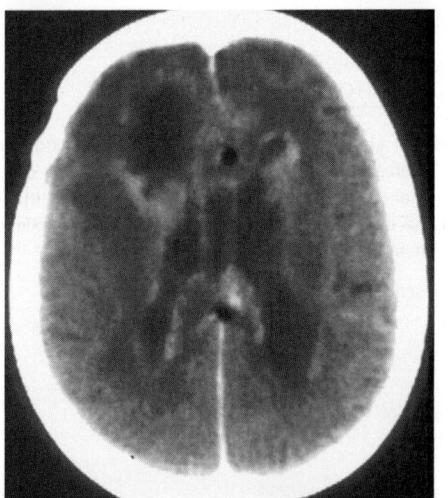

◀ **Lymphoma adjacent to right occipital horn (T1+C).**

Ependymal tumour seedlings

Cerebrospinal fluid spread and ependymal seeding occur with several malignancies including: ependymoma, glioma, and medulloblastoma. Lesions may be solitary and mimic intraventricular mass lesions. More typically multiple lesions or diffuse spread are seen. Lesions typically enhance, calcification is rare prior to treatment.

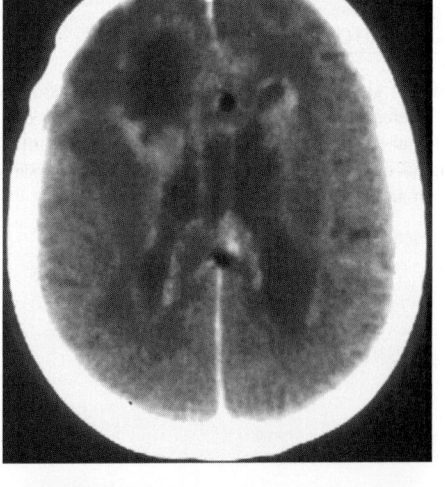

◀ **Extensive ependymal seeding of primary astrocytoma (CT with contrast).**

Hamartomas

Subependymal nodules (SEN) are a feature of tuberous sclerosis (TS). Occur in 95% of TS patients. Two-thirds seen near the head or body of the caudate nucleus; 88% of SEN eventually calcify. Lesions are non-calcified in the neonate and appear isointense to white matter on T2-weighted images. In older children they become hypointense due to calcification. Other stigmata of TS will be seen.

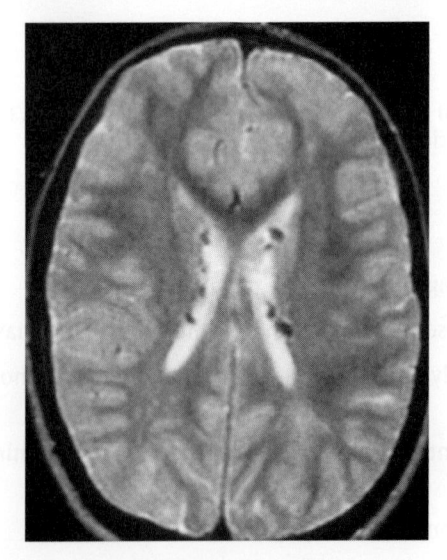

◀ **Multiple calcified hamartomas in tuberous sclerosis (T2).**

Periventricular lesions

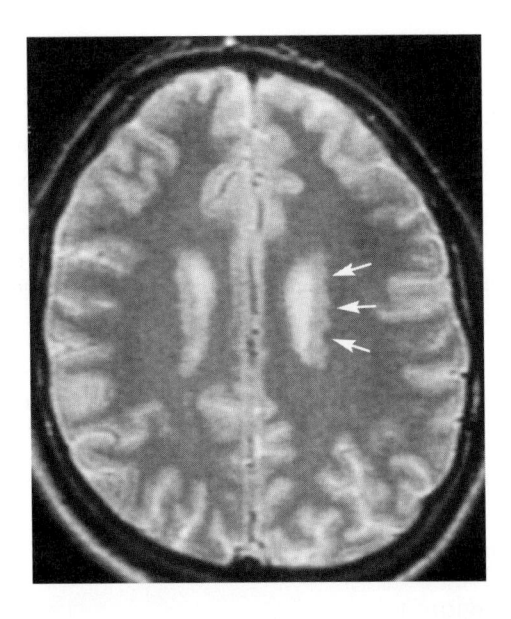

Grey matter heterotopias

Arrest of the normal migration of neuronal tissue during the brain's development results in the deposition of disordered clumps of otherwise normal grey matter. These are common in the subependymal area and are isointense to normal grey matter on all modalities.

Heterotopia may be laminar, or nodular, focal or diffuse. Although present from birth heterotopias may be seen at all ages.

◀ Periventricular grey matter heterotopias (arrowed, T2).

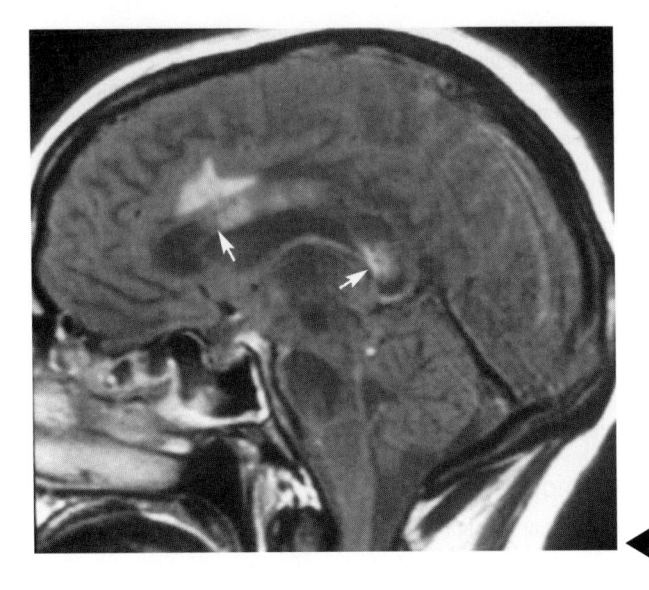

Multiple sclerosis

Multiple sclerosis is the commonest cause of periventricular abnormality in adults. Inflammation occurs preferentially around penetrating veins so that lesions are commonly seen at cerebrospinal fluid boundaries. Common sites include the lateral part of the lateral ventricles, the centre of the lower border of the corpus callosum (calloso or septal lesion), the floor of the fourth ventricle and the anterior surface of the brainstem.

◀ Extensive callosal (arrows) and periventricular high signal in multiple sclerosis (FLAIR).

Remember

1 Periventricular abnormality is common in patients with AIDS (acquired immunodeficiency syndrome) and can result from cytomegalovirus infection, HIV (human immunodeficiency virus) encephalitis, Kaposi's sarcoma, lymphoma, progressive multifocal leukoencephalopathy (PML) or toxoplasmosis.

Extra-axial: Sellar and parasellar lesions

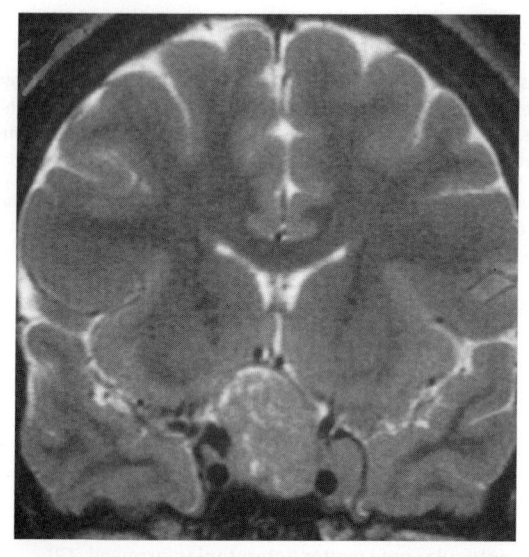

Pituitary masses

Physiological

Physiological enlargement of the pituitary gland may occur in pregnancy or as a result of end-organ failure (e.g. hypothyroidism).

Congenital

Benign pituitary cysts occur relatively rarely. They are usually colloid or Rathke's pouch cysts. They are thin walled, non-calcifying and non-enhancing.

Neoplastic

Pituitary adenomas are classified as microadenoma (<10mm) or macroadenoma. Macroadenomas commonly extend into the suprasellar region and show internal necrosis, haemorrhage and cyst formation. All adenomas enhance but contrast administration is seldom needed to establish the diagnosis.

◀ **Pituitary adenoma (T2).**

Meningioma

Meningioma is the second commonest suprasellar neoplasm. Rarely it presents as a purely intrasellar mass. En-plaque spread is a common and helpful diagnostic feature best seen on post-contrast images. CT may demonstrate local hyperostosis; however, other typical features of meningioma such as oedema and calcification are relatively unusual at this site.

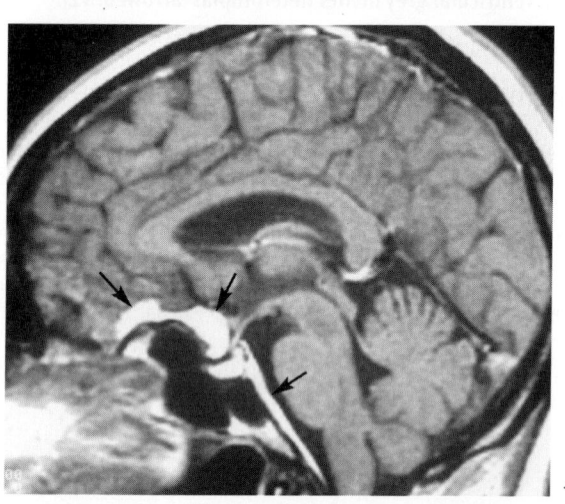

◀ **En-plaque meningioma of the olfactory groove, tuberculum sella and clivus (T1+C).**

Craniopharyngioma

Occur at all ages but account for 50% of suprasellar tumours in children; 80–90% show calcification and cyst formation. All show enhancement. They commonly extend up into the brain and third ventricle and may erode down into or through the skull base. Cysts may appear bright on CT and T1-weighted MRI.

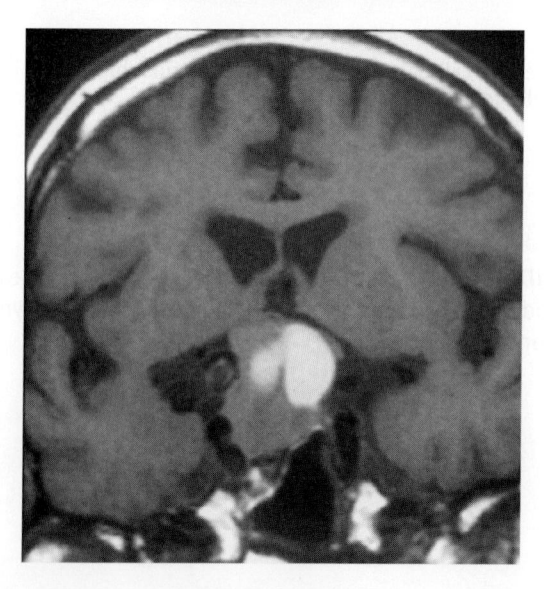

◀ **Craniopharyngioma with high signal internal cyst (T1).**

Extra-axial: Sellar and parasellar lesions

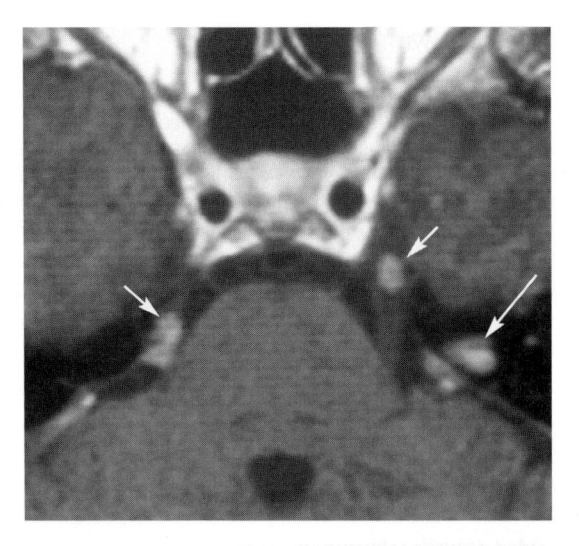

Nerve sheath tumours

Schwannomas of the cranial nerves in the cavernous sinus may present as a parasellar mass. Vth nerve origin is most common and the pattern of growth from Meckel's cave, into the lateral wall of the cavernous sinus is distinctive. They may be bilateral or multiple in type 2 neurofibromatosis. They are well defined, follow the route of the nerve and show marked enhancement.

Plexiform neurofibromas are also rarely seen in the parasellar region. They most commonly arise from the trigeminal nerve, especially the ophthalmic division.

◀ **Multiple bilateral trigeminal schwannomas (arrows) and left acoustic neuroma (long arrow) in patient with neurofibromatosis (T1+C).**

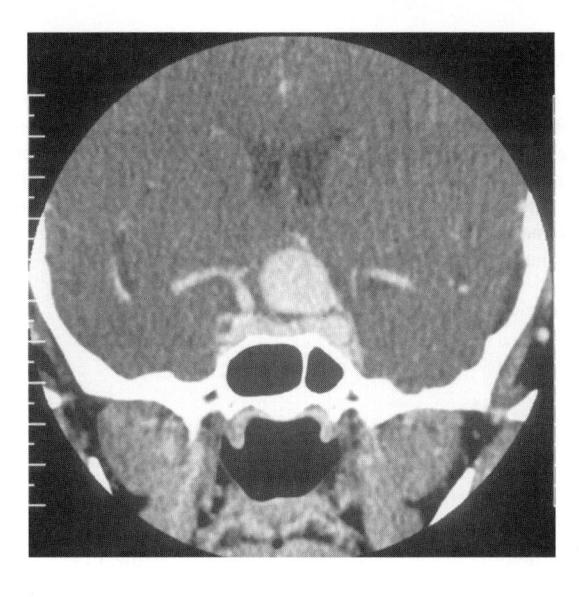

Aneurysm

Aneurysms of the basal arteries may mimic other parasellar mass lesions. This is an important differential diagnosis and must be considered in all cases in order to avoid inappropriate surgery. Large aneurysms may appear hyperdense on unenhanced CT and show homogenous enhancement. Although they are usually eccentric they may be entirely midline. Bone excavation and remodelling are common features. Calcification in the aneurysm wall may provide a clue but is not always present. MRI classically demonstrates an area of signal void although layers of maturing thrombus may be visible.

◀ Large suprasellar aneurysm (CT with contrast).

Remember

1. The range of pathologies in this area is particularly wide (Chapter 3).
2. Skull base lesions such as cephalocoeles, dermoid cysts and chordoma may extend into the sellar and parasellar regions.

Extra-axial: Infratentorial

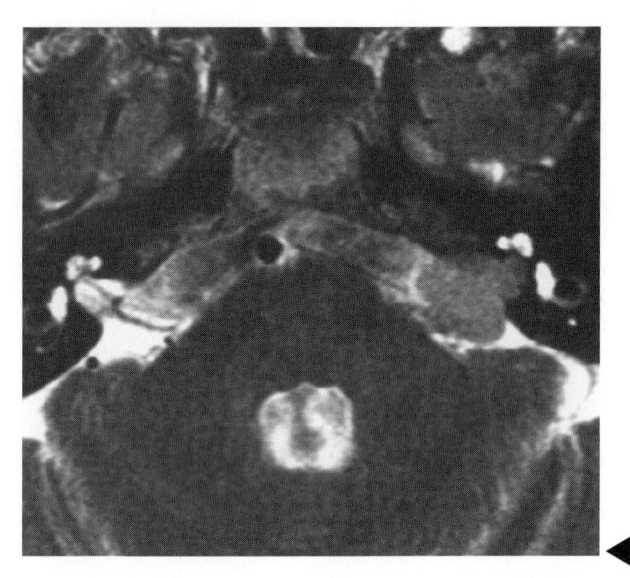

Acoustic schwannoma

The commonest benign tumour of the posterior fossa. Acoustic schwannoma (AS) arises from the VIIIth cranial nerve and is seen in or adjacent to the internal auditory meatus (IAM). Small lesions may be entirely intracannalicular. Larger AS grow into the cerebellopontine angle and have a distinctive 'ice cream cone' shape. All enhance, none calcify. Larger lesions may show cyst formation and necrosis. Bilateral lesions are diagnostic of type 2 neurofibromatosis.

Schwannomas of other cranial nerves (particularly V and VIII) are also seen. They have similar imaging characteristics and are distinguished by their location.

◀ Left-sided acoustic schwannoma (T2)

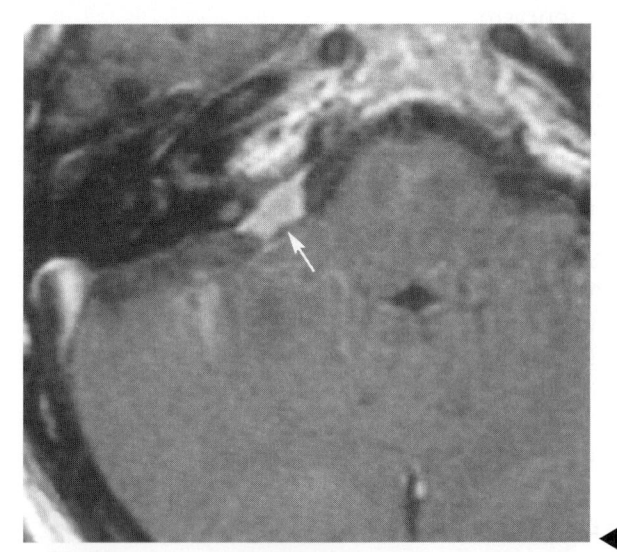

Meningioma

Second commonest benign tumour in the posterior fossa. They are most commonly found on the clivus around the cerebellopontine angle (CPA) or foramen magnum. In the region of the CPA they are commonly mistaken for acoustic schwannoma. In fact they may overly the internal auditory meatus (IAM) but are seldom centred there. Intrameatal extension does occur but is rare. En-plaque growth is common and calcification is occasionally seen.

◀ Meningioma of the cerebellopontine angle (arrow, T1+C).

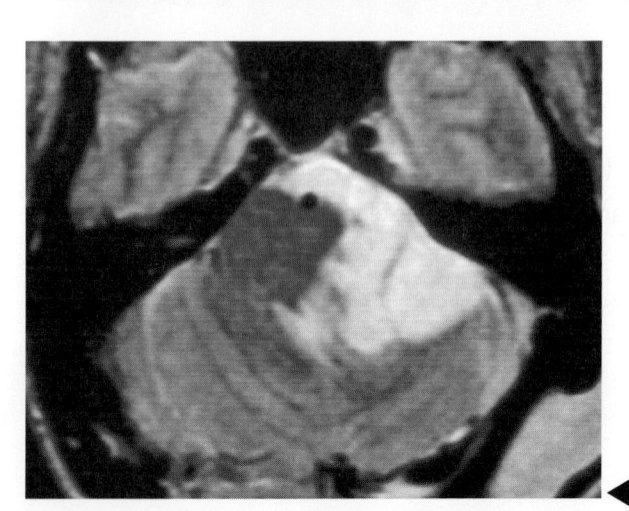

Epidermoid tumour

These benign lesions have distinctive CT and MR appearances. Most commonly seen in the cerebellopontine angle they tend to fill available CSF spaces. They are low attenuation on CT and are often indistinguishable from CSF. On MRI they also show similar signal characteristics to CSF on T1- and T2-weighted images but are usually hyperintense to CSF on proton density weighted images. They do not calcify and mild enhancement is seen rarely.

Commonly occur between 20 and 60 years.

◀ Left cerebellopontine angle epidermoid (T2).

Extra-axial: Infratentorial

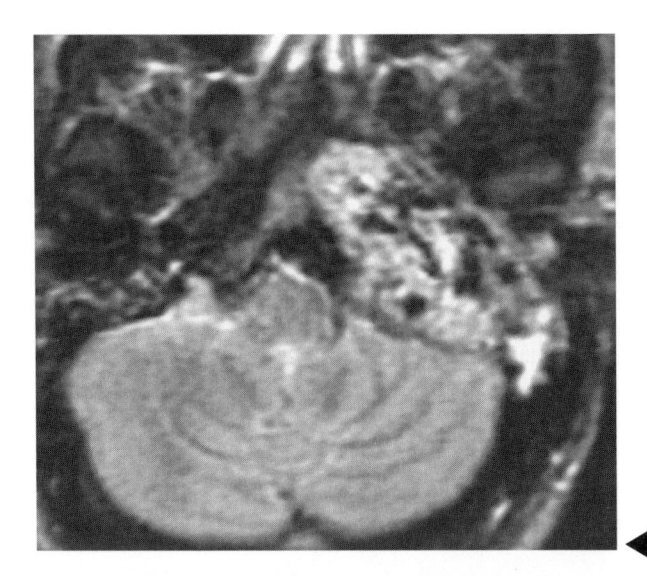

Paraganglioma (Glomus tumour)

Paragangliomas are skull base tumours which may extend into the posterior fossa. They usually arise in the petrous bone, either in the jugular canal or middle ear cavity. They are bone destructive lesions producing well demarcated defects in the skull base. Intracranial extension is invariably through the internal jugular foramen. They are highly vascular and non-enhanced MRI shows a heterogeneous appearance with multiple signal voids. They enhance markedly. They commonly grow into and occlude the jugular vein.

◀ Large left-sided glomus jugulare (T2).

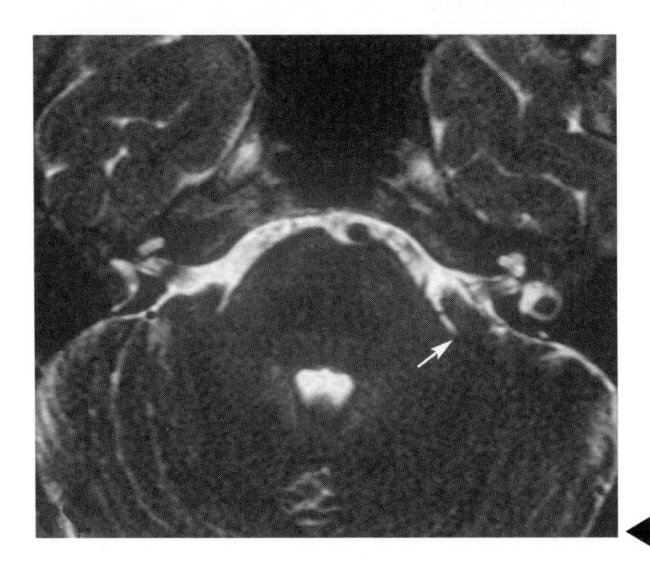

Normal structures

A number of normal structures in the posterior fossa can cause confusion if the anatomy is not appreciated. These include

1 The jugular bulb: can be large and dehiscent and may extend into the posterior fossa or middle ear.
2 The flocculus of the cerebellum extends anterolaterally into the cerebellopontine angle. It has the same imaging characteristics as normal brain and can be seen to extend from the cerebellum on lower images.
3 The vertebral and basilar arteries can become ectatic and dilated. They commonly distort normal structures.
4 The vermis of the cerebellum normally extends into the fourth ventricle and must not be mistaken for abnormal tissue.

◀ Flocculus of cerebellum (arrow); note normal nerves entering internal auditory meatus (T2).

Remember

1 Any destructive skull base lesion may present as a posterior fossa mass lesion.
2 Arachnoid cysts are commonly found in the posterior fossa (see Extra-axial: Supratentorial lesions, pp. 36–37).
3 Cerebrospinal fluid flow rates in the posterior fossa are significant and may produce flow voids on T2-weighted images. This is particularly common in the pre-pontine cistern around the basilar artery.

Extra-axial: Supratentorial

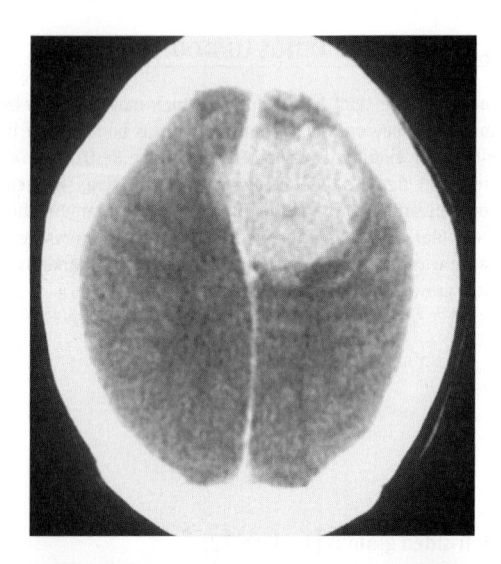

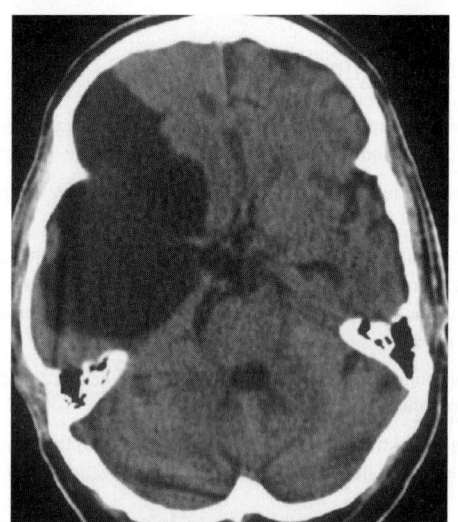

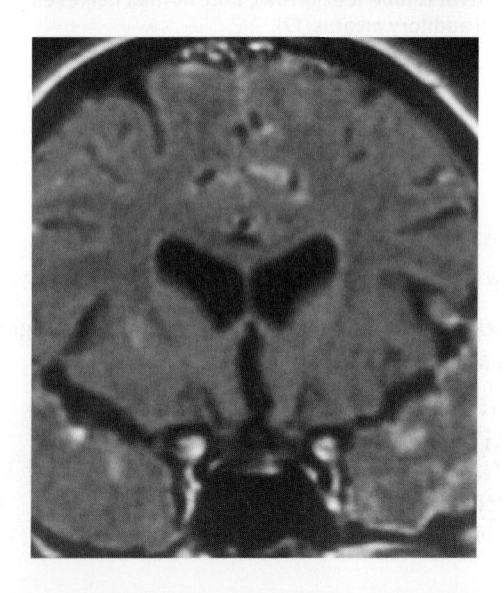

Meningiomas

Commonest brain tumour in adults; arise from meninges and may grow as focal masses or more unusually as diffuse infiltrating plaques. Most have a broad base on the meningeal surface which often tapers giving rise to the 'tail sign'. Tend to grow along meningeal surfaces and may engulf major vessels and nerves. May cause bone erosion or regional hyperostosis. Over 50% associated with profound oedema which can give a misleading impression of an intra-axial lesion. Meningiomas enhance intensely and often calcify. Areas of internal necrosis may be seen. Meningiomas are multiple in 5% of cases. On unenhanced MRI signal intensity is similar to normal brain and they may be difficult to identify.

Seen at all ages but commonest in adults and increase in frequency with age.

◀ **Large parafalcine meningioma (CT with contrast).**

Arachnoid cysts

These are common benign congenital CSF filled cysts which arise as a result of maldevelopment of the dura. They displace brain and cause thinning and re-modelling of the overlying skull vault. They do not enhance and show signal void on FLAIR sequences. They can occur anywhere but sites of predilection are the anterior middle cranial fossa, parasellar cistern and over the convexity. In the posterior fossa they are commonly seen in the cerebellopontine angle, the quadrigeminal cistern and behind the cerebellum.

◀ **Large right-sided temporal arachnoid cyst (CT).**

Diffuse meningeal disease

Diffuse meningeal disease is seen as the result of a number of disorders. Idiopathic meningeal thickening is occasionally seen and is typified by diffuse meningeal thickening and enhancement. Similar but localized changes can be seen as a sequelae of trauma, radiotherapy and surgery. Neoplastic causes include diffuse meningiomatosis, melanoma, metastasis, lymphoma, leukaemia, and all tumours which seed via the cerebrospinal fluid. Metastases are most commonly seen with primary tumours of breast, lung and gastrointestinal tract. Inflammatory causes include sarcoidosis and histiocytosis.

Meningeal disease can be difficult to identify and is usually best seen on contrast-enhanced MRI images.

◀ **Diffuse meningeal thickening and enhancement due to malignant melanoma (T1+C).**

Extra-axial: Supratentorial

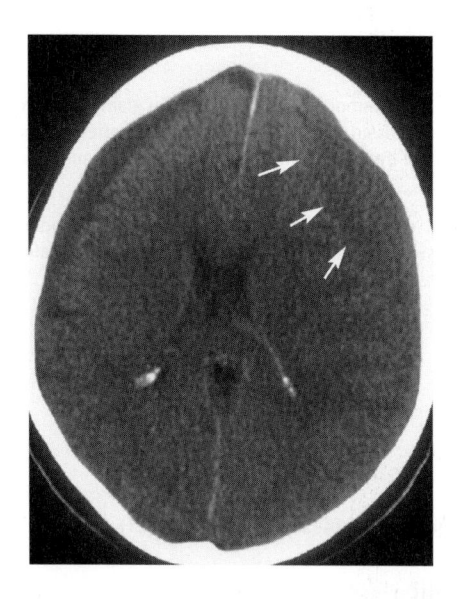

Extradural and subdural haemorrhage

Usually occur as a result of trauma. Extradural haematoma is usually an acute clinical presentation. They are biconvex collections with an acute angle at their leading edges which seldom cross suture lines where the dura is more tightly adherent. They may separate dural venous sinuses from underlying bone. Subdural haematoma results from venous bleeding and may be associated with minimal trauma. It is commoner in the elderly, in alcoholics and following ventricular shunting. They are often extensive and classically have a concave inner surface over the convexity. They may extend along the falx cerebri and tentorium cerebelli. CT and MRI appearances vary with the age of the collection and subacute subdural collections may be isodense to brain on CT images.

◀ Bilateral chronic subdural haematomas: isodense on left (arrows, CT).

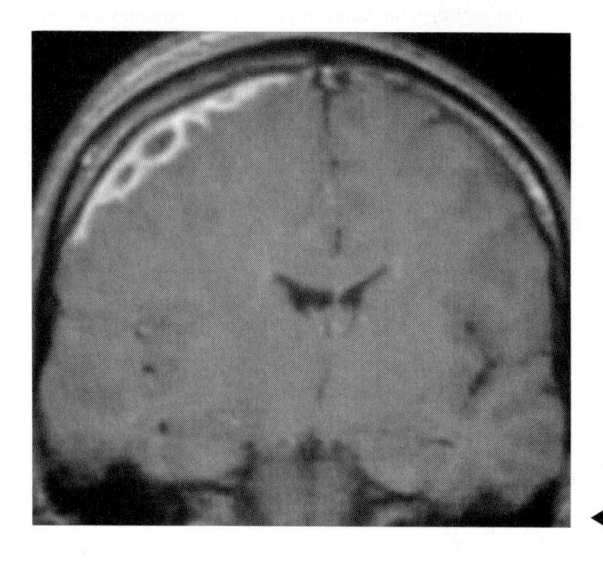

Extradural and subdural empyema

Infective collections arise as a complication of meningitis, systemic sepsis or local infections such as osteomyelitis or sinusitis.

Morphologically they have similar characteristics to haemorrhagic collections. However they are usually small and are frequently multiple or loculated. They are characterized by marked enhancement in the solid components. They can be associated with adjacent cerebral oedema and cerebritis and may cause dural venous sinus thrombosis. Contrast-enhanced scans are required to adequately delineate the extent of disease.

◀ Right-sided enhancing subdural empyema (T1+C).

Remember

1 Acute haemorrhagic extra and subdural collections may occur as a consequence of bleeding from cerebral arteriovenous malformations or circle of Willis aneurysms.

Calcification

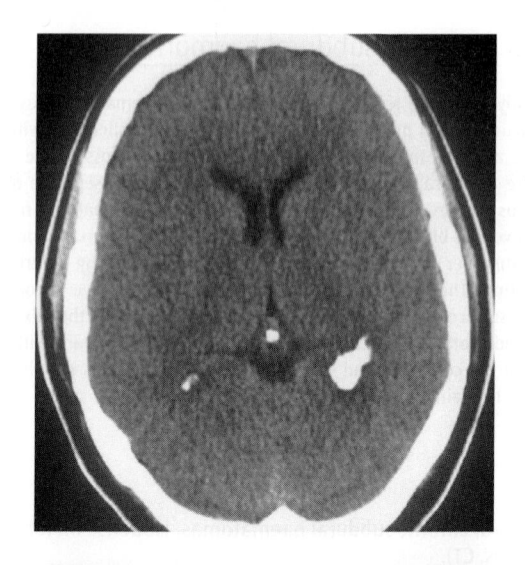

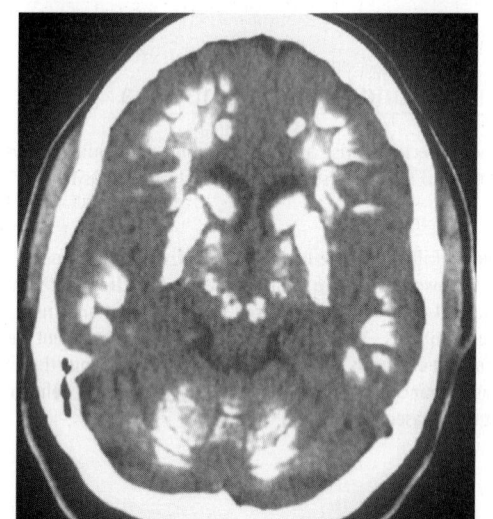

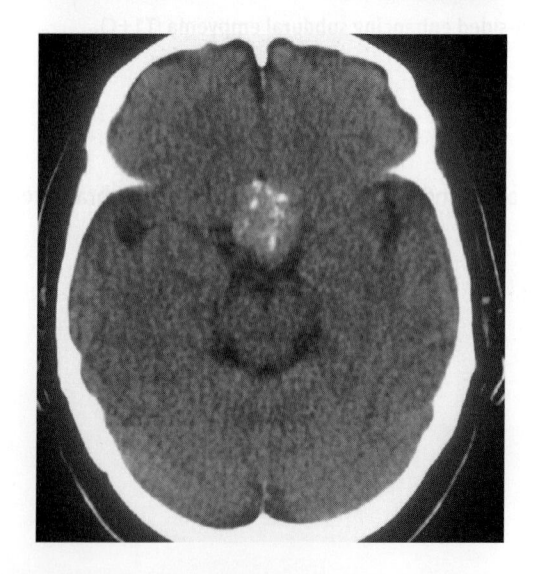

Physiological

Calcification is commonly seen in the pineal gland, the falx and tentorium, the choroid plexus and in major arteries in the elderly. Calcification of the basal ganglia and dentate nuclei may also occur in the elderly.

Exaggerated calcification in a physiological distribution is seen in some disease processes (e.g. dense choroid plexus calcification in neurofibromatosis).

◀ **Pineal and choroid plexus calcification (CT).**

Metabolic

Calcium deposition in the brain and cerebral membranes is a feature of many metabolic disorders including: systemic hypercalcaemia, primary and secondary hyperparathyroidism, hypoparathyroidism, pseudohypoparathyroidism, lead encephalopathy and carbon monoxide poisoning.

◀ **Extensive parenchymal calcification in metabolic disease (CT).**

Neoplastic

Calcification is seen in almost any cerebral tumour with a great variation in frequency. For example: oligodendroglioma and craniopharyngioma (90%), ependymoma and primitive neuroectodermal tumour (PNET) (50–60%), meningioma (25%), astrocytoma (15–25%).

Dystrophic calcification can be seen as a consequence of hypercalcaemia or as a non-neoplastic syndrome in association with a range of non-cerebral tumours (e.g. small cell lung tumours).

◀ **Parenchymal calcification in craniopharyngioma (CT).**

Calcification

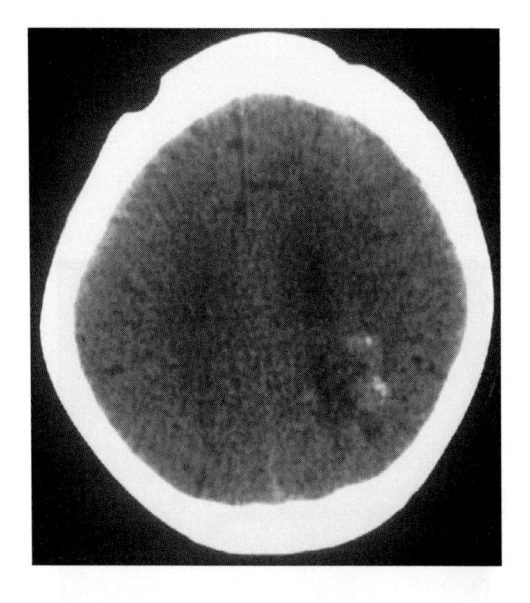

Vascular

Calcification may be seen in the walls of cerebral aneurysms (5%), arteriovenous malformations (25%) and atherosclerotic vessels.

Calcification of cortex and subcortical white matter is seen adjacent to the angioma in Sturge–Weber syndrome.

Dense calcification occurs in chronic subdural and parenchymal haematomas.

◀ Calcification in a parenchymal arteriovenous malformation (CT).

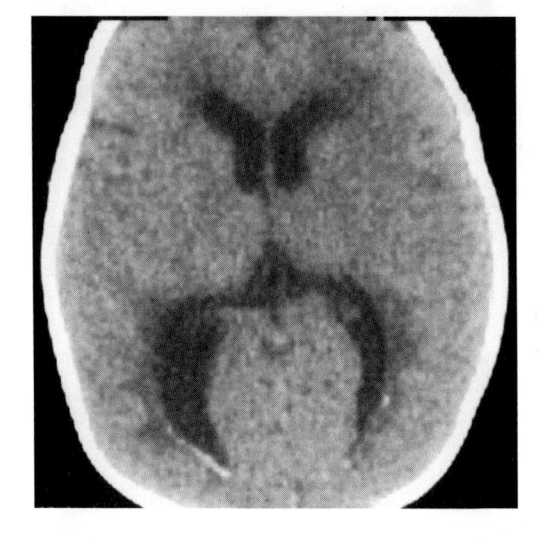

Inflammatory

Calcification of inflammatory tissue is a feature of the TORCH infections (Toxoplasmosis, Rubella, CMV and Herpes simplex). Calcification is seen as multiple small areas and as more diffuse periventricular, cortical and basal ganglia calcification.

Calcification occurs in tuberculous and fungal granulomas and may be seen in some parasitic infestations (e.g. cysticercosis and echinicoccus).

◀ Periventricular calcification in cytomegalovirus (CT).

Remember

1 Calcification is significantly more difficult to detect on MRI than CT.
2 Substantial foci of calcification appear as areas of signal void on MRI but smaller areas may be undetectable.
3 Gradient echo techniques are more sensitive than spin echo in detecting calcification.
4 Microcalcification may have a bright signal on T1-weighted images.

Appearances of parenchymal haematoma

T1

T2

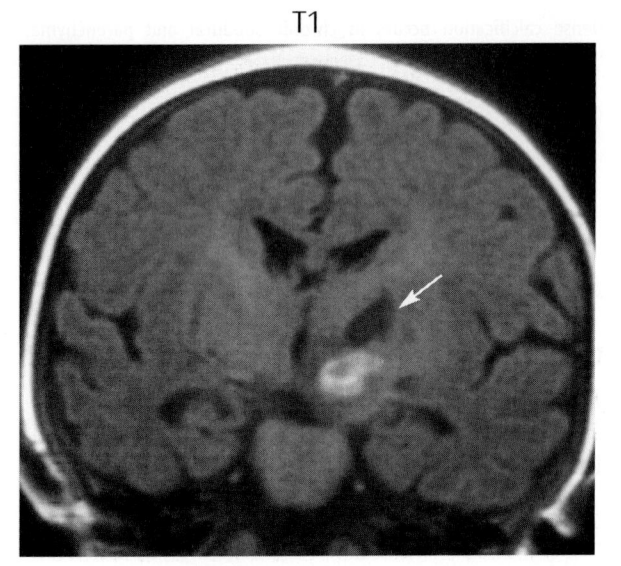

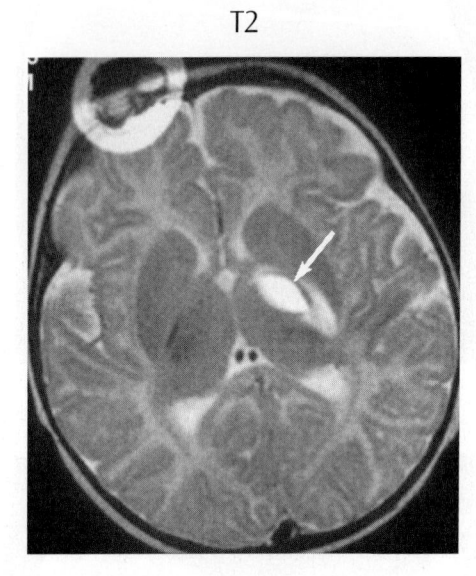

Hyperacute

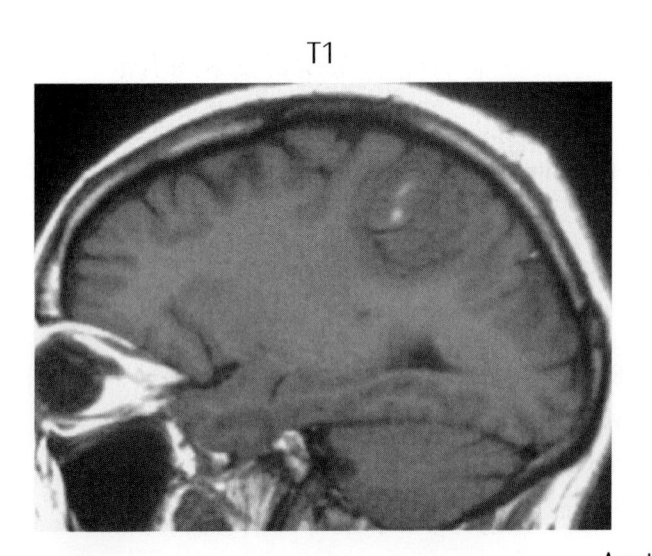

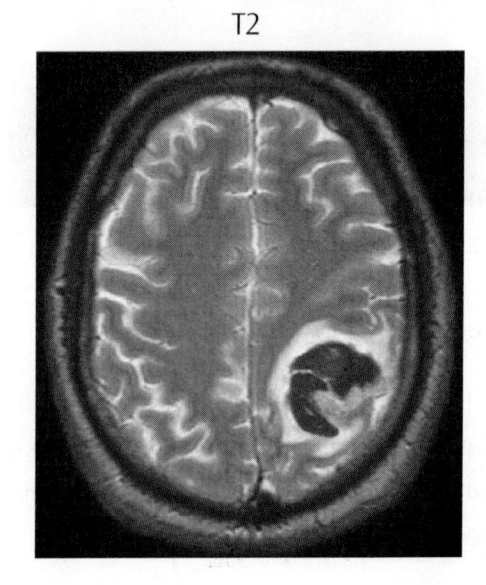

T1

T2

Acute

Appearances of parenchymal haematoma

T1　　　　　　　　　　　　T2

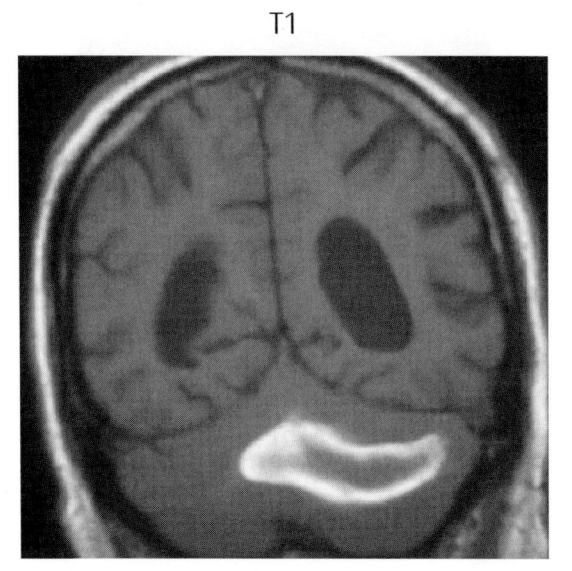

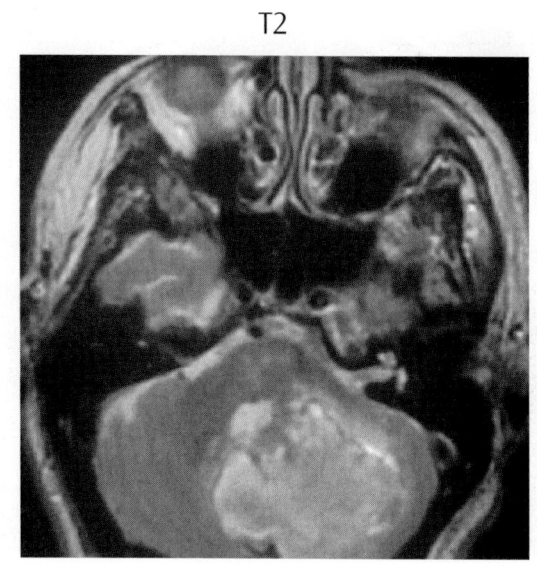

Subacute

T1　　　　　　　　　　　　T2

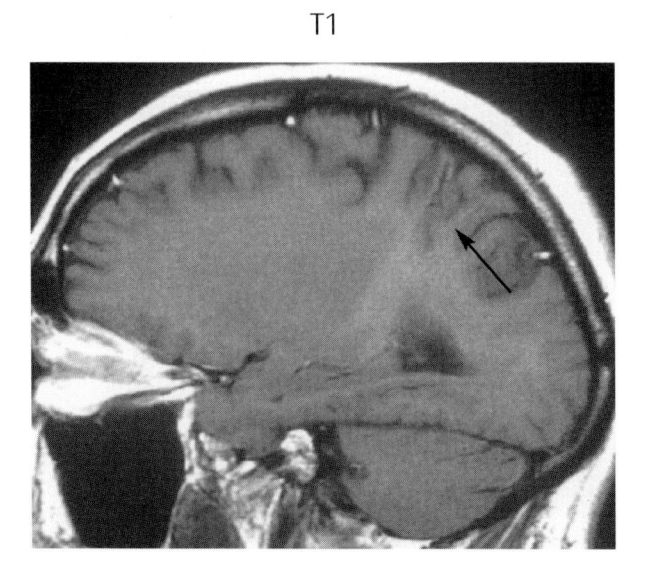

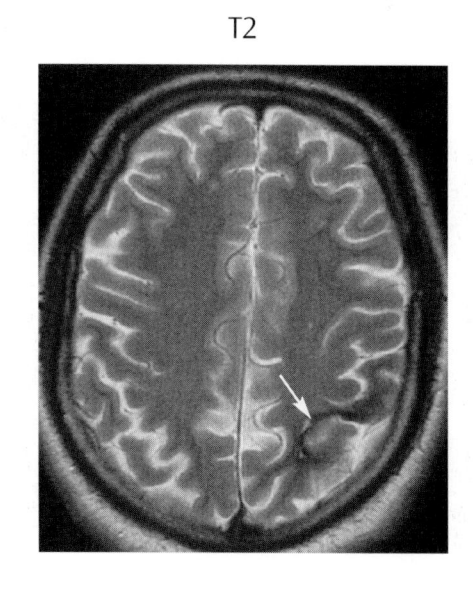

Chronic

Appearances of subdural haematoma

T1

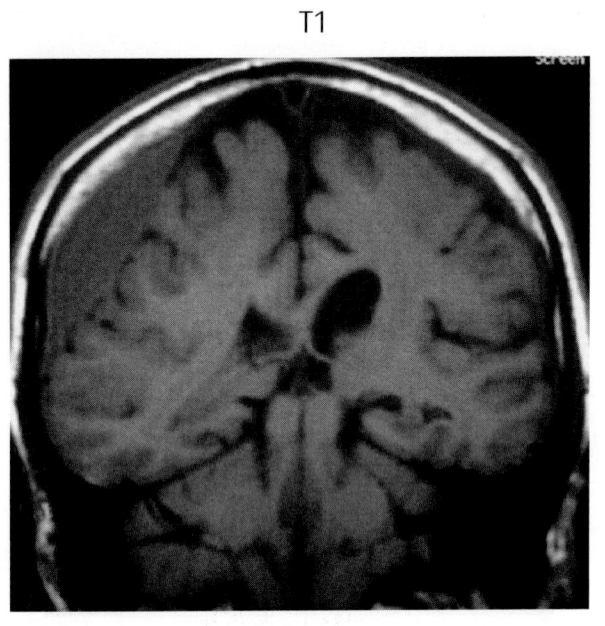

T2

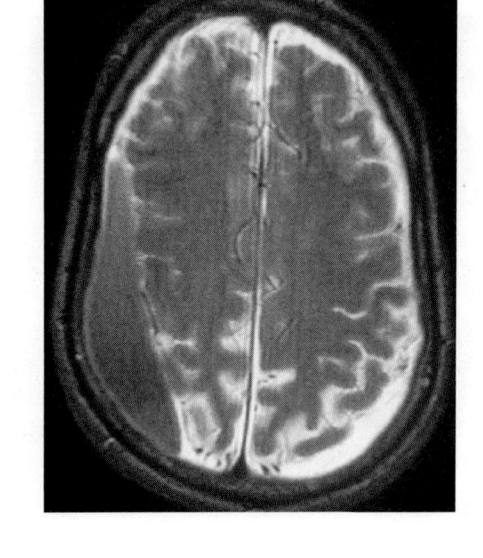

Acute

T1

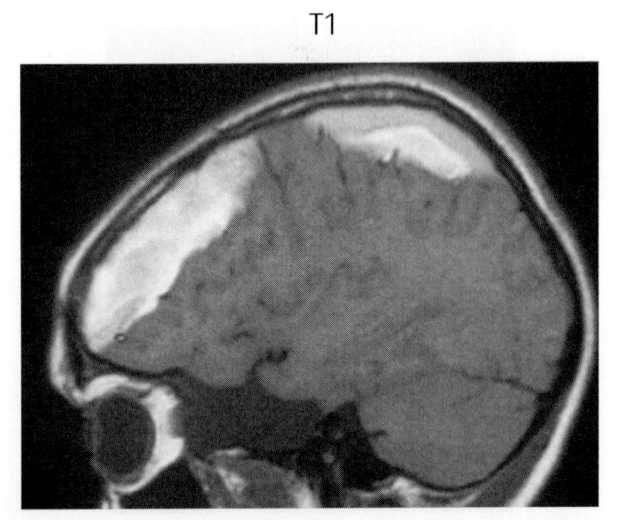

T2

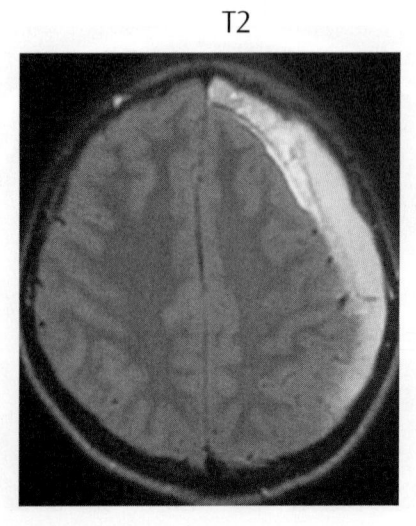

Subacute/chronic

Appearances of parenchymal/subdural haematoma

	Haemoglobin state	T1-Weighted appearances	T2-Weighted appearances
Hyperacute (4–6 hours)	Oxyhaemoglobin, intracellular	Isointense	Hyperintense
Acute (6 hours–3 days)	Deoxyhaemoglobin, intracellular	Isointense	Hypointense
Early subacute (4–7 days)	Methaemoglobin, intracellular	Hyperintense	Hypointense
Late subacute (1–4 weeks)	Methaemoglobin, extracellular	Hyperintense	Hyperintense
Chronic (months–years)	Haemosiderin and ferritin	Hypointense	Hypointense

Remember

1 Most haematomas will have a mixture of appearances since evolution of clot proceeds at slightly different rates in different areas.
2 Evolution of changes generally occurs earlier in the periphery.
3 Haemosiderin is rarely seen in chronic subdural haematomas which more commonly show layers of haemorrhage, of differing areas, due to repeated re-bleeding.
4 On T1 30% of chronic subdural haematomas become iso or hypointense.
5 Acute subarachnoid haemorrhage is difficult to detect on conventional MR sequences but may be seen on FLAIR acquisitions.

Part 3

1

Congenital abnormalities

JAMES E GILLESPIE

Introduction		Disorders of cellular migration	62
MR and CT imaging techniques	44	Disorders of myelination	70
Disorders of dorsal induction	44	References	71
Disorders of ventral induction	47	Further reading	72
Disorders of neuronal proliferation, differentiation and histogenesis	52		

INTRODUCTION

Congenital anomalies are often a difficult and perplexing group of abnormalities to decipher on imaging. Even within specialist paediatric units most of these abnormalities are encountered very infrequently so building up significant experience in this field is difficult. As interpretation is helped by having some knowledge of how the brain develops the abnormalities will be discussed using the basic classification framework proposed by Van Der Knaap and Valk[1] which lists the abnormalities according to the time of onset during gestation of the developmental disruption. Each category of abnormality will be proceeded by very brief highlights of the normal development process occurring at that chronological stage. Although these processes are described separately there is considerable overlap in their time scales and so the presence of one congenital anomaly should trigger a search for other co-existing anomalies.

MR AND CT IMAGING TECHNIQUES

Magnetic resonance (MR) is undoubtedly the imaging technique of choice for the investigation of virtually all congenital anomalies. In neonates, transcranial ultrasound may well demonstrate that major structural anomalies are present but even in these circumstances MRI is usually undertaken to further evaluate the child. My basic MR brain protocol consists of a sagittal T1-weighted spin echo sequence and an axial T2-weighted sequence, usually obtained as a long TR (repetition time) spin echo sequence with a short and long TE (echo time) giving proton density weighted and T2-weighted images. An occasional alternative is a fast spin echo T2-weighted sequence. In practice, I find images in the three orthogonal planes extremely useful and usually essential when investigating congenital anomalies and therefore to this protocol I add a coronal T1-weighted sequence, usually a spin echo sequence or, if I am particularly interested in looking at grey matter structure, a fast inversion recovery sequence. In children under the age of 18 months, an axial T1-weighted spin echo sequence is also extremely useful when assessing early white matter maturation (for those under 6 months of age) and for brain structure (particularly 12- to 18-month olds).[2] Another approach to obtaining multiplanar T1-weighted images is to perform a three-dimensional (3-D) data acquisition using a spoiled GRASS (Gradient Recalled Acquisition in Steady State) (SPGR) type sequence allowing a large number of very thin slices to be reconstructed and subsequently reformatted into any desired image plane. Intravenous contrast–enhancement with a gadolinium-based contrast–medium is essential when investigating most of the neurocutaneous disorders (phakomatoses). Otherwise, contrast–enhancement is only occasionally required when investigating congenital anomalies and these are mentioned where relevant. Throughout this chapter the phrases 'T1-weighted images' and 'T2-weighted images' will be shortened to T1WI and T2WI respectively.

Computed tomography (CT) generally plays a supplementary role in the investigation of congenital brain anomalies. Its strength is in the detailed evaluation of cortical bone structure particularly with cephaloceles and in the investigation of craniofacial anomalies. Spiral CT acquisition methods are useful in these circumstances as they allow thin, overlapping slices to be reconstructed, ideal for subsequent 2-D multiplanar or 3-D surface reformations. These images are best reconstructed using a bone algorithm.

Spiral CT scanning techniques have reduced the problem of movement with infants and young children but when high resolution bone images for reformatting are being obtained or, more usually, MRI is being performed, sedation or anaesthesia may have to be considered. Neonates may lie still long enough for good quality scanning shortly after a feed. Oral sedation can be undertaken with a variety of different agents depending upon local preference; in our hospital triclofos, sometimes supplemented by trimeprazine are often successful for shorter MR or CT examinations. However, our paediatric anaesthetists prefer a general anaesethetic to heavy doses of sedative agents when a longer, more detailed examination is required. It is essential that departmental policy on sedation, anaesthesia and patient monitoring be drawn up in consultation with the local anaesthetic department.

In the following sections on individual anomalies, details of imaging technique will only be mentioned when it varies from the above general protocol or when specific imaging requirements exist.

DISORDERS OF DORSAL INDUCTION

Dorsal induction is the process leading to the formation of the neural tube. The brain and spinal cord develop from a thickening of neuroectoderm which forms the neural plate. The neural plate contains a central neural groove, surrounded on each side by the elevated neural folds. As the neural groove deepens, the neural folds then fuse in the midline resulting in the formation of the neural tube. Neuroectoderm cells from the margins of the neural folds separate from the folds before fusion occurs to form the neural crest which surrounds the neural tube. The neural crest will eventually give rise to the dorsal root ganglia, cranial nerves and autonomic ganglia and parts of the adrenal medulla. Neural tube closure commences in the area which will eventually become the neck of the embryo with closure conventionally thought to proceed cranially and caudally from this point. This process of neural tube formation is called *neurulation* and has been divided into primary and secondary neurulation. Primary neurulation refers to neural tube formation from about L1-L2 upwards, the region from which the brain and spinal cord will develop and occurs in the 3rd and 4th week of gestation. Secondary neurulation describes the development of the lower spine which occurs between the 4th and 7th week of gestation. Disorders of secondary neurulation result in spinal dysraphism, a description of which is outside the scope of this book.

Disorders of primary neurulation can result in severe deformities, incompatible with life, such as anencephaly. The main abnormalities of primary neurulation which will be discussed here are cephaloceles and Chiari malformations.

Cephaloceles

These are defects in the skull and dura allowing the intracranial contents to extend outside the skull. Cephaloceles are usually mid line masses located at suture lines or the junction of several adjoining bones.[2,3] The incidence of these abnormalities is 0.8–3 per 10 000 births. A notable geographical variation in the incidence of different types of cephaloceles exists with occipital cephaloceles being most common in Europe and North America while in South East Asia cephaloceles in the nasal region predominate. Cephaloceles are described according to their contents: *meningoencephaloceles* which contain brain in addition to cerebrospinal fluid (CSF) and meninges, while *meningoceles* contain CSF and meninges but no brain. Cephaloceles can protrude through the skull vault convexity or through the skull base, and are named according to their location.

Some of the commoner or more notable sites include:

a. *Occipital* These make up 80% of all cephaloceles occurring in Europe or North America. They may contain brain contents from above or below the tentorium as well as portions of the ventricular system and venous sinuses (Fig. 1.1).
b. *Frontoethmoidal* In the normal process of development a projection of dura passes through the foramen caecum (located between the developing nasal cartilage and bone) which then gradually regresses.[4] Failure of regression can result in a number of abnormalities. Protrusion of brain through the dural projection results in a cephalocele. Dermoid and epidermoid tumours can also form along this tract or a nasal glioma can form which is dysplastic brain tissue no longer connected to the brain. Dermal sinus tracts are marked by a skin dimple due to the non-regressed dura attaching to the overlying skin. Frontoethmoidal cephaloceles can be associated with a variety of other developmental disorders including craniofacial anomalies with hypertelorism.
c. *Parietal* These make up about 10% of cephaloceles and present as small hairless midline masses through a small calvarial defect. Because of their position, they may involve the superior sagittal sinus.
d. *Nasopharyngeal* These make up probably no more than 1% of all cephaloceles but are notable because they may remain clinically silent for many years, patients presenting with difficulty with nasal

46 Congenital abnormalities

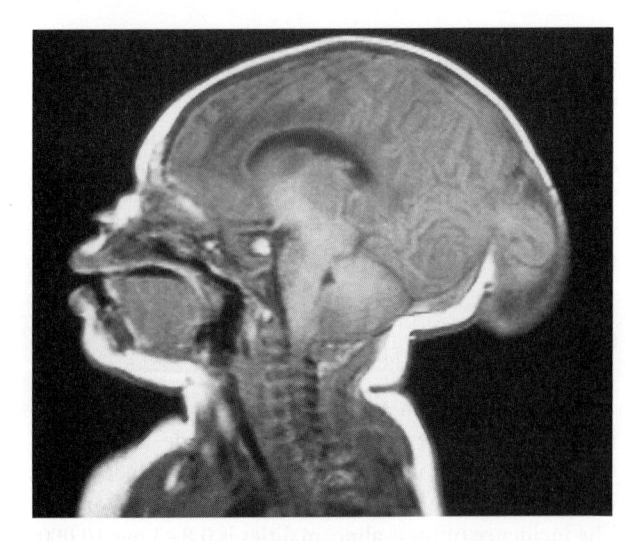

Figure 1.1 *Occipital meningoencephalocele. Sagittal T1WI showing herniated occipital lobe within the CSF sac. (Courtesy of Professor P Griffiths, Sheffield.)*

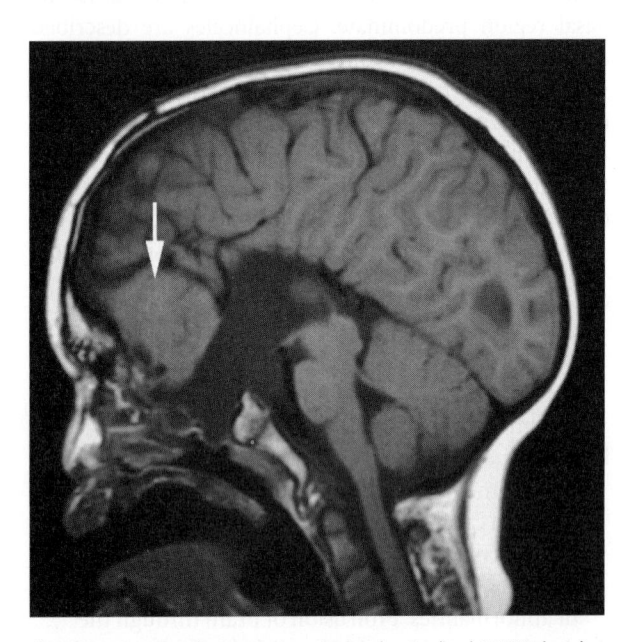

Figure 1.2 *Nasopharyngeal cephalocele. Sagittal T1WI showing a large CSF sac extending down through the sphenoid bone into the upper nasopharynx. The anterior portion of the sac contains dysplastic-looking brain tissue (arrow). Very attenuated optic nerves/chiasm can just be identified within the sac. Note complete absence of the corpus callosum.*

breathing. Among the contents of the cephalocele there may be portions of the optic nerves and chiasm, third ventricle and the hypothalamic/pituitary axis, resulting in hypoplastic optic discs and abnormalities of hypothalamic/pituitary function. Agenesis of the corpus callosum is a very common association (Fig. 1.2).

Chiari malformations

a. *Chiari I* This is defined as downward displacement of the cerebellar tonsils below the foramen magnum into the cervical spinal canal without brainstem herniation and with a normally positioned fourth ventricle.[5] Cerebellar tonsillar ectopia is a term often used for mildly descended cerebellar tonsils unassociated with clinical symptoms, as opposed to a Chiari I malformation causing signs and symptoms.[6] The distinction between these two conditions has been the subject of much discussion. Distance of the tonsils below the mid point of the anterior and posterior lips of the foramen magnum (basion and the opisthion) is a commonly used criterion and several studies have related this distance with the likelihood of clinical symptoms. Up to 3 mm below is considered normal while more than 5 mm below this line is considered abnormal in adults. Up to 6 mm below the foramen magnum, however, is considered normal in children between the ages of 5 and 15 years.

Other criteria often denoting significant tonsillar descent include a pointed inferior configuration to the tonsils (Fig. 1.3) and an associated syrinx within the cord. Whether or not the foramen magnum region looks 'tight' is often a subjective assessment used to decide whether surgical decompression is warranted. Objective

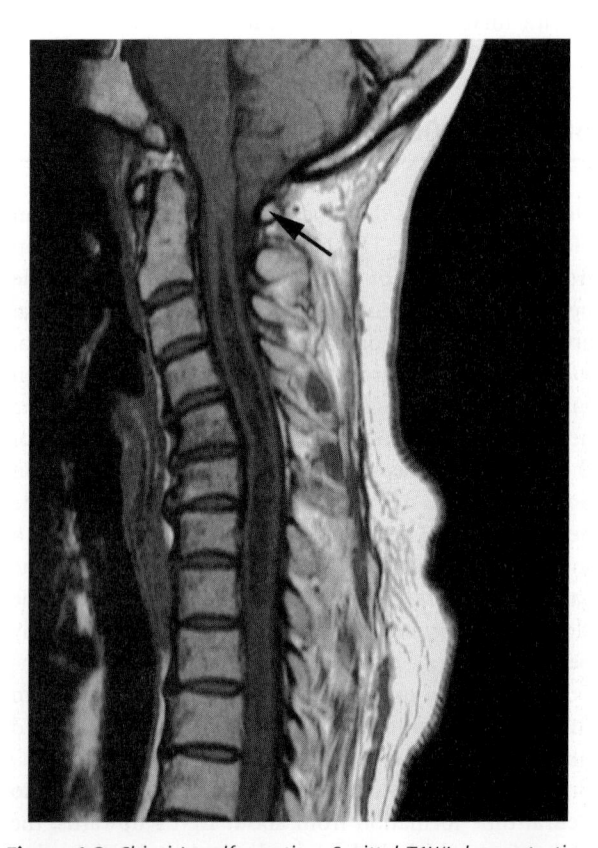

Figure 1.3 *Chiari I malformation. Sagittal T1WI demonstrating abnormally descended cerebellar tonsils reaching the lower margin of C1 with an associated distended cervicothoracic syrinx. Note the brainstem and fourth ventricle are normal in position.*

studies of CSF flow through the foramen magnum may, in the future, help the surgeon decide whether or not to operate.

Chiari I malformations have a number of postulated causes including intrauterine hydrocephalus (resulting in tonsilar descent where they remain following myelination); developmental anomalies of the craniocervical junction; acquired skull base abnormalities (including basilar invagination); and intracranial mass lesions. With the latter, tonsilar descent may be reversible following removal of the mass.

The estimated incidence of associated syringomyelia has gradually decreased with increasing availability of MRI. Currently, syringomyelia is said to occur in about 25% of cases. Associated skeletal anomalies at the craniocervical junction including platybasia, the Klippel–Feil syndrome and occipitalization of the atlas occur in between 23% and 45% of cases.

b. *Chiari II (also known as the Arnold–Chiari malformation)* This is a hind brain dysgenesis characteristically associated with a myelomeningocele.[5] Conceptually, it has been described as a normal cerebellum developing within a small posterior fossa with a low tentorial attachment.

Consequently the cerebellar vermis and tonsils as well as the lower brainstem (medulla) lie within the upper cervical canal (Fig. 1.4). The fourth ventricle typically becomes flattened and lies in an abnormally low position and the cervicomedullary junction displays a kink as downward displacement of the cervical cord is restricted by the dentate ligaments. The cerebellum can become wrapped around the brainstem and the tectal plate may assume a 'beaked' appearance, probably due to side-to-side compression by the temporal lobes and cerebellar hemispheres.

Hydrocephalus, is seen in over 90% of patients and hydromyelia of the cervical cord develops in 50–90% of cases. Occasionally the fourth ventricle can become trapped or 'encysted' and appear of a relatively normal size. Uncommonly, the cerebellum may be small or virtually absent due to degeneration. Supratentorial anomalies are present in up to 90% of patients including corpus callosum anomalies. Aqueduct stenosis can occur as well as neuronal migration anomalies. In keeping with the small posterior fossa concept, scalloping of the petrous bones and clivus, posteriorly, may be noted, most evident on CT.

c. *Chiari III and IV malformations* Both are rare. The Chairi III malformation consists of a cephalocele protruding through a posterior spina bifida at C1–C2 containing the posterior fossa contents while the Chiari IV malformation is described as severe cerebellar hypoplasia but with no posterior fossa contents below the foramen magnum.

DISORDERS OF VENTRAL INDUCTION

Ventral induction takes place between the 5th and 10th weeks of gestation and results in formation of the brain and facial structures. The process occurs at the cephalic end of the neural tube which expands to form the lamina terminalis from which the hindbrain, midbrain and forebrain develop. Table 1 summarizes the embryological names of these divisions and the structures they will eventually become. The main disorders of ventral induction to be discussed in this section are holoprosencephaly, septo-optic dysplasia, disorders of the posterior fossa and craniosynostosis.

Holoprosencephaly

This disorder involves the failure of the prosencephalon to divide into distinct cerebral hemispheres and the transverse division of the prosencephalon into the diencephalon and telencephalon is also disordered[7] (see Table 1.1). Holoprosencephaly therefore results in varying degrees of fusion across the midline of the cerebral hemispheres and other midline structures, including the basal ganglia and thalami as well as abnormalities of the third and lateral ventricles. Additionally, as the optic and olfactory systems begin development about 1 week after cerebral hemisphere division, associated abnormalities of the optic and olfactory systems are common.

The condition affects males and females equally and can be seen in trisomy 13 and 18 syndromes. Patients usually have micrencephaly except in the milder forms and there is a strong association with facial deformities involving hypotelorism and midline clefts. Generally,

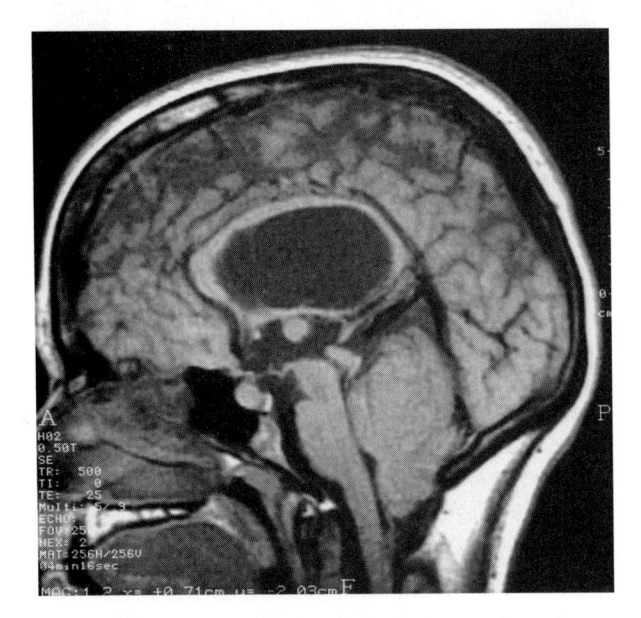

Figure 1.4 *Chiari II malformation. Sagittal T1WI shows descent of the lower cerebellum and most of the medulla into the upper cervical canal. The fourth ventricle is flattened and in an abnormally low position. Hydrocephalus is present.*

Table 1.1 *Embryological brain divisions and their final derivatives*

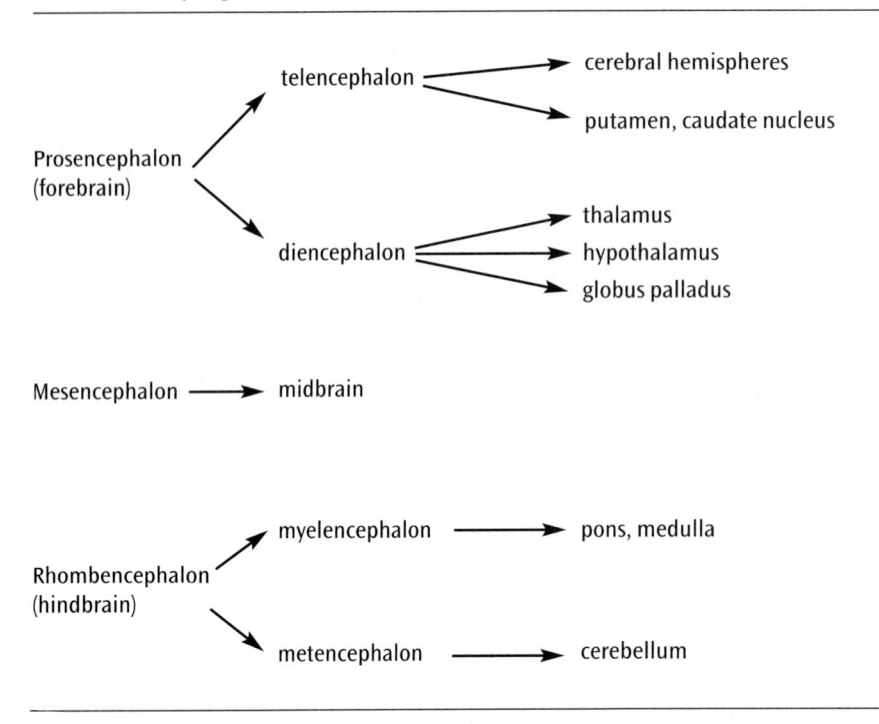

```
                          ┌─→ telencephalon ──┬─→ cerebral hemispheres
Prosencephalon           │                    └─→ putamen, caudate nucleus
(forebrain)              │
                          └─→ diencephalon ───┬─→ thalamus
                                              ├─→ hypothalamus
                                              └─→ globus palladus

Mesencephalon ──→ midbrain

Rhombencephalon          ┌─→ myelencephalon ──→ pons, medulla
(hindbrain)              │
                          └─→ metencephalon ───→ cerebellum
```

severity of facial deformity mirrors severity of intracranial development with cyclopsia in the most severe cases and normal facies in the mildest cases. Although holoprosencephaly is traditionally divided into three categories, these should be regarded as a spectrum in which forebrain development is more severely affected anteriorly than posteriorly.

a. *Alobar* This is the most severe form in which there is no interhemispheric fissure, falx or corpus callosum. The thalami and basal ganglia are fused and so there is no third ventricle present. The fused cerebrum lies in the most anterior part of the skull, in an inverted U shape, posterior to which is a large single ventricle (holoventricle) continuous with a large posteriorly positioned fluid-filled cyst which occupies most of the supratentorial space (Fig. 1.5). Posterior fossa contents are usually normal. In most cases babies are still born or survive only a brief length of time.

b. *Semilobar* In this less severe form, the structures anteriorly are still fused but there is some division seen in the posterior portions of the fore brain. The posterior portions of the interhemispheric fissure and falx can be identified and as there is partial separation of the thalami, a small third ventricle may be seen (Fig. 1.6). Some temporal horn formation occurs but the dorsal cyst is usually still present. The septum pellucidum (which usually lies between the normally divided lateral ventricles anteriorly) is absent as it is in all forms of holoprosencephaly. The posterior part of the corpus callosum (the

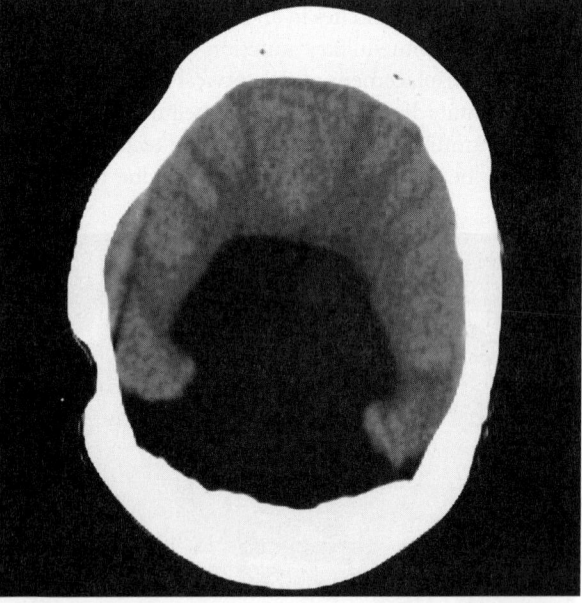

Figure 1.5 *Alobar holoprosencephaly. Axial CT section demonstrating the characteristic U shape of the fused cerebrum anteriorly posterior to which is the large holoventricle. (Courtesy of Dr T Jaspan, Nottingham.)*

splenium) can be present, a configuration which is unusual in developmental conditions since the corpus callosum develops in the anterior to posterior direction.

c. *Lobar* This is the mildest variety in which anterior forebrain division is more advanced so that a hypoplastic

(a)   (b)

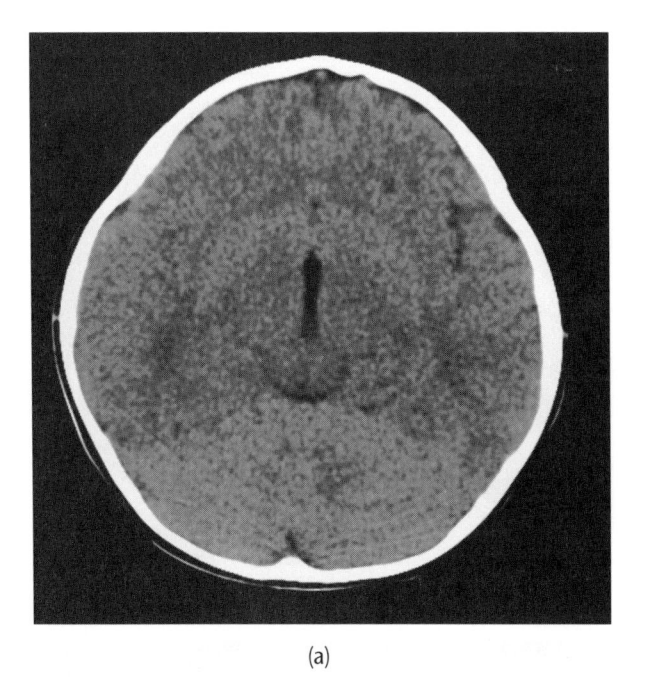

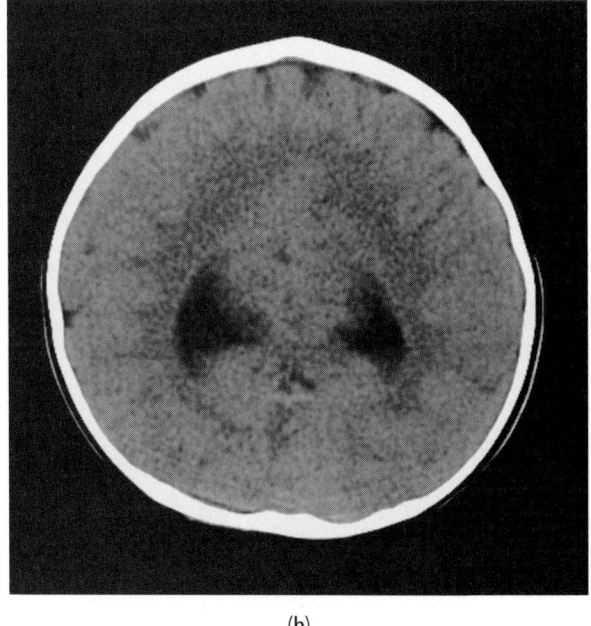

Figure 1.6 *Semilobar holoprosencephaly. Axial CT sections. Anteriorly the cerebral hemispheres are fused but there is formation of a well defined third ventricle (a), posterior portions of the lateral ventricles and there is a falx posteriorly (b). The level of brain development in this case lies along the spectrum between semilobar and lobar holoprosencephaly.*

anterior falx may be present along with some frontal horn development. There is a greater degree of callosal development but the septum pellucidum remains absent and the frontal lobes may be hypoplastic. There is a third ventricle and usually no dorsal cyst. There are some similarities between this mild group of holoprosencephaly and septo-optic dysplasia.

Septo-optic dysplasia

This disorder is characterized by hypoplasia of the optic nerves and aplasia or hypoplasia of the septum pellucidum.[7] Two-thirds of patients have dysfunction of the hypothalamic/pituitary axis (with reduced growth hormone and thyroid stimulating hormone) resulting in growth retardation. Patients may present with decreased visual acuity and nystagmus but vision can also be normal. Ophthalmological examination will detect hypoplasia of the optic discs and MRI may show hypoplasia of the optic nerves and chiasm if sufficiently severe (Fig. 1.7) (about 50% of patients) but look normal in milder cases. The frontal horns are continuous across the mid line due to the absence of the septum pellucidum and assume a box-like configuration although they are usually more pointed inferiorly. The pituitary gland and infundibulum may be small or absent, depending upon severity of involvement (Fig. 1.8) but the falx and interhemispheric fissure are usually normal.

In addition to septo-optic dysplasia and holoprosencephaly, the septum pellucidum may be absent in a number of other developmental conditions,[8] including dysgenesis of the corpus callosum, schizencephaly, lissencephaly, Apert syndrome (a variety of craniofacial synostosis) and Chiari II malformation. The septum pellucidum may also be damaged by acquired disease including longstanding hydrocephalus, leptomeningitis and trauma.

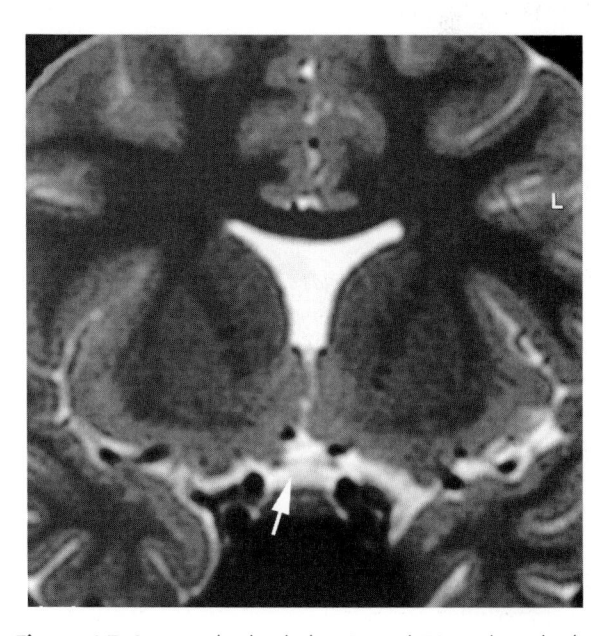

Figure 1.7 *Septo-optic dysplasia. Coronal T2WI through the pituitary gland shows absence of the septum pellucidum with the frontal horns continuous across the midline. The optic chiasm is hypoplastic (arrow).*

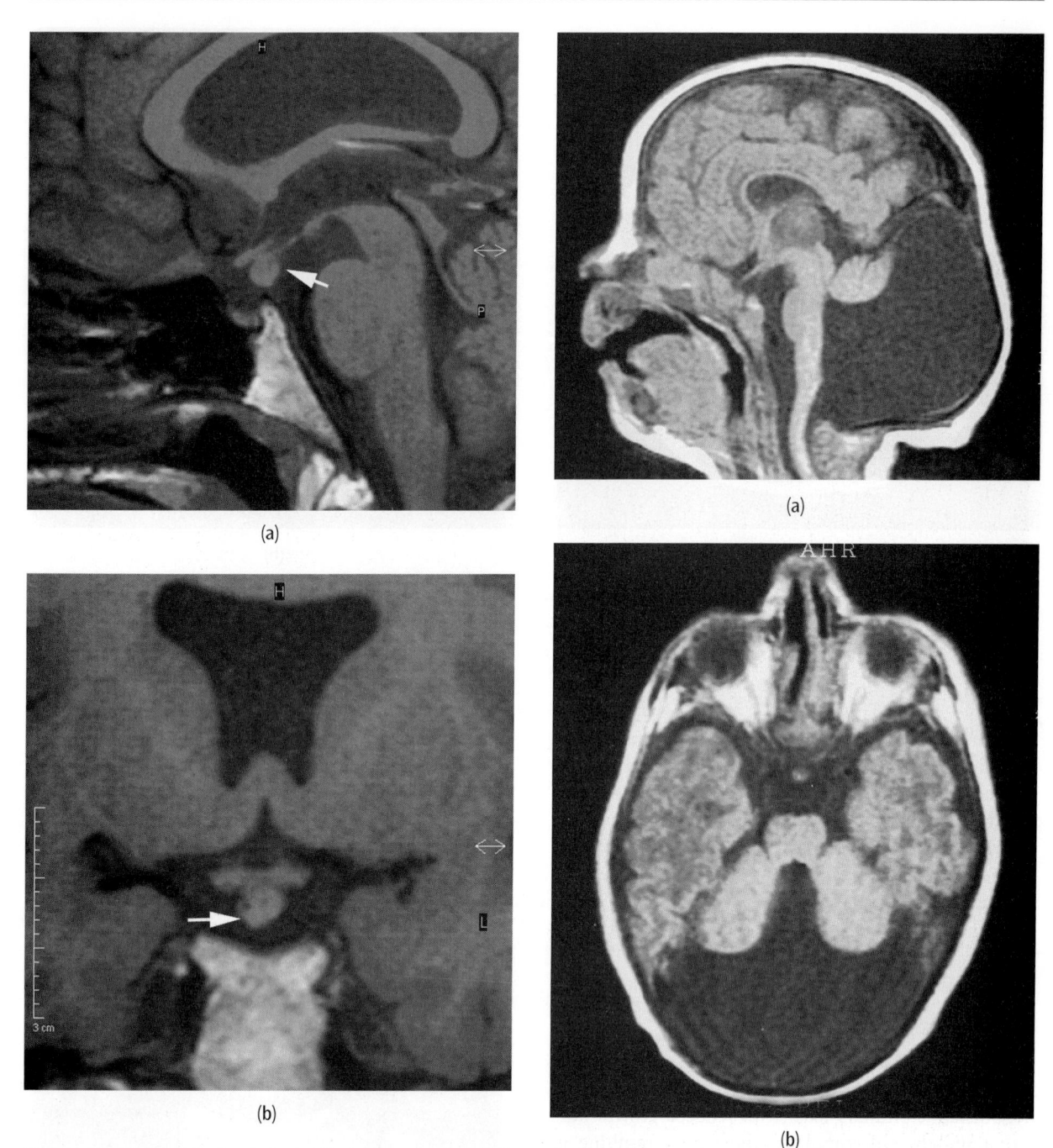

Figure 1.8 *Septo-optic dysplasia. Sagittal (a) and coronal (b) T1WI. The pituitary gland is small and there is absence of the usual high signal posterior pituitary. The lower infundibulum is absent but there is a soft tissue nodule in the position of the upper infundibulum probably representing a hamartoma (arrow). Normal optic chiasm. Note the lack of separation of the frontal horns and the characteristic box-like shape with pointed inferior margins.*

Figure 1.9 *Dandy–Walker malformation. Sagittal (a) and axial (b) T1WI. There is a huge cyst occupying an enlarged posterior fossa. The vermis is absent and the cerebellar hemispheres are hypoplastic. Note continuity between the cyst and fourth ventricle posteriorly.*

Dandy–Walker complex

The Dandy–Walker malformation consists of an enlarged posterior fossa with a high tentorium and torcular, hypoplasia or aplasia of the cerebellar vermis, hypoplasia of the cerebellar hemispheres and a cystic dilatation of the fourth ventricle which fills most of the posterior fossa space[5] (Fig. 1.9). The Dandy–Walker variant is a less severe version of the malformation with less enlargement of the posterior fossa, a hypoplastic vermis and an enlarged fourth ventricle. The mega cisterna magna is the least severe form with a normal fourth ventricle and vermis and with a prominently enlarged cisterna magna, which communicates at some point with the fourth ventricle (Fig. 1.10). The latter communication distinguishes the mega cisterna magna from an arachnoid cyst in which the CSF collection does not communicate with the fourth ventricle (Fig. 1.11). In practice it is often difficult to clearly categorize a patient into one of these distinct syndromes and this has led to the concept of the Dandy–Walker complex[9] where these entities are part of a spectrum of posterior fossa cystic malformations.

Hydrocephalus, though not usually present at birth, is seen in 75% of patients by 3 months of age and in 90% at the time of diagnosis. Other associated anomalies include hypoplasia of the corpus callosum in 32%, polymicrogyria or grey matter heterotopia in 5–10% and occipital cephaloceles in 16%. The degree of developmental delay in these patients is related to the presence of these other supratentorial anomalies and how well the hydrocephalus is controlled.

Non-cystic posterior fossa anomalies

a. *Joubert syndrome* This consists of vermian hypoplasia or aplasia in the absence of any posterior fossa cyst, distinguishing it from the Dandy–Walker complex. The cerebellar hemispheres become apposed in the mid line and the superior cerebellar peduncles are nearly horizontal in orientation. The fourth ventricle, viewed axially, has a bat-wing shape superiorly and a triangular shape in its mid section (Fig. 1.12).
b. *Rhombencephalosynapsis* In this disorder, the cerebellar hemispheres and superior cerebellar peduncles are fused with a small or absent vermis.

Craniosynostosis

Premature fusion of cranial sutures can occur as a developmental anomaly (primary) or from causes such as intrauterine skull compression, teratogens or poor brain growth (secondary).[10] Craniosynostosis can be classified as either simple or isolated when only one suture is involved, or compound or multiple when more than one suture is involved. Premature fusion of the suture causes: a) bony bridging and heaping of bone along the affected suture line with narrowing of the suture space which becomes indistinct and, b) compensatory growth at other non-fused sutures which can result in widening of the subarachnoid space beneath the areas of growth but with subarachnoid space effacement underlying those areas where growth has ceased prematurely.

Isolated sagittal synostosis is the commonest variety and results in a long narrow head termed *scaphocephaly* or *dolichocephaly* (Fig. 1.13a), while metopic synostosis results in a prominent rather wedge shaped forehead, termed *trigonocephaly* (Fig. 1.13b). Unilateral coronal or lambdoid suture synostosis results in an asymmetric skull shape termed *plagiocephaly* and both may occur together; this needs to be distinguished from the more common postural asymmetry causing occipital flattening (Fig. 1.14).[11] Unilateral coronal synostosis results in a relatively shallow anterior cranial fossa and orbit on the affected side with uplifting of the orbital roof resulting in the so called 'harlequin eye deformity'.

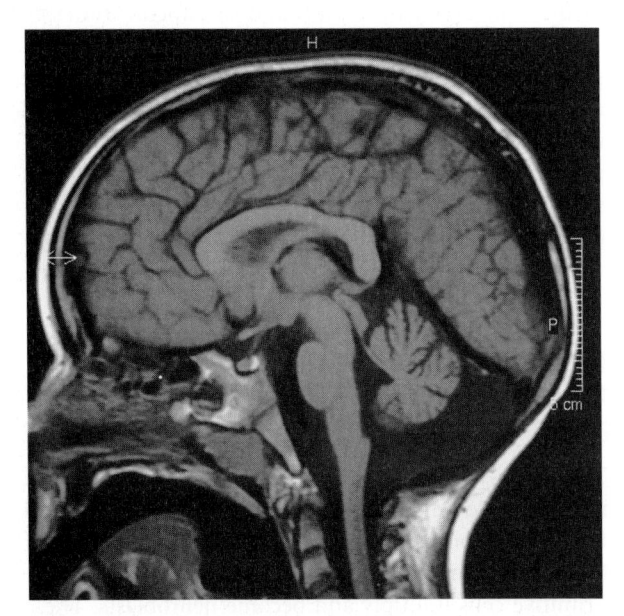

Figure 1.10 *Mega cisterna magna. Sagittal T1WI demonstrating a prominent CSF collection communicating with the fourth ventricle through widened inferior outlet foramina. Note scalloping of the inner table of the occiput.*

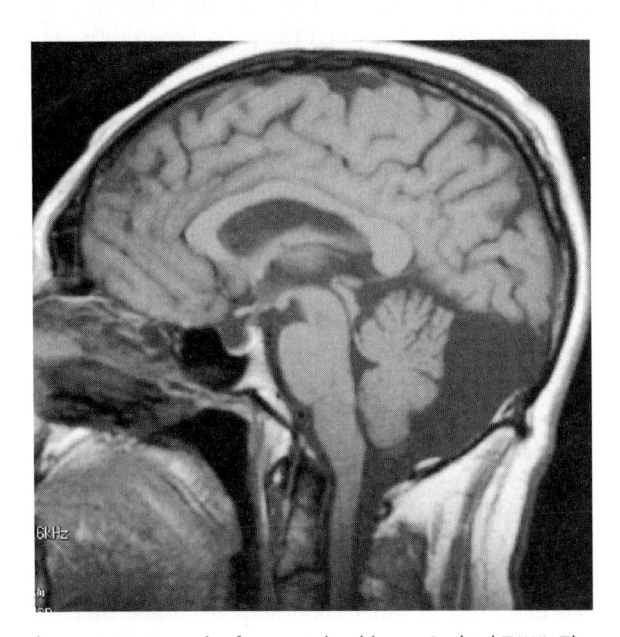

Figure 1.11 *Posterior fossa arachnoid cyst. Sagittal T1WI. There is no direct communication between the CSF collection and the fourth ventricle. There is thinning of the overlying occipital bone and slight flattening of the posterior surface of the vermis. Distinction between this entity and a mega cisterna magna is often not straightforward.*

Disorders of neuronal proliferation, differentiation and histogenesis

bone expansion between the fused sutures. Multiple or compound synostosis may be associated with syndactaly or polydactaly and congenital brain anomalies.[12]

IMAGING IN CRANIOSYNOSTOSIS

Skull X-rays may suffice in simple cases. However, the fusion may occur only over a small portion of the suture or the fusion may be fibrous and so difficult to detect. The technique of choice is CT for more difficult or complex cases with the images reconstructed using a bone algorithm. Spiral CT techniques can be usefully applied in this situation, reconstructing multiple thin overlapping slices; these data can also be usefully presented in surface rendered 3-D format. MRI is essential for multiple or compound synostosis syndromes to look for associated brain anomalies.

DISORDERS OF NEURONAL PROLIFERATION, DIFFERENTIATION AND HISTOGENESIS

This process occurs simultaneously with the phase of cell migration (to be described later) and occurs in the 2nd to the 5th months of gestation. Lining the periphery of the ventricular system is the germinal matrix where primitive cells multiply and become neuroblasts. These cells will eventually migrate peripherally to form the cerebral and cerebellar cortex. They reach their final destination by migrating along radial glial fibres, (see section: DISORDERS OF CELLULAR MIGRATION (p. 62). Abnormalities of cellular proliferation, differentiation and histogenesis arise when there has been destruction of the germinal matrix, the migrating neurons or the radial glial fibres, which guide the neurons. These abnormalities may also involve the formation of the cerebral vasculature, subarachnoid spaces and result in primitive cellular elements persisting. The conditions to be described in this section are megalencephaly/unilateral megalencephaly and the phakomatoses.

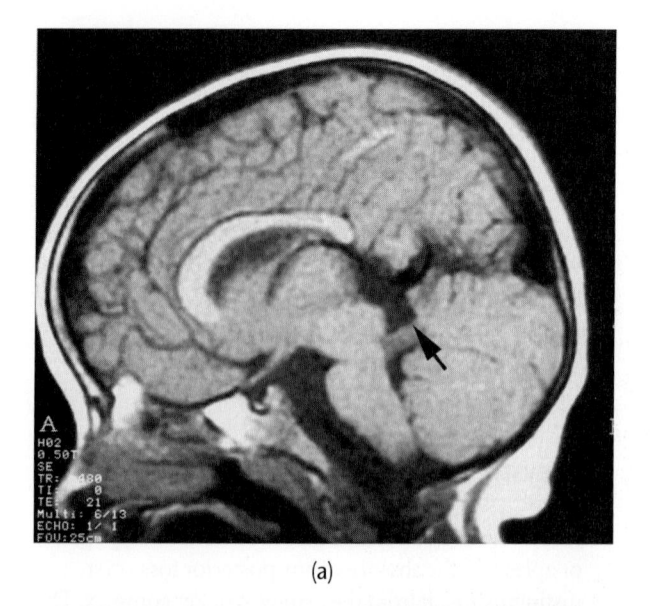

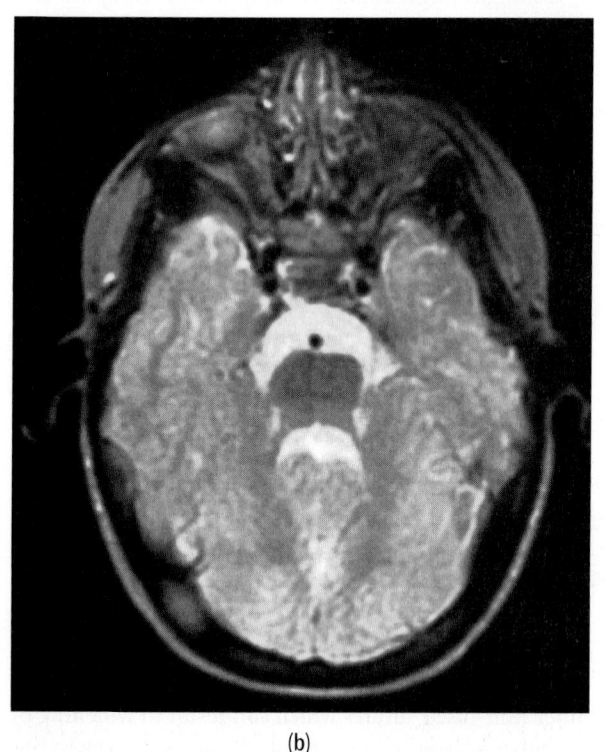

Figure 1.12 *Joubert syndrome. Sagittal T1WI (a) and axial T2WI (b) MRI. The cerebellar hemispheres are apposed in the mid line. Note the 'bats-wing' configuration of the fourth ventricle in (b) and the horizontal superior cerebellar peduncle (arrow) in (a). (Courtesy of Professor Paul Griffiths, Sheffield.)*

The compound or multiple synostosis syndromes are usually genetic in nature and bilateral coronal involvement is the most common. The term *acrocephaly* is applied when all the sutures are involved or the coronal sutures plus one other suture (Fig. 1.15). The 'clover leaf skull' (kleeblattschadel) deformity is a result of bilateral coronal and sagittal synostosis, with or without bilateral lambdoid involvement and is a result of membranous

Megalencephaly/unilateral megalencephaly

The term megalencephaly refers to enlargement of all or part of the cerebral hemispheres. Megalencephaly is seen in those conditions causing an accumulation of abnormal metabolites including the mucopolysaccharidosis, leukodystrophies (Alexander disease and Canavan disease) and gangliosidoses (Tay-Sachs disease). It has also been described in other conditions including tuberous sclerosis, achondroplasia and neurofibromatosis.

Unilateral megalencephaly is a rare disorder in which there is enlargement of all or part of a cerebral hemisphere.[13] Patients clinically can present with seizures, hemiplegia and significant developmental delay. Pathologically, the affected hemispheres can

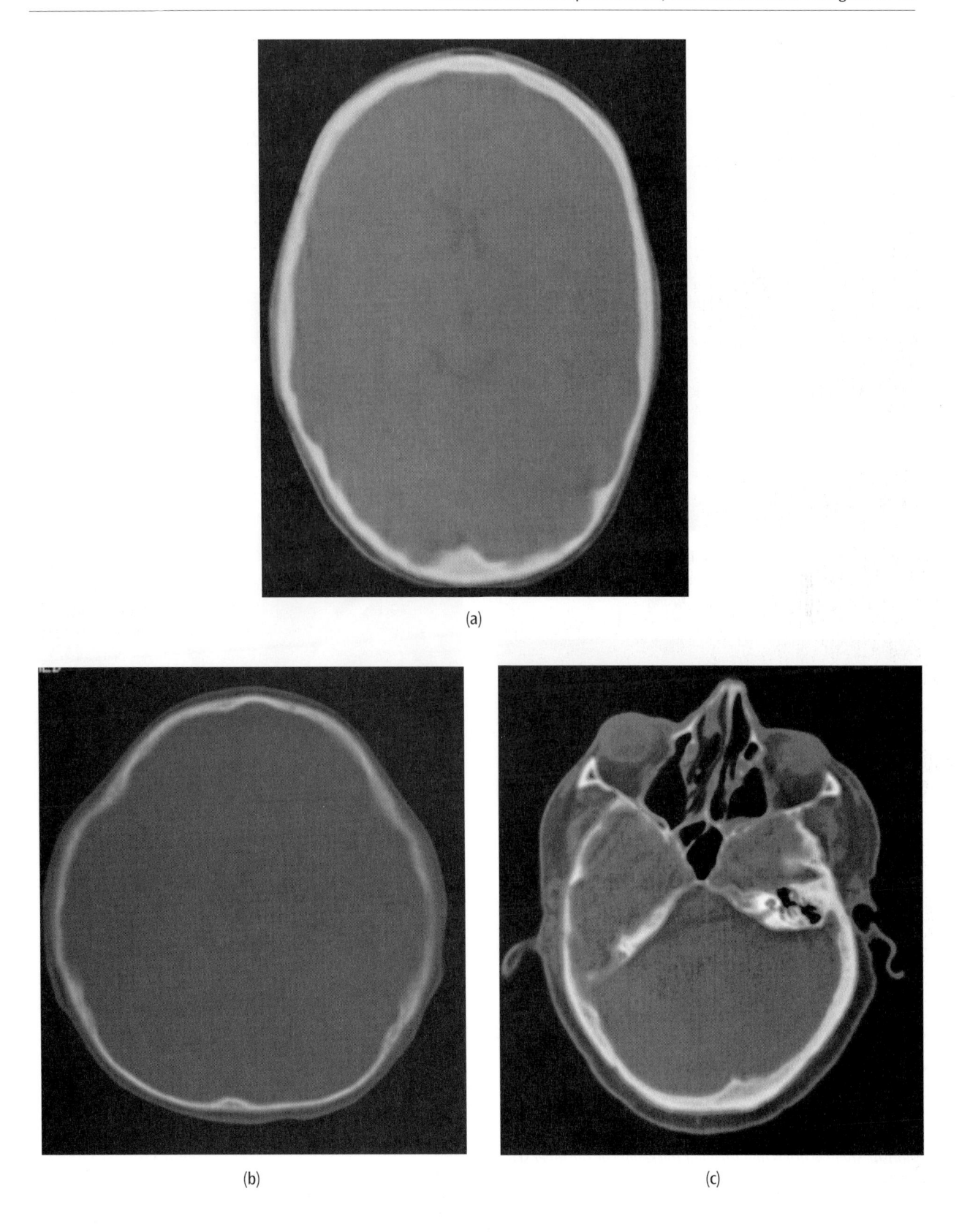

Disorders of neural proliferation, differentiation and histogenesis   53

Figure 1.13 *Craniosynostosis. Axial CT scans demonstrating scaphocephaly (a), trigonocephaly (b), and plagiocephaly (c).*

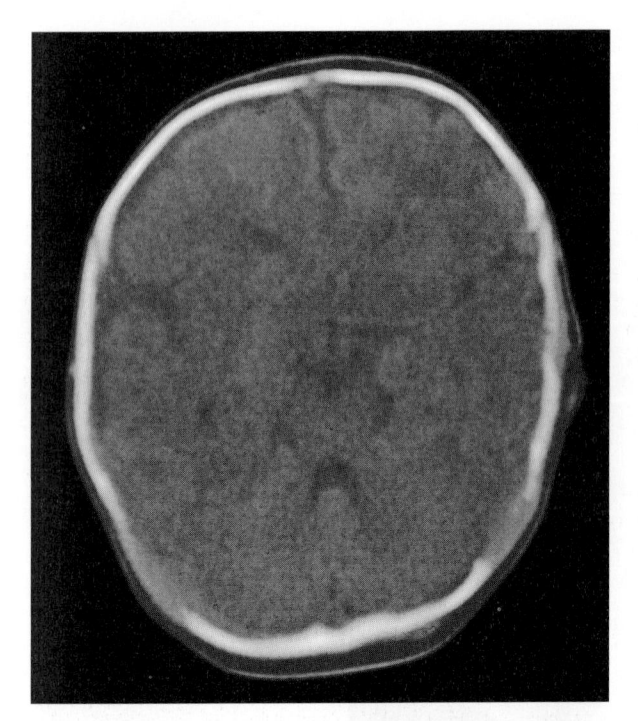

Figure 1.14 *Postural occipital flattening. Axial CT showing posterior head asymmetry with relative flattening of the left occiput in the absence of premature suture fusion.*

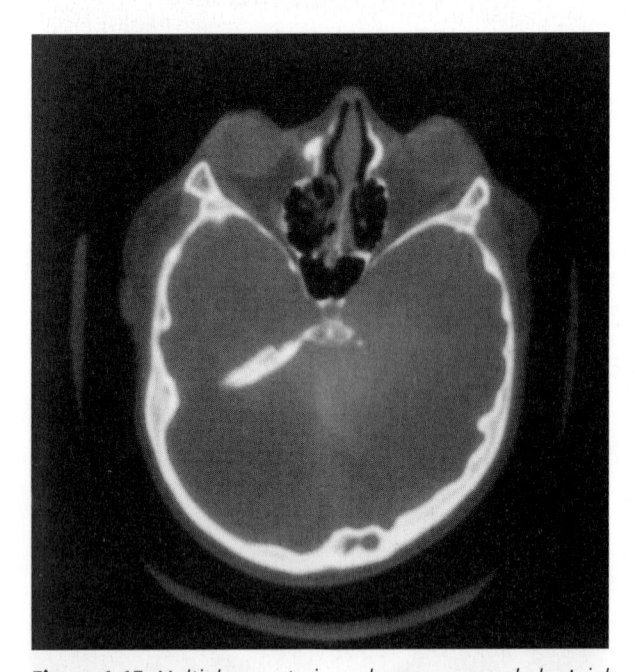

Figure 1.15 *Multiple synostosis syndrome – acrocephaly. Axial CT slice from a child with Apert syndrome demonstrating hypertelorism, shallow orbits and irregular thickening of the inner skull table.*

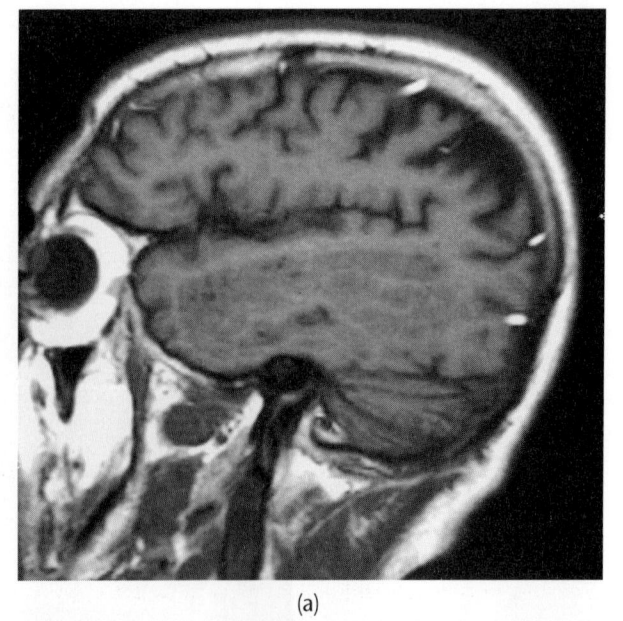

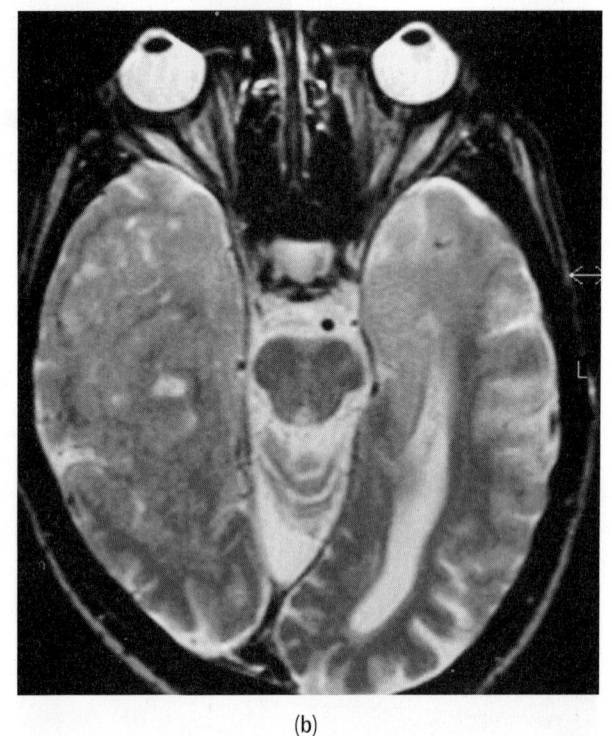

Figure 1.16 *Unilateral megalencephaly. Sagittal T1WI (a) and axial T2WI (b) MRI. An enlarged grossly disorganized right temporal lobe is evident with complete absence of normal grey/white matter differentiation.*

demonstrate pachygyria, polymicrogyria, areas of heterotopia, white matter gliosis and neuronal migration abnormalities.

On MRI, affected white matter shows a decrease in signal intensity on T1WI and increased signal on T2WI due to heterotopias and gliosis, these areas appearing as decreased density on CT. The grey–white matter interface may be indistinct and rarely the affected brain may have a grossly disorganized, hamartomatous appearance (Fig. 1.16). The lateral ventricle and the affected hemisphere are enlarged proportionately and the frontal horn may have an almost straight, pointed configuration. Treatment involves removal of the affected portions of the cerebral hemisphere if the seizures become intractable, the involved brain having no useful function.

Phakomatoses (neurocutaneous syndromes)

These disorders are characterized by abnormalities involving the skin and central nervous system. The lesions are dysplasias or neoplasias derived mainly from embryonic ectoderm (which gives rise to the skin and the central and peripheral nervous system) but abnormalities can also affect organs derived from mesoderm (including blood vessels and bone) and endoderm (including the gastrointestinal tract epithelium).

NEUROFIBROMATOSIS

The two major types of neurofibromatosis, NF1 and NF2 are now regarded as two separate diseases.[14,15] NF1 (Von Recklinghausen disease) is a result of a defect on chromosome 17, where as NF2 (formerly called 'central neurofibromatosis') is associated with a defect on chromosome 22. The primary manifestations of NF2 are seen in the central nervous system with few cutaneous signs. In Table 1.2 the characteristic radiological manifestations of NF1 and NF2 are compared.

NEUROFIBROMATOSIS TYPE 1

Neurofibromatosis type 1 has a prevalence of about 1 per 4000 of the population with 100% penetrance and a 50% spontaneous mutation rate.

The principal intracranial manifestations are:

a. *Optic glioma* This is the most common intracranial tumour in NF1 and occurs in 5–15% of patients. Pathologically these tumours are pilocytic astrocytomas and are therefore usually well defined, stable childhood tumours compatible with long

Table 1.2 *Radiological features of NF1 and NF2*

Neurofibromatosis type 1
Optic nerve glioma.
Cerebral gliomas
Focal high-signal lesions of supratentorial grey and white matter, brainstem and cerebellum on T2WI (sometimes also on T1WI in basal ganglia)
Spinal gliomas and neurofibromas
Plexiform neurofibromas
Dural ectasia
Skeletal and vascular dysplasias

Neurofibromatosis type 2
Bilateral acoustic schwannomas
Other cranial nerve schwannomas
Intracranial meningiomas
Spinal canal schwannomas and meningiomas
Spinal cord ependymomas

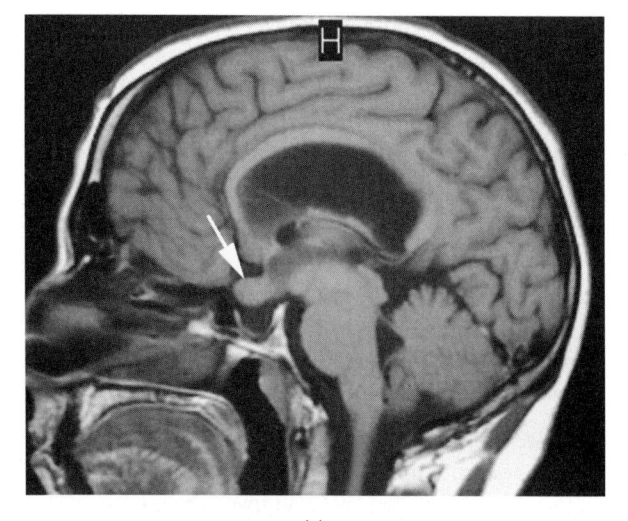

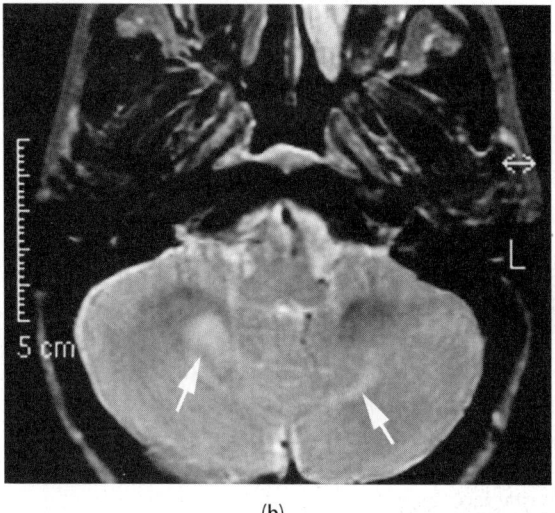

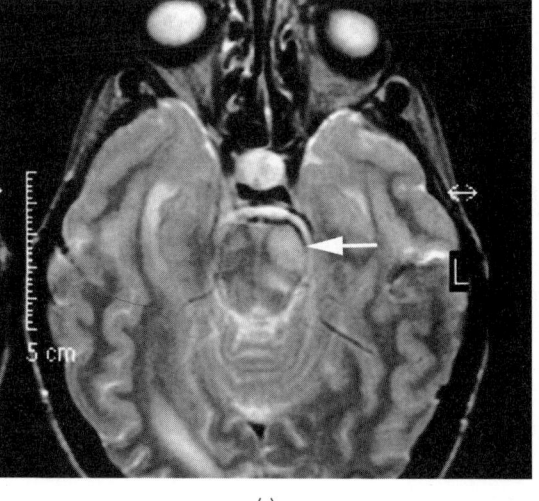

Figure 1.17 *NF1. Sagittal T1WI (a) and axial T2WI (b,c) MRI. There is an optic nerve glioma involving the optic chiasm (arrow) (a). Typical UNOs are present in the cerebellum (b) and brainstem (c) (arrows).*

survival. Optic gliomas can involve the optic nerves, chiasm and optic tracts and are demonstrated on MR as hypo- or isointense on T1WI and mildly to strongly hyperintense on T2WI (Fig. 1.17a). Of all patients with optic gliomas, 25% will be suffering from NF1.

b. *Other gliomas* These can occur in the brainstem and hypothalamus and are also usually relatively benign pilocytic astrocytomas. More diffuse gliomas in the cerebrum or cerebellum are uncommon. Enhancement will occur in both the more benign and malignant varieties of glioma and so is not a good discriminator between them.

c. *Unidentified neurofibromatosis objects* (UNOs) These occur in up to 80% of patients and are high signal foci identified on T2WI involving the cerebellum, brainstem, internal capsule, basal ganglia, thalamus and supratentorial white matter (Fig. 1.17b,c). They tend to be more common in those with optic nerve gliomas. White matter UNOs are isointense to surrounding brain on T1WI with no mass effect or enhancement. The most common sites in decreasing frequency are the cerebellum, brainstem and internal capsule.

In childhood their number and size may increase but have a tendency to disappear with increase in age. Lesion enlargement in children over the age of 10 years should prompt close observation in case a glioma is present rather than a UNO. The explanations offered for white matter UNOs have included low-grade tumours, areas of heterotopia, hamartomas and areas of abnormal myelination.[16] Areas of vascular or spongiotic change have been shown pathologically in one recent study.[17] The UNOs involving basal ganglia resemble the white matter lesions on T2WI. On T1WI, however, increased signal can be seen in the globus pallidus and there may be some mass effect identified. This T1 shortening may evolve over a different time course and later than the increased T2-weighted signal. Postulated causes for the T1-weighted signal changes, which may not regress over time, include remyelination and calcification.[18]

d. *Other lesions* Aqueduct stenosis, internal auditory meatus ectasia and sphenoid wing dysplasia (resulting in a 'bare orbit') (Fig. 1.18) can all occur without associated mass lesions. Extracranial plexiform neurofibromas also occur.

The principal spinal manifestations are:

a. *Neurofibromas* which arise as intradural, extramedullary lesions but can extend into an extradural location, via the spinal exit foramina, resulting in a 'dumb-bell' or 'hour glass' configuration. These lesions are usually benign.

b. *Intramedullary gliomas* These have similar imaging characteristics to spinal cord gliomas in non-NF1 patients.

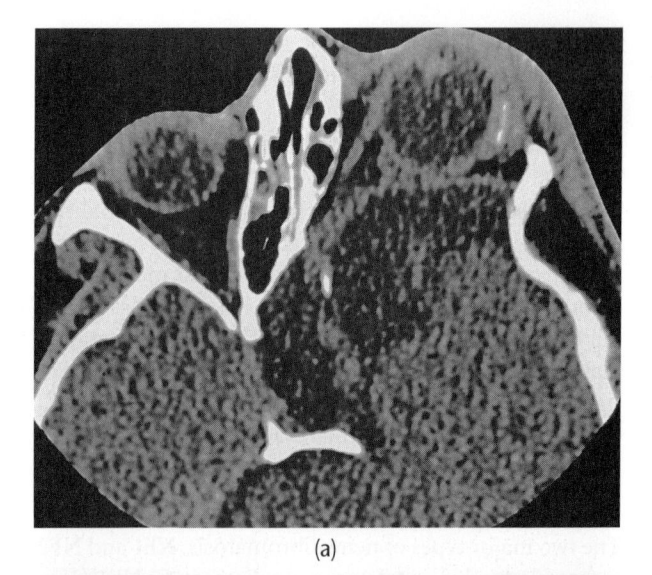

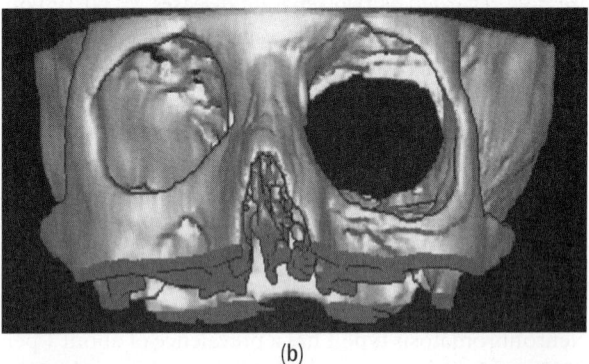

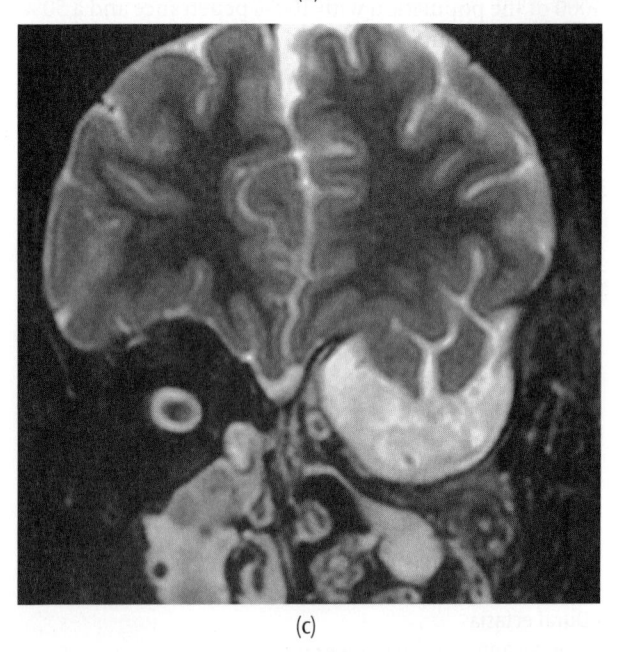

Figure 1.18 *NF1. Axial CT (a), 3-D CT surface reconstruction (b), and coronal T2-weighted MRI (c) demonstrating the classic 'bare-orbit' of NF1. The left-sided sphenoid wing dysplasia is clearly shown in (a) and (b). There is direct communication between the intracranial cavity and the orbit with CT showing a cystic collection causing left-sided proptosis. Coronal MRI (c) confirms the presence of a CSF sac containing brain, effectively a meningoencephalocele.*

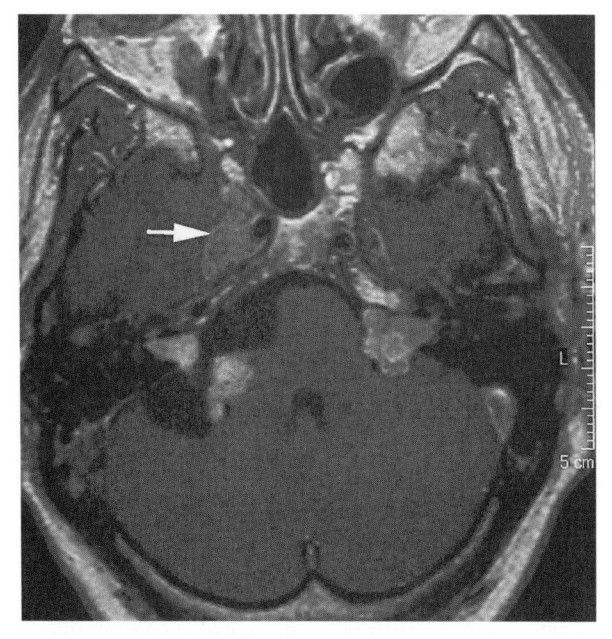

Figure 1.19 NF2. Axial contrast-enhanced T1WI scans showing bilateral acoustic schwannomas and a right trigeminal schwannoma. The right-sided acoustic schwannoma is partially solid and partially cystic and is causing significant compression of the brainstem. The right-sided trigeminal schwannoma is causing asymmetric expansion of the cavernous sinus (arrow).

Imaging in NF1

In addition to a standard brain examination T1WI before and after intravenous contrast, usually in the axial plane, are normally required to characterize areas of increased signal on the T2WI. Coronal images through the orbits and chiasm are recommended for assessing the optic nerves, particularly in association with fat suppression. Spinal canal imaging requires contrast-enhanced T1WI with T2WI as necessary, similar to the protocol recommended for NF2 screening (see next section).

NEUROFIBROMATOSIS TYPE 2

Neurofibromatosis type 2 is an autosomal dominant condition with a prevalence of approximately 1 per 50 000 of the population and therefore much less common than NF1.[14,15] Patients usually present to the radiologist in two main groups. Most commonly patients come with a definite or suspected clinical/genetic diagnosis of NF2 for screening of the neural axis to define the number and type of lesions present. Occasionally patients will present simply with sensorineural deafness and in the course of investigation will be found to have bilateral acoustic schwannomas or other suspicious combination of abnormalities.

The principle intracranial lesions of NF2 are:

a. *Cranial nerve schwannomas* These may affect any cranial nerve from III to XII with the VIIIth nerve being the commonest site of involvement. Virtually all

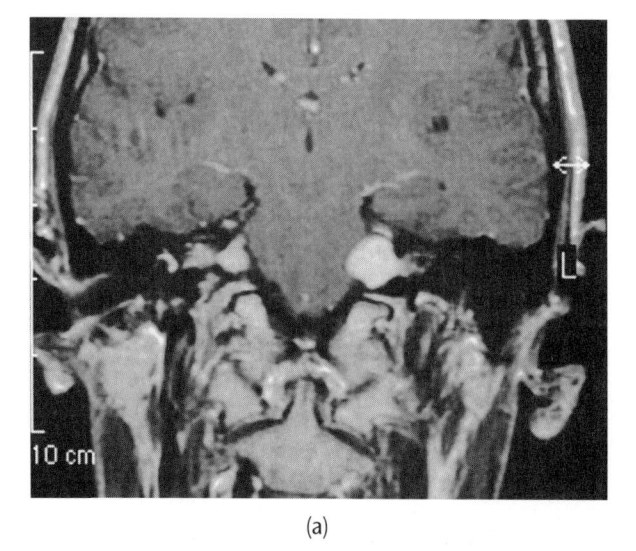

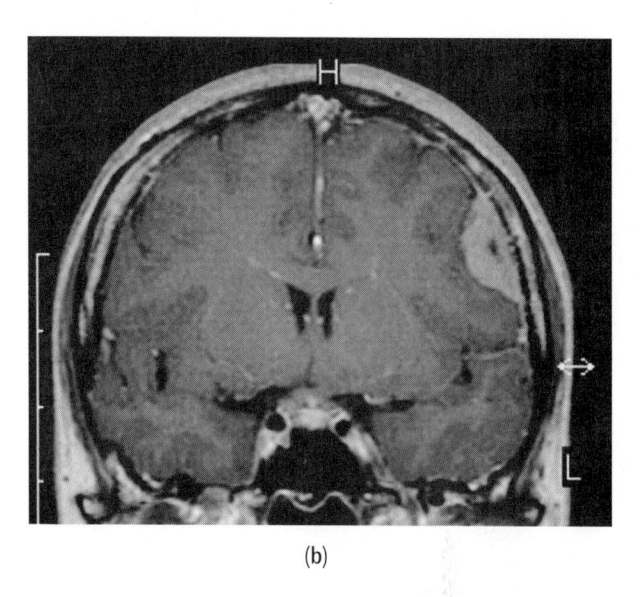

Figure 1.20 NF2. Contrast-enhanced coronal T1WI. This patient has bilateral acoustic schwannomas (a) and a left convexity meningioma (b). Note the labyrinthine schwannoma on the right in (a).

NF2 patients develop bilateral acoustic schwannomas at some stage of their disease though not necessarily synchronously either clinically or radiologically. The trigeminal nerve is the next commonest site of involvement. (Fig. 1.19). Cranial nerve schwannomas in NF2 have the same imaging characteristics as those occurring in non-NF2 patients (Fig. 1.20) (see Chapter 4 by Hourihan). Abnormalities of the VIIth and Vth nerves can occur either from direct compression of an enlarging VIIIth nerve schwannoma or from schwannomas affecting these nerves themselves. Brainstem and fourth ventricular compression can be particularly severe with bilaterally enlarging lesions. Labyrinthine schwannomas are very uncommon but are being increasingly recognized (Fig. 1.20a); they are known to be more common in NF2 patients than non-NF2 patients.[19]

b. *Meningiomas* These benign dural based tumours can be either solitary or multiple. As with non-NF2 patients, meningiomas are most commonly seen involving the falx, cerebral convexities, sphenoid ridge, cerebellopontine angle cistern, olfactory groove and planum sphenoidale (Fig. 1.20b). They may also be intraventricular in location, particularly related to the trigone of the lateral ventricle. Their imaging characteristics do not differ from those in non-NF2 patients.

Spinal canal involvement in NF2 has previously been underestimated with the incidence of occult tumours being as high as 89% (Fig. 1.21).[20]

The principal spinal manifestations of NF2 are:

a. *Schwannomas* The number of these detected can vary from one up to dozens. Like spinal neurofibromas, from which they are indistinguishable, these are extramedullary intradural lesions which can extend through the exit foramina into an extradural location. MR signal and enhancement characteristics are similar to those of intracranial schwannomas.

b. *Meningiomas* These are most commonly seen in the thoracic canal and are usually confined to the spinal canal itself. However, they may extend out through the exit foramina and assume a 'dumbbell' appearance similar to schwannomas. Bony erosion can occur. Both schwannomas and meningiomas may compress the cord and, in practice, distinguishing between these two entities on MR scanning is usually not possible.

c. *Ependymomas and astrocytomas* Most of the intrinsic cord tumours which have been examined histologically have proven to be ependymomas. Although ependymomas and astrocytomas can be difficult to distinguish radiologically, ependymomas tend to be better defined and more focal than astrocytomas which tend to be diffusely infiltrating lesions. In practice, diffuse spinal cord neoplasms with MR features strongly suggesting an astrocytoma are often not treated surgically or verified histologically. Both lesions on MRI will expand the cord and are usually iso/hypointense on T1WI and hyperintense on T2WI. They can be homogeneous or heterogeneous in texture and be associated with cyst formation, necrosis or, in the case of ependymomas, haemorrhage. Contrast enhancement is necessary to differentiate solid from cystic or necrotic segments and to distinguish a tumoural cyst from an associated syrinx.

Radiological screening in NF2 patients

It is mandatory to examine not only the intracranial cavity but also the entire spinal axis with contrast-enhanced T1WI being the corner stone of this examination. Our protocol is shown in Table 1.3.[21]

TUBEROUS SCLEROSIS

This is an autosomal dominant condition consisting of dysplasias and neoplasias of ectoderm, mesoderm and endoderm.[14] Incidence has been estimated to be between 1 in 10 000 and 50 000 of the population and abnormalities of chromosome 9 and 11 have been implicated in some patients. The cerebral abnormalities in tuberous sclerosis

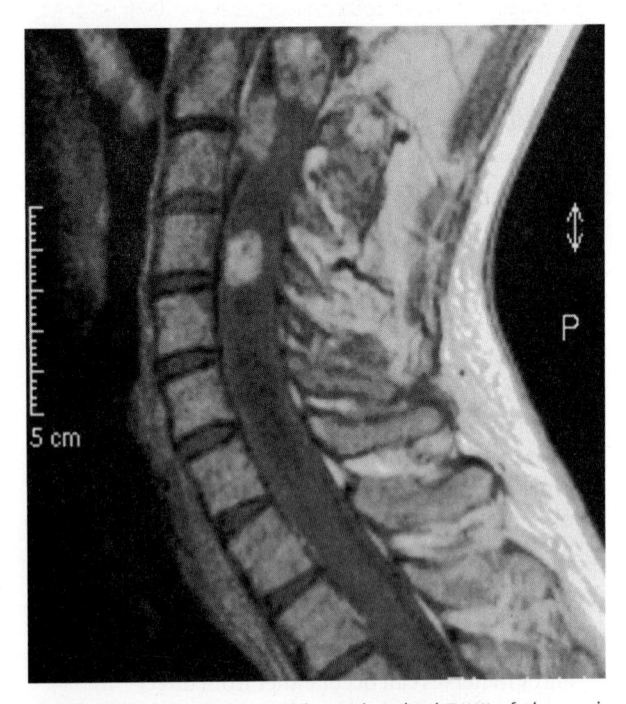

Figure 1.21 *NF2. Contrast-enhanced sagittal T1WI of the cervical spine. Two intradural, extramedullary presumed schwannomas are evident at C2 level distorting the cord. The cervical cord itself is expanded with decreased signal centrally within which there is a prominently enhancing nodule opposite C4. This is likely to represent an ependymoma.*

Table 1.3 *MRI Screening protocol in NF2*

Brain: pre-contrast (5mm slices)
Sagittal T1 SE
Axial T2 TSE or GRASE

Brain: post-contrast (5mm-slices)
Axial T1 SE (3mm through CPA; 5mm to vertex)
Coronal T1 SE

Spinal canal: post-contrast (5mm slices)
Sagittal and coronal T1 SE
Axial T1 SE (selected levels only)
Sagittal T2 TSE (optional if intrinsic cord mass)

SE: spin echo; GRASE: gradient spin echo; TSE: turbo (or fast) spin echo may be the result of abnormal migration of dysgenetic cells. Diagnosis relies upon demonstration of the radiological hallmarks as less than half of sufferers will have the classical clinical triad of adenoma sebaceum (papular facial nevus), seizures and mental retardation. Four main varieties of brain abnormality are described:

a. *Cortical tubers* These hamartomas are identifiable in 95% of patients on MRI. In order of decreasing frequency, they are located in the frontal, parietal, occipital and temporal lobes and the cerebellum.[22] Although 80% of cortical tubers are identified only by their abnormal signal, 20% may cause some gyral distortion. On MRI the appearances differ according to whether or not myelination has occurred. In the premyelinated neonatal or infant brain the lesions are hyperintense on T1WI and hypointense on T2WI in relation to premyelinated white matter. In the myelinated older child or adult brain they are usually hypointense on T1WI and hyperintense on T2WI (Fig. 1.22). Tubers do not undergo malignant degeneration and enhancement is seen in less than 5%.
On CT, cortical tubers evolve from being areas of peripheral lucency through an isodense phase through to calcification. The incidence of calcification increases with age, being rare in infancy whereas by the age of 10 years, 50% of patients have some calcified tubers.

b. *White matter lesions* The four patterns described (in order of decreasing frequency) are: straight or curvilinear bands extending from the ventricle to the cortex, wedge-shaped lesions, conglomerate or 'tumefactive' foci, and cerebellar radial bands. These lesions have no mass effect and 12% enhance. The T1W1 and T2WI characteristics are identical to those described above for cortical tubers.

c. *Subependymal nodules (SENs)* These hamartomas occur in 95% of patients with two-thirds located near the caudate nucleus just behind the foramen of Monro with others occurring in the atria and temporal horns of the lateral ventricles. They very uncommonly occur in relation to the third and fourth ventricles. The SENs range in size from 1mm up to 12mm and are shown on MR as irregular nodules projecting into the CSF. Signal intensity is variable but they are usually iso- or hypointense to both grey and white matter (due to calcification) (Fig. 1.23). Heterogeneity of signal can occur and between 30% and 50% enhance but enhancement does not indicate neoplastic transformation. On CT, calcification is well demonstrated (Fig. 1.24). As with cortical tubers the incidence of calcification increases with age, being unusual in infants but present in almost 100% of young adults. Imaging follow-up is required for lesions near the foramen of Monro in case a lesion in this location represents a subependymal giant cell astrocytoma (SGCA).

d. *Subependymal giant cell astrocytomas* These occur in approximately 15% of patients with tuberous sclerosis. They most commonly occur near the foramen of Monro and consequently patients present with obstructive hydrocephalus. Most patients present between approximately 5 and 18 years of age. More than one lesion may be present with size range commonly between 2 and 5cm. On MRI the lesions are usually heterogeneous and iso- to hypointense on T1WI and hyperintense on T2WI (Fig. 1.25). Signal voids due to intratumour vessels or areas of calcification may be noted. Enhancement is intense but heterogeneous.

e. *Other central nervous system (CNS) lesions* These include retinal hamartomas (in 50%), mild non-obstructive hydrocephalus (in 25%) and vascular anomalies including a dysplasia causing occlusion of craniocervical vessels. The disease also causes a progressive degeneration in large elastic arteries such as the aorta, leading to aneurysm formation and other non-CNS manifestations are also well described.

Radiological screening in tuberous sclerosis
Cranial CT or MRI is recommended every 1–2 years particularly between the ages of 8 and 18 years, the peak ages for SCGA presentation.

VON HIPPEL–LINDAU DISEASE

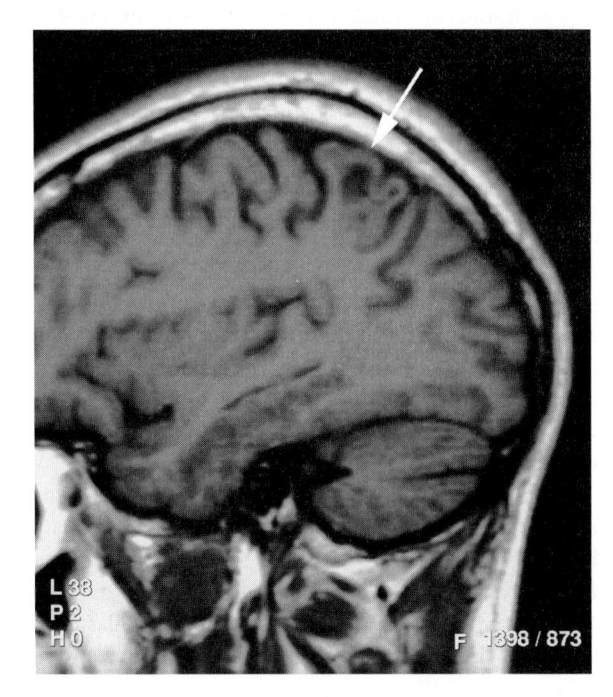

Figure 1.22 *Tuberous sclerosis–cortical tuber. T1WI demonstrating an area of hypointensity within a distorted gyrus in an adult patient.*

Von Hippel–Lindau (VHL) disease is an autosominal dominant condition with incomplete penetrance. It is

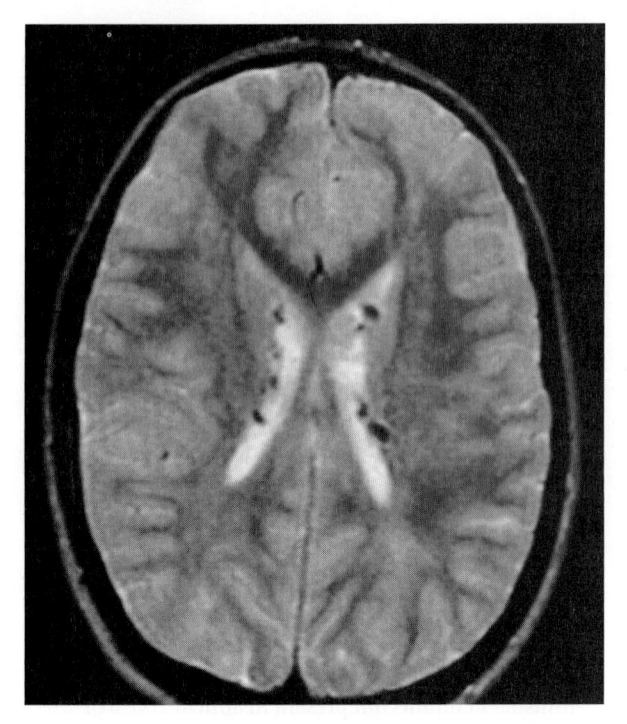

Figure 1.23 *Tuberous sclerosis–subependymal nodules. Axial T2WI shows numerous focal areas of marked hypointensity representing calcified (SENs) projecting into the high-signal CSF of the lateral ventricles.*

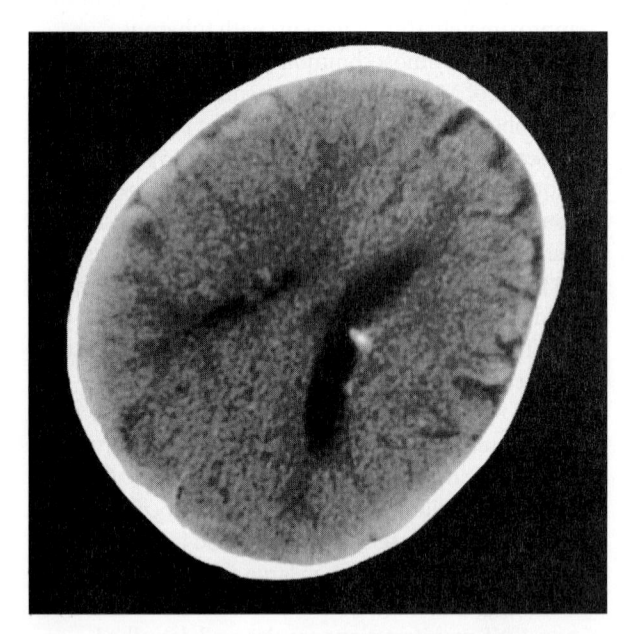

Figure 1.24 *Tuberous sclerosis–subependymal nodules. Axial non-contrast CT section demonstrating calcified SENs.*

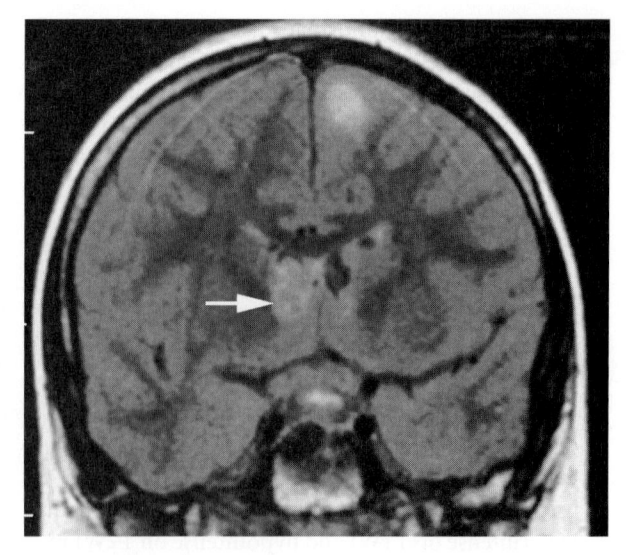

Figure 1.25 *Tuberous sclerosis–subependymal giant cell astrocytoma. Coronal FLAIR (fluid attenuated inversion recovery sequence) section at the level of the foramina of Monro shows an SGCA on the right side (arrow). Several SENs are visible projecting into the left lateral ventricle. Note also the high signal cortical tuber at the left vertex.*

linked to a defect on chromosome 3 and has a prevalence of 1 per 35 000–40 000. The characteristic lesion is the haemangioblastoma involving the cerebellum, lower brainstem or spinal cord.[23,24] In VHL patients the peak of haemangioblastoma occurrence is at 32 years whereas they occur generally later in non-VHL patients, during the fifth and sixth decades. Other causes of morbidity in VHL include retinal haemangioblastomas, renal cell carcinoma and pheochromocytomas. Death is usually due to cerebellar haemangioblastoma (53%) or renal cell carcinoma (32%).

The typical appearance of a haemangioblastoma is a cyst containing a vascular mural nodule (Fig. 1.26) but 20% of lesions are solid, without any surrounding cyst. The cysts may contain high concentrations of erythropoietin. Haemangioblastomas always reach the pial surface and so tend to be fairly superficial although surface infolding can result in a deeper location. The posterolateral surface of the cerebellar hemisphere is the most common location with the vermis less often involved; 5% of patients will have involvement of the lower medulla (area postrema). Although a solitary haemangioblastoma may be seen at presentation, multiple lesions are common. Supratentorial locations are rare but haemangioblastomas may be seen in the pituitary/hypothalamic region, optic nerve, within the walls of the ventricles (third and temporal horn) the frontal and temporal lobes, and the meninges.

Spinal cord involvement is common (13–59%) particularly the lower cervical and lower thoracic cord and they are associated with cysts in the majority of cases (80%). Nerve root or extradural locations are rare. Whereas only 5–30% of cerebellar haemangioblastomas occur in VHL cases, 80% of spinal haemangioblastomas are associated with the disease.

On MRI, the tumour nidus or mural nodule is hypo- to isointense on T1WI and hyperintense on T2WI. Cysts are slightly hyperintense on T1WI and hyperintense on

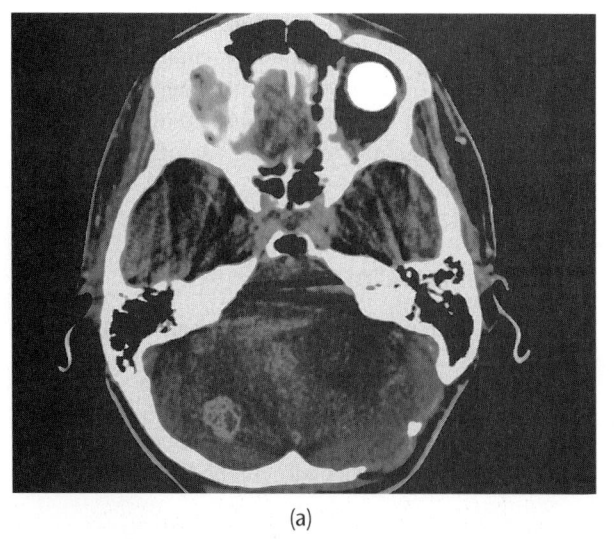

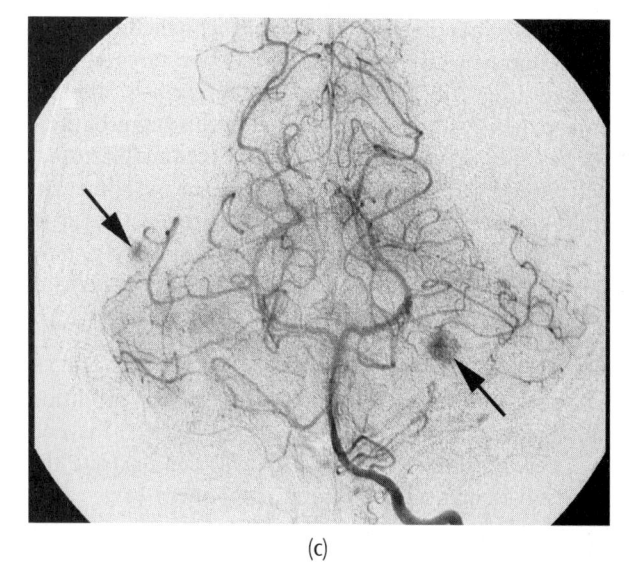

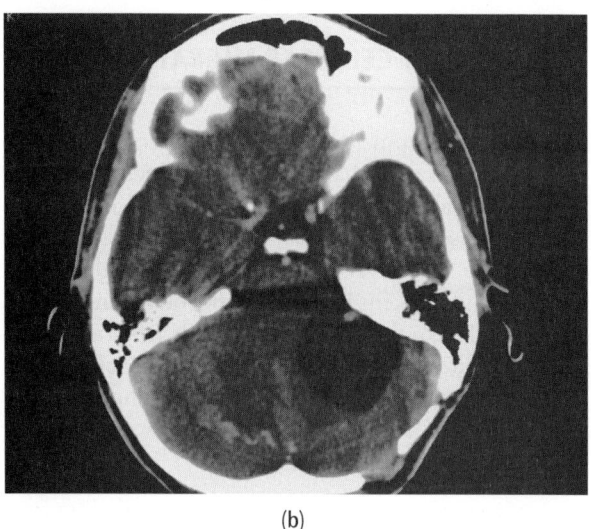

Disorders of neural proliferation, differentiation and histogenesis 61

Figure 1.26 Von Hippel–Lindau disease. Axial contrast-enhanced CT sections (a),(b). There is a left occipital craniotomy from previous surgery. Two haemangioblastomas are present, the one on the left side being predominantly cystic with a small enhancing mural nodule seen just behind the left petrous bone (b); the right-sided tumour is a solid lesion with some surrounding oedema (a). Note the cortical vessel in (b) extending to the solid nodule. A vertebral angiogram (c) in the same patient shows the intense blush typical of haemangioblastomas (arrows) though contrast-enhanced MRI has superseded angiography in this situation.

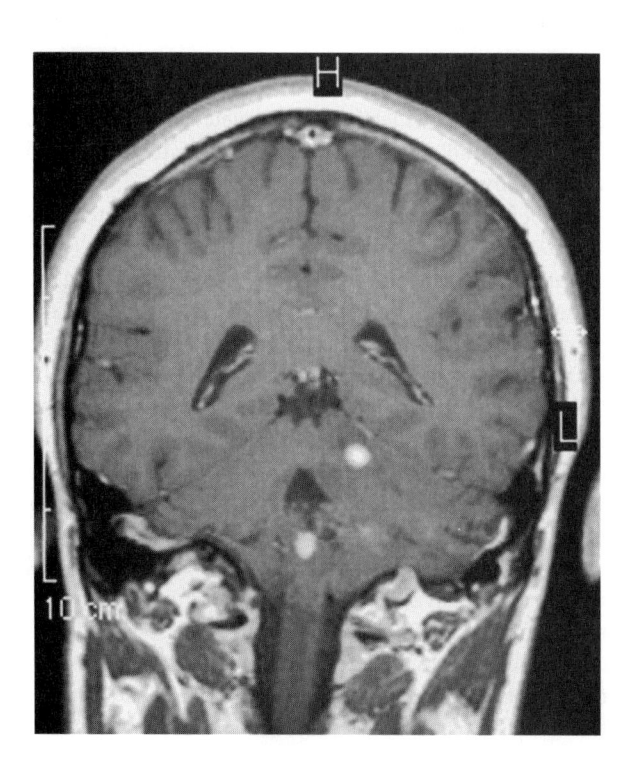

Figure 1.27 Von Hippel–Lindau disease. Coronal contrast-enhanced T1WI demonstrating two enhancing haemangioblastomas in the cerebellum.

T2WI. Haemangioblastoma nodules enhance intensely with contrast which is mandatory if lesions are not to be missed (Fig. 1.27). Adjacent cortical vessels may be enlarged, a feature which may help distinguish these lesions from cystic astrocytomas or medulloblastomas which tend to be less vascular lesions. In the spine, the solid component has imaging characteristics similar to those in the posterior fossa. The tumoural cysts have poorly defined, enhancing margins and a signal intensity on T1 and T2WI greater than CSF.

Radiological screening in VHL

Contrast-enhanced MRI is mandatory in this condition as considerably more small lesions will be seen than on CT. Cerebral angiography, which will demonstrate the intense vascularity of the solid component (Fig. 1.26), has largely been superseded by MRI. Screening recommendations are annual retinal examination from the age of 5 years, annual to biennial abdominal CT and contrast enhanced MRI of the CNS from the age of 20 years.

STURGE–WEBER SYNDROME

Though occasionally familial, most cases arise sporadically. The two major features of the Sturge–Weber syndrome are:

a. *A cutaneous vascular nevus (port-wine nevus)* of the face usually in the distribution of the first division of the trigeminal nerve.
b. *Leptomeningeal (pial) angiomastosis* of the ipsilateral occipital lobe with variable parietal and temporal lobe extension.[23,25]

Other brain features include cortical calcification, hemi-atrophy and patchy gliosis, and demyelination. Much of the damage seen to the involved brain is thought to be due to disordered venous drainage, resulting from occlusion of deep veins.

Clinically, patients present with seizures (in 90%), homonymous hemi-anopsia, and hemiparesis on the opposite side to the leptomeningeal abnormality in about two-thirds of cases. Other features include hemi-sensory deficit, mental dysfunction and, rarely, subarachnoid or intracerebral haemorrhage.

On imaging (Fig. 1.28) non-contrast MRI may appear normal and so intravenous contrast injection is mandatory to demonstrate the enhancing thickened leptomeninges; T2WI will show areas of high signal resulting from areas of gliosis and demyelination in the white matter. Both CT and MRI will demonstrate angiomatous changes of the ipsilateral choroid plexus which show evidence of enlargement and enhancement as well as associated calvarial changes with hyperpneumatization of the paranasal sinuses and mastoid, elevation of the petrous ridge and widening of the diploic space on the affected side.

Associated hemi-atrophy will also be visible. The characteristic feature on CT is calcification in the involved cortex. This calcification is progressive during childhood, becoming stationary at the end of the second decade. The leptomeningeal enhancement demonstrable on MRI is difficult to see on CT because of the overlying calcification. Magnetic resonance angiography (MRA) may show a pial blush.

OTHER PHAKOMATOSES

Two other groups of uncommon phakomatoses are described:[22]

a. *Vascular* including Osler–Weber–Rendu disease, ataxia telangiectasia, and meningioangiomatoses.
b. *Melanocytic* including neurocutaneous melanosis.

DISORDERS OF CELLULAR MIGRATION

In normal development, the cells of the germinal matrix migrate along radial glial fibres to their final destination in the cerebral cortex.[26] The normal cortex contains six layers of cells with the first layer being the most superficial and the sixth layer being the deepest. As the cortex develops and thickens it becomes convoluted in order to fit within the confines of the skull vault. The radial glial fibres involute and later become astrocytes. Some disorders of migration such as polymicrogyria and closed lip schizoncephaly are probably the result of vascular insults to the already formed cortex.

Lissencephaly

This term means 'smooth brain' but has come to encompass both agyria which is the complete lack of any gyral formation, and pachygyria which refers to broad gyri with shallow sulci.[27]

In the most severe agyric form imaging demonstrates a thickened cortex with a smooth brain surface, with abnormal, vertically orientated sylvian fissures giving the brain a figure of 8 appearance when viewed in the axial plane (Fig. 1.29). The amount of white matter is reduced with a smooth grey-white matter interface. There may be callosal agenesis as well as a hypoplastic brainstem due to lack of formation of the corticospinal and corticobulbar tracts. Pachygria is less severe and results in the formation of a few broad, flat gyri and can occur focally or more diffusely. Both forms of abnormal cortex can coexist with agyria predominating in the parieto-occipital region, and pachygyria being more common in the frontotemporal area. Lissencephaly can be associated with congenital eye malformations (Walker–Warburg syndrome) and congenital cytomegalovirus (CMV) infection.

Disorders of cellular migration 63

(a)

(b)

(c)

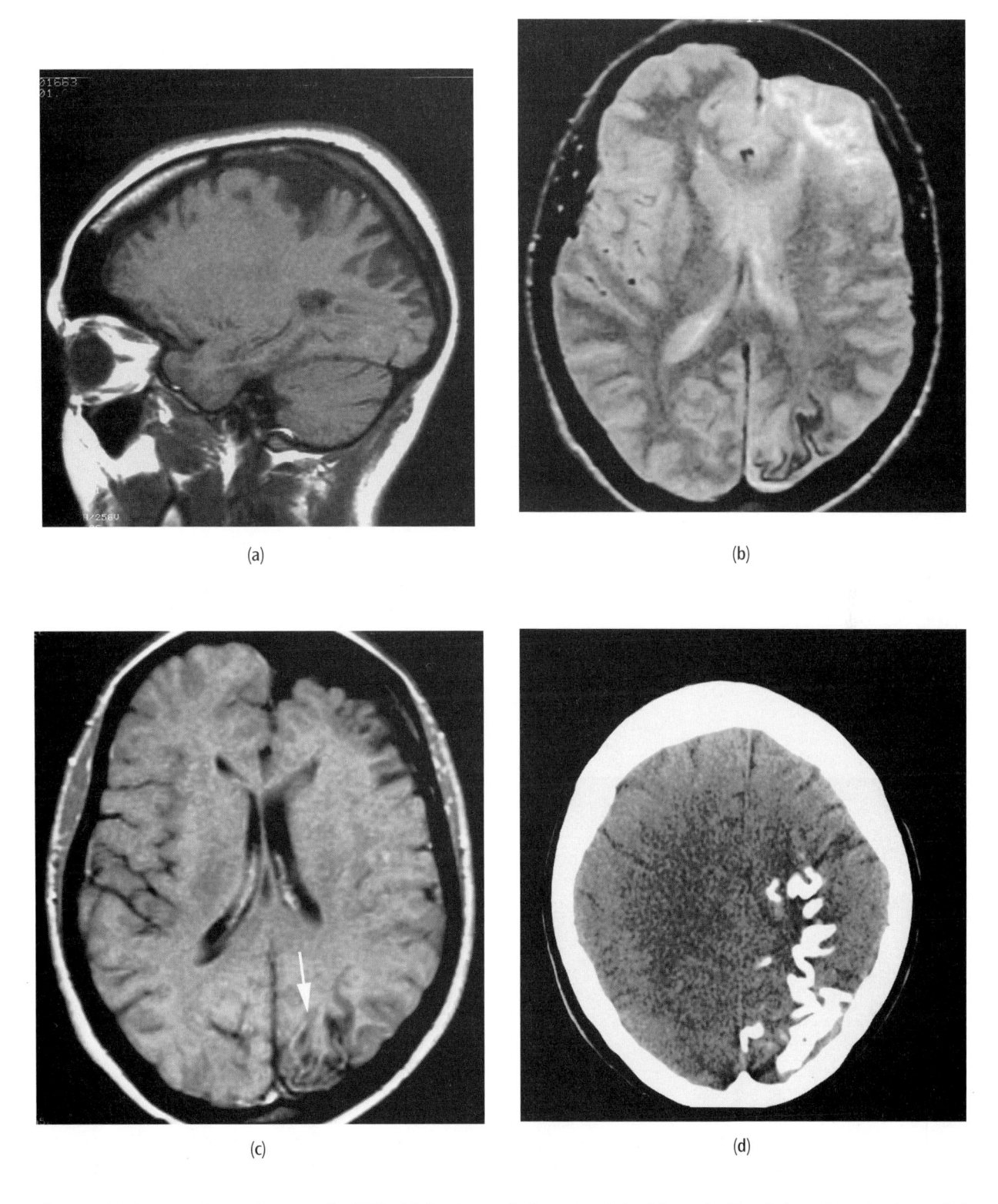

(d)

Figure 1.28 *Sturge–Weber syndrome. Sagittal T1WI (a) showing marked atrophy of the right cerebral hemisphere. Note also the marked diploic space widening within the frontal bone and gross enlargement of the frontal paranasal sinus. Axial T2W (b), post-contrast T1W (c) and plain CT (d) scans in a different patient. In (b) there is left frontal gliosis while in the left posterior parietal lobe low sign gyral calcification is evident. The post-contrast images (c) at the same level highlights the atrophy in both affected areas and subtle leptomeningeal enhancement (arrow). CT (d) taken 7 years later shows gross gyral calcification.*

64 Congenital abnormalities

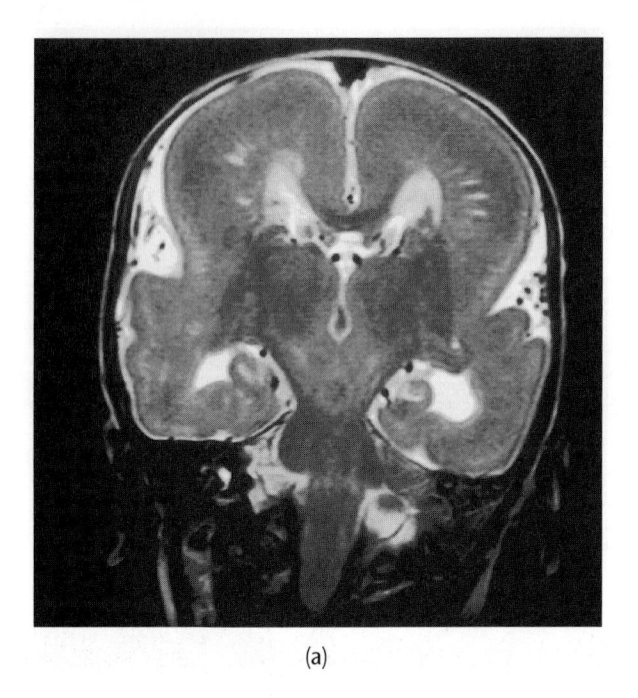

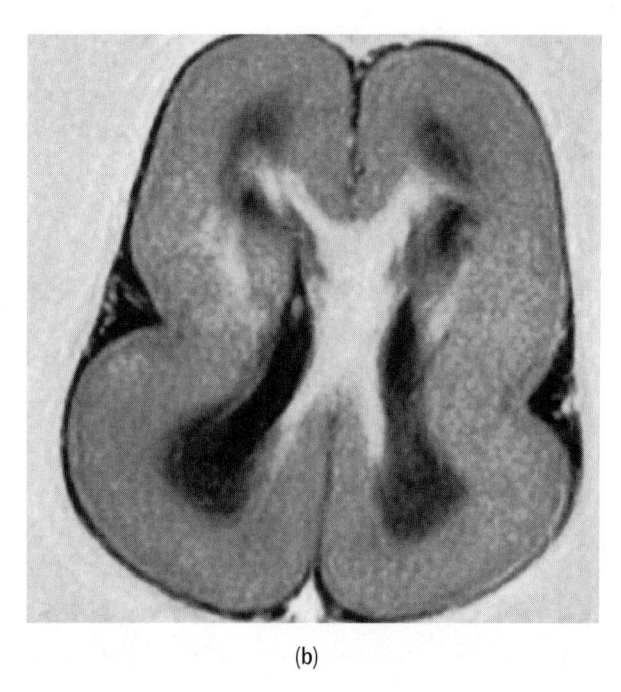

Figure 1.29 Lissencephaly. Coronal T2WI (a) and axial T1W inversion-recovery turbo-spin echo image (b) demonstrating the typical smooth figure of 8 configuration of the most severe agyric from of lissencephaly. Note the thickness of the cortex. (Courtesy of Dr Scott Shepard, Emory University Hospital, Atlanta.)

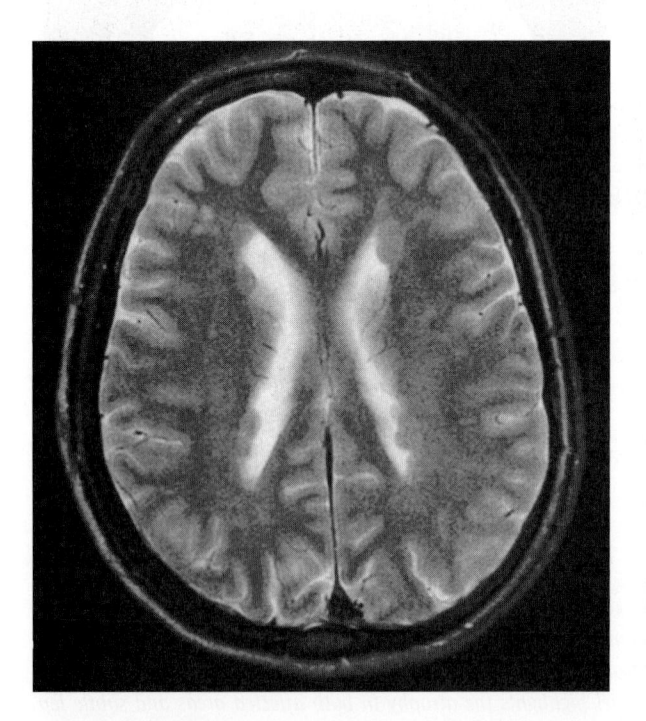

Figure 1.30 Grey matter heterotopia. Axial T2WI showing multiple areas of subependymal heterotopia. The nodules of ectopic grey matter are of identical signal intensity to the cortical grey matter and are projecting into and are highlighted by high signal CSF within the lateral ventricles.

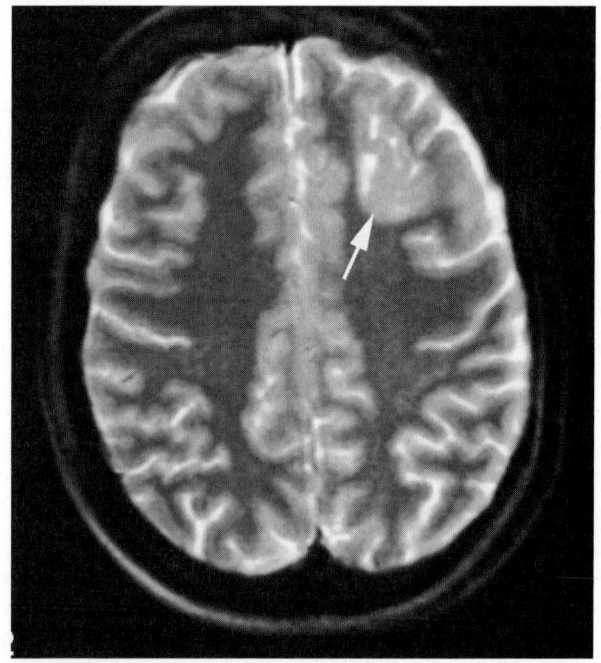

Figure 1.31 Grey matter heterotopia. Axial T2WI demonstrating a focal subcortical heterotopion in the left anterior parietal region (arrow). The 'mass' is mainly of normal grey matter signal within which there are multiple areas of CSF signal due to cortical infolding. Note there is no mass effect on the adjacent sulci.

Disorders of cellular migration 65

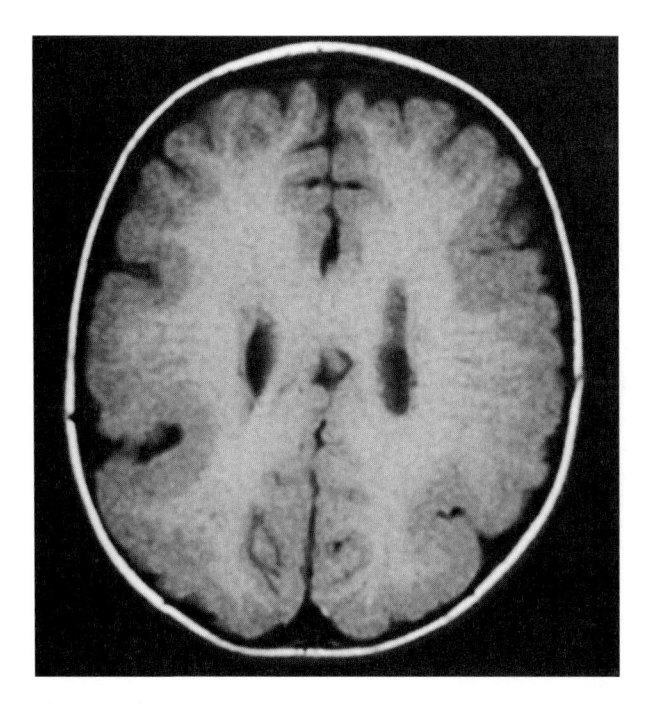

Figure 1.32 *Polymicrogyria (cortical dysplasia). Axial T1WI showing bilaterally abnormal parietal lobes with a thickened cortex and paucity of normal sulci. The superficial surface of the cortex has a finely irregular appearance typical of polymicrogyria. This example is virtually indistinguishable from pachygyria. (Courtesy of Professor P Griffiths, Sheffield.)*

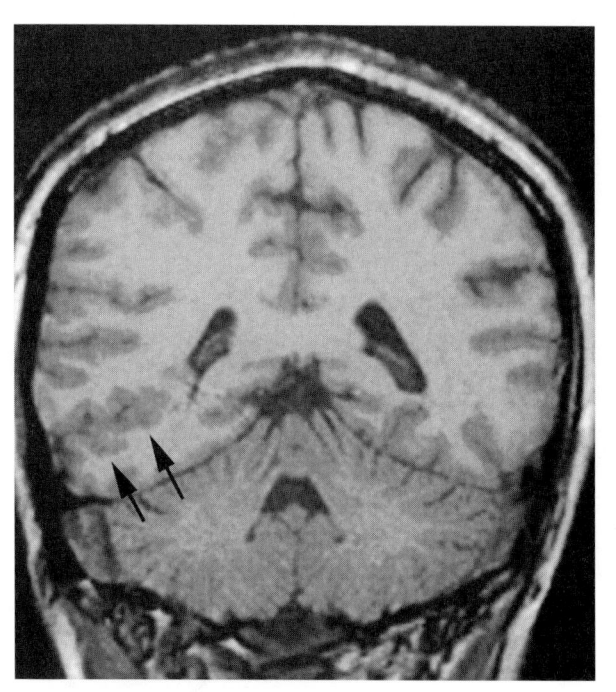

Figure 1.34 *Schizencephaly – closed lip variety. Coronal T1WI from a 3-D volume acquisition showing a band of ectopic grey matter extending to the right lateral ventricular margin (arrows). Portions of an elongated narrow sulcus can be seen within this.*

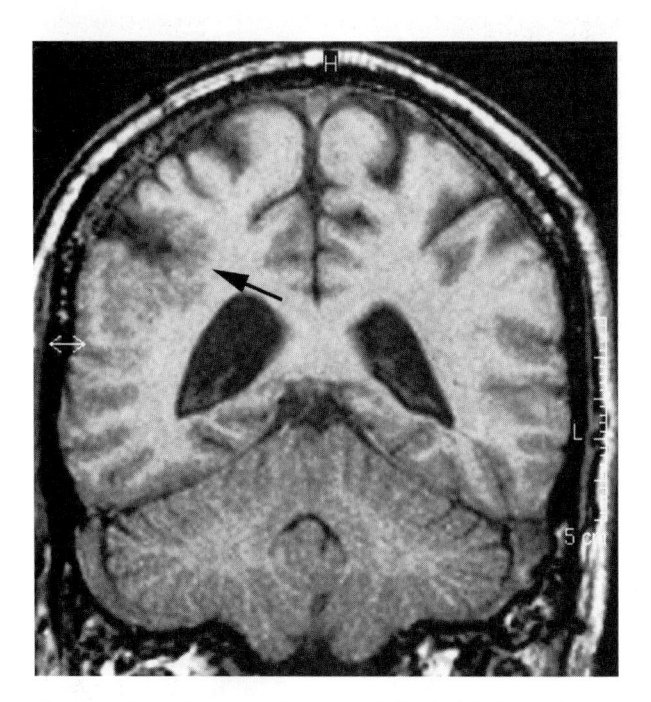

Figure 1.33 *Polymicrogyria (cortical dysplasia). Coronal T1WI showing a prominent area of cortical dysplasia over the right cerebral convexity (arrow). There is a widened sulcus with an irregularly thickened surrounding cortex. This is one slice from a high resolution 3-D volume acquisition.*

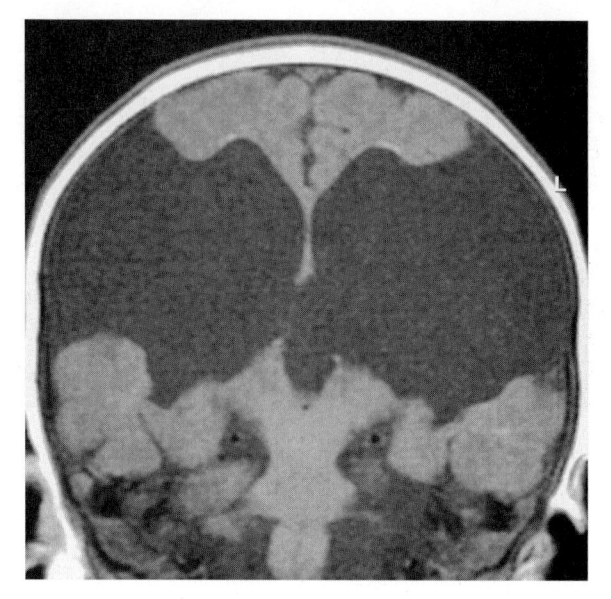

Figure 1.35 *Schizencephaly – open lip variety. Coronal T1WI demonstrates large bilateral symmetric CSF clefts extending from the cortex into the lateral ventricles.*

Grey matter heterotopia

When the normal migration of nerve cells to the cortex is arrested, the cells are left in abnormal locations, and are known as areas of heterotopia.[28] On imaging they

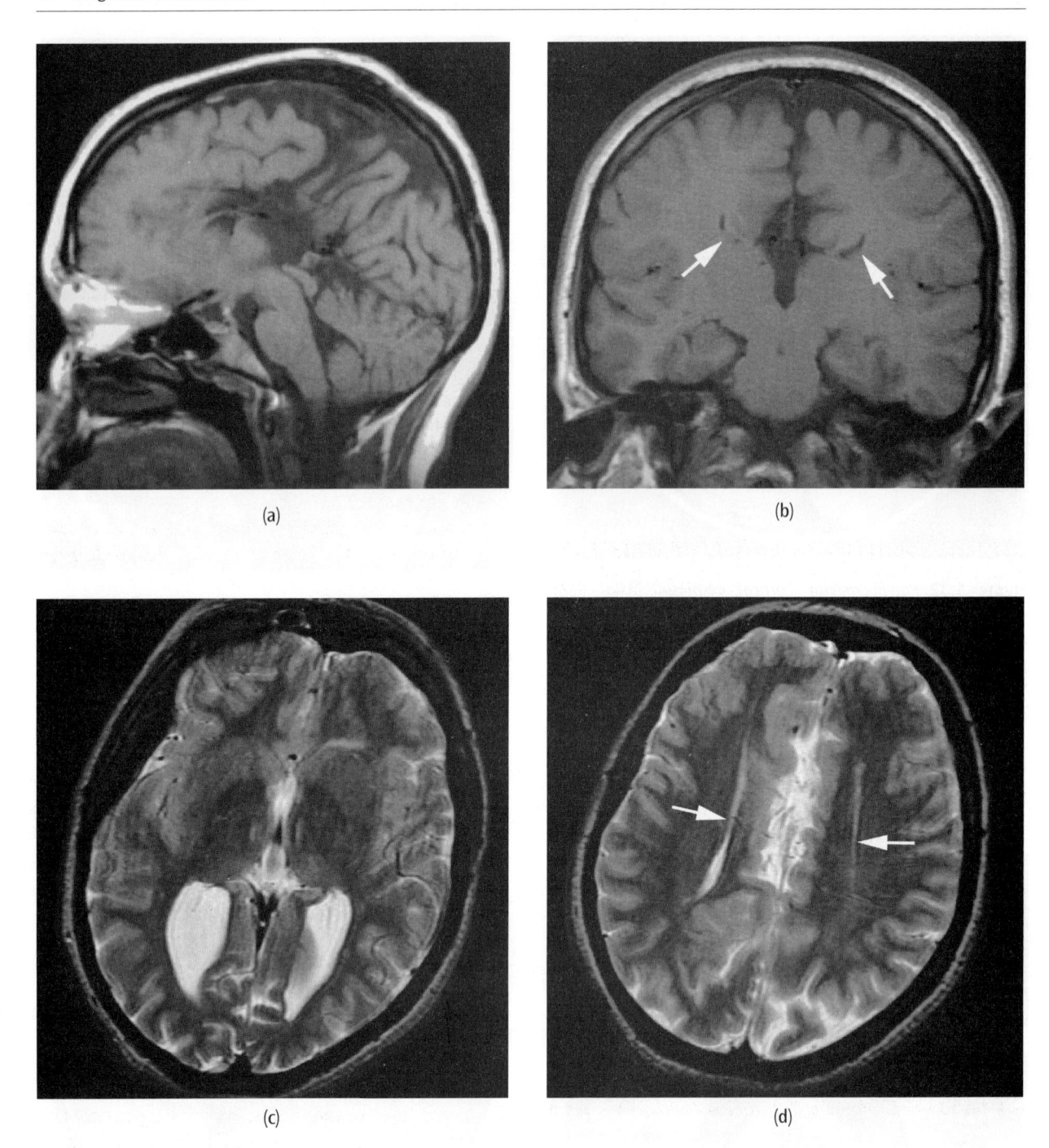

Figure 1.36 Complete agenesis of the corpus callosum. Sagittal and coronal T1WI (a,b) and axial T2WI (c,d). The lateral ventricular bodies are widely separated and parallel in orientation (arrows in b and d). An enlarged third ventricle extends upwards between the lateral ventricles and merges with the interhemispheric fissure. Note the abnormal configuration of the lateral ventricles in (b) which are convex inferolaterally and concave superomedially. Colpocephaly of the trigones and occipital horns is shown in (c).

appear as nodular or broad areas of tissue characteristically isointense with normal cerebral grey matter on all pulse sequences. No enhancement occurs and they are not associated with cerebral oedema. Patients usually present with seizures and may have developmental delay.

Three varieties of heterotopia are described according to their location. With *subependymal heterotopia*, imaging demonstrates smooth ovoid nodules projecting into the lateral ventricle (Fig. 1.30) *Focal subcortical heterotopia* can be larger collections of cells and may contain vessels and CSF due to cortical infolding next to the heterotopion and exert some mass effect on adjacent CSF spaces (Fig. 1.31). In *diffuse grey matter* or *'band' heterotopia*, imaging will demonstrate a circumferential band

Disorders of cellular migration 67

of grey matter deep to the cortex from which it is separated by a layer of normal white matter resulting in a double cortex appearance.

Polymicrogyria (cortical dysplasia)

In this condition, the migrating neurons have reached the cortex but their organization is abnormal resulting in the formation of multiple small gyri.[29] It is most commonly seen around the sylvian fissure but can affect any cortical location. Symptoms depend upon the amount of brain involved, with bilateral involvement (or more than half of a single side involved) correlating with developmental delay and motor dysfunction. Polymicrogyria, along with schizencephaly[30] and hydrancephaly may form a spectrum of disorders due to a vascular insult. It can also be seen in congenital CMV infection.

On imaging, an irregular bumpy inner and outer cortical surface is typical. It may be indistinguishable from pachygria (Fig. 1.32) or can look so subtle that very high resolution slices from a 3-D volume acquisition may be required for detection.[27] The abnormally organized cortical cells are isointense to normal grey matter on all sequences although areas of hyperintensity in adjacent white matter can be seen in 20% of cases and calcification has been identified in a very small minority on CT. The areas of cortical dysplasia can parallel the normal cortical arc or have a more focal infolded appearance (Fig. 1.33). If this infolding extends to the ventricular surface then the abnormality is virtually an area of schizencephaly (see below). Anomalous venous drainage may affect the dysplastic cortex.

Schizencephaly

These are defined as grey matter lined clefts extending from the ependyma of the lateral ventricle to the pia of the cortex, thus extending through the entire width of the cerebral hemisphere.[31] The clefts are divided into those with fused or closed lips, where the opposite walls are apposed with no intervening CSF (Fig. 1.34), or those with separated or open lips with CSF filling the gap in between (Fig. 1.35). In either type, the grey matter lining of the cleft is dysplastic. Clinical disability depends upon the amount of involved brain and can result in development delay with seizures and hemiparesis. A third of cases may have blindness due to optic nerve hypoplasia. On imaging, the dysplastic grey matter lining the cleft will be isointense to normal grey matter on all sequences. Adjacent cortex may be dysplastic and subependymal heterotopia may be seen at the ventricular end of the cleft. Closed lip clefts may have a dimple on the ventricular wall. Areas of cortical dysplasia may affect the opposite cerebral hemisphere and the septum pellucidum is absent in between 80% and 90% of cases.

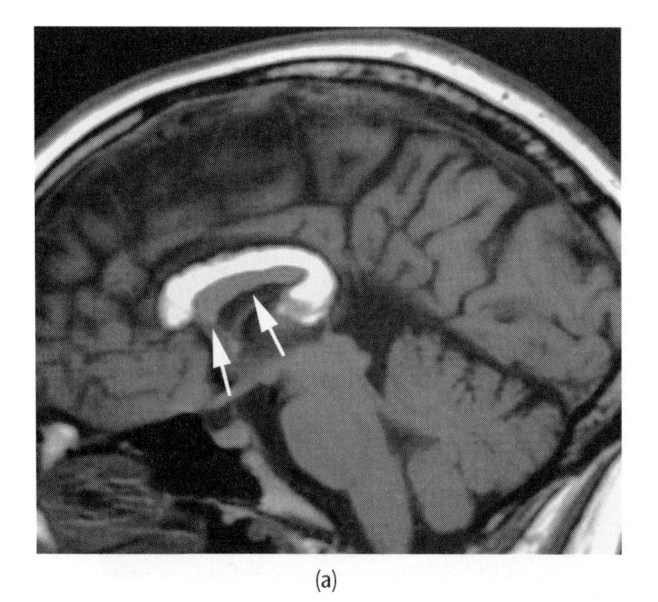

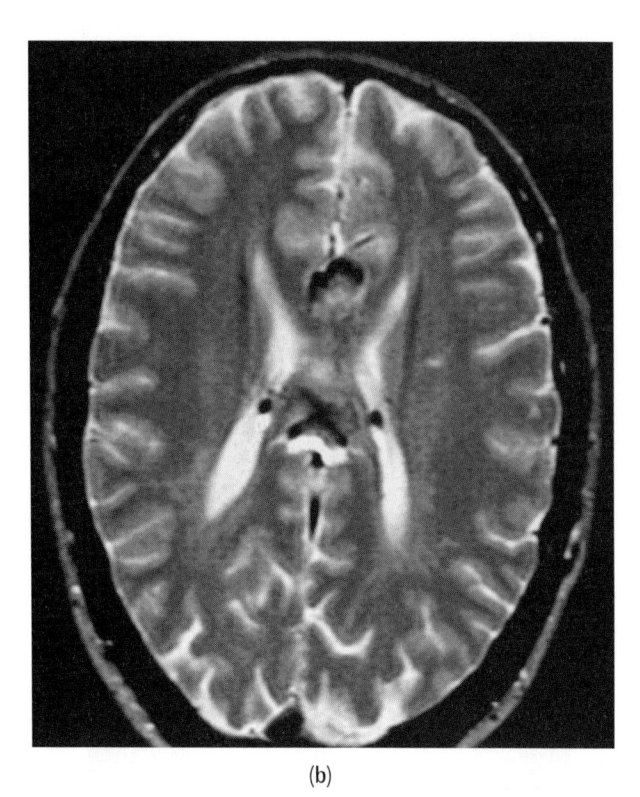

Figure 1.37 *Hypoplasia of the corpus callosum with associated lipoma. The genu and body of the corpus callosum are present (arrows) but the rostrum (anteroinferior) and splenium (posteriorly) are missing (a). There is a well defined curvilinear shaped lipoma overlying the callosum best identified because of its very bright signal on the T1-weighted sequence. In (b) the anterior portions of the lateral ventricles do show some convergence towards the mid line but the posterior bodies are widely spaced. Note that the lipoma is less clearly seen as it is now the same intermediate signal as the subcutaneous fat but is highlighted by a very prominent chemical shift artefact (adjacent low and high signal bands).*

68 Congenital abnormalities

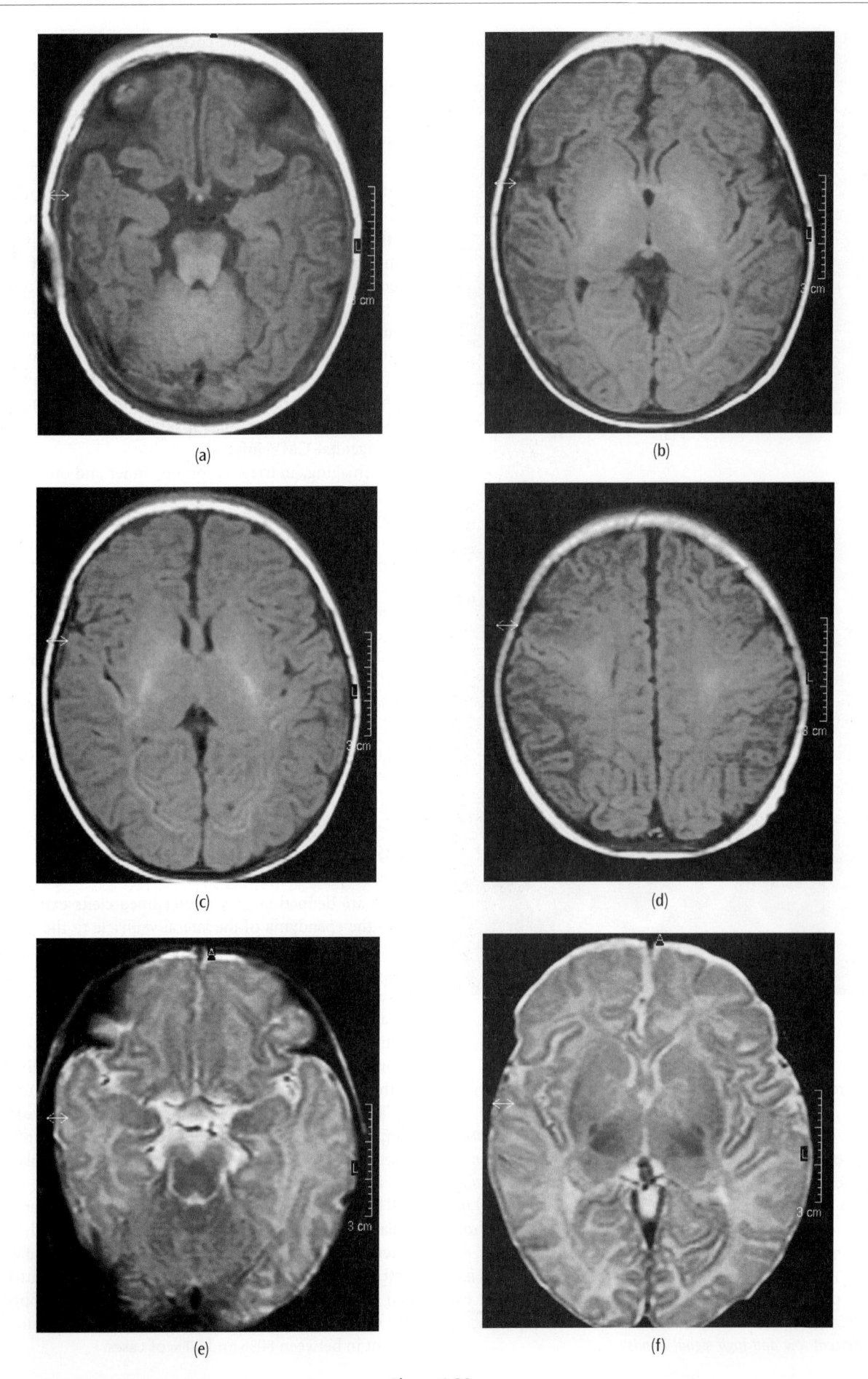

Figure 1.38

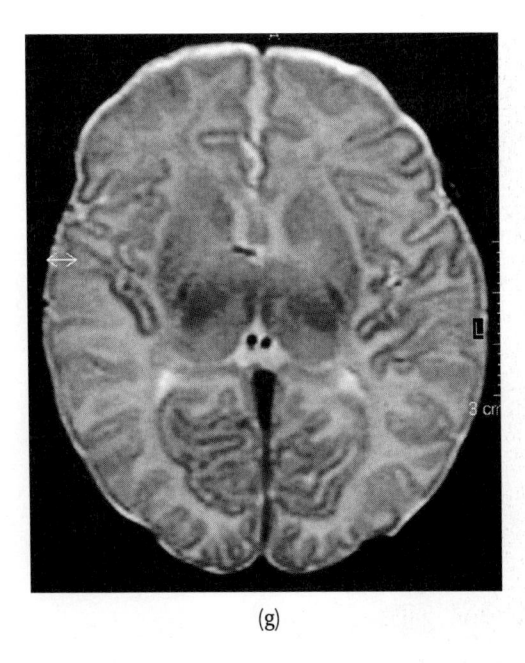

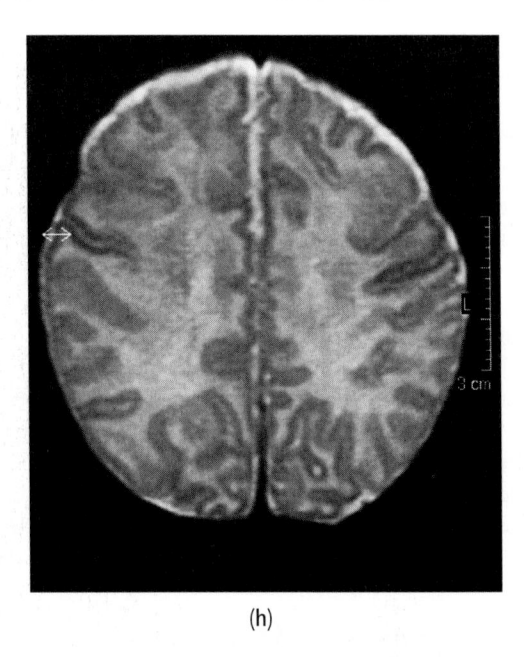

Figure 1.38 a–f (facing page), (g–h above) *Normal myelination pattern in a 9-day-old infant. Axial T1-weighted spin echo images (a–d) and T2-weighted spin echo images (e–h) performed at 1.5T. In this child myelination (shown as areas of developing hyperintensity on T1WI and hypointensity on T2WI) is evident in the dorsal brainstem, posterior limbs of the internal capsule and lateral thalami, optic radiations, the central corona radiata and around the central sulcus. The signal changes are easier to appreciate on the T1WI. Note that on the T2WI there is a predominantly infantile pattern with most white matter brighter than grey matter.*

Abnormalities of the corpus callosum

Normal corpus callosal development proceeds in an anterior to posterior direction i.e. genu, body, splenium, but with the rostrum (anteroinferior portion) forming last; callosal myelination proceeds in the posterior to anterior direction.[27] Because of this developmental pattern a corpus callosum in which there is a splenium but little or no genu or body implies that a destructive process has occurred following initial development (exceptions to this rule include holoprosencephaly, porencephaly and schizencephaly).

Developmental anomalies of the corpus callosum can be complete or partial. When complete or nearly complete (Fig. 1.36), axial CT and MRI will demonstrate widely displaced parallel lateral ventricles with the interhemispheric fissure running in continuity between the lateral ventricles from front to back. The third ventricle extends upwards between the lateral ventricles to merge with the interhemispheric fissure. The frontal horns are convex shaped laterally but have indentations medially due to indentation by axonal fibres unable to cross the midline (bundles of Probst). Expansion of the posterior aspect of the lateral ventricles into adjacent white matter may be seen (colpocephaly). In milder cases where only the posterior callosum is deficient, the frontal horns and anterior portions of the lateral ventricular bodies will have a more normal configuration but the posterior ends will be abnormally widely separated (Fig. 1.37). MRI particularly in the sagittal plane, best depicts areas of callosal agenesis or hypogenesis and may be the only method of detecting milder degrees of underdevelopment. Coronal and sagittal MRI will also demonstrate absence of the cingulate sulcus and everted cingulate gyri which are normally immediately above the callosal body. Because the corpus callosum develops over a relatively long period (2–5 months), many associated anomalies may be seen, some of which are listed in Table 1.4. Interhemispheric lipomas, if present, are nearly always associated with callosal anomalies and are very evident on T1WI as areas of very high signal which gradually decrease on longer TR sequences (Fig. 1.37).

Table 1.4 *Congenital abnormalities associated with maldevelopment of the corpus callosum*

Neuronal migration anomalies (including agyria, pachygyria, heterotopias)
Encephaloceles
Dandy–Walker malformation
Chiari II
Holoprosencephaly
Septo-optic dysplasia
Interhemispheric lipoma
Trisomy 13–15 and 18
Aicardi syndrome (chorioretinopathy and infantile spasms)

DISORDERS OF MYELINATION

Normal myelination patterns

Brain myelination, in general, proceeds from inferior to superior, posterior to anterior and central to peripheral. Chronologically it commences around the 5th month of fetal life starting with the cranial nerves, and at birth evidence of myelination is seen in the medulla, dorsal midbrain, the inferior and superior cerebellar peduncles and the posterior limb of the internal capsule. This process proceeds rapidly and is nearly complete by 18 months to 2 years of age. The process, however, continues slowly throughout adult life with some association centres remaining unmyelinated until 30 years of age.

Imaging of normal myelination

Imaging by MR offers an excellent means of following the normal pattern of myelination and the use of serial scanning can help distinguish between those children whose white matter maturation is delayed (but proceeding) from those with retarded myelination. Within the first 6 months of life myelination is more easily detected on T1WI rather than T2WI and is shown by areas of increasing signal intensity (Fig. 1.38). Between 6 and 18 months of age T2WI are preferable with myelination being shown as a progressive decrease in white matter signal intensity. Dietrich and colleagues[31] have analysed myelination patterns using T2-weighted spin echo images and found three distinct patterns:

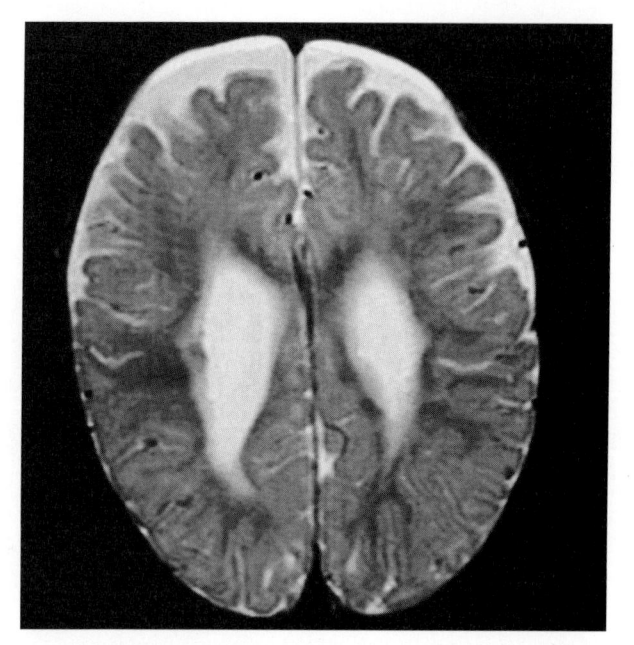

Figure 1.39 *Periventricular leucomalacia and delayed myelination. Axial T2-weighted spin echo image in a 15-month-old child born premature. The lateral ventricular bodies are enlarged with undulating margins and some periventricular high signal typical of PVL. Although some myelination is present the degree of 'arbourization' of the myelinated white matter into the subcortical regions is delayed and more typical of a 12-month-old child.*

a. *Infantile* where white matter is brighter than grey matter and occurs in children up to 6 months of age;
b. *Isointense* where grey and white matter are of similar intensity occurring in children between 8 and 12 months of age;

Table 1.5 *Normal brain myelination – ages when changes appeared*

Anatomic region	Age when changes of myelination appeared	
	T1-Weighted images	T2-Weighted images
Middle cerebellar peduncle	Birth	Birth to 2 months
Cerebellar white matter	Birth to 4 months	3–5 months
Posterior limb internal capsule		
Anterior portion	Birth	4–7 months
Posterior portion	Birth	Birth to 2 months
Anterior limb internal capsule	2–3 months	7–11 months
Genu corpus callosum	4–6 months	5–8 months
Splenium corpus callosum	3–4 months	4–6 months
Occipital white matter		
Central	3–5 months	9–14 months
Peripheral	4–7 months	11–15 months
Frontal white matter		
Central	3–6 months	11–16 months
Peripheral	7–11 months	14–18 months
Centrum semiovale	2–4 months	7–11 months

T1-weighted sequence was SE 600/20 (TR ms/TE ms); T2-weighted sequence was 2500/70. (Reproduced from Ref. 32, with permission.)

c. *Early adult* where white matter is of lower signal intensity than grey matter (the normal adult pattern) and occurs in children between 12 and 31 months of age.

Barkovich and colleagues, using a 1.5T magnet, documented the ages at which normal myelination was detected in a variety of key anatomical sites on both T1WI and T2WI (Table 1.5).[32] Delayed myelination has been associated with a wide variety of conditions including various ischaemic or infective insults to the perinatal brain (Fig. 1.39), hydrocephalus, and systemic illness including respiratory insufficiency, renal failure and malnutrition.

REFERENCES

1. Van Der Knapp MS, Valk J. Classification of congenital abnormalities of the CNS. *Am J Neuroradiol* 1988; **9**:315–26.
2. Barkovich AJ. Normal development of the neonatal and infant brain, skull and spine. In: *Pediatric Neuroimaging* 2nd edn, pp. 9–54. New York: Raven Press, 1995.
3. Naidich TP, Altman NR, Brauffman BH, McLone DG, Zimmerman RA. Cephaloceles and related malformations. *Am J Neuroradiol* 1992; **13**:655–90.
4. Barkovich AJ, Vandermarck P, Edwards MSB, Cogen PH. Congenital nasal masses: CT and MR imaging features in 16 cases. *Am J Neuroradiol* 1991; **12**:105–16.
5. Naidich TP, Brauffman BH, Altman NR, Birchansky SB Malformations of the posterior fossa and craniovertebral junction. *Rivista Neuroradiol* 1997; **10**(Suppl 1):55–71.
6. William S, Ball MD JR, Crone MD. Chiari I malformations: from Dr Chiari to MR imaging. *Radiology* 1995; **195**:602–4.
7. Fitz CR. Holoprosencephaly and septo-optic dysplasia. Neuroimaging clinics of North America. *Pediat Neuroradiol* 1994; **4**:263–81.
8. Sarwar M. The septum pellucidum: normal and abnormal. *Am J Neuroradiol* 1989; **10**:989–1005.
9. Barkovich AJ, Kjos BO, Norman D, Edward MS. Revised classification of posterior fossa cysts and cystlike malformations based on the results of multiplanar MR imaging. *Am J Neuroradiol* 1989; **10**:977–88.
10. Benson ML, Oliverio PJ, Yue NC, Zinreich SJ. Primary craniosynostosis: imaging features. *Am J Radiol* 1996; **166**:697–703.
11. Jones BM, Hayward R, Evans R, Britto J. Occipital plagiocephaly: an epidemic of craniosynostosis? *Br Med J* 1997; **315**:693–4.
12. Tokumaru A, Barkovich AJ, Ciricillo SF, Edwards MSB. Skull base and calvarial deformities: association with intracranial changes in craniofacial syndromes. *Am J Neuroradiol* 1996; **17**:619–30.
13. Barkovich A, Chuang SH. Unilateral megalencephaly. *Am J Neuroradiol* 1990; **11**:523–31.
14. Brauffman B, Naidich TP. The phakomatoces: Part I Neurofibromatosis and tuberous sclerosis. Neuroimaging clinics of North America: *Pediat Neuroradiol* 1994; **4**:299–324.
15. Aoki S, Barkovich AJ, Nishimura K, Kjos BO, Machida T *et al*. Neurofibromatosis Type 1 and 2: cranial MR findings. *Radiology* 1989; **172**:527–34.
16. Sevick RJ, Barkovich AJ, Edwards MSB, Koch T, Berg B, Lempert T. Evolution of white matter lesions in neurofibromatosis Type 1: MR findings. *Am J Radiol* 1992; **159**:171–5.
17. DiPaolo DP, Zimmerman RA, Rorke LB, Zackai EH, Bilaniuk LT, Yachnis AT. Neurofibromatosis Type 1: pathologic substrate of high-signal-intensity foci in the brain. *Radiology* 1995; **195**:721–4.
18. Terada H, Barkovich AJ, Edwards MSB, Ciricillo SF. Evolution of high-intensity basal ganglia lesions on T1-weighted MR in neurofibromatosis Type 1. *Am J Neuroradiol* 1996; **17**:755–60.
19. O'Keefe LJ, Camilleri AE, Gillespie JE, Cairns A, Ramsden RT. Primary tumours of the vestibule and inner ear. *J Laryngol Otol* 1997; **111**:709–14.
20. Mautner VF, Tatagiba M, Lindenau M, Funsterer C, Pulst SM *et al*. Spinal tumours in patients with neurofibromatosis Type 2: MR imaging study of frequency, multiplicity and variety. *Am J Radiol* 1995; **165**:951–5.
21. Gillespie JE. Imaging in neurofibromatosis Type 2: screening using MRI. *Ear Nose Throat J* 1999; **2**:102–9.
22. Braffman BH, Bilaniuk LT, Naidich TP, Altman NR, Post JD *et al*. MR Imaging of tuberous sclerosis: pathogenesis of this phakomatosis, use of gadopentetate dimeglumine and literature review. *Radiology* 1992; **183**:227–38.
23. Braufmann B, Nidich TP. The phakomatoces: Part II Von Hippel–Lindau disease, Sturge-Weber syndrome, and less common conditions. Neuroimaging clinics of North America: *Pediat Neuroradiol* 1994; **4**:325–48.
24. Choyke PL, Glenn GM, Walther MM, Patronas NJ, Linehan WM, Zbar B. Von Hippel–Lindau disease: genetic, clinical and imaging features. *Radiology* 1995; **194**:629–42.
25. Marti-Bonmati L, Menor F, Poyatos C, Cortina H. Diagnosis of Sturge–Weber syndrome: comparison of the efficacy of CT and MR imaging in 14 cases. *Am J Radiol* 1992; **158**:867–71.
26. Barkovich AJ, Chuang SH, Norman D. MR of neuronal migration anomalies. *Am J Neuroradiol* 1987; **8**:1009–17.
27. Barkovich AJ. Congenital malformations of the brain and skull. In: *Pediatric Neuroimaging* 2nd edn, pp. 177–275. New York: Raven Press, 1995.
28. Barkovich AJ, Kjos BO. Gray matter heterotopias: MR characteristics and correlation with development and neurologic manifestations. *Radiology* 1992; **182**:493–9.
29. Barkovich AJ, Kjos BO. Nonlissencephalic cortical dysplasias: correlation of imaging findings with clinical deficits. *Am J Neuroradiol* 1992; **13**:95–103.
30. Barkovich AJ, Kjos BO. Schizencephaly: correlation of clinical findings with MR characteristics. *Am J Neuroradiol* 1992; **13**:85–94.

31 Dietrich RB, Bradley WG, Zaragoza EJ, Otto RJ, Taira RK *et al*. MR Evaluation of early myelination patterns in normal and developmentally delayed infants. *Am J Neuroradiol* 1988; **9**:69–76.
32 Barkovich AJ, Kjos BO, Jackson DE, Normal D. Normal maturation of the neonatal and infant brain: MR imaging at 1.5T1. *Radiology* 1988; **166**:173–80.

FURTHER READING

1 Barkovich AJ. *Pediatric Neuroimaging* 2nd edn. New York: Raven Press 1995.
2 Castillo, M, Mukherji, SK. *Imaging of the Pediatric Head, Neck and Spine.* Philadelphia, New York: Lippencott–Raven Publishers, 1996.

2

Trauma

DONALD M HADLEY, EVELYN M TEASDALE

Introduction	73	Primary injury	77
Classification of injuries	73	Secondary consequences	90
The role of plain films	74	Late sequelae	94
Brain injury	76	Conclusion	96
Indications for CT	76	References	96
MRI in head injury	77	Further reading	97
SPECT in head injury	77		

INTRODUCTION

Cerebral trauma represents a major and frequently underrated cause of death and disability especially in young and otherwise healthy people. Two-thirds of serious head injuries are sustained by men usually in their second or third decade. Although road engineering, vehicle design, seat belt, alcohol and crash helmet safety legislation has helped to reduce hospital admissions, road traffic accidents still cause the largest proportion of serious head injuries. Falls, assaults and sports injuries are, however, increasing and now result in a substantial workload for emergency and neurosurgical departments.[1,2]

So far preventative measures have had only limited success and these patients still require urgent and continuing efficient evaluation at the site of the accident, during transport to the emergency department and when admitted to the hospital ward. Improving an individual's clinical outcome depends on accurately defining the extent of the initial trauma, developing a better understanding of the pathophysiology of the different types of injury and with that knowledge instituting more focused and effective means of treatment, support and rehabilitation. Neuroimaging plays a crucial role in the triage of these patients when admitted and in their continuing care and assessment following therapeutic interventions.

The development of X-ray computed tomography (CT) in the early 1970s showed directly for the first time the extent and complexity of lesions resulting from head injuries (see Figs 2.7, 2.10, 2.13, 2.18, 2.30) and has largely replaced plain radiographs (in all but the triage of minor injuries) and more invasive imaging. The increasing availability of high resolution rapid acquisition CT scanners ensures their place as the first line investigation. Magnetic resonance imaging (MRI) is more sensitive to the presence of minute amounts of oedema and blood degradation products enabling the demonstration of lesions invisible to CT (Figs 2.4, 2.9, 2.11). This makes MRI particularly useful in the subacute and chronic stages once the patient has been stabilized.

Although plain radiography and CT are excellent for demonstrating fractures of the spinal column, MRI is unique in its ability to show lesions of the spinal cord and adjacent soft tissue associated with acute head trauma, especially when the patient is paralysed and ventilated.

Functional imaging with single photon emission computed tomography (SPECT) or positron emission tomography (PET) is currently used in research to assess abnormalities of cerebral perfusion and metabolism which are common with brain injury and are potentially reversible. This provides both a challenge and a measure of the effectiveness of the emerging neuroprotective therapies and pharmacologic manipulations now being developed.

CLASSIFICATION OF INJURIES

By combining clinical and imaging data injuries may be classified into primary lesions, secondary consequences and late sequelae[3] (Table 2.1). Primary lesions are due to

Table 2.1 *Classification of blunt head injury*

Primary injury	Secondary consequences	Late sequelae
Skull fracture	Pneumocephalus	Cerebromalacia
Diffuse axonal injury	Raised intracranial pressure	CSF fistula
Contusions and lacerations	Ischaemic damage	Vascular lesions
Haemorrhage	Vascular injury	Hydrocephalus
intracerebral	Infection	Infection
intraventricular		Cerebral atrophy
subarachnoid		Epilepsy
subdural		Post-concussion syndrome
extradural		

damage occurring at the moment of impact and its immediate complications. They include skull fractures, diffuse axonal injury, contusions, cerebral lacerations and intracranial haemorrhage which may be found in both intra- and extracerebral locations. Secondary consequences occur later, separated in time from the primary impact and include brain swelling, raised intracranial pressure, ischaemic damage and infarction due to brain herniation or vascular injury. Late sequelae include cerebromalacia, cerebral atrophy, hydrocephalus, cerebrospinal fluid (CSF) fistula, infection and vascular lesions. Penetrating injuries, usually caused by a bullet, knife or a bone fragment form a subgroup of primary and secondary injury while child abuse associated with non-accidental injury is an increasingly recognized cause of paediatric primary brain damage.

THE ROLE OF PLAIN FILMS

Assessing the skull

Since nearly all general hospitals have CT scanners the indications for skull radiographs and CT scanning in general hospitals are undergoing reappraisal. This is still an evolving debate and only broad recommendations can be given.

The indications for skull films need to be considered in the context of the criteria for CT scanning. If urgent neurosurgical referral or CT is already deemed necessary on clinical grounds, performing a skull X-ray will only delay appropriate management and give no additional information. The time will be better spent ensuring that there are no other major injuries to the chest, abdomen and pelvis which could cause hypotension, and to stabilize the patient prior to transfer. If this is not the case then immediate skull radiographs should be considered. Unless the Glasgow Coma Score (GCS) is 15, CT or plain skull films are mandatory. In those patients with a minor head injury (GCS of 15) skull films may be performed to identify those in whom a fracture is present. As these patients have a 1:35 risk of a surgically significant intracranial lesion they can be placed under observation and scanned electively within the following 4 hours.[4,5]

Teleradiology with image transfer to specialists for diagnosis and management advice is increasingly available and its use has been shown to improve patient care.[6,7] All general hospitals should have this facility to maximize the benefit from local CT and MRI.

Patients without a fracture who have a normal conscious level and who do not have post-traumatic amnesia are at minimal risk of a significant cerebral injury (1:31 300).

In remote communities other factors must be taken into account when considering the usefulness of skull films as a triage tool. Where CT is not available the finding of a skull fracture (carrying an increased risk) may influence the decision to evacuate a patient. However, if a helicopter or a plane is needed even to obtain skull

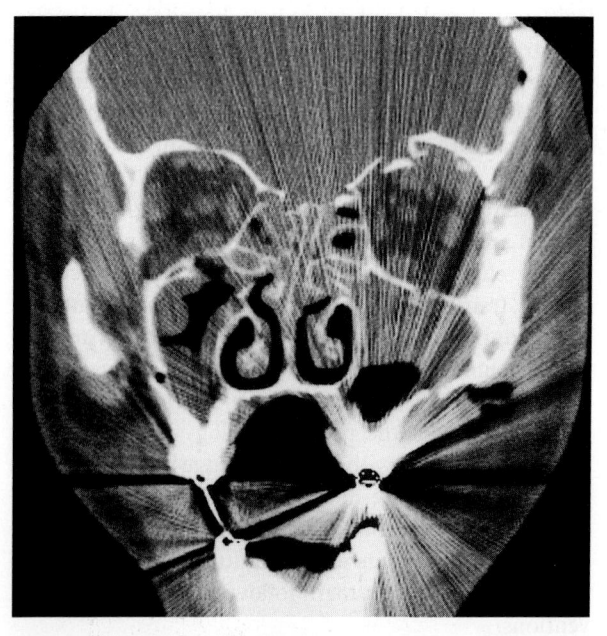

Figure 2.1 *Direct coronal CT of the orbits and facial bones showing complex fractures of the orbital walls and ethmoids with superior intraorbital haemorrhage and inferior tagging. They are clearly seen despite streak artefacts from dental fillings.*

Assessing the facial skeleton

Plain films and ideally direct coronal CT are used to assess complex facial fractures (Fig. 2.1). These can be delayed for up to 48 hours or carried out when corrective surgery is imminent.[8] By this time the patient will have been stabilized and will be fit enough to co-operate with the positioning for direct coronal CT. Three-dimensional (3-D) surface reconstruction of a stack of CT sections gives the surgeon an interactive dynamic interpretation of the image highlighting bony displacements or distortions (Fig. 2.2). Although superficially attractive the algorithms used in the production of 3-D surface rendering can obscure or falsify fracture lines and their value in patient management is therefore limited. However, 3-D protocols can be used to plan detailed reconstructions and make accurate acrylic or metallic prostheses.

Assessing the cervical spine

In the head-injured patient with a severely impaired conscious level it is frequently impossible to exclude a cervical spine injury without radiology[9] (Fig. 2.3).

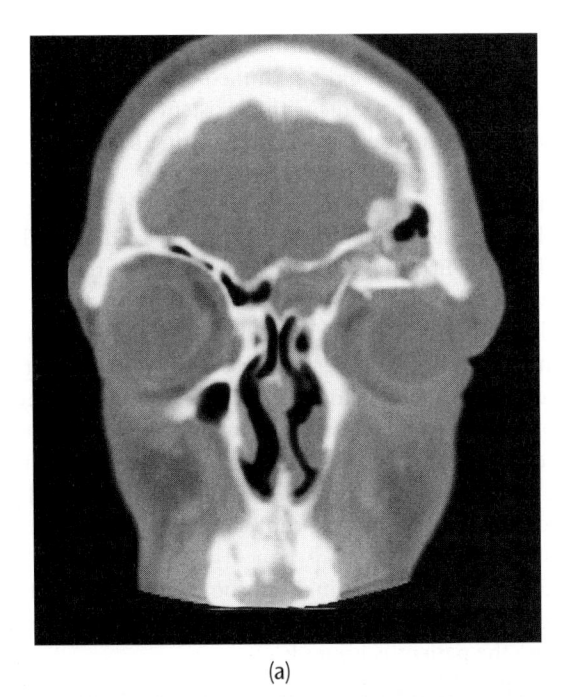

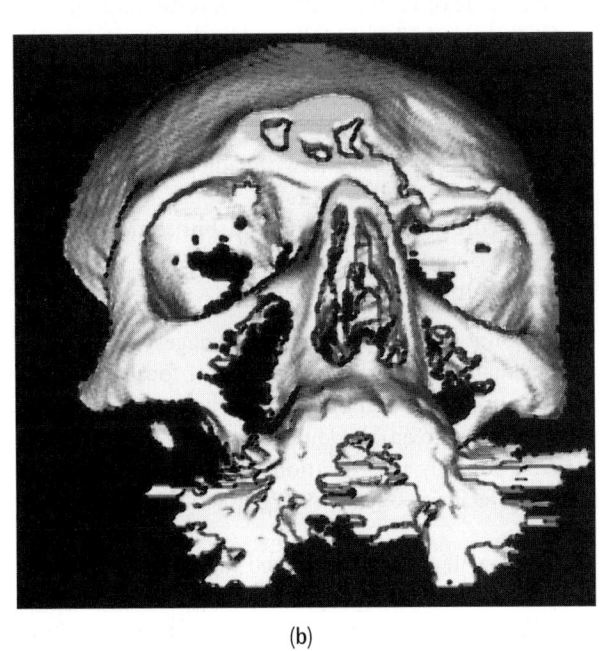

Figure 2.2 *Left facial and frontal fractures with ethmoidal haemorrhage. (a) Direct coronal CT; (b) 3-D CT reconstruction with surface rendering shows the extent of the deformation.*

films then it is more appropriate to arrange transfer to a centre with a CT scanner and neurosurgical facilities.

For demonstrating depressed or comminuted skull fractures, CT is excellent, although those fractures parallel to the plane of section may be missed. If required, skull base fractures including those of the temporal bone can be demonstrated on thin sections (1.5–2.5mm) and should be reconstructed with specific bone algorithms for optimal visualization.

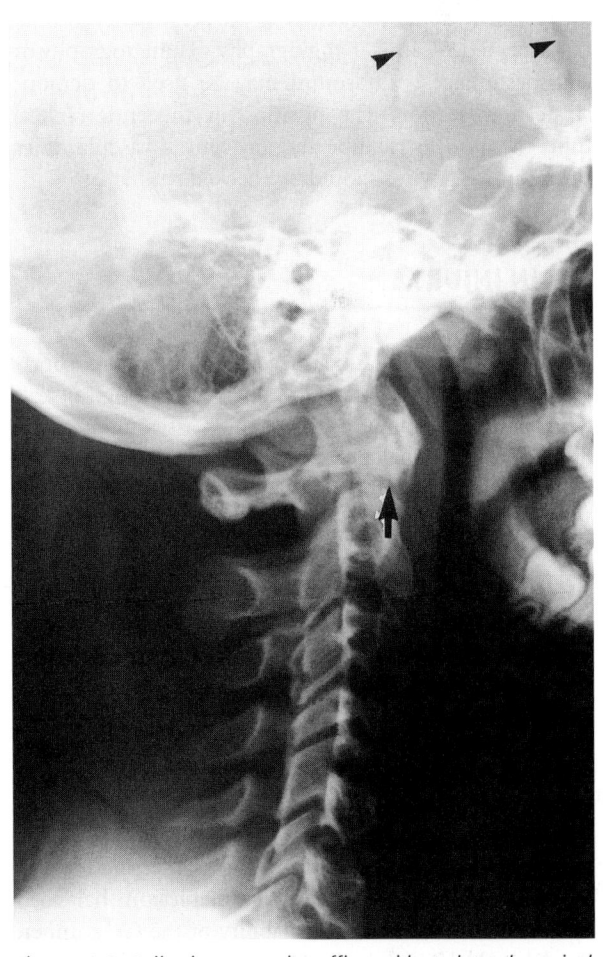

Figure 2.3 *Following a road traffic accident, lateral cervical spine radiograph in the neutral position shows a type II fracture of the odontoid peg (arrow), in addition to frontal fractures (arrowheads).*

Lateral and frontal films which include the craniocervical junction and the first thoracic vertebra must be obtained. As the cervicothoracic region is frequently not satisfactorily imaged on the acute lateral films an anterior oblique anteroposterior (AP) view may suffice. If not, thin section CT from CV6 to TV2 should be carried out axially with midline and oblique parasagittal reformations to show any fractures or subluxation present. This can be done at the same time as the brain CT. Views carefully taken in flexion and extension are sometimes needed to show instability in the assessment of ligamentous injury in the conscious patient without a fracture, but MRI may still be required to demonstrate or exclude soft tissue injury involving the cord, ligaments, paraspinal tissues or potentially treatable acute disc prolapse.

Assessing the chest

A frontal supine chest X-ray should be carried out to exclude a treatable cause of hypoxia. If there is widening of the upper mediastinal shadow, if a small apical pleural effusion is present or if there is a fracture of the posterior aspect of the upper ribs injury to the great vessels should be suspected.[10] Catheter angiography, CT angiography or transoesophageal ultrasound may be used to demonstrate a dissection. The position of the endotracheal tube, the nasogastric tube and any central vascular lines or monitoring wires should be checked.

BRAIN INJURY

For assessing acute brain damage and deciding appropriate therapy CT is the most valuable radiological test, while MRI contributes to the detailed assessment of the damage and is particularly sensitive to diffuse injuries. MRI is most often used in the subacute stage; SPECT and PET have a role in research.

INDICATIONS FOR CT

In the acute stage a CT scan can answer the key clinical question – is there evidence of structural intracranial damage? The decision to obtain a scan requires an assessment of the advantages and disadvantages for the individual patient. This relates to the benefit of confirming or excluding the clinical diagnosis (i.e. the level of risk of finding a *significant* intracranial lesion) balanced by the ease of access and availability of the CT scanner, the delay, the hazards and costs of transfer to the scanner and the potential risk of the general anaesthetic sometimes needed to obtain clinically useful images of the head. Patients who have a bleeding diathesis or are taking anticoagulants have an increased risk of intracranial haematoma and should be scanned. Scanning is reasonable if a patient presents with persistent headache unresponsive to simple analgesia, or vomiting following even a minor head injury without a fracture.

There are several groups in the UK who have addressed this problem and have issued guidance. They include the British Society of Neurological Surgeons, the Royal College of Surgeons, London and the Royal College of Radiologists.[5] Rationalizing these ideas in conjunction with recent research the Scottish Intercollegiate Guideline Network (SIGN) development group took the view that CT scanning would be justifiable as the primary investigation when the risk of finding an abnormality on CT was at least 10% and of finding a surgically significant abnormality was at least 1%.[11]

Emergency CT examinations should be carried out on any patient with the following features, irrespective of where the patient is injured:

- GCS score of 12 or less after initial resuscitation;
- GCS score of 13 or 14 followed by deterioration or by failure to improve during the course of a period of clinical observation, irrespective of the presence or absence of a skull fracture;
- GCS score of 13, 14 or 15 with radiological/clinical evidence of a skull fracture;
- GCS score of 15 with no fracture but clinical concern during observation;
- focal neurological signs.

When the initial clinical features suggest an intracranial haematoma (e.g. the emergence of focal signs, or a fall in conscious level not explained by extracranial factors such as hypoxia), it would be sensible to transfer the patient promptly to a location which not only has CT scanning facilities but an emergency neurosurgical service.

Patients will usually be scanned supine but if restless a lateral decubitus position may settle them long enough to enable a diagnostic scan to be carried out without sedation or anaesthetic. Intermittent incremental 1 second exposures timed to the patient's movements offer better quality than spiral acquisitions from a moving subject.[12] The scan should extend from the foramen magnum to the vertex and be angled parallel to the line between the floor of the frontal fossa and the foramen magnum to avoid irradiating the lens of the eye.[13] A compromise has to be made between slice thickness, the signal-to-noise ratio and contrast resolution. Contiguous 10mm sections may exclude a neurosurgically significant haematoma but will not allow an assessment of the true extent of the brain damage which requires the identification of the type of injury present and any secondary complications. In the posterior fossa the slice thickness should not exceed 5mm in order to minimize partial volume averaging which can obscure small but potentially significant haematomas and contusions. Soft tissue, intermediate and bone window images can be obtained from the same data set and 3-D reconstructions should be possible although they are rarely needed.

MRI IN HEAD INJURY

Now that MRI-compatible cardiorespiratory monitoring and support equipment are available, critically ill patients can be imaged safely at any stage after a head injury.[14,15] However, if the patient is not unconscious or paralysed and ventilated, a much higher degree of co-operation is required than for CT. These patients may have sustained multiple injuries and careful screening is required to exclude ferrometallic foreign bodies or electronic implants.

With appropriate choice of sequence the contrast between normal and pathological tissues can be many times that of CT. Routinely, a long TR (repetition time) spin echo dual echo set of axial sections provide T2-weighted and proton density weighted contrast while a further set of short TR spin echo or inversion recovery sections demonstrate T1-weighted contrast differences. Gradient echo T2*-weighted sequences highlight changes in magnetic susceptibility making them very sensitive to acute and chronic haemorrhage[16] (Fig. 2.4).

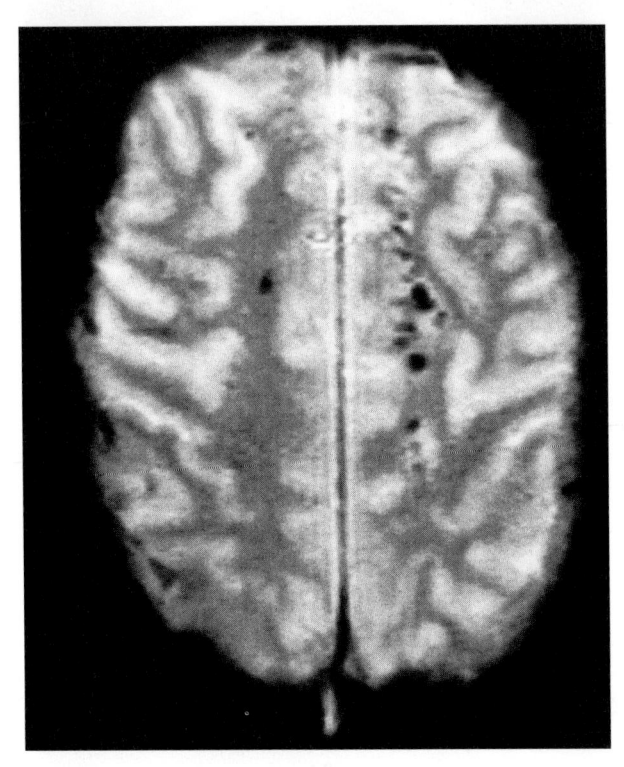

Figure 2.4 *A 26-year-old passenger thrown from a car. Gliding contusions only shown on T2* gradient echo sections. The hypointense susceptibility effects of the petechial haemorrhage are highlighted by this sequence.*

Fast or Turbo spin echo sequences have been developed which are three to four times faster than conventional spin echoes and are now in routine use. The increased speed of acquisition can be used to carry out a quicker study in children or severely injured patients. Alternatively a larger number of acquisitions can be obtained in the same time as a conventional scan to improve anatomical detail. Unfortunately because of its multiple 180° pulses this sequence is less sensitive to the magnetic susceptibility effects of acute and chronic haemorrhage[16,17] but give the advantage of better imaging close to air–bone–brain interfaces.

Gradient echo sequences produce the highest sensitivity to acute and chronic haemorrhage but are degraded by artefact around the skull base and frontal sinuses. Fluid attenuated inversion recovery (FLAIR) sections are most useful to show contusions at brain-CSF borders where the usual hyperintensity of CSF obscures small cortical lesions.[18]

Ultrafast echo planar imaging with cerebral diffusion, perfusion and functional sequences will soon compete with the lower resolution data from SPECT and PET.[19] Magnetic resonance spectroscopy is possible now but so far it is only used as a research tool with no direct effects on patient management.[15,20]

SPECT IN HEAD INJURY

In the routine clinical setting SPECT scanning with agents such as ^{99m}Tc hexamethyl propylene amine oxime (^{99m}Tc-HMPAO) is used to map regional cerebral blood flow (rCBF). After intravenous injection of ^{99m}Tc-HMPAO, its delivery to the brain is proportional to rCBF. As it is lipophilic it crosses the blood–brain barrier where it is rapidly converted into a hydrophilic compound and is trapped for several hours. This distribution is mapped using either rotating gamma cameras or dedicated head imagers (Fig. 2.5). These cerebral perfusion maps have improved our understanding of the long-term link between cerebral blood flow and brain function. Clinically this can provide objective correlates for the behavioural and psychometric abnormalities found following head injury especially in individuals who have normal results on structural imaging.[21]

PRIMARY INJURY

This is the damage which occurs at the moment of impact and its immediate complications.

Diffuse axonal injury

Diffuse axonal injury is a pathological diagnosis and

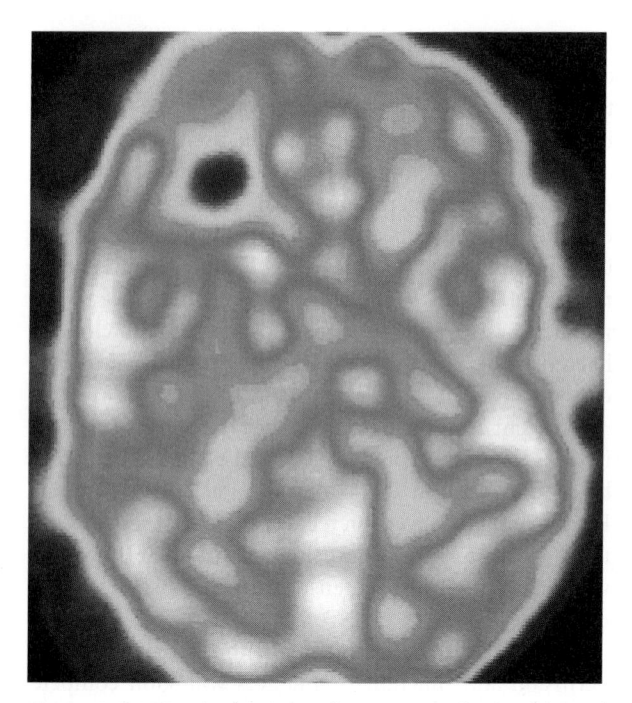

Figure 2.5 SPECT in the early subacute stage of a head-injured 35-year-old man shows hypoperfusion adjacent to a right frontal contusion but also shows unexpected hypoperfusion of the left frontal lobe where there was no evidence of injury on CT. This illustration appears as Plate 1 in the colour plate section.

what is seen radiologically is the vascular injury and oedema associated with the shearing forces that disrupt axons and capillaries. These shearing forces in the brain are caused by the differential acceleration and deceleration of the grey/white matter, and blood vessels with the brain at the moment of injury. There are varying degrees of white matter tract disruption usually with involvement of adjacent capillaries as well as axons. It has recently been shown that these lesions may not be complete immediately and so a treatment may be developed to limit the extent of damage. This makes the recognition of the associated acute radiological pattern of diffuse axonal injury crucial although sometimes the damage may only inferred by finding diffuse atrophy at follow-up CT or MRI (Fig. 2.6).

Axonal damage occurs in a 'top down' pattern. With a mild concussive injury small lesions with increased water content are seen paramedially at the junction of the cortical grey/white matter on MRI (Fig. 2.4) while on CT these lesions are rarely visible.[22,23] They represent the 'gliding contusions' described neuropathologically although direct correlation is not available as these lesions are not on their own fatal. With increasing severity other lesions become apparent in the corpus callosum and extend downward into the rostral brain stem. MRI is very sensitive to these lesions especially when using

(a)

(b)

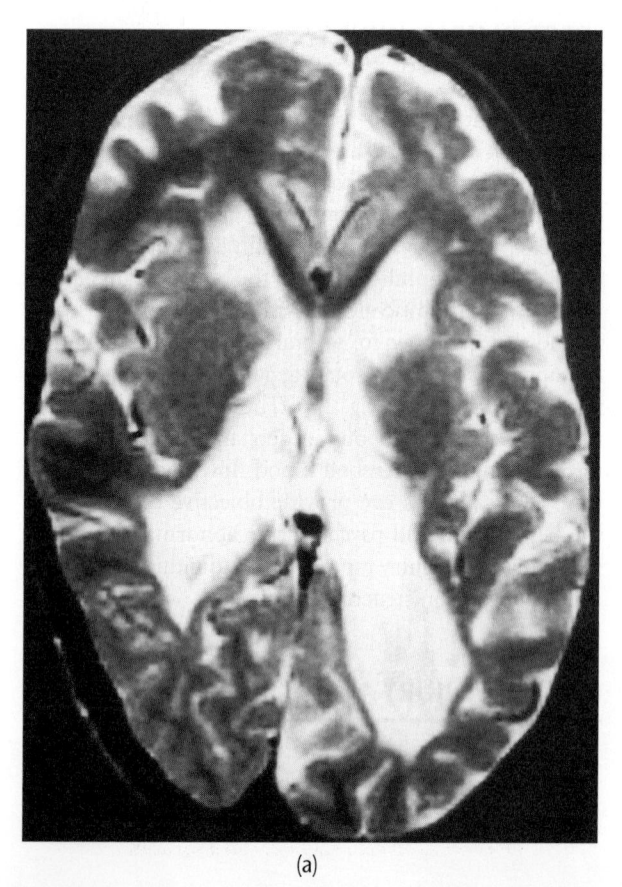

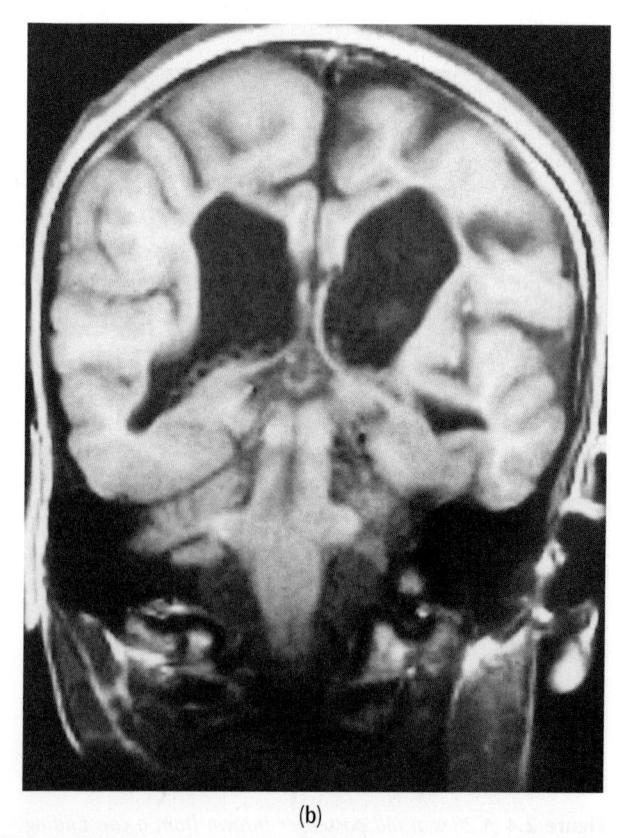

Figure 2.6 Diffuse atrophy at follow-up may be the only sign of diffuse axonal injury. (a) T2-weighted axial; (b) T1-weighted coronal sections showing irregular diffuse atrophy with loss of white matter and ex-vacuo enlargement of the ventricles and sulci on follow-up at 3 months in an 11-year-old passenger involved in a road traffic accident.

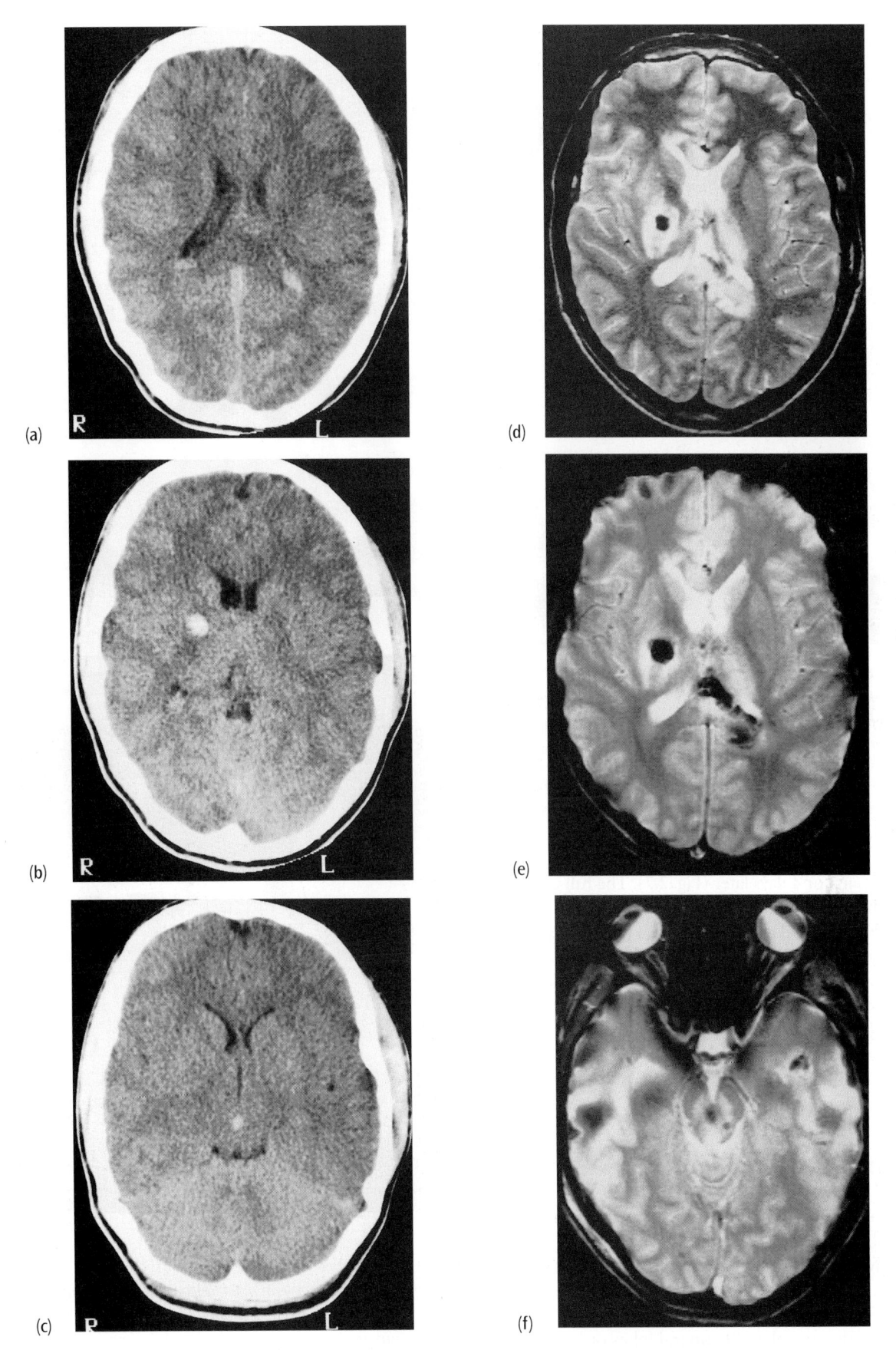

Figure 2.7 CT and MRI consistent with diffuse axonal injury in the 23-year-old driver of a crashed stolen car. (a, b, c) CT shows apparently non-haemorrhagic corpus callosum contusion, right basal ganglial haematoma and brainstem haemorrhage while similar (d) T2-weighted and (e), (f) T2*-weighted axial sections show the full extent of the hypointense acute haemorrhage and surrounding hyperintense oedema.

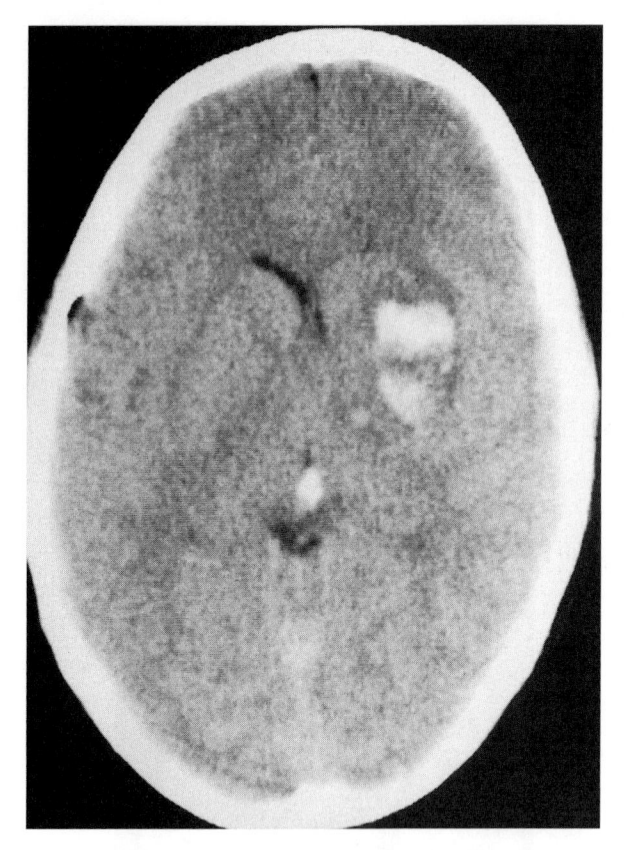

Figure 2.8 *CT with left putaminal and posterior internal capsular marginal haemorrhage, typically associated with diffuse axonal injury.*

gradient echo sequences (Fig. 2.7) even in the absence of macroscopic associated haemorrhage. This almost always has to be present before they are visualized on early CT although areas of reduced attenuation are frequently seen 3 or 4 days later (Fig. 2.7). The full classical triad of haemorrhage in the brainstem, the corpus callosum and the cortical grey/white matter junction is rarely found on CT or MRI. Intraventricular haemorrhage and small primary haemorrhages in the basal ganglia or at the internal capsular margins are associated shearing injuries (Fig. 2.8) but are not part of the pathological definition of diffuse axonal injury. If it is necessary to document diffuse axonal injury in the subacute or late phase MRI is required (Fig. 2.9).

Contusions and lacerations

Contusions are bruises of the brain formed by coalescing petechial haemorrhages caused by acute cerebral deformation following direct contact with the inner table of the skull. They are the most common of all the traumatic brain lesions and are seen most frequently on the under surfaces of the frontal and temporal lobes or lie deep to fractures. Lacerations are due to tearing of the brain by penetrating sharp objects such as bone spicules, bullets or stabbing. They can also occur in the immature brain

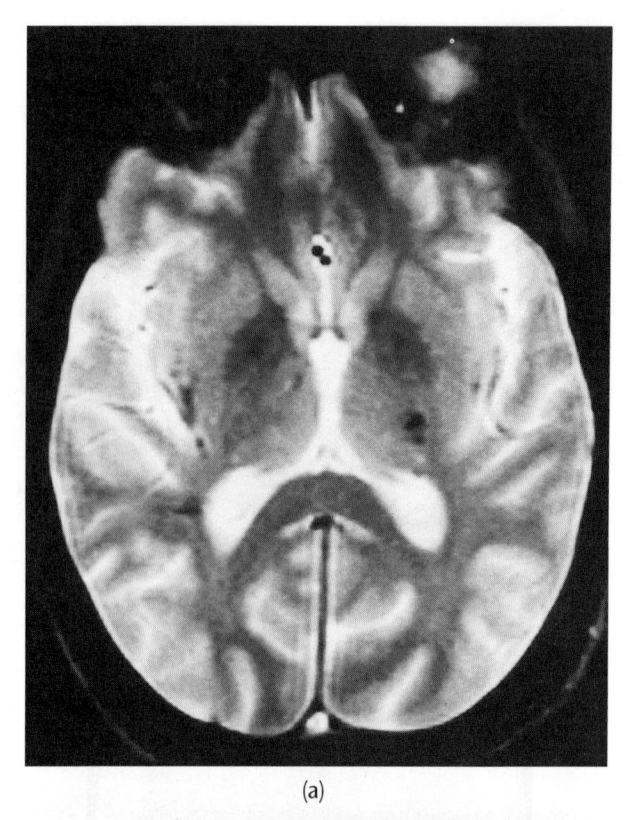

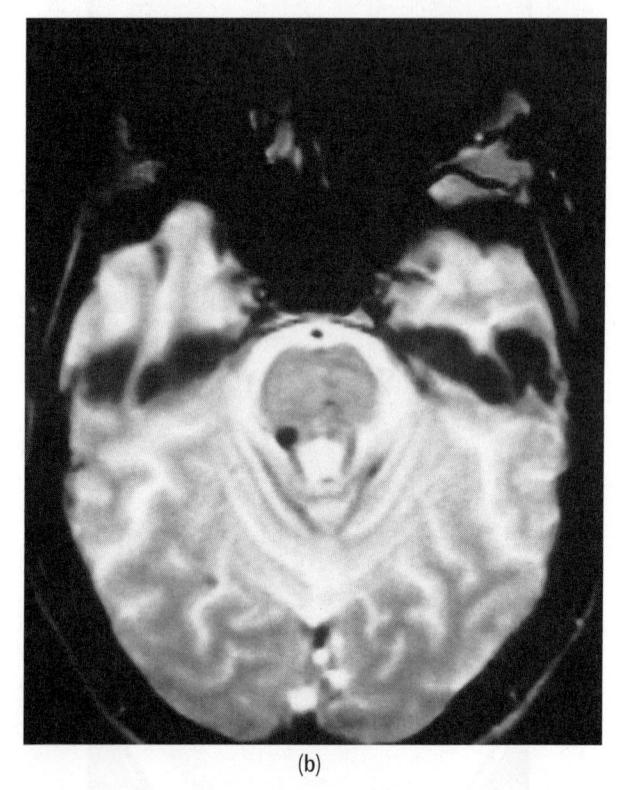

Figure 2.9 *A 26-year-old painter who fell three stories. CT was normal but the patient remained unconscious and ventilated. (a), (b) T2*-weighted axial sections show evidence of diffuse axonal injury in the early chronic stage with haemosiderin in the internal capsule and posterolateral quadrant of the upper brainstem with additional flecks of hypointense mature haemorrhage in the right trigone, occipital lobe and vermis.*

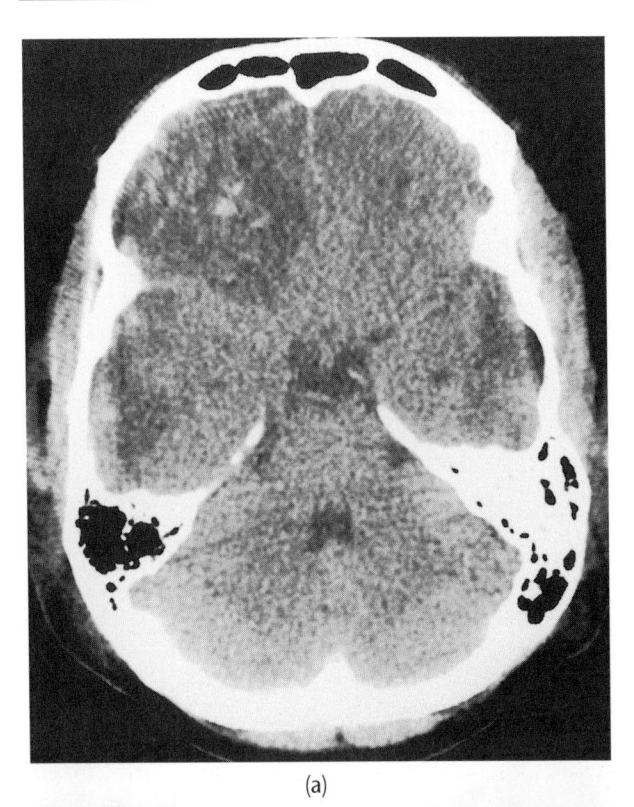

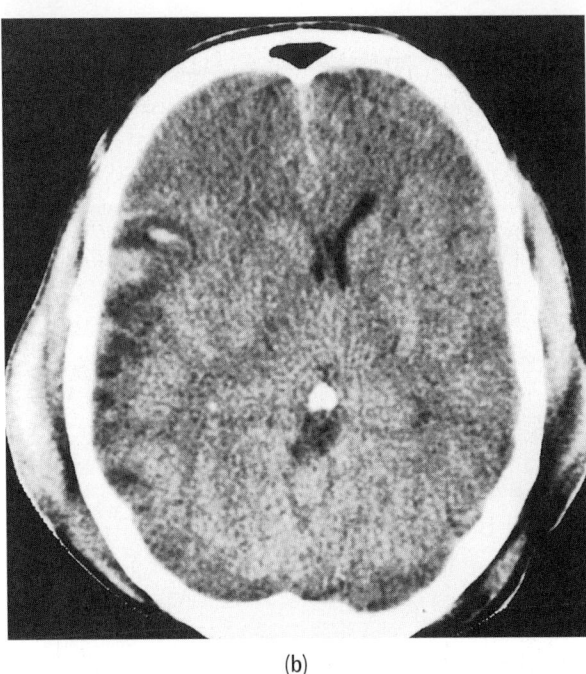

Figure 2.10 *Admission CT shows (a) frontal and (b) temporal contusions with petechial haemorrhage and mass effect causing right lateral ventricular compression, obliteration of the third ventricle and 5mm of right to left midline shift.*

without penetration when associated with non-accidental paediatric injury. Surrounding the contusion or laceration is a variable amount of ischaemic brain which further enlarges the area of swelling. The blood–brain barrier breakdown can be demonstrated in this surrounding ischaemic area in the subacute healing phase

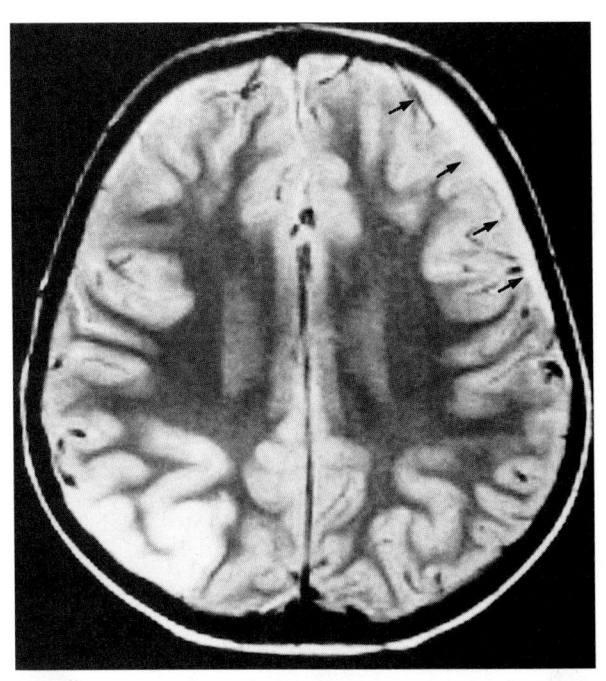

Figure 2.11 *A 33-year-old who fell down stairs. Acute MR: T2-weighted axial section shows a right parietal non-haemorrhagic hyperintense gyral contusion and thin left frontal subdural haemorrhage (arrows); CT was normal.*

by contrast enhancement on CT, MRI[24,25] or radionuclide uptake on SPECT. This adds nothing to the diagnosis and since contrast is potentially neurotoxic it may further damage the brain and should be avoided unless there is a therapeutic issue.

The CT and MRI appearances of contusions are varied (Figs 2.10 to 2.15) but specific and their progression over time is predictable. Haemorrhage is always present pathologically but may be microscopic and undetectable on CT. The most minor contusions will be seen only as an area of dark low attenuation. The amount of blood present varies from a small quantity on the surface to substantial collections extending deeply into the subcortical white matter. The associated oedema may increase over the first 5 to 7 days following the injury and may precipitate a delayed clinical emergency. This is especially so for bifrontal lesions (Fig. 2.15). Contusions are associated with focal neurological deficits but if uncomplicated do not result in alteration in conscious level. Follow-up CT should be performed only if there is clinical decline. Contusions heal with maturation of the haemorrhage and gliosis resulting in shrinkage of a variable volume of white matter and loss of cortex (Fig. 2.33). This is termed cerebromalacia.

Haemorrhage

INTRACEREBRAL HAEMATOMA

Most intracerebral haematomas develop as a complication of a contusion (Fig. 2.15) but some occur because a

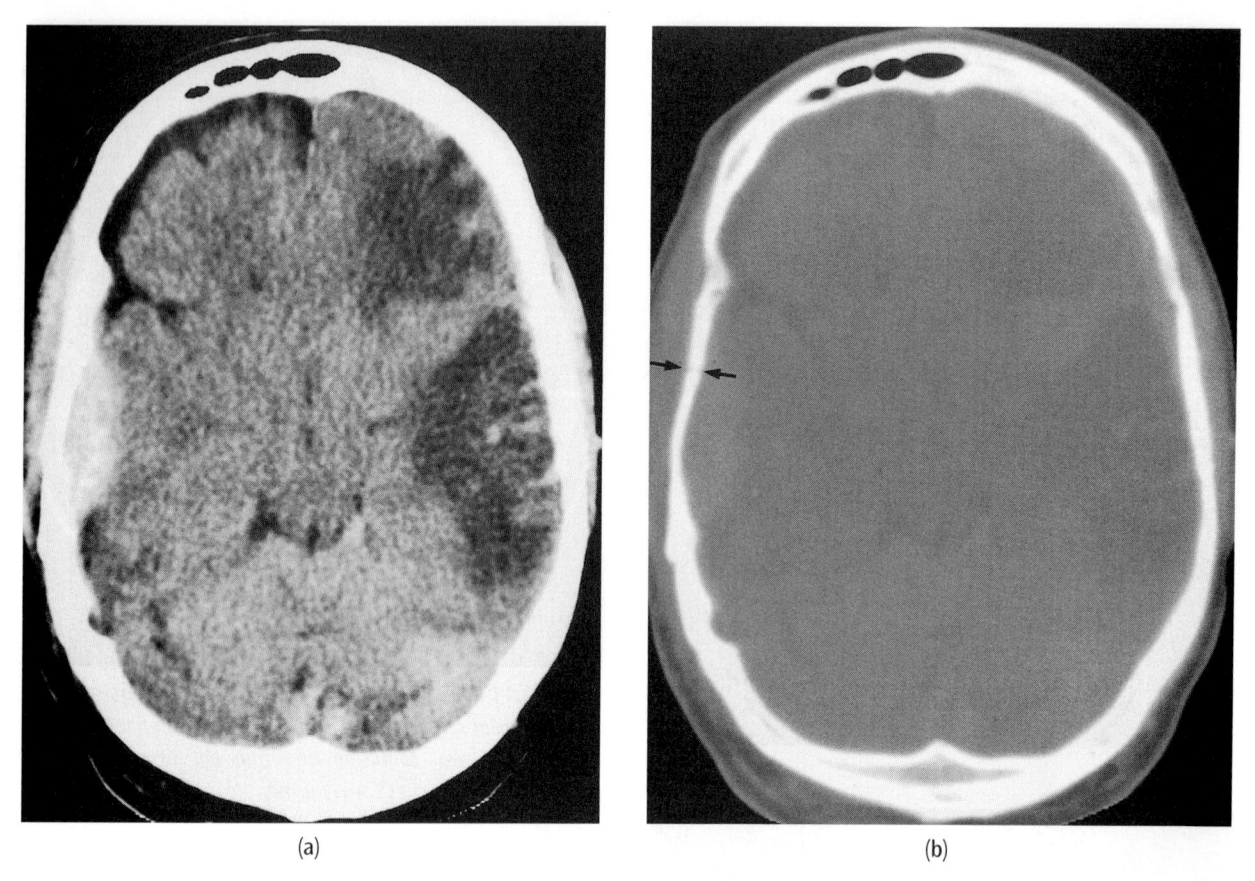

Figure 2.12 CT shows left frontal and temporal contusions with small right extradural haemorrhage (a). Bone windows (b) demonstrate the fracture (arrows) which caused the extradural haemorrhage.

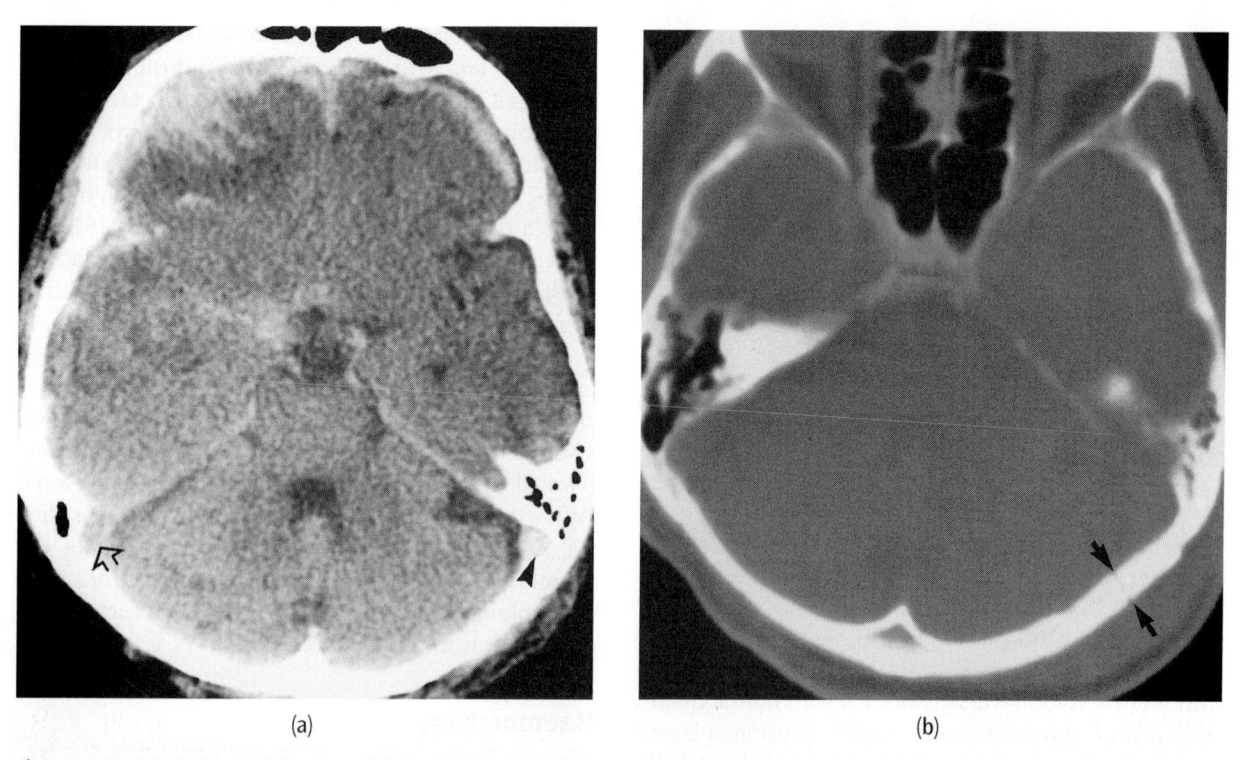

Figure 2.13 Admission CT following a fall from height. (a) Soft tissue; (b) bone windows. A right-sided burst frontal lobe (contusion with adjacent subdural haemorrhage), diffuse right-sided subarachnoid haemorrhage and undisplaced fracture of the left occipital bone at the point of impact (arrows). The fracture has involved the left transverse venous sinus resulting in thrombosis. Compare in (a) the attenuation of the right sinus – low attenuation – open arrow and the left sinus – high attenuation – arrowhead).

Primary injury 83

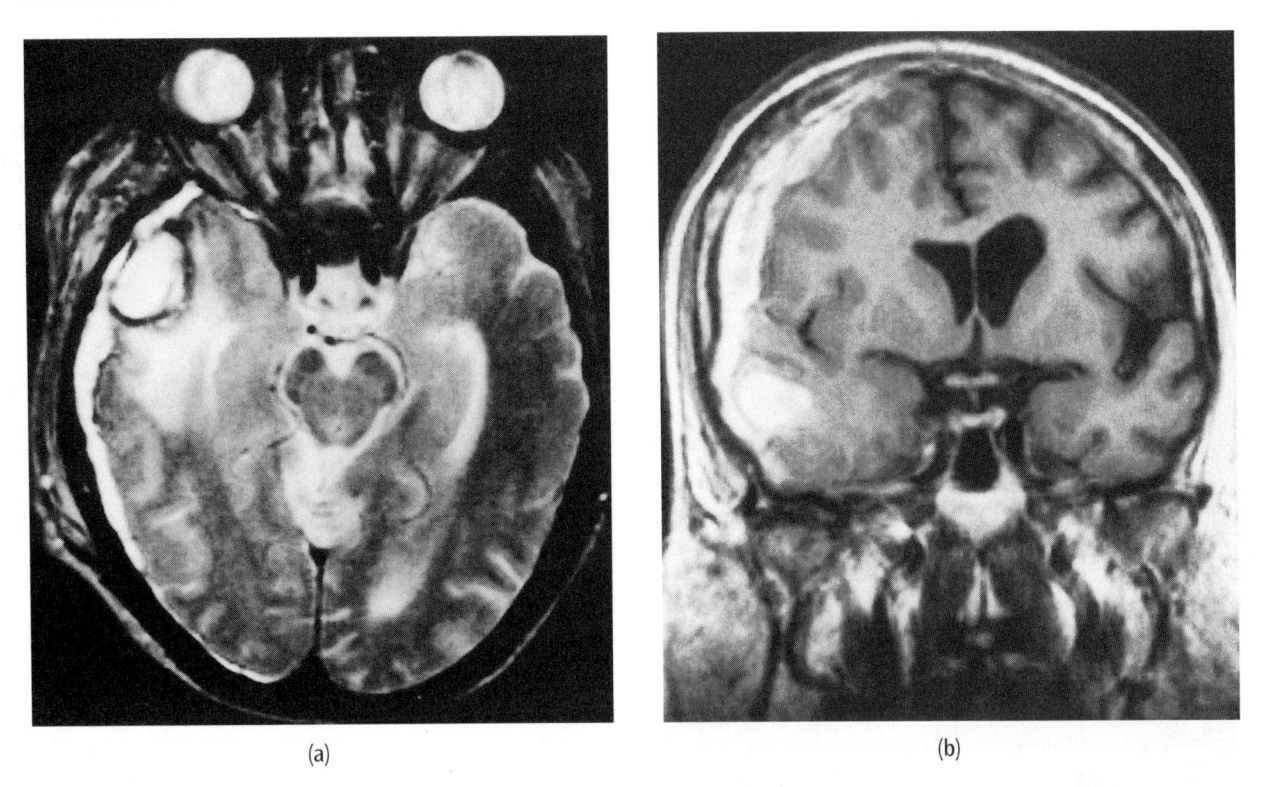

(a) (b)

Figure 2.14 *A 55-year-old following an assault: late subacute temporal haemorrhagic contusion with subdural haemorrhage. (a) T2-weighted axial and (b) T1-weighted coronal sections show mass effect with sulcal effacement and lateral ventricular compression.*

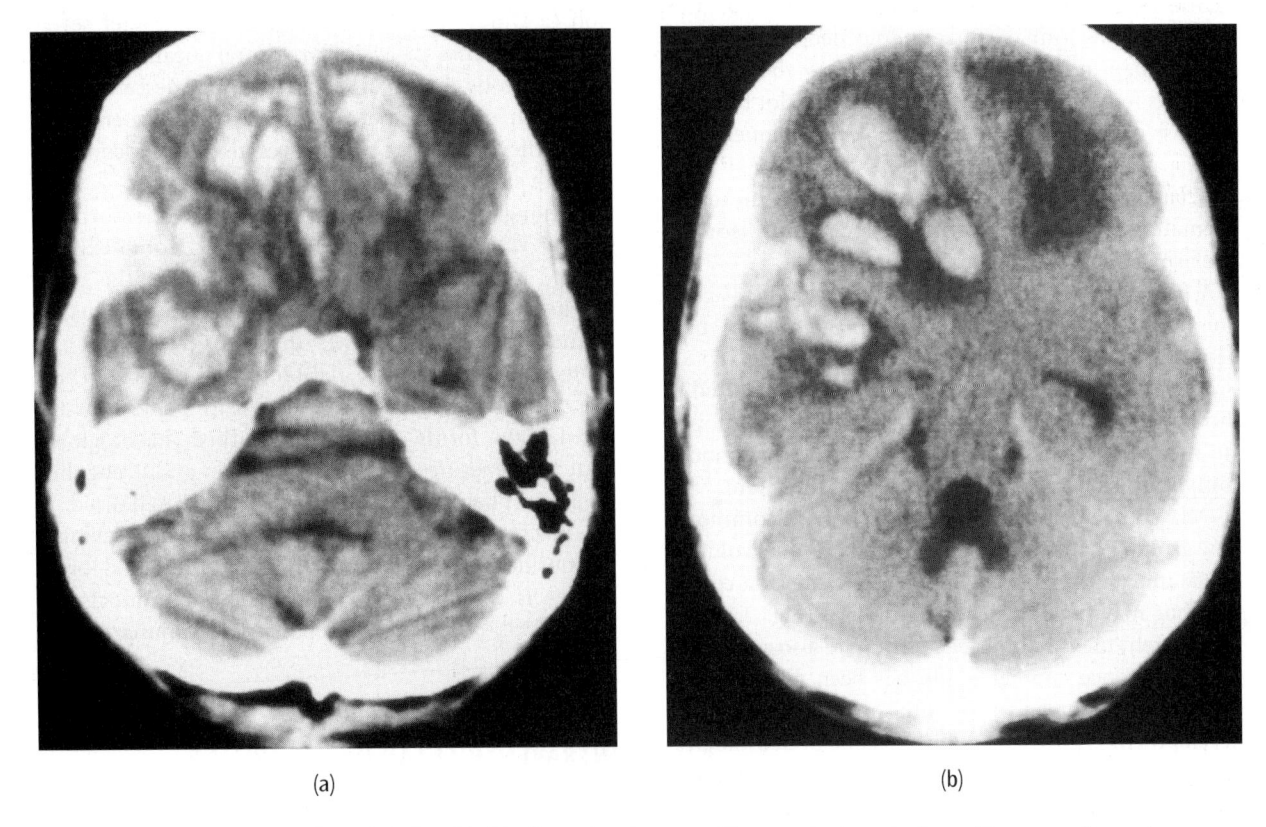

(a) (b)

Figure 2.15 *CT 4 days after admission. (a), (b) Bifrontal and temporal haemorrhagic contusions with surrounding oedema.*

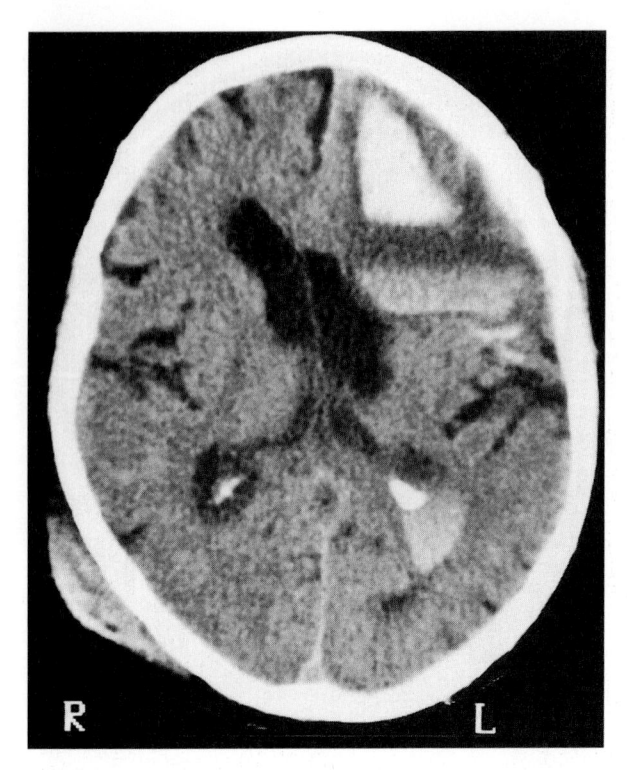

Figure 2.16 *A 50-year-old alcoholic found lying in the street. CT shows fluid levels in a right frontal haemorrhage which has broken into the ventricles.*

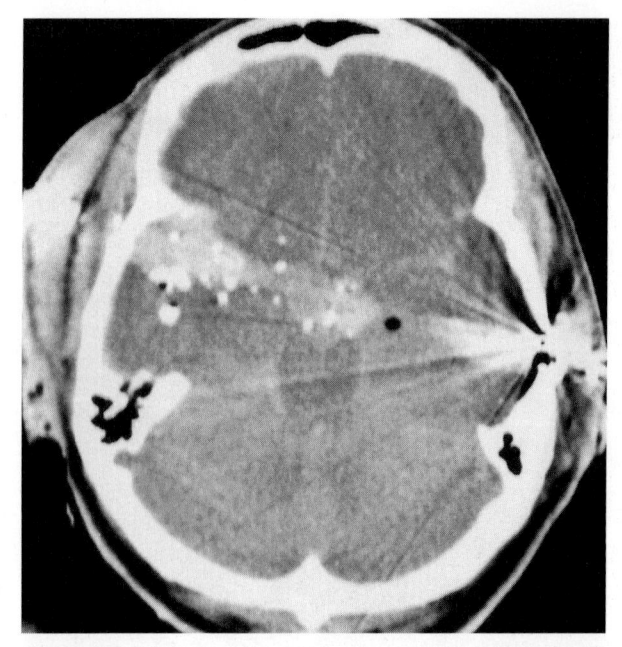

Figure 2.17 *Penetrating gunshot wound shows as linear haemorrhagic lacerations with dense foreign bodies caused by the fragmenting bullet.*

vessel within the brain substance is torn. On CT, acute haemorrhage is seen as an area of increased attenuation with a narrow rim of surrounding oedema which is darker than normal brain. As it ages the oedema increases for approximately 4 days and the clot becomes isodense with the brain over several weeks. Liquefaction is indicated if a fluid level develops (Fig. 2.16). This is associated with a worse prognosis and is common in haematomas associated with coagulation disorders (wafarin and alcohol-related trauma).[26]

A penetrating injury should be suspected if a laceration is demonstrated and haemorrhage is seen in a peripheral-to-deep linear orientation or if a foreign body is present (Fig. 2.17). Urgent angiography is required to show any associated vascular injury and allow appropriate therapy to avoid further haemorrhage or embolic complications from a dissection or false aneurysm.[27]

Delayed haematomas are being seen more commonly now as more patients are scanned early in the evolution of the injury. They usually occur at the site of a contusion but may develop in the extradural (Fig. 2.18) or, more rarely, the subdural space. They are also seen more frequently once another lesion has been resected (e.g. subdural haemorrhage) or after resuscitation. Their development is associated with a decline in neurological status.[28] Very early CT scanning within 2 hours of injury may therefore give a false sense of security and patients seen with small lesions should not be discharged.[29]

Brainstem haematomas are found in three circumstances: lying in the rostral brainstem lateral or anterolateral to the fourth ventricle when associated with diffuse axonal injury (Figs 2.7, 2.9), centrally in the pons and mesencephalon when secondary to tentorial herniation (a Duret haematoma) (Fig. 2.19) and after severe primary trauma in a similar central location. This is thought to be due to an acute transient descent of the brainstem at the time of the impact stretching and rupturing the perforating pontine vessels and is incompatible with survival.

Although MRI is more sensitive to haemorrhage than CT, the appearances are more complex and depend on multiple factors. These include the paramagnetic form of haemoglobin present, clot matrix formation, changes in erythrocyte hydration and changes in the degree of red blood cell packing. There is a characteristic sequence of intensity patterns as the haematoma forms, serum is absorbed, haemoglobin matures, denatures to methaemoglobin and is engulfed by macrophages. Methaemoglobin is metabolized in the macrophages which then die eventually leaving a haemosiderin-lined cleft. By this time the blood–brain barrier is intact and these degradation products are trapped.[14,30,31] This evolving pattern is summarized in Table 2.2.

INTRAVENTRICULAR HAEMORRHAGE

Even in severe head injury intraventricular haemorrhage is unusual (3%) most commonly occurring

Figure 2.18 *Delayed extradural haemorrhage in a 14-year-old boy hit by a golf club. (a) On admission CT there is a tiny temporal extradural haemorrhage; (b) following clinical deterioration at 6 hours CT shows the enlarged extradural haemorrhage; (c) on bone windows temporal fracture seen (arrow).*

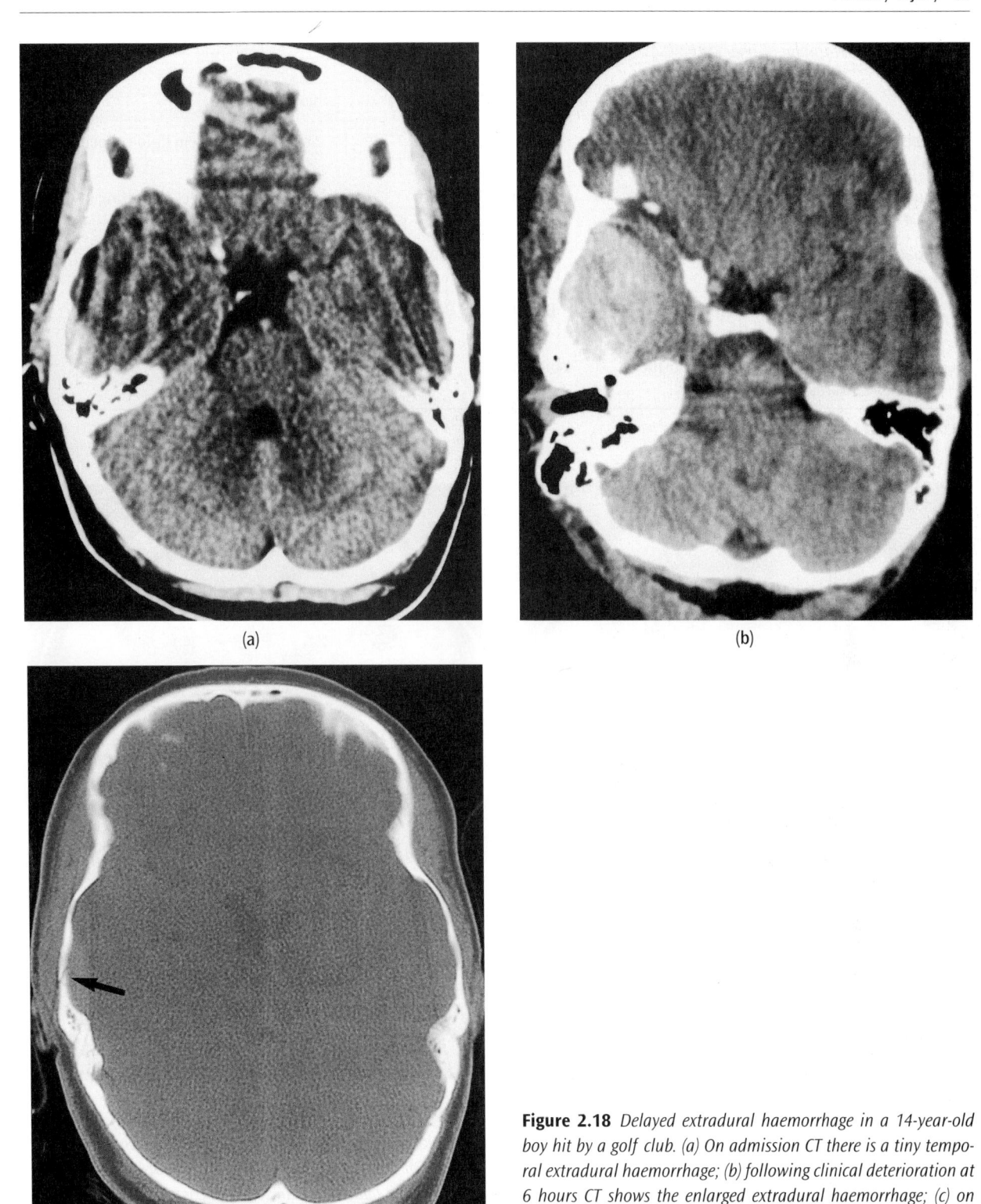

when an intracerebral haemorrhagic contusion or haematoma breaks into the ventricle. In this situation it indicates a poorer prognosis especially if there is a large amount of clot.[32] Intraventricular haemorrhage is commonly associated with a callosal tear and so, in the correct clinical setting, intraventricular haemorrhage can act as one of the markers for diffuse axonal injury.[33] In elderly patients intraventricular haemorrhage can sometimes occur as an isolated finding where it is likely to be due to rupture of a subependymal vein. In this situation it has little prognostic value except that it increases the likelihood of secondary hydrocephalus which is commoner in patients with intraventricular haemorrhage from any cause.

Table 2.2 *The maturation of haemorrhage on MRI*

Stage	Biochemistry	T1	T2	Comments
1. Hyperacute up to 2–3h	Oxyhaemoglobin	Dark	Bright	Simple high protein fluid collection
2. Acute 3h–4 days	Deoxyhaemoglobin	Isointense	Dark	Susceptibility effect of clotting RBCs
3. Subacute: early 4–7 days	Methaemoglobin	Bright	Dark	Intact RBCs in clot
4. Subacute: late 6 days–8 weeks	Methaemoglobin	Bright	Bright	RBC lysis, loss of susceptibility effect
5. Chronic 8 weeks–onwards	Ferritin/haemosiderin	Isointense	Dark	Marked susceptibility

RBC: Red blood corpuscle

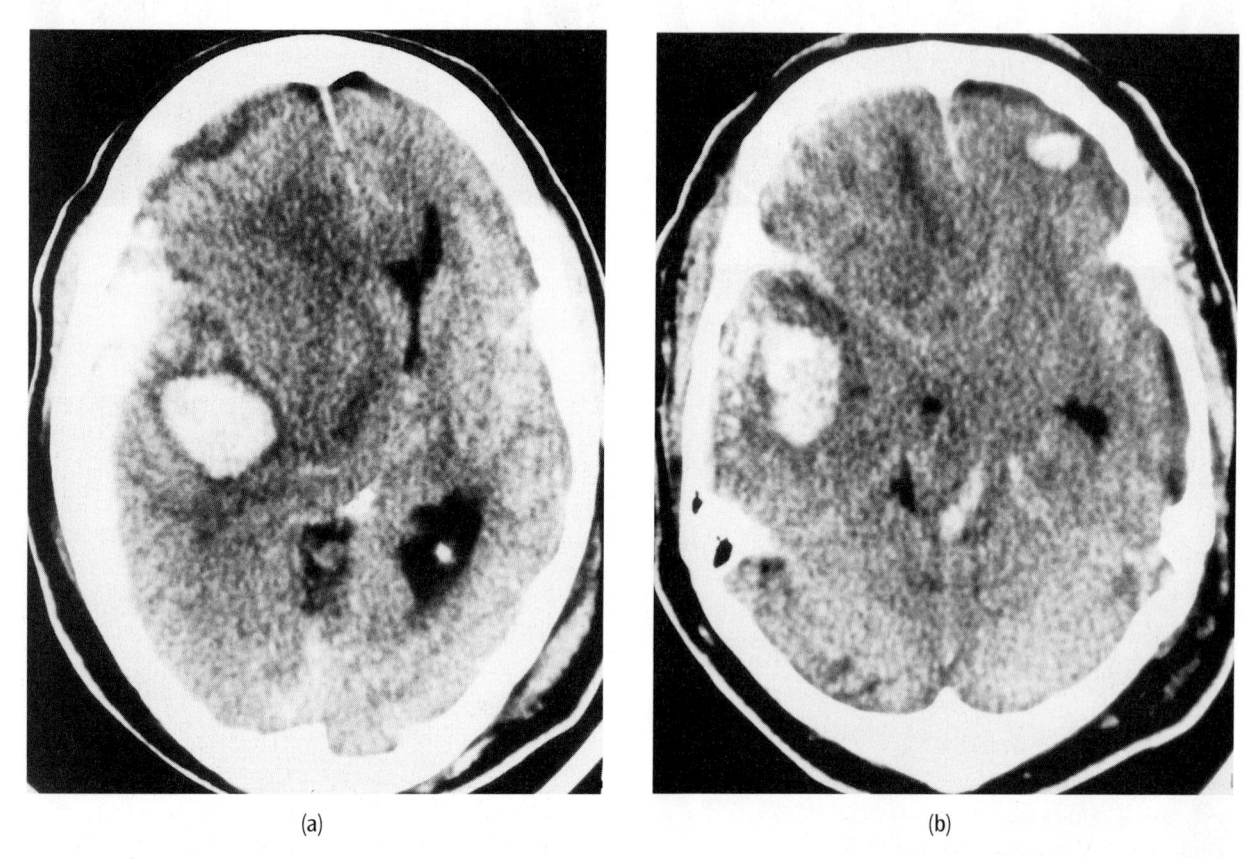

(a) (b)

Figure 2.19 *This patient fell down stairs drunk. Glasgow Coma Score was 3 with fixed and dilated pupils. CT on admission (a) subdural haemorrhage, haemorrhagic temporal contusion and massive shift associated with severe compression of the ipsilateral ventricle, dilatation of the contralateral trigone and rotation of the midbrain and upper brainstem indicating transtentorial coning. This has resulted in a (b) brainstem haematoma and herniation of the medial temporal lobe.*

SUBARACHNOID HAEMORRHAGE

Up to a third of severely head-injured patients have associated subarachnoid haemorrhage. It is clearly shown by good quality CT in the first 24 hours following trauma. If it is extensive it correlates with a poorer state on admission.[34,35] It may co-exist with any type of traumatic lesion but usually found isolated in the basal cisterns after a skull base fracture while subarachnoid haemorrhage over the hemispheres may be related to a vault fracture, local haemorrhage or cerebral contusion (Fig. 2.20). Subarachnoid haemorrhage occurs without overt evidence of an increase in ischaemic events and so does not seem to cause marked vasospasm. Occasionally

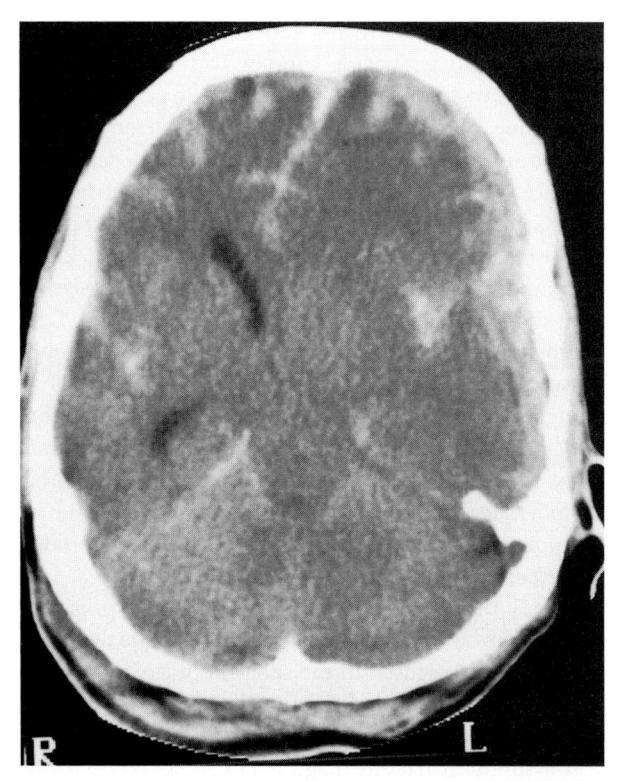

Figure 2.20 *A 58-year-old, who fell from a crane, had a subdural haemorrhage with extensive subarachnoid haemorrhage and severe compression of the left lateral ventricle resulting in transtentorial coning.*

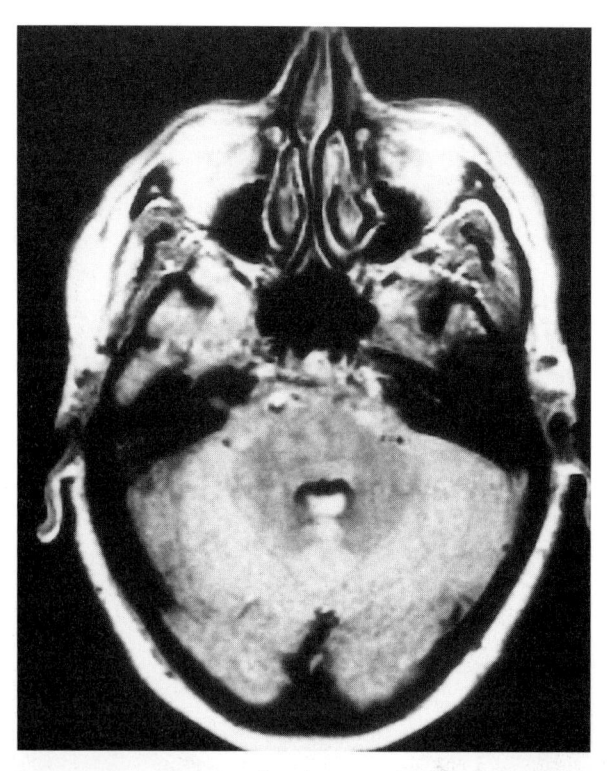

Figure 2.21 *FLAIR MR section shows acute subarachnoid haemorrhage in the prepontine cistern and fourth ventricle where the normally hypointense cerebrospinal fluid has become hyperintense due to its increased protein content.*

angiography may be required to exclude aneurysm rupture if the history is not clear.

Subarachnoid haemorrhage can only be shown by MRI in the acute stage if additional sequences such as FLAIR are used[36,37] (Fig. 2.21). If there is sufficient clot left in the subarachnoid space it will be seen as hyperintense on T1WI. As the haemorrhage associated with trauma is not usually extensive or recurrent, the haemosiderin laden macrophages from maturing clot are washed away and the build-up of superficial or ependymal siderosis giving its hypointense pencilled outline on T2WI is rare, only being occasionally seen with the recurrent trauma associated with alcoholics or epileptics.

SUBDURAL HAEMORRHAGE

These collections lie in the potential space between the arachnoid membrane and the inner meningeal layer of the dura most significantly over the convexity of the brain but they are also common along the falx and the tentorium. They are usually caused by tearing of the relatively unsupported veins which cross the subdural space but can also form directly from adjacent severe contusions and subarachnoid lacerations. When severe contusions are associated with an adjacent subdural haemorrhage the lesion is termed a 'burst lobe' (Figs 2.13, 2.14).

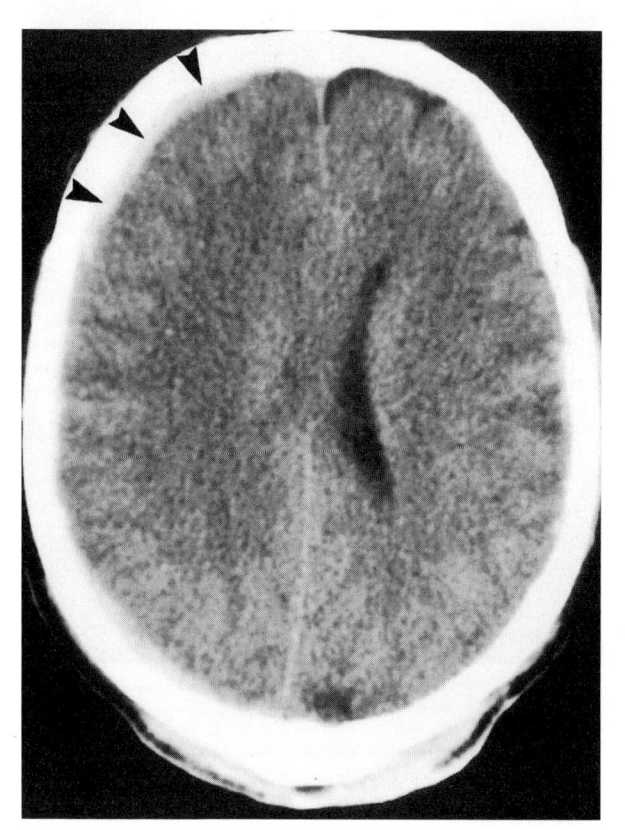

Figure 2.22 *CT showing effacement of the right frontal sulci (cf left) raising suspicions of a thin subdural haemorrhage (arrowheads).*

It is important to review any CT examination in a trauma patient with wide window widths and specific bone window images to distinguish hyperdense clot from bone. Occasionally a thin subdural haemorrhage may be suspected only from the compressive pattern it produces on the lateral ventricle (Fig. 2.22). The lack of bone artefact on MRI has shown that small subdural haemorrhages are almost universally present (Fig. 2.11) with moderate to severe contusions but surgically significant subdural haemorrhage will not be missed on CT. In the hyperacute stage subdural haemorrhage may rarely be seen as mixed, iso- or hypodense on CT. This is thought to be due to acute anaemia and haemodilution associated with resuscitation from multiple injuries and a clot which has yet to consolidate (Fig. 2.23). Subdural haemorrhage is limited by the dural reflections and so will not cross the midline but may track along the sides of the falx or on either surface of the tentorium.

SPECT may demonstrate diffuse cortical hypoperfusion deep to subdural haemorrhage. This tissue may well become hyperperfused in the subacute stage due to loss of autoregulation and if severe will predict loss of that tissue at follow-up.

If a subdural haemorrhage is not removed or if the patient presents a week or more after the trauma a more mature clot will be shown: the haematoma becoming isodense with brain at approximately 7–10 days and

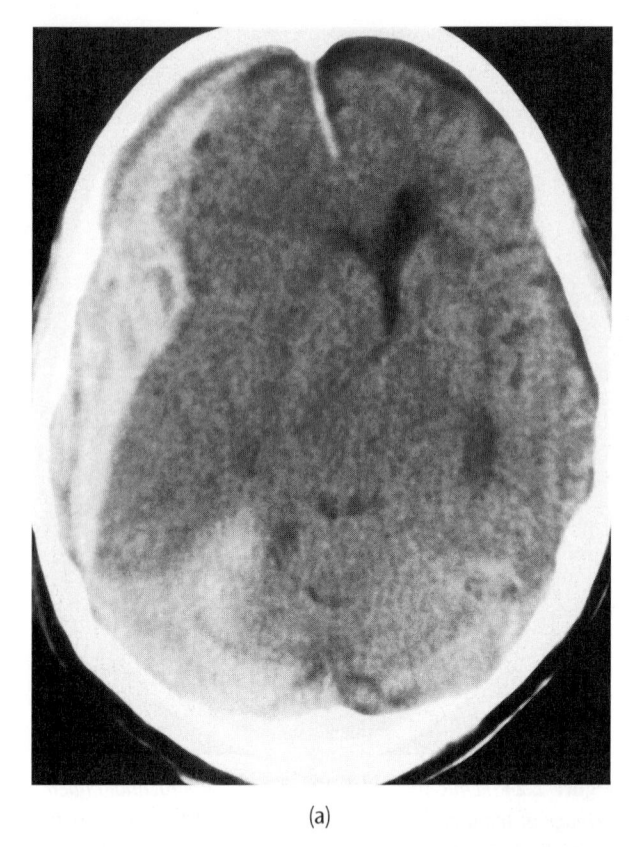

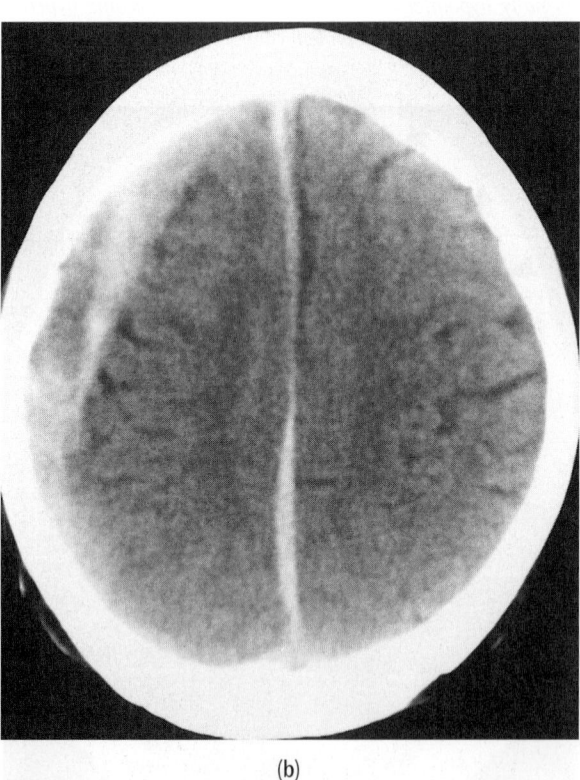

Figure 2.23 *A 78-year-old who fell from a stepladder. Admission CT. (a), (b) A large right-sided acute subdural haemorrhage with areas of hyperacute low attenuation unclotted haematoma within it. Parafalcine and supratentorial subdural haemorrhage is also noted. This is causing massive shift (1.7cm) and ventricular compression which is resulting in a transtentorial pressure cone.*

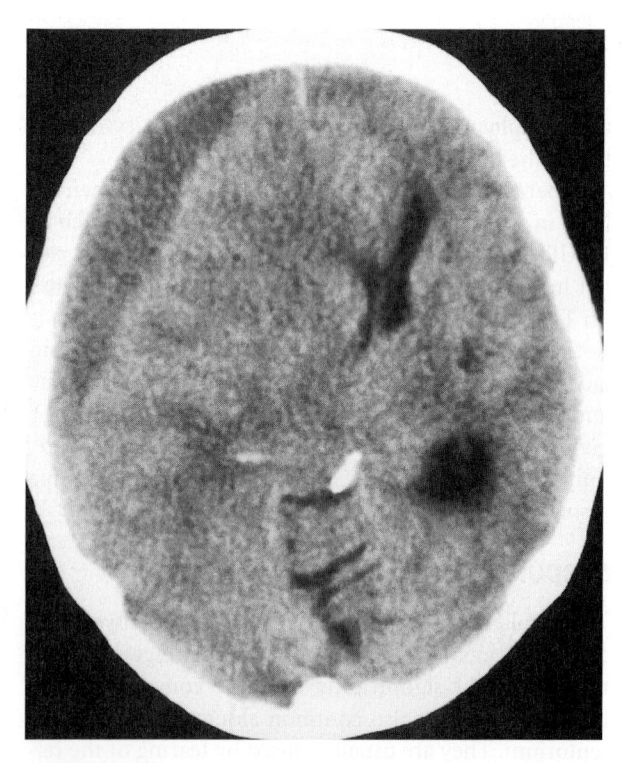

Figure 2.24 *A 54-year-old man who presented 3½ weeks after 'bumping his head on a door', with a Glasgow Coma Score of 5. CT shows chronic low attenuation right frontal subdural haemorrhage causing mass effect, severe ipsilateral lateral ventricular compression, midline shift (2cm), contralateral trigonal dilatation and incipient coning.*

Primary injury 89

Figure 2.25 *CT on admission. (a), (b) Large left hemisphere chronic subdural haemorrhage containing high attenuation recent acute haemorrhage. The acute component of the haemorrhage is likely to be the cause of the patient's sudden deterioration in conscious level.*

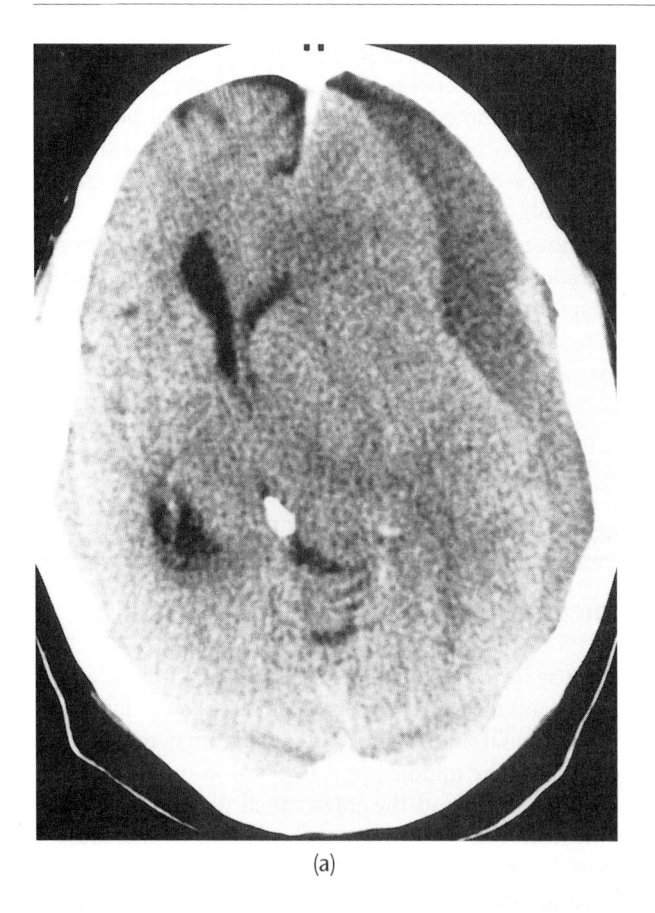

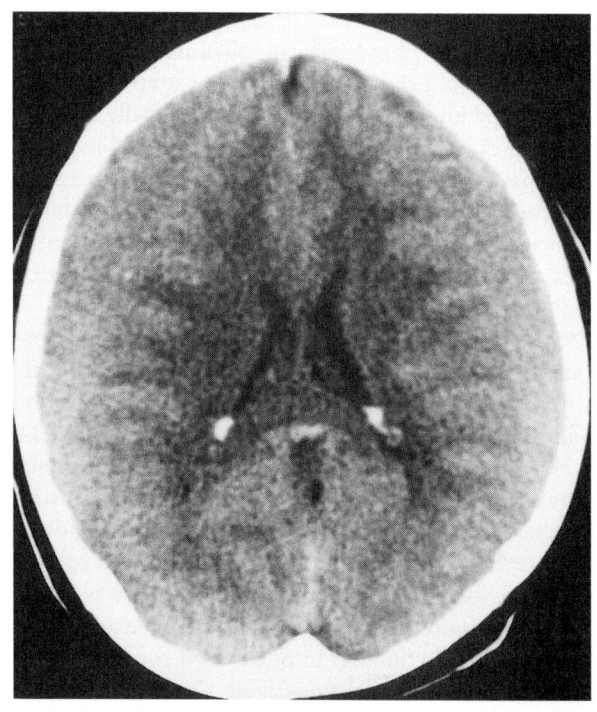

Figure 2.26 *Bilateral subdural haemorrhages approximately 10 days after a fall in an 89-year-old. The haemorrhage has the same attenuation as grey matter giving it a thickened appearance with compression of both lateral ventricles.*

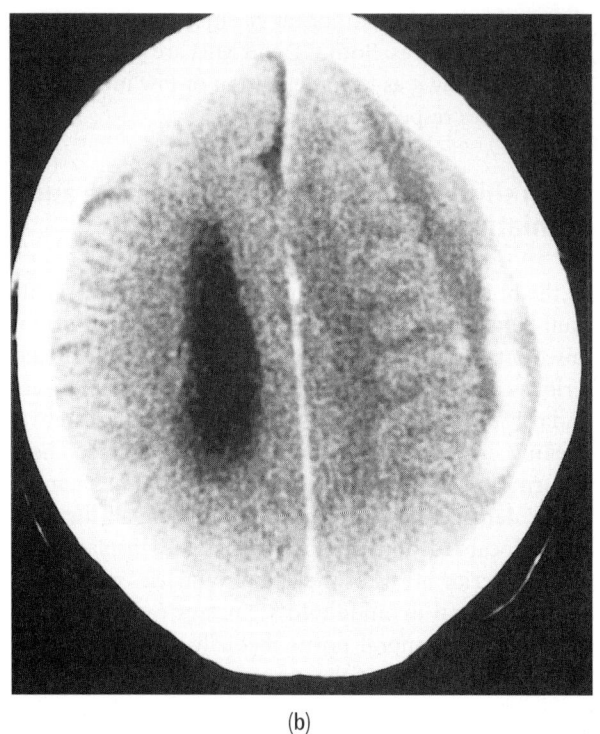

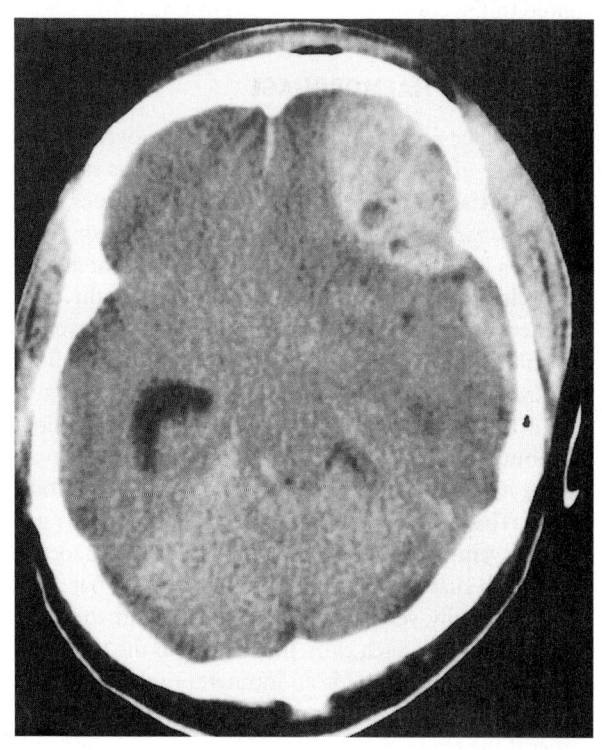

Figure 2.27 *Acute left frontal extradural haemorrhage with loculi of hyperacute unclotted blood giving a low attenuation. A posterolateral quadrant brainstem haematoma is also noted. The mass effect of the extradural haemorrhage has caused uncal herniation with contralateral temporal horn enlargement.*

hypodense by 21–30 days (Fig. 2.24). Fresh haemorrhage can also occur within a subacute subdural haemorrhage which will produce a mixed or layered pattern (Fig. 2.25) of high and low attenuation clot.[38] Occasionally isodense bilateral subdural haemorrhage without midline shift may make diagnosis more difficult. An increase in apparent cortical thickness (Fig. 2.26), symmetrical posterior displacement of the anterior horns of the lateral ventricles and compression or absence of the third ventricle will alert one to the correct diagnosis.

MRI will always show a subdural haemorrhage separate from the underlying brain. If at least two sequences with different weighting are carried out the collection will have a signal different to that of brain[14] (Figs 2.14, 2.29). The sharply delineated, low intensity dura lying between the haematoma and the displaced brain distinguishes an extradural haematoma from a subdural haemorrhage which is associated with displaced cortical pial veins demarcated by flow voids. If there is doubt about the compartment involved or the full extent of an extra-axial collection has to be assessed coronal MRI is ideal (Fig. 2.14). Collections lying along the falx, the peritentorial space and along the floor of the middle fossa are clearly demarcated while the volumetric perception of those lying over the convexity is more accurately assessed. Subdural collections thicker than a few millimetres are ovoid rather than crescentic when viewed in the coronal plane by MRI or CT.

EXTRADURAL HAEMORRHAGE

Haemorrhage occurs in this potential space between the inner table of the skull and the dura when it is stripped off in association with a fracture. The blood comes from the skull marrow, from torn meningeal arteries or veins or from a laceration of the dural sinuses. The clot is usually limited by the adjacent skull sutures where the dura is tethered but if there is a dural sinus tear it may cross the midline. Classically CT shows a uniformly high attenuation biconvex lesion based against the skull vault (Fig. 2.12). As more patients are being scanned within a few hours of their injury many extradural clots are now seen as mixed (Fig. 2.27) or even mainly low attenuation lesions. This is because the blood is still liquid, clot is still forming, and does not yet resemble the usual dense dehydrated mature haematoma. An extradural haemorrhage is usually very obvious unless it lies in the axial plane of the scan. Such clots, in the floor of the temporal fossa, can be mistaken for an intratemporal lesion (Fig. 2.18) and those on the vertex of the skull missed altogether if the scan is not continued to the top of the head.

On MRI extracerebral haematomas (subdural and extradural haemorrhages) age in a similar way to intracerebral haemorrhage, but their appearance is modified in the acute and subacute stages by decreased reabsorption of serum and varying degrees of liquefaction. They therefore appear to mature more quickly than their intracerebral counterparts. If air enters the collection through a compound fracture (extradural haemorrhage), attempted aspiration or surgery, the process of oxidative reduction of deoxyhaemoglobin to methaemoglobin is accelerated giving an earlier hyperintense signal on T1WI.

Unlike haemorrhage into the subdural space a chronic extradural haemorrhage is rare. It shows a similar low or mixed attenuation pattern with dural marginal enhancement after contrast on either CT or MRI. Unusually an extradural haemorrhage will develop as a delayed clot at a site previously unsuspected to be injured.

SECONDARY CONSEQUENCES

Pneumocephalus

Air may lie in the subarachnoid space or within the ventricles and this usually follows a basal fracture involving the paranasal sinuses, most often the frontal, the mastoid air cells or the middle ear. A CSF leak commonly develops (see later) and the intracranial pressure is usually low. If no CSF escapes air will accumulate and cause a mass lesion, often in the subdural space or rarely as a pneumatocele in the brain itself. Small bubbles of air are frequently seen in extradural haemorrhage associated with basal fractures. Both CT and MRI are very sensitive to air and show it as low attenuation or low intensity on all sequences respectively (Fig. 2.28).

Brain shift, raised intracranial pressure and herniation

As the brain is enclosed within the rigid confines of the skull between the dural folds of the falx and tentorium raised intracranial pressure >20mmHg is a frequent and serious complication of head injury. Displacements secondary to focal mass lesions, generalized cerebral swelling or hydrocephalus can be demonstrated. These in turn can cause additional ischaemic or even haemorrhagic damage. If a focal mass lesion is small the shift will be localized: anterior contusions cause displacement of the anterior horns of the lateral ventricles posteriorly while temporal or middle fossa masses cause displacement of the temporal horns medially. Contusions will cause local swelling of the gyri with obliteration of the overlying sulci.

Large supratentorial masses produce lateral and downward herniation (Figs 2.19, 2.23, 2.25, 2.27). There is compression of the ipsilateral ventricle, shift of the midline structures below the falx to the contralateral side and dilatation of the contralateral trigone and temporal horn of the lateral ventricle once the foramen of Monro is occluded. This dilatation is often associated with some

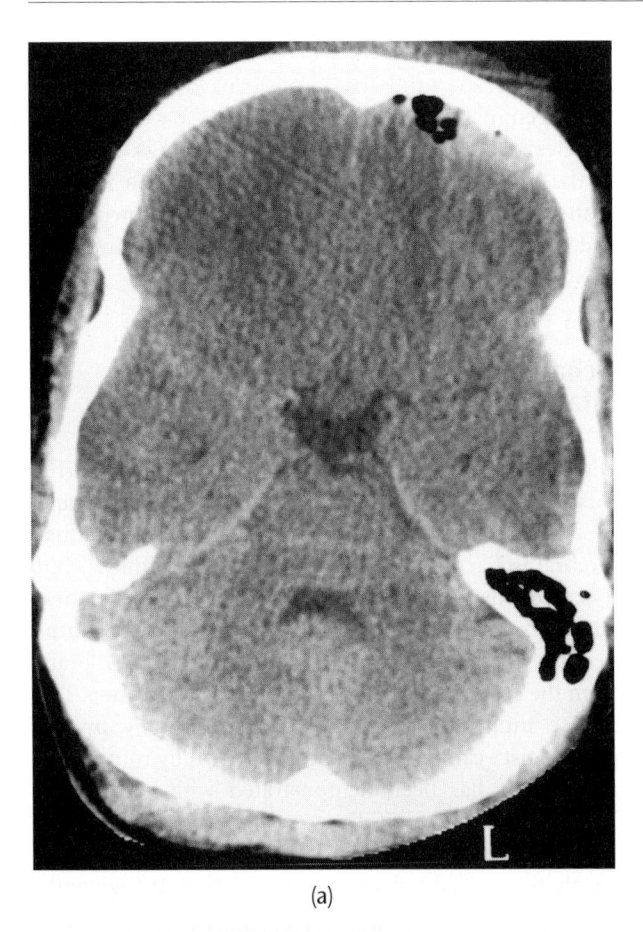

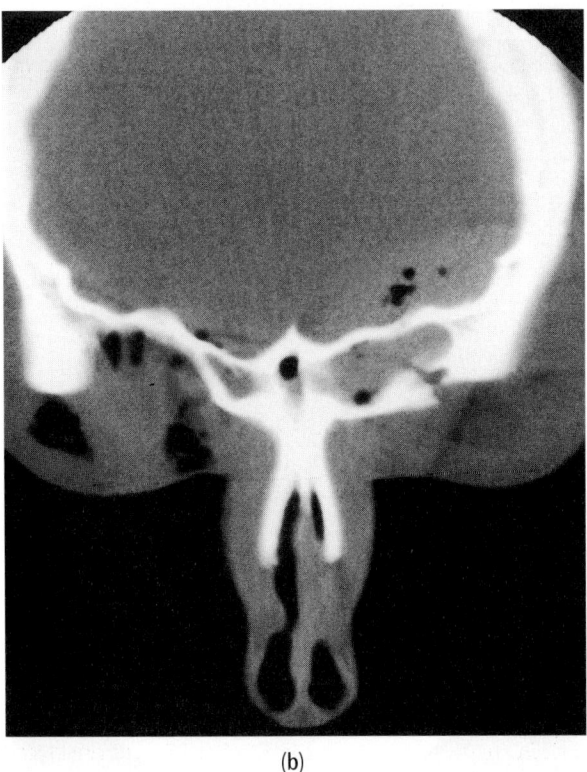

Figure 2.28 *An 18-year-old boy assaulted with a brick. CT (a) axial and (b) direct coronal section with bone windows shows the fracture through the left ethmoid sinus and supraorbital rim with an associated frontal contusion and pneumocephalus.*

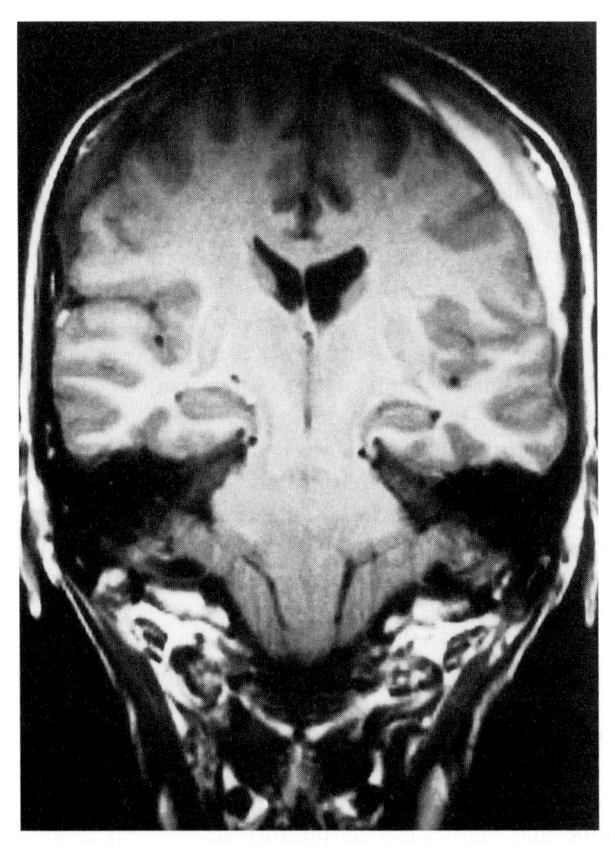

Figure 2.29 *A 52-year-old who fell down steps: T1-weighted coronal section shows a left-sided mixed intensity subdural haemorrhage with bilateral herniation of the medial aspects of the temporal lobes. (Note the flow voids of the posterior cerebral arteries and their relation to the herniation.)*

periventricular oedema. The third ventricle will be obliterated by the time this stage is reached. These additional signs correlate with clinical signs of brainstem compression indicative of transtentorial herniation.[39] With CT, in the absence of underlying atrophy, it is usually not possible to identify the herniated uncus because the basal cisterns, which normally provide the CT contrast between these structures, are already obliterated. An increase in oedema in the cortex of the medial aspect of the temporal lobe shown by hyperintensity on axial T2-weighted MRI indicates that herniation is occurring while on coronal T1-weighted sections the anatomical distortion is easily demonstrated (Fig. 2.29). It is this downward shift which produces the damage secondary to increased intracranial pressure. Severe lateral shift can be tolerated if there is no downward shift and the third ventricle and the basal cisterns remain patent as in patients with older atrophic brains. With the multiplanar sections available from MRI, subcallosal and uncal herniation can be more easily appreciated (Fig. 2.29).

The fourth ventricle should also always be seen, central and symmetrical in any reasonably well positioned axial scan. If it is displaced or compressed a local cause for this should be sought and a thin infratentorial extracerebral collection excluded by interrogating the scan at different window levels or carrying out MRI. Significant posterior fossa injury is always associated with occipital basal skull fracture.

Tonsillar herniation cannot be shown directly by CT although it is clearly demonstrated by sagittal sections on MRI. Isolated masses within the posterior fossa can cause an acute obstructive hydrocephalus of the third and lateral ventricles by compressing the fourth ventricle. The earliest sign of developing hydrocephalus is dilatation of the temporal horns which in normal young people are seen only as narrow curved slits. Upward tentorial herniation is unusual because isolated infratentorial traumatic lesions are uncommon. On CT it can be inferred from a pattern comprising obliteration of the basal and supracerebellar cisterns with associated triventricular hydrocephalus. Sagittal and coronal MRI again demonstrates this shift pattern directly.

When there are bilateral similar sized mass lesions or if there is general swelling of the hemispheres then the midline may remain undisplaced but a significant downward herniation can still be present with an associated raised intracranial pressure. If either the third ventricle or the basal cisterns are obliterated with <5mm of midline shift the intracranial pressure lies between 20 and 30mmHg. If both are obliterated, it is >30mmHg.[40]

Normally it should always be possible to identify the third ventricle and basal cisterns (ambient and quadrigeminal) as low attenuation CSF spaces. It is still not clear whether hyperaemia or ischaemia is the cause of the generalized hemisphere swelling which is commonest in children and young adults. Following the widespread use of seatbelts this type of head injury is now seen less commonly.

Ischaemic damage, vascular injury and infarction

On CT ischaemia (reversible) and infarction (irreversible) are both indicated by reduced attenuation and so cannot be differentiated in the acute phase. Diffuse cerebral ischaemia is universal in fatal head injuries but it is rarely demonstrated by CT in life. The commonest pattern is seen when low attenuation surrounds a contusion but it is impossible to separate the necrotic brain from the co-existent cytotoxic oedema of ischaemia. The diffuse multifocal ischaemia seen commonly by the pathologist[41] cannot be specifically shown by routine CT although it has been demonstrated with subtraction Xenon CT and on SPECT.[42]

Arterial vascular territory ischaemia is the most commonly recognized ischaemic complication. It frequently

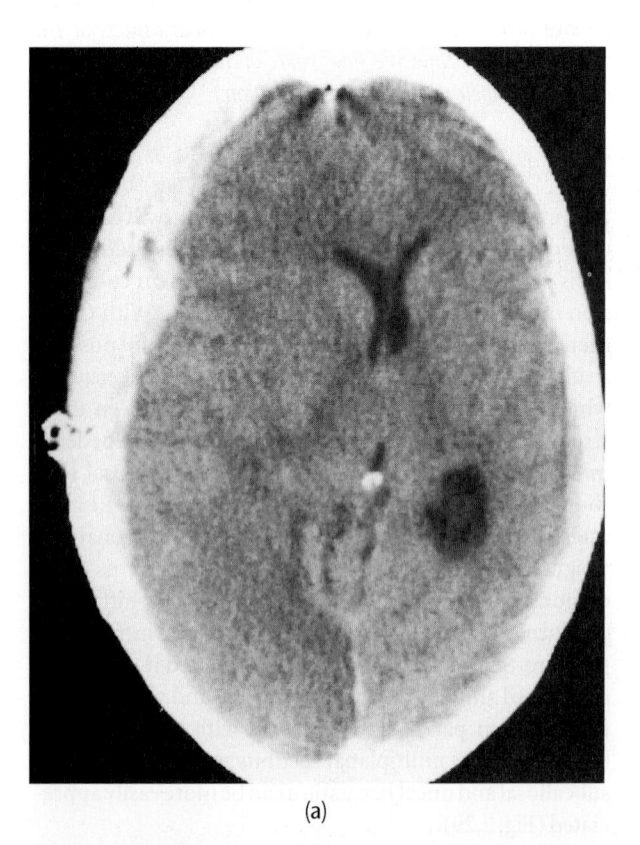

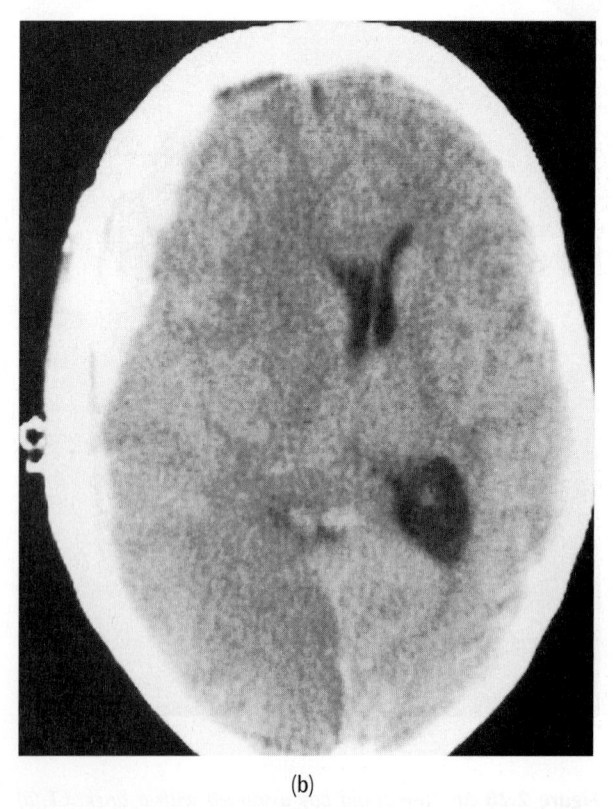

Figure 2.30 *Following transfer from a general hospital, CT on admission to neurosurgery. (a), (b) Extensive right-sided acute subdural haemorrhage with mass effect causing coning. This has resulted in an ipsilateral low attenuation posterior cerebral artery territory infarct.*

involves the posterior cerebral artery ipsilateral to a mass lesion causing severe midline shift (Fig. 2.30). Pericallosal artery ischaemia can be produced in a similar way.

If middle cerebral territory ischaemia is present on CT or MRI it suggests that there has been damage to the carotid artery in the neck or skull base, local dissection or embolic thrombosis from more proximal dissection (Fig. 2.31). Early angiography will identify lesions which can be treated surgically although treatment for small vessel dissection or thrombosis remains controversial in trauma. Ischaemia in the basilar territory causes diffuse low attenuation in the brainstem and midbrain usually contrasted against the preserved normal density pattern of the cerebellum. Vertebral dissection may show only as an infarction in the ipsilateral PICA (posterior inferior cerebellar artery) territory.

All ischaemia is much better visualized with MRI, especially that in the posterior fossa and medial aspects of the temporal lobes. Well defined focal regions of hyperintensity on T2- and proton density-weighted sequences with corresponding less prominent areas of hypointensity on T1-weighted sections will be seen.

Watershed ischaemia can develop after a period of global hypotension. On CT areas of reduced attenuation will be seen while on MRI there is hyperintensity on T2- and proton density-weighted images with hypointensity on T1WI. These changes are seen in the frontal region at the watershed between the anterior and middle cerebral artery territories, in the parafalcine region and posterosuperiorly in the parietal region between the middle and the posterior cerebral artery territories.

Profound persistent hypotension, ischaemia or a generally elevated intracranial pressure results in loss of the normal grey/white matter differentiation on CT and MRI. This usually involves both hemispheres and is associated with an apparent increase in the attenuation or intensity of the normal cerebellum and tentorium. These appearances are limited to children and young adults and are pathognomonic of a non-perfused cerebrum.

Cortical venous infarction can be caused by a fracture involving a major venous sinus (Fig. 2.13) or secondary infection which results in dural venous sinus thrombosis.[43] It is similar to an arterial infarction but is less well defined with a pseudovasogenic pattern of oedema involving the white matter usually with some haemorrhage.

SPECT is more sensitive to perfusion changes than CT or MRI and often shows regions of abnormally high and abnormally low cortical blood flow in the same patient. All focal traumatic mass lesions such as contusions and intracerebral haematomas show zones of severely reduced rCBF which can persist for days to months in the oedematous surrounding area. In the subacute stage if the brain is compressed by extraaxial lesions it often shows a paradoxical increase in perfusion presumed to be due to loss of autoregulation. Occasionally the

Figure 2.31 *Following craniotomy and removal of a right-sided subdural haemorrhage the CT shows swelling and low attenuation in the territories of the middle cerebral artery branches (with preservation of the perforators), anterior cerebral artery and posterior cerebral artery. This represents infarction.*

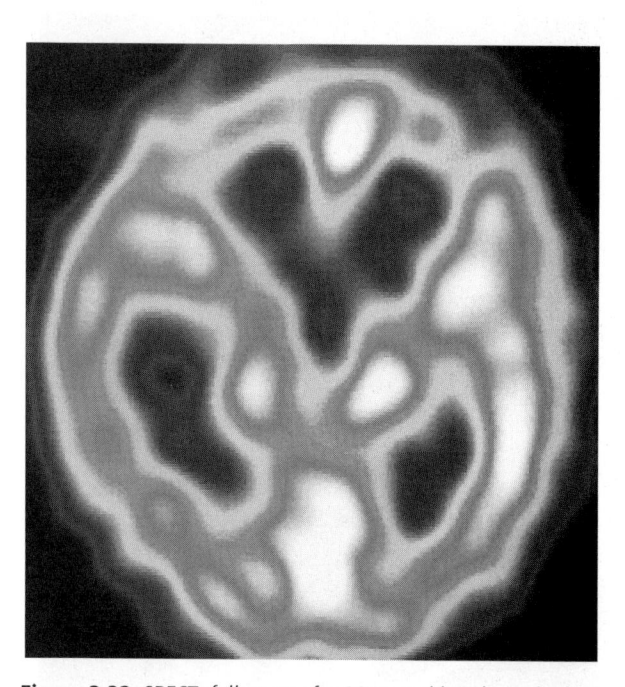

Figure 2.32 *SPECT: follow-up of a 28-year-old patient who had a severe diffuse axonal injury. Perfusion pattern shows markedly reduced functioning cortex with a pattern consistent with diffuse atrophy. This illustration also appears as Plate 2 in the colour plate section.*

abnormal perfusion pattern persists over several months although the structural appearance on CT or MRI returns to normal. This may correlate with some of the late neuropsychological sequelae found after head injury[21] (Fig. 2.32).

LATE SEQUELAE

Cerebromalacia

As contusions heal by progressive degradation and maturation of haemorrhage with eventual gliosis they shrink to leave a low attenuation area on CT with loss of cortex and the underlying involved white matter. This lesion is termed cerebromalacia. It is typical in appearance and classically found in a subfrontal and/or temporal area.

On MRI the border zone adjacent to the macrocystic cerebromalacia of a healed region of haemorrhagic contusion where there was persistent vasogenic oedema may show an irregular relatively narrow border of hyperintensity on T2WI and isointensity to grey matter on T1- and proton density weighted images. This represents a region of microcystic cerebromalacia or gliosis which often contains foci or a rim of hypointensity on T2WI representing residual haemosiderin. The acute space-occupying effect resolves and an *ex-vacuo* effect supervenes with enlargement of adjacent sulci and ventricles (Fig. 2.33).

Cerebrospinal fluid fistula

An overt CSF leak is present in about 25% of patients with CT diagnosed pneumocephalus but in the majority there is spontaneous cessation within 7–10 days. If the leak persists or if there is evidence of late post traumatic meningitis then a search for the fracture site should be made. Direct coronal high resolution CT of the anterior fossa is used to investigate CSF rhinorrhoea and similar sections of the petrous bones in patients with CSF otorrhoea (Figs 2.1, 2.2). If this fails to demonstrate a fluid or soft tissue density adjacent to a bone defect the examination should be repeated following contrast opacification of the cisternal CSF by instillation of 5ml of a suitable 300mg% non-ionic contrast medium via a lumbar puncture. The contrast is then run up to the basal cisterns and positioned over the appropriate portion of the skull base and direct coronal CT performed. The dural defect associated with the fracture can then be surgically repaired.

Although there were initial hopes that heavily T2-weighted thin section MRI would non-invasively show CSF leaking through the defect, the technique has proved insensitive when so many of the population suffer from incidental sinusitis.[44,45]

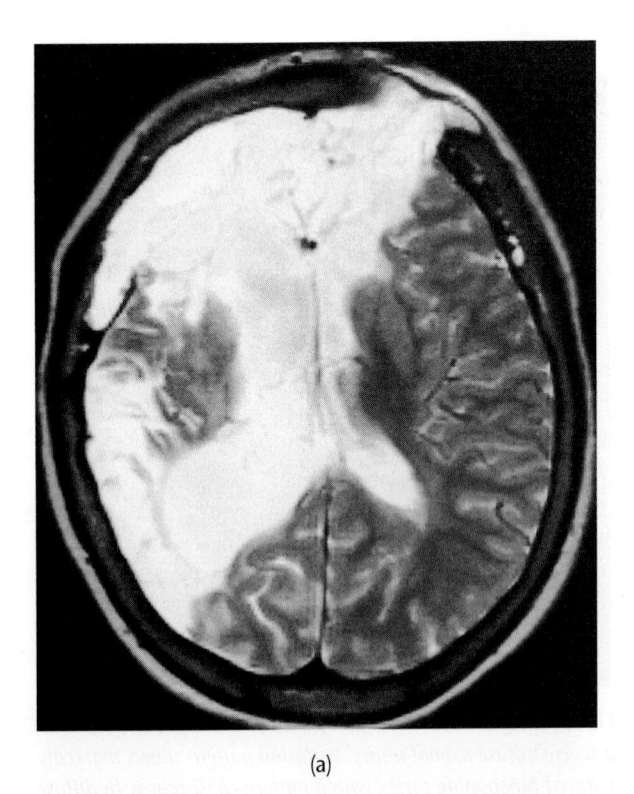

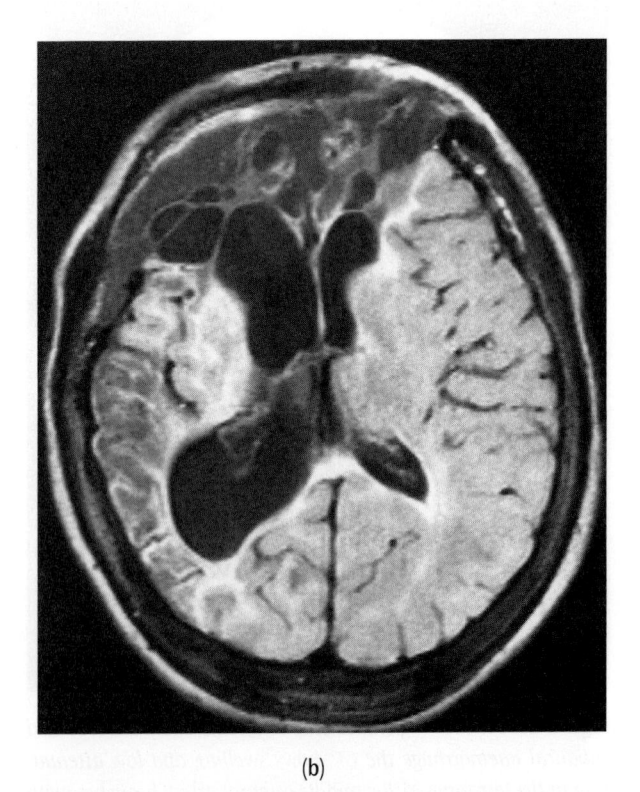

Figure 2.33 *Follow-up after severe bifrontal and right temporal contusions. (a) T2-weighted axial; (b) matching T1-weighted axial sections show macrocystic and microcystic (gliosis) cerebromalacia with* ex-vacuo *enlargement of the adjacent ventricle.*

Vascular lesions

Penetrating injuries have been mentioned above. They must be recognized in the acute stage and any associated vascular damage demonstrated by urgent angiography. Arteriovenous fistula or pseudoaneurysm can form secondary to a skull fracture and tearing of the meningeal vessels. Delayed or recurrent intracranial haematomas can follow rarely. When the intracavernous segment of the carotid artery is damaged with or without an overt skull base fracture a carotico-cavernous fistula can form with unilateral or bilateral pulsing exophthalmos or much less commonly a pseudoaneurysm may form (Fig. 2.34). Although these can present at the time of injury they are commoner after several weeks have elapsed. Angiography is required for the full definition of the vascular components but the dilated veins and abnormal vascular contours will be shown on enhanced CT and MRI. An endovascular approach with embolization is the treatment of choice to occlude a fistula; however, false aneurysms of the internal carotid artery require permanent vessel occlusion.

Hydrocephalus

Hydrocephalus in the acute episode has already been discussed. Localized atrophic dilatation of a ventricle may be seen adjacent to a large area of cerebromalacia but generalized hydrocephalus is unusual and most often follows intraventricular or subarachnoid haemorrhage where there is disproportionate ventricular enlargement compared with the cortical sulci and cisterns and when severe, periventricular white matter oedema can be shown on CT or MRI. Although the temporal horns should be involved, care has to be taken as their enlargement can also be a local complication of cerebromalacia. This active hydrocephalus with increased intracranial pressure must be differentiated from the progressive ventricular dilatation associated with enlarged cortical sulci and cisterns which may be seen 4–6 months after an injury due to cerebral atrophy and may be the only sign of diffuse axonal injury.

Infection

Nowadays infection is still a serious problem but is usually pre-empted and often treated prophylactically. The radiology of infection is discussed in Chapter 1.

Meningitis is a common complication of compound skull fractures. It is diagnosed clinically and a CT or plain film usually just confirms the fracture site. If CT or MRI is carried out after IV contrast in the acute phase they can be normal but if untreated, generalized meningeal enhancement will be seen; MRI is more sensitive to these changes than CT but lumbar puncture with bacteriological analysis of CSF is the optimal test.

Cerebral abscess may present late as an intracranial mass. It is most often associated with a penetrating injury or a foreign body although the primary breach in the dura may not have been suspected.

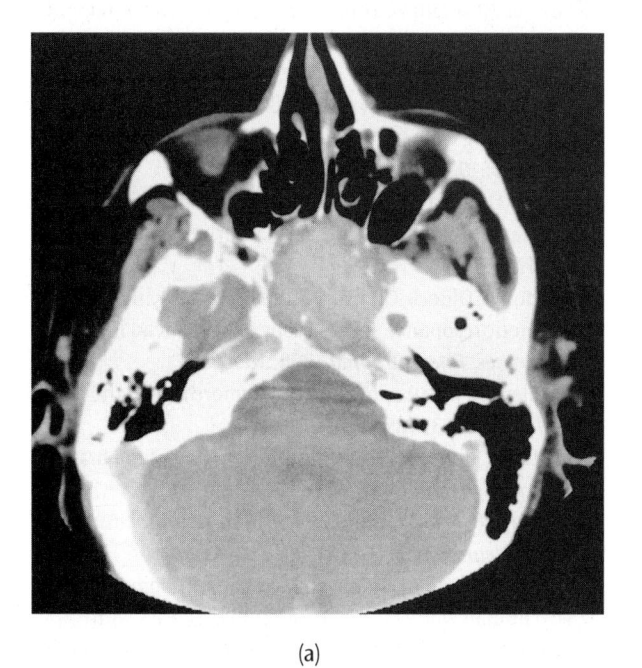

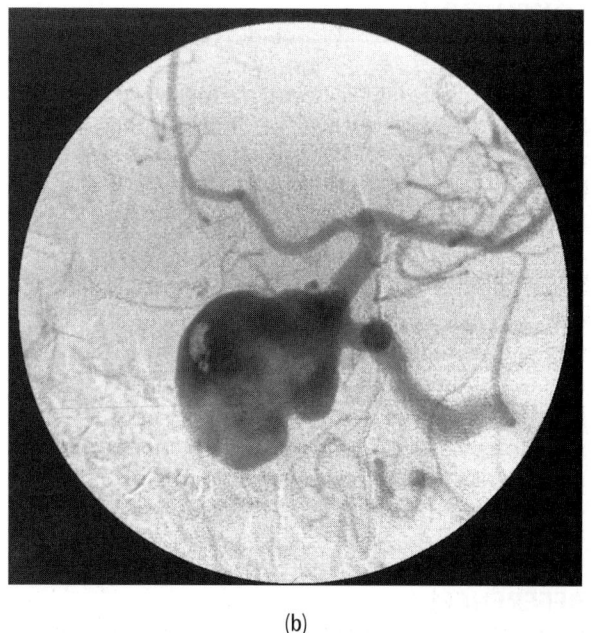

Figure 2.34 *A 43-year-old complained of intermittent nose bleeds. A sphenoidal mass was found. An attempt at biopsy with an endoscope in the general hospital resulted in more haemorrhage. CT (a) showed high attenuation enhancing mass bulging out of the sphenoid sinus; (b) subsequent selective internal carotid artery angiogram showed the mass to be a pseudoaneurysm of the carotid siphon. A history of a head injury 8 months previously was finally elicited.*

Bone infection is unusual and is seen most frequently in association with a craniotomy bone flap or an infected scalp wound. Plain films, CT or MRI will all show the abnormalities once the infection is established.

Cerebral atrophy

This can develop rapidly in patients in a vegetative state but more usually can be appreciated around 4 months after a head injury. It may be progressive with ventricular dilatation and enlarged sulci and cisterns (Fig. 2.33).

Epilepsy

Epilepsy is most common in patients who have fits in the acute phase, have had a depressed fracture or a craniotomy. Other than establishing that a cerebral injury has occurred radiology only rarely has a role.[46]

Post-concussion syndrome

This syndrome is being increasingly recognized and comprises symptoms such as headache, dizziness, lack of concentration and poor memory. Although it may relate to minor diffuse cerebral injury CT, MRI and SPECT show similar proportions of abnormalities in these patients as in patients with no complaints following head injury.[47]

CONCLUSION

The first choice for detecting surgically significant lesions in the first few hours after injury is still CT. If diffuse axonal injury is suspected and CT is normal the higher sensitivity of MRI may well show underlying haemorrhagic or non-haemorrhagic lesions although it cannot exclude the presence of microscopic axonal tears. In the subacute and chronic stages MRI is superior to CT especially in the posterior and middle fossae or if the history of head injury is not forthcoming. SPECT is a practical test in these difficult patients and can give valuable information about cerebral perfusion. Each of these modalities has helped to refine the treatment and prognostic assessment of the head injured patient.

REFERENCES

1. Jennett B, Teasdale GM, Galbraith S et al. Severe head injuries in three countries. *J Neurol Neurosurg Psychiat* 1977; **40**: 291–8.
2. Waxweiler R, Gautile T, Klauber MR et al. Monitoring the impact of traumatic brain injury: a review and update. In: *Traumatic Brain Injury: Bioscience and Mechanics* pp. 1–8. Bandak FA, Eppinger RH, Ommaya AK (Eds), New York: MA Liebert, 1996.
3. Teasdale G, Teasdale E, Hadley D. Computed tomographic and magnetic resonance imaging classification of head injury. *J Neurotrauma* 1992; **9**: 249–57.
4. Teasdale G, Murray G, Anderson E et al. The risks of intracranial haematoma after head injury in adults and children. *Br Med J* 1990; **300**: 363–7.
5. RCR Working Party. *Making the Best Use of a Department of Clinical Radiology* 4th edn. London: The Royal College of Radiologists, 1998.
6. Spencer JA, Dobson D, Hoare M et al. The use of a computerized image transfer system linking a regional neuroradiology centre to its district hospitals. *Clin Radiol* 1991; **44**: 342–4.
7. Lewis M, Boyd Moir AT. Medical telematics and telemedicine: an agenda for research evaluation in Scotland. *Hlth Bull* 1995; **53**: 129–37.
8. Trott J, David DJ. Definitive management principles, priorities and basic technique. pp. 233–50. In: *Craniomaxillofacial Trauma.* David DJ, Simpson DA (Eds), Edinburgh: Churchill Livingstone, 1995.
9. Harris MB, Waguespack AM, Kronlage S. 'Clearing' cervical spine injuries in polytrauma patients: is it really safe to remove the collar? *Orthopedics* 1997; **20**: 903–7.
10. White CS, Mirvis SE. Pictorial review: imaging of traumatic aortic injury. *Clin Radiol* 1995; **50**: 281–7.
11. Scottish Intercollegiate Guidelines Network (SIGN). *Head Injury*. Edinburgh: SIGN (in press).
12. Bahner ML, Reith W, Zuna I et al. Spiral CT vs incremental CT: is spiral CT superior in imaging of the brain? *Eur Radiol* 1998; **8**: 416–20.
13. MacLennan AC, Hadley DM. Radiation dose to the lens from CT scanning in a neuroradiology department. *Br J Radiol* 1994; **68**: 19–22.
14. Hadley DM, Teasdale GM, Jenkins A et al. Magnetic resonance imaging in acute head injury. *Clin Radiol* 1988; **39**: 131–9.
15. Condon B, Oluoch-Olunya D, Hadley D et al. Early 1H magnetic resonance spectroscopy of acute head injury: Four cases. *J Neurotrauma* 1998; **15**: 563–71.
16. Bradley WG Jr. MR appearance of hemorrhage in the brain. *Radiology* 1993; **189**: 15–26.
17. Jolesz FA, Jones KM. Fast spin-echo imaging of the brain. *Topics Magn Reson Imag* 1993; **5**: 1–13.
18. Ashikaga R, Araki Y, Ishida O. MRI of head injury using FLAIR. *Neuroradiology* 1993; **39**: 239–42.
19. Makris N, Worth AJ, Sorensen AG et al. Morphometry of *in vivo* human white matter association pathways with diffusion-weighted magnetic resonance imaging. *Ann Neurol* 1997; **42**: 951–62.
20. Cecil KM, Hills EC, Sandel ME et al. Proton magnetic resonance spectroscopy for detection of axonal injury in the splenium of the corpus callosum of brain-injured patients. *J Neurosurg* 1998; **88**: 795–801.

21 Wilson JTL, Mathew P. SPECT in head injury. In: *SPECT Imaging of the Brain* pp. 69–93. Duncan R (Ed), London: Kluwer Academic Publishers, 1997.
22 Jenkins A, Teasdale G, Hadley MDM *et al*. Brain lesions detected by magnetic resonance imaging in mild and severe head injuries. *Lancet* 1986; **ii**: 445–6.
23 Mittl RL, Grossman RI, Hiehle JF *et al*. Prevalence of MR evidence of diffuse axonal injury in patients with mild head injury and normal head CT findings. *Am J Neuroradiol* 1994; **15**: 1583–9.
24 Lang DA, Hadley DM, Teasdale GM *et al*. Gadolinium DTPA enhanced magnetic resonance imaging in acute head injury. *Acta Neurochirurgica* 1990; **51**: 293–5.
25 Kushi H, Katayama Y, Shibuya T *et al*. Gadolinium DTPA-enhanced magnetic resonance imaging of cerebral contusions. *Acta Neurochirurgica Suppl (Wien)* 1994; **60**: 472–4.
26 Katayama Y, Tsubokawa T, Kinoshita K *et al*. Intraparenchymal blood-fluid levels in traumatic intracerebral haematomas. *Neuroradiology* 1992; **34**: 381–3.
27 Bula WI, Loes DJ. Trauma to the cerebrovascular system. *Neuroimag Clin N Amer* 1994; **4**: 753–72.
28 Stein SC, Spettell C, Young G *et al*. Delayed and progressive brain injury in closed-head trauma: radiological demonstration. *Neurosurgery* 1993; **32**: 25–31.
29 Gentleman D, Nath F, Macpherson P. Diagnosis and management of delayed traumatic haematomas. *Br J Neurosurg* 1989; **3**: 367–72.
30 Gomori JM, Grossman RI. Head and neck hemorrhage. In: *Magnetic Resonance Annual* pp. 71–112. Kressel HY (Ed), New York: Raven Press, 1987.
31 Gomori JM, Grossman RI, Hackney DB *et al*. Variable appearances of subacute intracranial hematomas on high-field spin-echo MR. *Am J Neuroradiol* 1987; **8**: 1019–26.
32 LeRoux PD, Haglund MM, Newell DW *et al*. Intraventricular hemorrhage in blunt head trauma: an analysis of 43 cases. *Neurosurgery* 1992; **31**: 678–85.
33 Gentry LR, Thompson B, Godersky JC. Trauma to the corpus callosum: MR features. *Am J Neuroradiol* 1988; **9**: 1129–38.
34 Demircivi F, Ozkan N, Buyukkececi S *et al*. Traumatic subarachnoid haemorrhage: Analysis of 89 cases. *Acta Neurochirurgica* 1993; **122**: 45–8.
35 Kakarieka A, Braakman R, Schakel EH. Clinical significance of the finding of subarachnoid blood on CT scan after head injury. *Acta Neurochirurgica* 1994; **129**: 1–5.
36 Jenkins A, Hadley DM, Teasdale GM *et al*. Magnetic resonance imaging of acute subarachnoid haemorrhage. *J Neurosurg* 1988; **68**: 731–6.
37 Noguchi K, Ogawa T, Seto H *et al*. Subacute and chronic subarachnoid hemorrhage: diagnosis with fluid-attenuated inversion-recovery MR imaging. *Radiology* 1997; **203**: 257–62.
38 Kaminogo M, Moroki J, Ochi A *et al*. Characteristics of symptomatic chronic subdural haematomas on high-field MRI. *Neuroradiology* 1999; **41**: 109–16.
39 Stovring J. Contralateral temporal horn widening in unilateral supratentorial mass lesions: A diagnostic sign indicating tentorial herniation. *J Comput Assist Tomogr* 1977; **1**: 319–23.
40 Teasdale E, Cardosa E, Galbraith S *et al*. CT scan in severe diffuse head injury: physiological and clinical correlations. *J Neurol Neurosurg Psychiat* 1984; **47**: 600–03.
41 Graham DI, Adams JH, and Doyle D. Ischaemic brain damage in fatal non-missile head injury. *J Neurol Sci* 1987; **39**: 213–34.
42 Mitchener A, Wyper DJ, Patterson J *et al*. SPECT, CT, and MRI in head injury: acute abnormalities followed up at six months. *J Neurol Neurosurg Psychiat* 1997; **62**: 633–6.
43 Taha JM, Crone KR, Berger TS *et al*. Sigmoid sinus thrombosis after closed head injury in children. *Neurosurg* 1993; **32**: 541–5.
44 El Gammal T, Sobol W, Wadlington VR *et al*. Cerebrospinal fluid fistula: detection with MR cisternography. *Am J Neuroradiol* 1998; **19**: 627–31.
45 Shetty PG, Shroff MM, Sahani DV *et al*. Evaluation of high-resolution CT and MR cisternography in the diagnosis of cerebrospinal fluid fistula. *Am J Neuroradiol* 1998; **19**: 633–9.
46 Marks DA, Kim J, Spencer DD *et al*. Seizure localization and pathology following head injury in patients with uncontrolled epilepsy. *Neurology* 1995; **45**: 2051–7.
47 Kant R, Smith-Seemiller L, Isaac G *et al*. Tc-HMPAO SPECT in persistent post-concussion syndrome after mild head injury: comparison with MRI/CT. *Brain Injury* 1997; **11**: 115–24.

FURTHER READING

1 Osborne, AG. Craniocerebral Trauma. In: *Diagnostic Neuroradiology*, pp 199–247. London: Mosby 1944.
2 Gentry, LR. Head Trauma. In: *Magnetic Resonance of the Brain and Spine* 2nd edn pp 611–647. Ahas SW (Ed), Philadelphia: Lippincott-Raven, 1996.
3 Gean, AD. *Imaging of Head Trauma*. p. 557. New York: Raven Press, 1994.
4 Zee, CS, Go J. CT of head trauma. *Neuroimag Clin N Amer* 1998; **8**: 525–38.
5 Youmans, JR (Ed). *Neurological Surgery*. London: WB Saunders, 1995.

3

Supratentorial tumours

SHAWN FS HALPIN

Introduction	98	Extra-axial tumours	122
Basic scanning principles	98	Tumours of the sellar and parasellar region	126
Intra-axial tumours	99	References	136
Intraventricular tumours	114	Further reading	137
Pineal region tumours	119	Appendix	137

INTRODUCTION

The following two chapters deal with the neuroradiology of tumours above and below the tentorium, subdivided by site of origin. We hope to present a method for assessing computed tomography (CT) and magnetic resonance imaging (MRI) scans when common clinical scenarios suggest the presence of a tumour, as well as providing an overview of the range of appearances seen on scans.

As in all aspects of neurosciences, the first question is not 'what is the lesion?' but rather 'where is the lesion?', because by accurately positioning the tumour, the differential diagnosis is shortened. The size, position and extent of a tumour are in any event more likely to influence a surgeon's decision to operate than its histology. A histologically benign tumour in an eloquent site like the brainstem is likely to be inoperable, and eventually fatal, while a highly malignant metastasis in the non-dominant frontal lobe may be completely excised.

Therefore CT and MRI will have at least two roles: first to attempt a diagnosis, and second to provide the surgeon with as much information as possible prior to surgery. It is clear though that MRI will outperform CT in both these roles in the majority of cases, although by detecting calcification missed on MRI, sometimes CT may be better at predicting histology.

Although frequent mention will be given to post-contrast appearances, we emphasize that it is not always necessary to administer a contrast agent, particularly in MRI where the soft tissue contrast is so good. Generally, contrast medium injections are best reserved for when their administration will influence management, such as help-

ing to choose a site for biopsy, or detecting meningeal seeding, but they are of limited use in other situations. For example they will add no useful information when a pituitary microadenoma has been demonstrated on uncontrasted T1-weighted images (T1WI), or in the follow-up of an optic nerve glioma. In a unit which has access to CT and MRI, it may be possible to forgo the post-contrast CT scan if the patient is going to have an MRI scan for further evaluation. When following up tumours, however, enhanced scans will often suffice.

The approach of this chapter is primarily to describe typical radiological appearances of common tumours, but a scan will only reveal useful information if it has been targeted correctly, and so we have included imaging protocols for some common clinical presentations. Of course these should be amended to take account of the individual patient and the scan facility used.

BASIC SCANNING PRINCIPLES

Computed tomography

Generally, scans should be made from the foramen magnum, taking care to ensure that the lowest section shows cerebrospinal fluid (CSF) around the upper cervical cord, through the posterior fossa in thin contiguous 4–5mm sections and then through the rest of the cranium in 8–10 mm contiguous sections, ensuring that the uppermost slice is high against the vertex. Technical factors vary according to the particular machine in use, but often mAs values are greater in the posterior fossa to reduce beam-hardening artifact.

Coronal sections are useful to examine lesions near the vertex, around the sella and orbits or in the temporal lobes. Occasionally axial sections angled 20 degrees caudal to Reid's line will throw further light on a lesion low in the middle cranial fossa, but this is not routinely required in the search for a temporal lobe lesion. As a general rule, if an area is poorly demonstrated, or its anatomical relationships are unclear, then localized thin sections should be obtained. If iodinated contrast-medium is given, 50 ml of 300mgI$_2$/ml strength usually suffices as a bolus, but higher doses may be used in some situations, for example to seek an acoustic schwannoma. Pre-contrast scans are invaluable and although it is tempting only to perform contrast-enhanced scans in the investigation of a suspected tumour, there will be occasions when haemorrhage will mimic enhancement, or an infarct will enhance to isodensity, leading to misinterpretation. Obtaining a pre-contrast scan before each enhanced one will minimize reporting errors. Regrettably, the day-to-day reality of medical practice and workload may lead to compromises, and it is common for patients with suspected metastases to have post-contrast scans only. If this policy is adopted, then a low threshold for recalling the patient for a repeat unenhanced scan is vital.

MAGNETIC RESONANCE IMAGING

Most departments now use fast spin echo (FSE: turbo spin echo, or RARE are effectively synonyms) techniques as a routine. On a 1.5T machine acceptable technical factors will be TR (repetition time) 2500–4000, effective TE (echo time, TE/ef) 75–100, for a T2-weighted image (T2WI), using an echo train of 8. Spin (or proton) density (PD) images may be acquired either at the same acquisition, using TE/ef of around 20ms, or separately with a reduced echo train and TR to obtain better effective spin density weighting. Slice thickness of 5–6mm with minimal interslice gap and an acquisition matrix of 256 × 192 is usually adequate, although machines with fast gradients will provide higher resolution scans. Images in alternative planes, most commonly the coronal plane, are invariably helpful and T2-weighted coronal images are often used if a tumour is detected. Alternative supplementary strategies could include coronal inversion recovery scans (TR/TE/TI = 3500/30/650) – particularly useful in imaging a meningioma; or pre- and post-contrast conventional spin echo T1WI (600/15) with a bolus of a gadolinium chelate at 0.1–0.2mmol/kg body weight. Gradient echo T2*W scans may detect calcification or haemorrhage not shown by FSE because of their sensitivity to susceptibility effects, but CT remains a better technique for demonstrating subarachnoid blood and calcium. Fluid attenuated inversion recovery (FLAIR) scans are used by some to replace spin-density images: parameters for this sequence differ widely between different manufacturers.

In MRI, most lesions demonstrate 'usual' signal change i.e. hyperintense to grey matter on PD and T2WI, and hypointense to grey matter on T1WI. In order to save repetition, descriptions of the MRI appearances of various tumours in these two chapters will not make reference to their signal intensity, unless it differs substantially from the above.

Suggested CT and MRI scan protocols for a variety of common clinical presentations are listed at the end of this chapter in an appendix (pp. 137–9).

INTRA-AXIAL TUMOURS

Astrocytoma

This is the commonest of all cerebral tumours, accounting for up to 30% of cerebral tumours in adults. It may present at any age from the neonatal period onwards, but in adult life tends to present from the second to the fifth decade, with the exception of malignant lesions which present on average 10 years later. Presentation varies according to the aggressiveness of the tumour and its site of origin. At one extreme, an indolent tumour in a 'quiet' location may not present until it has reached massive proportions, while at the other, a small lesion in an eloquent position may present early with seizures or neurological deficit.

Astrocytomas are classified by the World Health Organization according to their malignancy into three groups: low grade astrocytoma, anaplastic, and the highest grade of malignancy as glioblastoma.[1] Astrocytoma is much more common than oligodendroglioma but a tumour may contain elements of both cell lines. It is a white matter tumour which can arise in any lobe but tends to spare the occipital lobes. Typically a glioma passes along white matter tracts and a deep seated tumour often traverses the corpus callosum to reach the contralateral hemisphere as a 'butterfly' glioma (Fig. 3.1). It can be very difficult to distinguish tumour margins from normal brain: the non-enhancing finger-like projections of white matter oedema which surround an aggressive lesion may contain tumour cells, and there is seldom a surgical plane of cleavage around a glioma. Tumour cells will be present in brain tissue which appears normal both macroscopically and on imaging. Calcification is seen in 20% of astrocytomas and 90% of oligodendrogliomas but may be poorly demonstrated or not seen on MRI. Since astrocytomas are much more common than oligodendrogliomas, a calcified glioma is more likely to be an astrocytoma than an oligodendroglioma.

Tumour cysts are common and have CT numbers or MR signal intensity identical to CSF, unless there has been haemorrhage into the cyst. High-grade lesions may

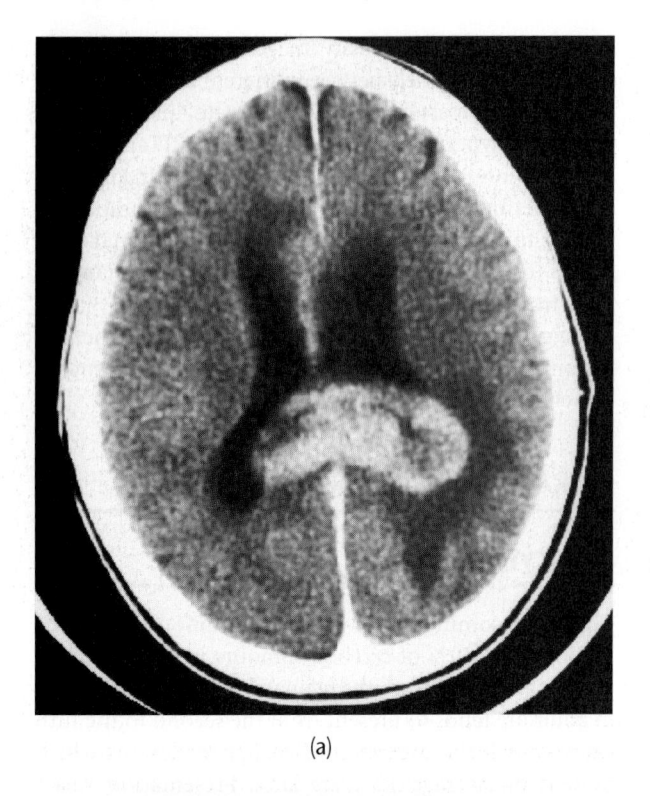

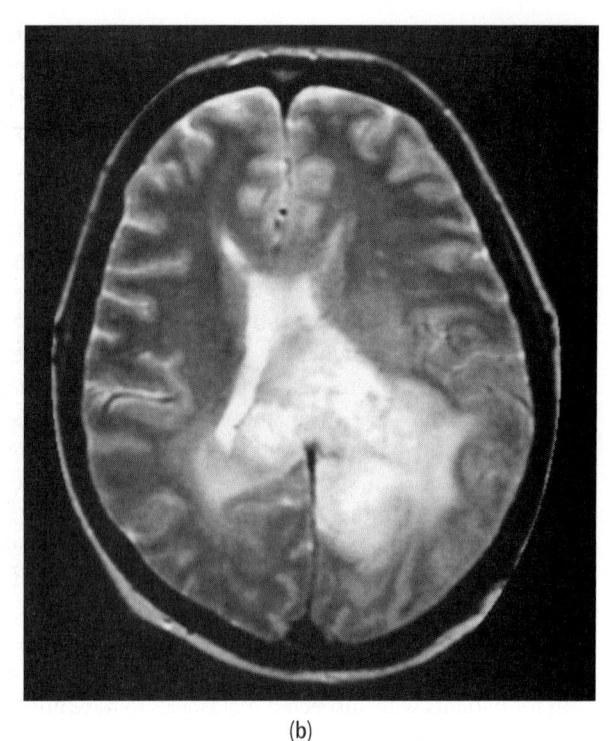

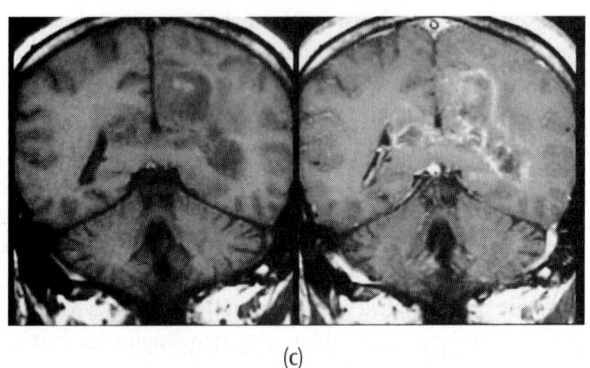

Figure 3.1. *(a) Contrast-enhanced CT; (b) T2-weighted; (c) T1-weighted MRI before and after gadolinium enhancement. Grade 3 astrocytoma straddling the corpus callosum, typical of a butterfly glioma. Oedema in the right parietal lobe does not show contrast enhancement but may contain tumour cells.*

present as the underlying cause for a cerebral haemorrhage. Mass effect is very variable. In low-grade glioma, there is often very little mass effect relative to the size of the tumour and mass may only be demonstrated by mild localized sulcal effacement (Fig. 3.2). Aggressive lesions usually have prominent mass effect, often with midline shift.[2] A tumour high in the brain may exhibit its mass by downward displacement of the lateral ventricles, a feature most easily seen on coronal images.

The best discriminator of the degree of malignancy is temporal change. It is characteristic of low-grade gliomas that they may show no discernible change in appearance over several years. Sometimes these lesions will apparently alter their character and turn from an indolent non-enhancing lesion into an aggressive high-grade tumour with necrosis, mass effect and rim enhancement (Fig. 3.3). It is rare for a glioma, however malignant, to metastasize, but erosion of bone is occasionally seen. If this occurs, direct spread outside the cranium may occur.

On CT, low-grade gliomas may appear of high, iso- or low density. If the latter are not isodense with CSF they should not be mistaken for cysts as they are usually of a rubbery consistency at surgery. High-grade tumours are nearly always inhomogeneous in density, due to necrosis and cyst formation, with an active rim of tumour which appears iso- or slightly hyperdense; these areas enhance after contrast medium administration (Fig. 3.4).

Nearly all gliomas will exhibit 'usual' signal intensities on MRI – i.e. hyperintense to grey matter on PD and T2WI, and hypointense to grey matter on T1WI. Intratumoral haemorrhage may, however, be evident as low signal on T2WI and/or high signal on T1WI. There is unfortunately no characteristic MRI signal pattern which is pathognomic of glioma. Often MRI will demonstrate thickening and signal change in grey matter which is not seen as density change on CT.

Contrast-enhancement within a glioma may be variable in amount and appearance and gadolinium enhancement is also sometimes present when none was

Intra-axial tumours 101

(a)

(b)

(c)

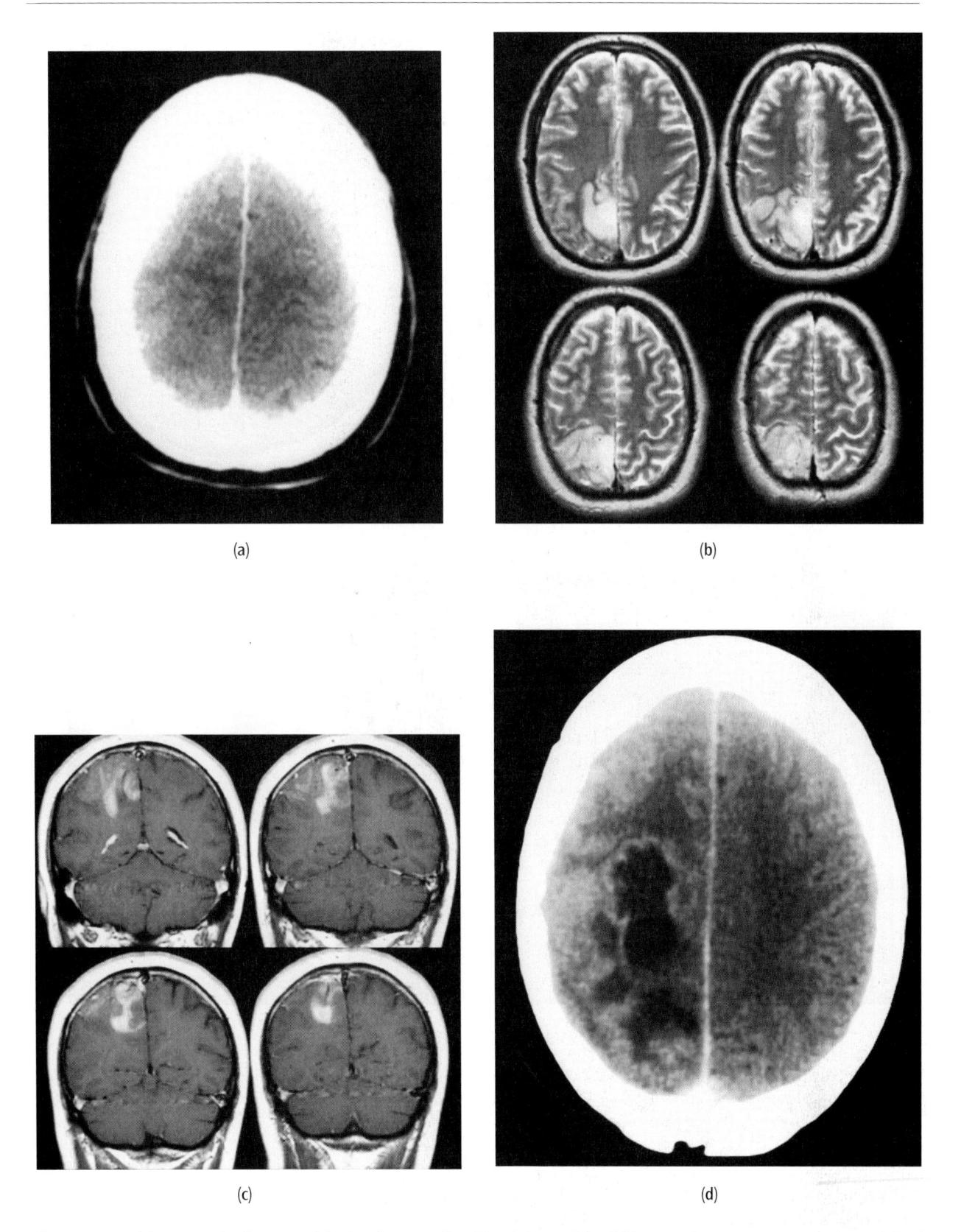

(d)

Figure 3.2. *Axial CT scans (a, d) separated in time by 5 months with axial T2-weighted (b) MRI and post-contrast coronal T1-weighted scans (c). The high right parietal mass was initially missed and demonstrates why CT scans must extend right up to the vertex. The lesion is much more obvious on MRI. The later CT (after biopsy) shows considerable enlargement of the lesion which is now more typical of aggressive glioma with cysts, oedema and irregular ring enhancement.*

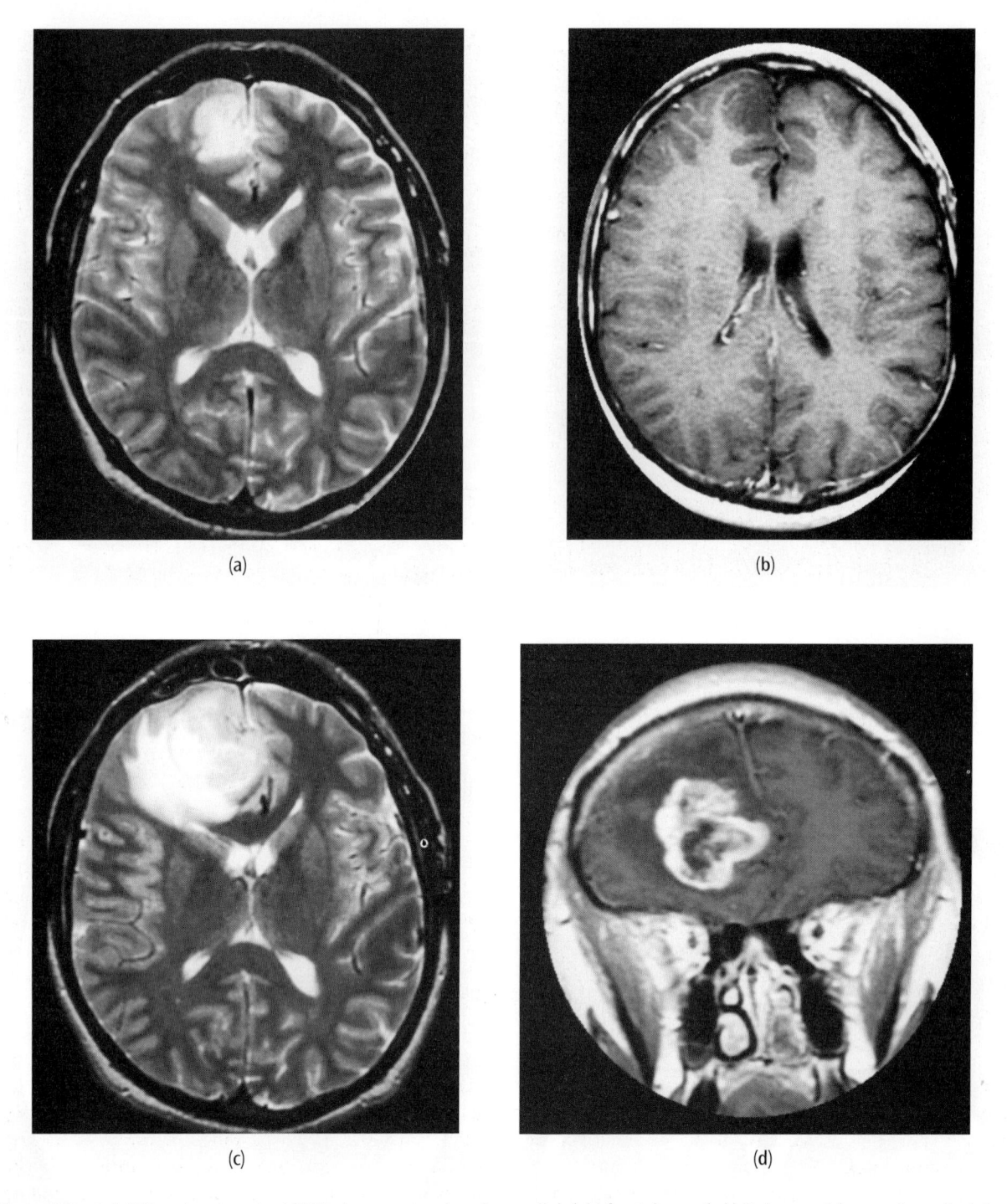

Figure 3.3. Axial T2 and post-contrast T1WI show a non-enhancing medial right frontal mass (a,b). Subsequent images 6 months later, the patient having refused biopsy, show that the lesion has changed its nature and there is now irregular contrast-enhancement, central necrosis and prominent oedema and mass effect (c,d). The lesion was glioblastoma at biopsy.

evident on CT. The most common pattern is ring enhancement; the enhancing rim is thick-walled and irregular, similar to that seen in a metastasis, but different from the smooth thin-walled rim seen in an abscess. Often, however, a glioma will not demonstrate contrast-enhancement, particularly (but not exclusively) if it is low grade; or the enhancement will be in a nodular, linear or diffuse pattern.

Low-grade tumours need to be distinguished from hamartomas and tubers, as well as vascular malformations, since true arteriovenous malformations and cavernous haemangiomas may present as calcified cerebral lesions. Vascular lesions will usually have a characteristic MRI appearance but hamartomas often cannot be distinguished radiologically from low-grade glioma. It is worth emphasizing that a lack of contrast-enhancement

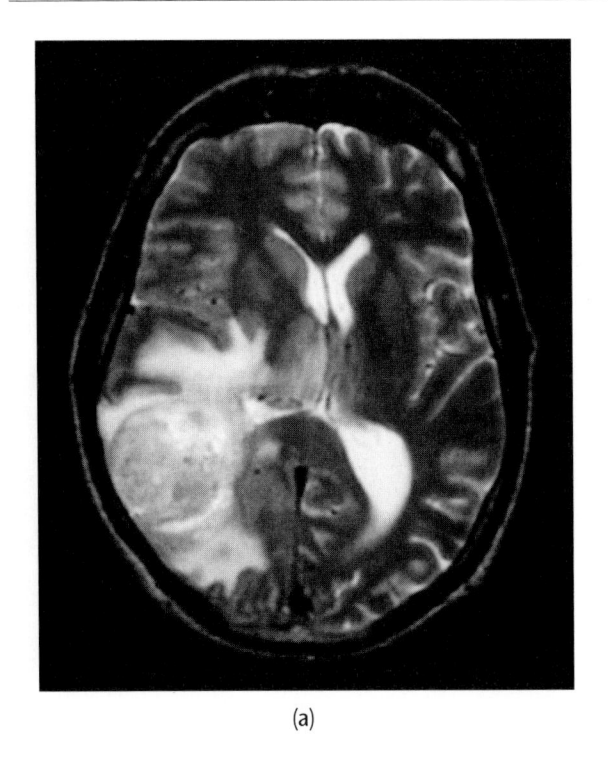

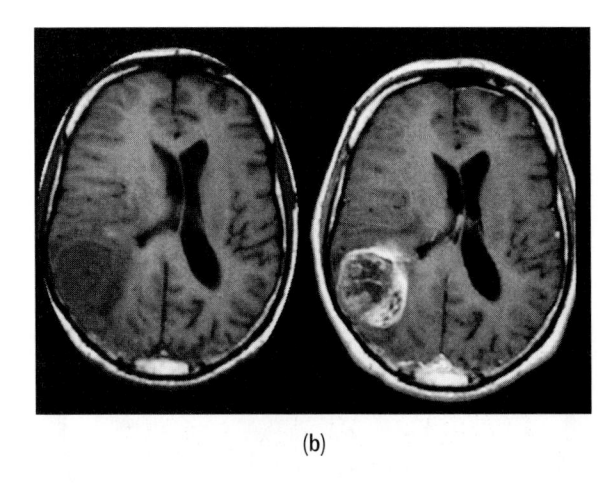

Figure 3.4. Axial T2 pre- (a) and post-contrast (b) axial T1-weighted scans. These are typical features of an agressive high grade glioma with mass effect, midline shift, compression of the trigone, oedema and thick-walled irregular ring-enhancement.

does not exclude glioma. Cerebral primitive neuroectodermal tumours (PNETs) can have identical appearances to gliomas, and the two can be inseparable, particularly in children. Dysembryoplastic neuroepithelial tumours (DNTs) have a typical location and imaging findings (see below) but in an unusual site may mimic a glioma. Primary cerebral lymphoma can usually be identified due to its site and characteristic appearance. Occasionally, a solitary large plaque of demyelination will mimic a tumour, and most surgical series of brain biopsy for tumour contain a few plaques of multiple sclerosis. Similarly, Behçet's and Whipple's disease may rarely mimic a tumour. Langerhans' histiocytosis can present with cerebral or cerebellar mass lesions which are usually multiple, iso- or hyperdense to grey matter, enhance homogenously and are periventricular in location (Fig. 3.5). The clinical picture almost invariably includes diabetes insipidus with an infundibular or hypothalamic mass.

High-grade glioma must be differentiated from abscess and metastasis, which are predominantly found at the grey/white boundary and are associated with a large amount of surrounding vasogenic oedema.

Abscesses have a smooth thin rim of contrast-enhancement, while metastases are irregular, thick-walled and usually multiple. Of course solitary metastasis and multifocal glioma are recognized findings so that primary and secondary brain tumours can sometimes be hard to separate.

It should, however, always be possible to distinguish an infarct by its characteristic distribution and prominent grey matter involvement. In those rare occasions where both the clinical presentation and the imaging findings cannot separate infarction from glioma, then a follow-up scan in 6–8 weeks time will demonstrate the typical evolution of an infarct.

Oligodendroglioma

Oligodendroglioma is a relatively uncommon tumour most usually found in a superficial position in the frontal or temporal lobes, but occurring also in the ventricles (cf central neurocytoma), cerebellum and rarely in the spinal cord. Up to half contain elements of other cell lines and are classified as 'mixed' tumours. On CT and MRI they exhibit a range of findings depending on their grade (Fig. 3.6).[3] Often on MRI their T2-weighted intensity is similar to grey matter – i.e. of somewhat lower signal than a 'typical' astrocytoma, but otherwise they mimic astrocytoma in the range of possible imaging appearances. A very indolent tumour may erode the overlying skull vault and this finding will often be more readily seen by CT than MRI. Cystic necrosis and haemorrhage are common in high-grade lesions. Linear or nodular calcification is seen in most and is more apparent on T2*WI than with spin-echo techniques. The calcification, when seen, is usually much heavier than that seen in an astrocytoma.

Other variants of glioma

Xanthoastrocytoma is seen in children and young adults. It is an indolent, cystic tumour, most often arising in temporal or parietal lobes, usually with an enhancing

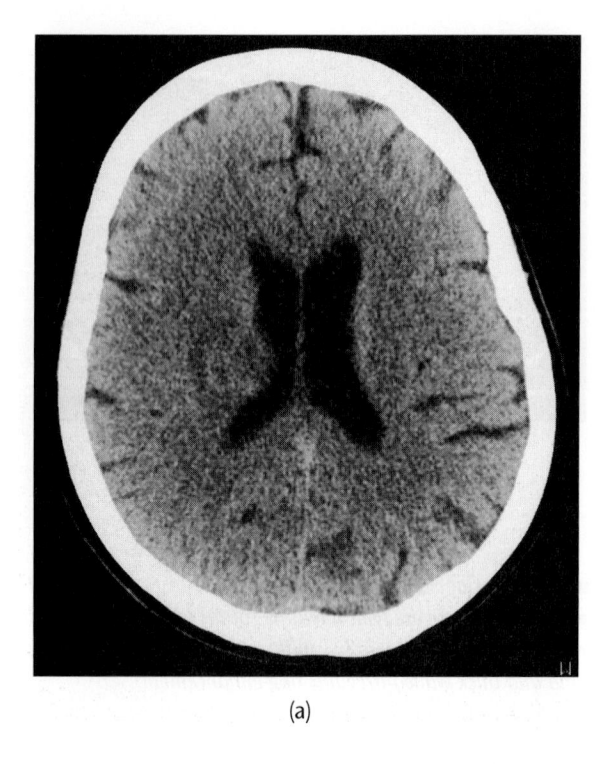

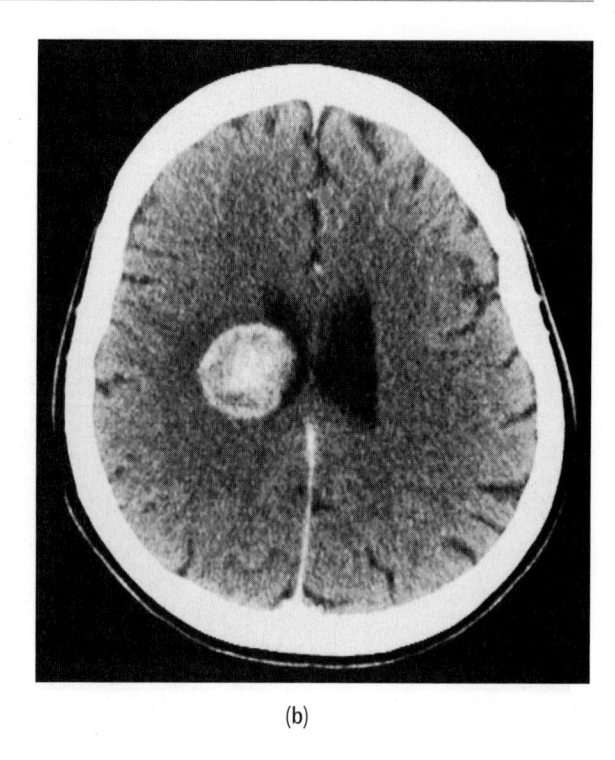

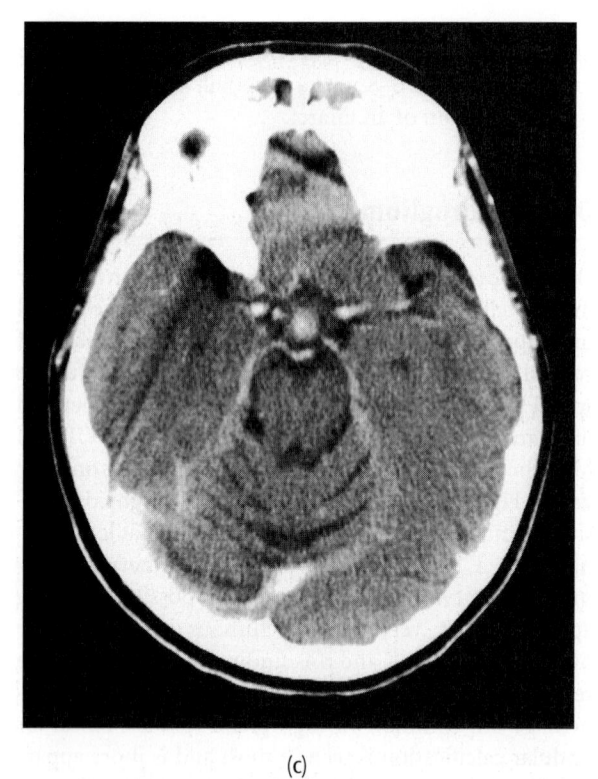

Figure 3.5. Pre- (a) and post-contrast (b),(c) CT images. Histocytosis. This characteristically involves the pituitary stalk which is the best clue to the otherwise non-specific appearance of the tumour.

mural nodule. Characteristically there is thinning of the overlying calvarium (Fig. 3.7), and there may be calcification. The lesion carries a relatively good prognosis and is sometimes completely excised.[4]

Giant cell astrocytoma arises exclusively in patients with tuberous sclerosis and represents neoplastic change within a tuber (Fig. 3.8). It characteristically arises at the foramen of Monro, causing hydrocephalus but may rarely grow within brain tissue. Typically it is hyperdense on CT scans and enhances brightly and almost uniformly. Calcification is present in the majority. The diagnosis is usually easy due to the coincident multiple lesions of tuberous sclerosis.

Gliomatosis cerebri usually presents between the second and fourth decades, but can be seen in children. Presentation is non-specific, often with personality and

Intra-axial tumours 105

(a)

(b)

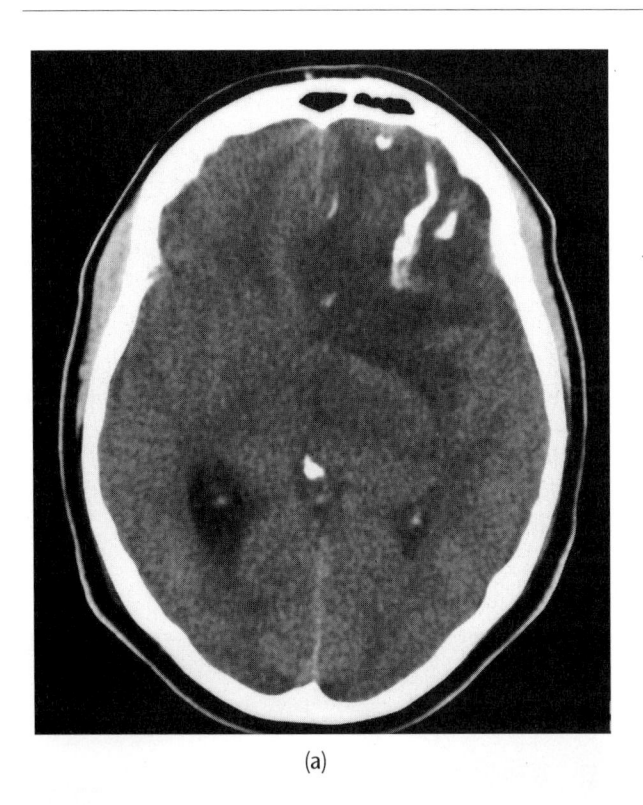

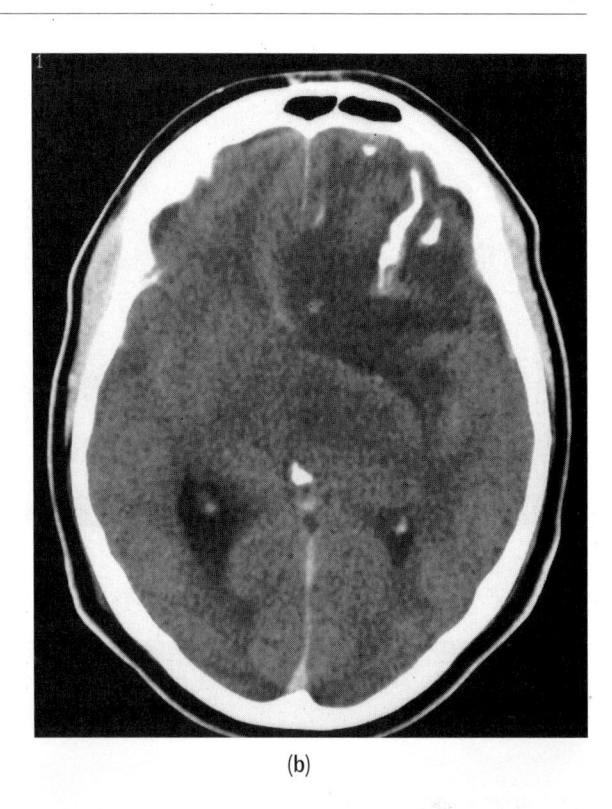

Figure 3.6. Axial pre- (a) and post-contrast (b) CT scans. There is a left frontal mass extending into the corpus callosum with prominent oedema and craggy calcification. There is a minimal contrast-enhancement. The calcification is typical of that seen in oligodendroglioma.

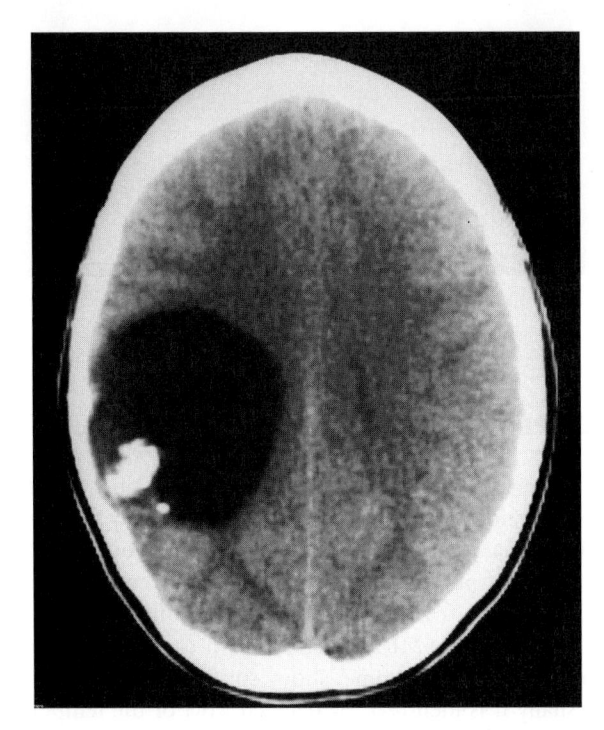

Figure 3.7. Axial-enhanced CT scan. There is a large mainly cystic intrinsic mass lesion with a calcified mural nodule. The overlying calvarium is thinned. Histology was of xanthoastrocytoma.

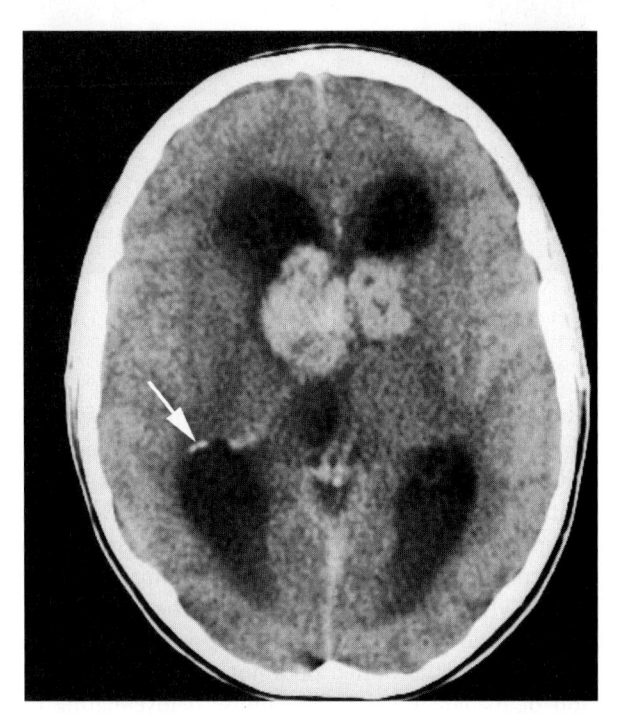

Figure 3.8. Axial-enhanced CT scan through the foramen of Monro. Giant cell astrocytoma. There is a lobulated patchily-enhancing mass at the foramen of Monro extending into both frontal horns. Patchy calcification is present on the uncontrasted scan. A calcified subependymal tumour is seen at the right trigone (arrow).

Figure 3.9. Coronal T1WI (a) (TR/TE = 500/25, 0.5T) and T2WI (b) (2400/95) weighted images. There is a mass within the mesial temporal lobe centred in grey matter around the collateral sulcus. There is mass effect and patchy, mainly rim, enhancement. This is a typical location and appearance of DNT.

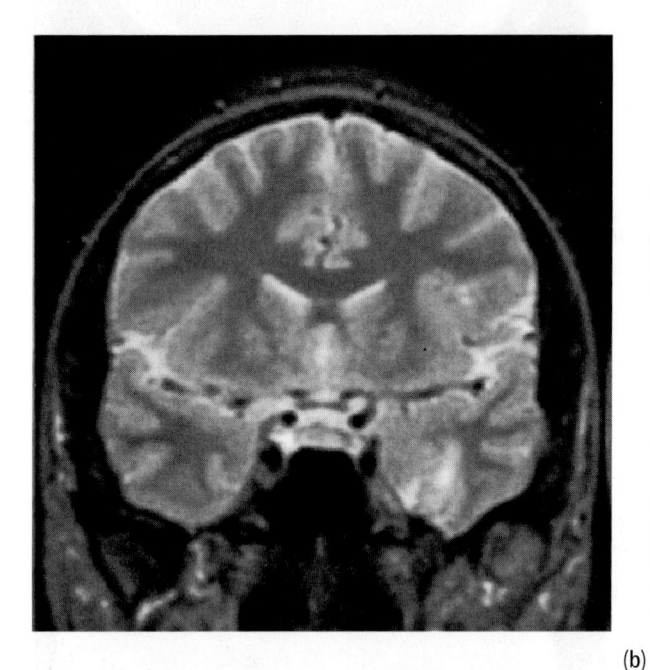

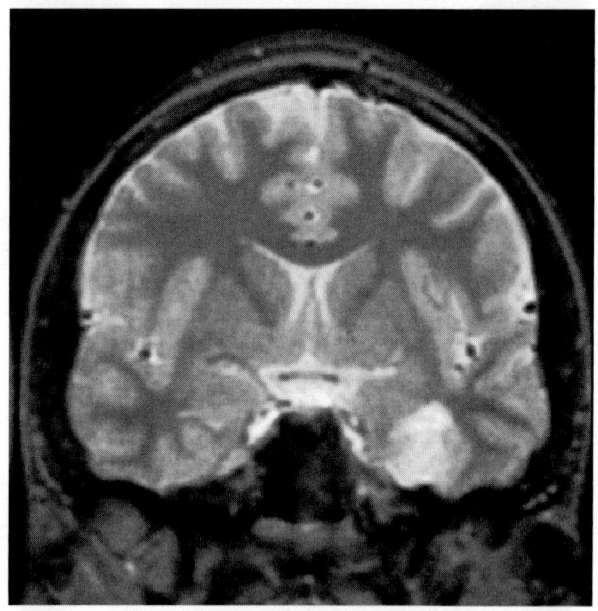

mental state change, and often symptoms and signs of raised intracranial pressure are absent. Pathologically and on imaging studies, the brain (both grey and white matter) is diffusely involved with relative preservation of the underlying structure and function. The basal ganglia are commonly involved. Mass effect is minimal and there is usually no contrast-enhancement.[5] The diagnosis is usually made at brain biopsy or autopsy, since the combination of features often does not raise clinical suspicion of malignancy – rather diffuse demyelinating or metabolic conditions are suspected.

Supratentorial pilocytic astrocytomas usually arise in the optic chiasm or hypothalamus. They have a heterogeneous appearance often with irregular contrast-enhancement and sometimes with small intralesional cysts.[6]

Dysembryoplastic neuroepithelial tumour

This recently recognized tumour has a distinct clinical picture, location and appearance.[7] It is usually found in the mesial temporal lobe of children and young adults suffering from long-term epilepsy, usually complex partial seizures. It is frequently small and often missed on CT and routine MRI scans. On CT it can be hypodense or calcified and some show contrast enhancement. Usually it is identified by detailed MRI of the temporal lobes. It is situated in grey matter, most commonly around the collateral sulcus. The cortex may appear thickened, or there may be a focal mass. The grey/white matter differentiation is usually blurred, evidence of the dysembryoplastic nature of the tumour, and contrast-enhancement may be seen, particularly in children (Fig.

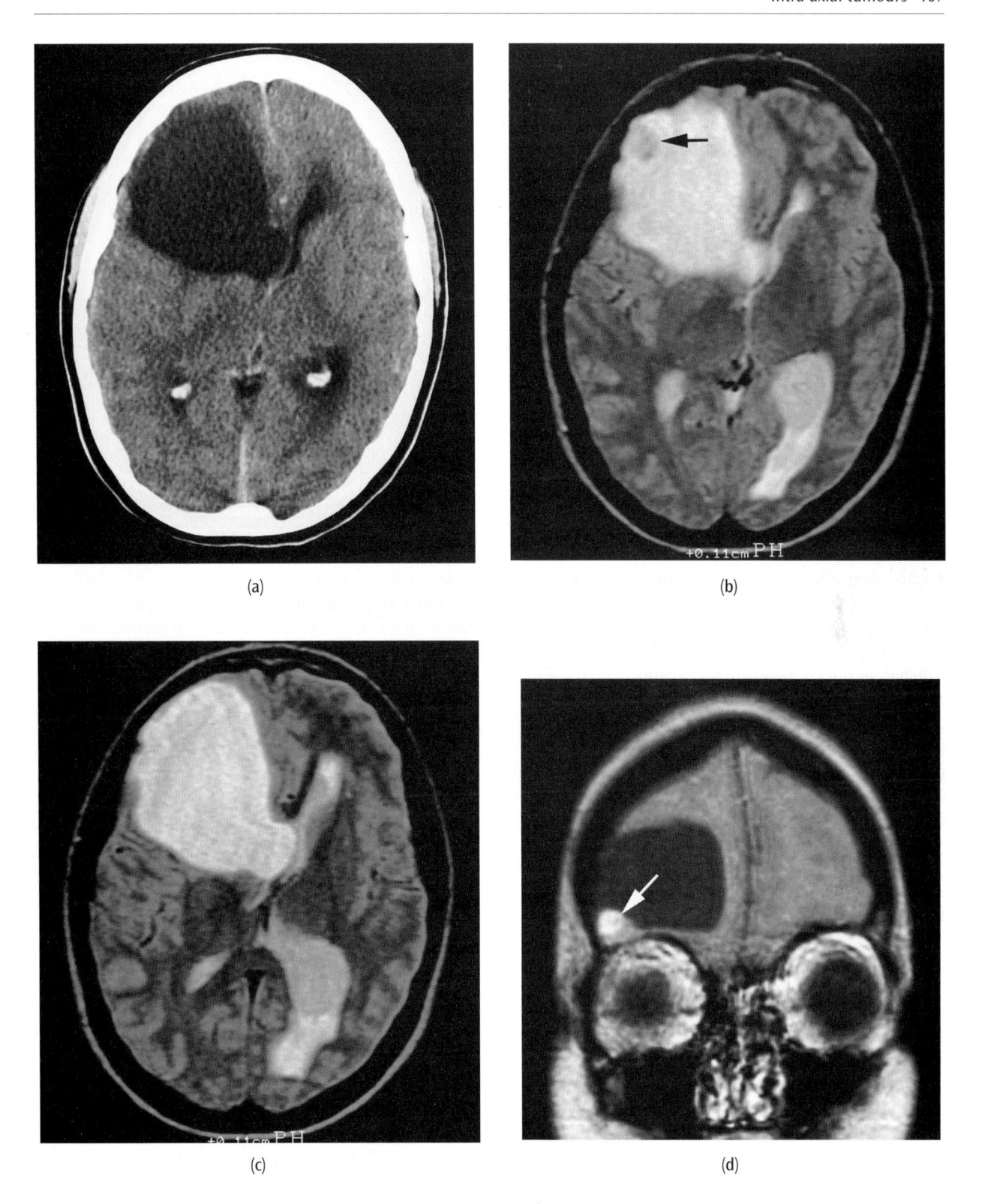

Figure 3.10. *Axial contrast-enhanced CT (a), axial T2-weighted (b),(c) and coronal T1-weighted post-contrast MRI (d). A large, mainly cystic frontal lobe ganglioglioma is demonstrated. There is a small solid nodule in the tumour base (arrow in (b) which enhances (arrow in (d)). Cyst signal/density is similar or slightly greater than CSF. Note hydrocephalus of the left lateral ventricle due to tumour compression of the foramen of Monro.*

3.9). The importance of the lesion is that it can nearly always be completely excised, and even incomplete excision will result in considerable improvement in seizure control. Many of these tumours have been called low-grade gliomas or hamartomas in the past but the success of surgery means that this lesion should be sought and recognized when present.

Ganglioglioma

This is a tumour of mixed cell type containing neural and glial elements. It presents in children and young adults typically in the temporal lobe but may arise in the spinal cord or posterior fossa as well as in the suprasellar region. It is almost always a well circumscribed lesion containing cysts and calcification. Mass effect is not a prominent feature and there is little or no surrounding vasogenic oedema. Irregular contrast-enhancement usually but not always occurs (Fig. 3.10).[8] Because they commonly occur in the temporal lobe, are well defined and have a benign nature, excision is often possible and so this tumour carries a relatively good prognosis.

The main differential lies between low-grade glioma and gangliocytoma, a rare variation on ganglioglioma which does not contain neural elements.[9] Often CT and MRI fail to differentiate these entities and the histological differences between ganglioglioma and gangliocytoma can be small. Neuronal heterotopia may rarely present as a mass lesion but its signal characteristics and CT density are always identical to grey matter and there is usually evidence of local failure of myelination and/or abnormal gyration.

Primitive neuroectodermal tumour

This is one of the two commonest cerebral tumours of childhood. In the cerebellar vermis PNET is known as medulloblastoma, but the term PNET is more common for cerebral tumours, although 'cerebral neuroblastoma' is sometimes also used.

When arising above the tentorium, the tumour is indistinguishable from an aggressive glioma, with variable CT density and MR signal intensity according to the amount of intratumoral haemorrhage, cyst formation or calcification present (Fig. 3.11).[10] Contrast-enhancement is to be expected but is not invariable and when present, may be patchy or inhomogeneous.

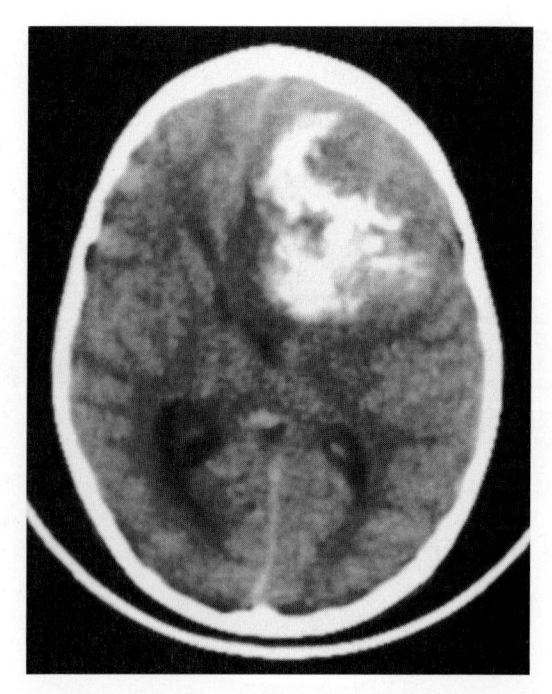

Figure 3.11. *Axial contrast-enhanced CT scan of PNET. There is a large heavily calcified left frontal tumour which extends into the genu of the corpus callosum. It has gross mass effect but the non-calcified portions of the tumour showed relatively little contrast-enhancement. This lesion is indistinguishable from glioma.*

Although around half arise in the first 5 years of life, an aggressive cerebral tumour in a young child is just as likely to be due to a glioma as a PNET. Spread outside the central nervous system (CNS), particularly to bone, is rarely seen but seeding within the subarachnoid space is common and best detected by contrast-enhanced MRI.

Lymphoma

Cerebral lymphoma may arise *de novo* in the brain or may spread usually to the meninges from lymphoma at other sites. Primary cerebral lymphoma is nearly always of the non-Hodgkin's type and occurs most commonly after the fifth decade.[11] Although rare, it is being seen more frequently in recent years in immunocompromised patients and is one of the defining criteria for the diagnosis of AIDS (acquired immunodeficiency syndrome). Most present as supratentorial masses and up to half are multiple. Primary lymphoma has a strong

Figure 3.12. (facing page) *Primary cerebral lymphoma. Axial pre- (a) and post- (b) CT scans; axial spin-density (c); T2-weighted (d); coronal T1WI pre- and post-contrast (e). There is a mass in the mesial temporal lobe extending medially to involve the optic chiasm. It is very slightly hyperdense to grey matter on pre-contrast scans and enhances brightly and homogeneously. The lesion is more obvious on spin density (c) than T2 (d) MR images, where its periventricular location and extent of the mass are apparent. Post-contrast coronal T1-weighted MR images demonstrate the medial spread of the tumour to involve hypothalamus and optic chiasm (arrow).*

Intra-axial tumours 109

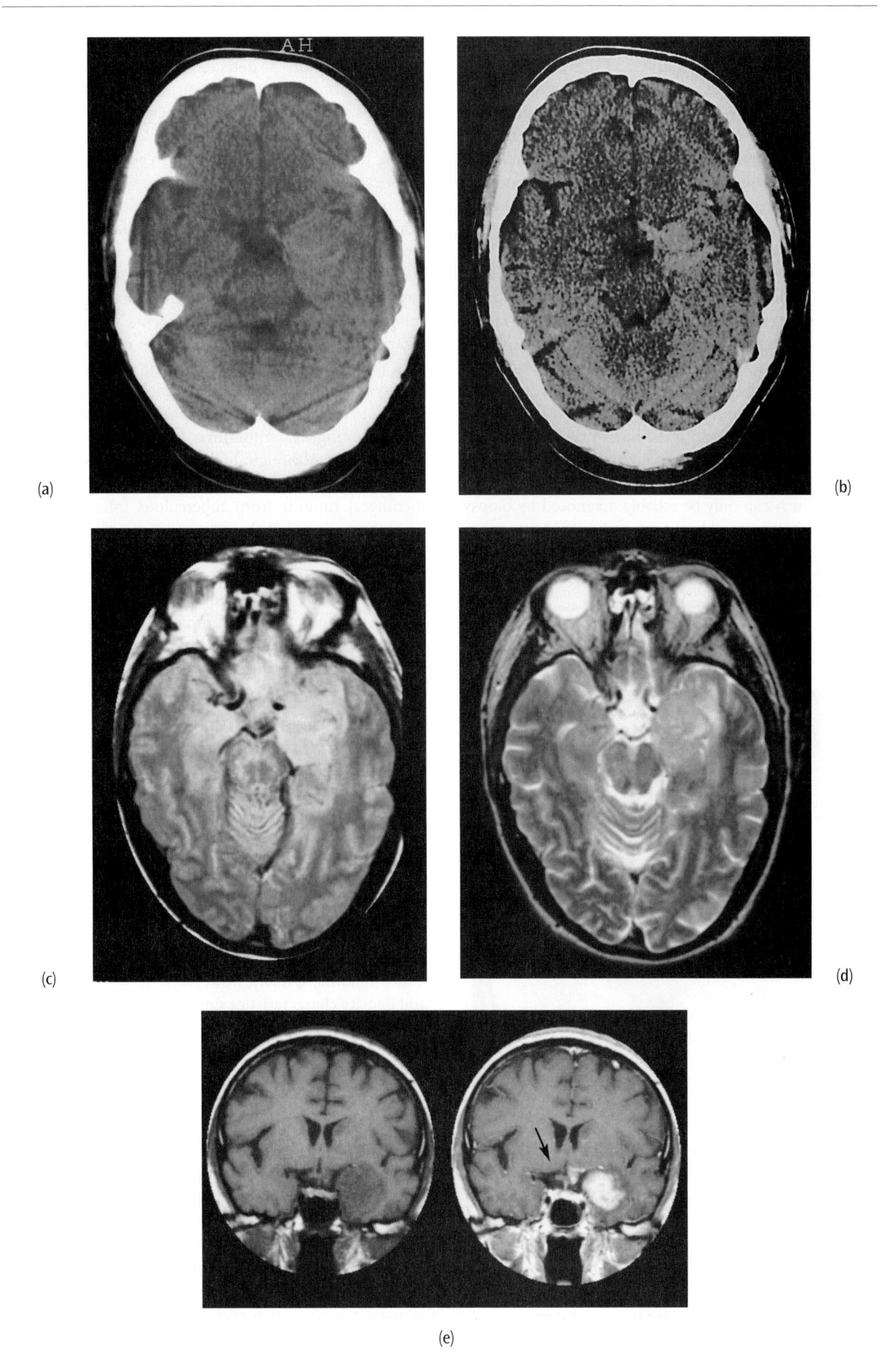

(a) (b)
(c) (d)
(e)

Figure 3.12

predilection for the periventricular white matter or may arise within the ventricles (Figs 3.12, 3.13). The deep grey matter and corpus callosum are also common sites. Characteristically, lymphoma is hyperdense to grey matter on CT, well defined, and enhances brightly and homogeneously. In AIDS patients, lymphoma may behave differently than in the general population and ring enhancement is the commonest pattern of enhancement. Calcification is not seen and surrounding oedema is not usually a prominent feature. While some lymphomas will be hyperintense to white matter on T1WI, they may also be isointense to grey matter on all sequences, or even markedly hyperintense to grey matter on T2WI. Intratumoral haemorrhage is rarely, if ever, seen. The diagnosis is usually clear in immune-competent patients but if there is immune compromise, the lesions cannot confidently be distinguished from infections such as toxoplasmosis. Failure of response of such a patient to standard toxoplasmosis chemotherapy within 2–3 weeks should raise the possibility of lymphoma which can only be reliably diagnosed by biopsy. Although corticosteroids can cause the rapid disappearance, even within hours, of cerebral lymphoma in the immune competent, this effect is not seen in the immune-compromised.

Metastatic lymphoma almost always involves the leptomeninges and is detected as abnormal contrast enhancement which coats the surface of the brain, brainstem or spinal cord (Fig. 3.14). Focal masses are far less common in metastatic disease.

The differential diagnosis of a hyperdense lesion on CT includes cavernous haemangioma which has characteristic appearances on MRI, while multiple lesions may mimic metastases. Meningeal-based lesions carry a differential diagnosis of leukaemia, and metastases (especially from breast and melanoma, both of which can have short relaxation times). Infection with syphilis, tuberculosis or other bacterial agents will cause leptomeningeal enhancement, often with infarction due to a localized arteritis of the penetrating small vessels, and rare syndromes such as neurocutaneous melanosis may present in this way. In AIDS, cryptococcal infection starts as a meningitis, sometimes extending into brain parenchyma. Although lumbar puncture will usually point to infection, it may not easily differentiate meningeal tumour from tuberculous infection. When presenting as a durally based mass, meningioma and sarcoid should be considered.

Dural enhancement, in the absence of other abnormality, should be interpreted with caution as it is a non-specific finding and is commonly seen after shunt insertion or even diagnostic lumbar puncture, with no pathological significance.

Aesthesioneuroblastoma

This tumour arises in or around the cribriform plate, from the olfactory nerves, bulb or mucosa. The cribriform plate is invariably involved on both sides but often in an asymmetric manner. Most often the bulk of the tumour is below it, but this lesion can present as a large frontal intracranial tumour which extends below the skull base. The characteristic location is the key to its recognition. Occasionally there can be local hyperostosis so that the intracranial portion of the tumour can mimic a meningioma. Usually, however, it appears with signal and density characteristics similar to other nasal or sinus tumours and shows bright homogeneous enhancement except in those portions of an aggressive lesion which have necrosed.[12]

Metastases

Brain metastases comprise about 20% of clinically detected cerebral tumours, but have been reported in almost 25% of patients with cancer at autopsy. Around 80% occur above the tentorium and present with symptoms and signs according to their anatomical location. Clinically silent metastases occur particularly with small cell or adenocarcinoma of the lung, and melanoma. It is clear from the literature that contrast-enhanced scans

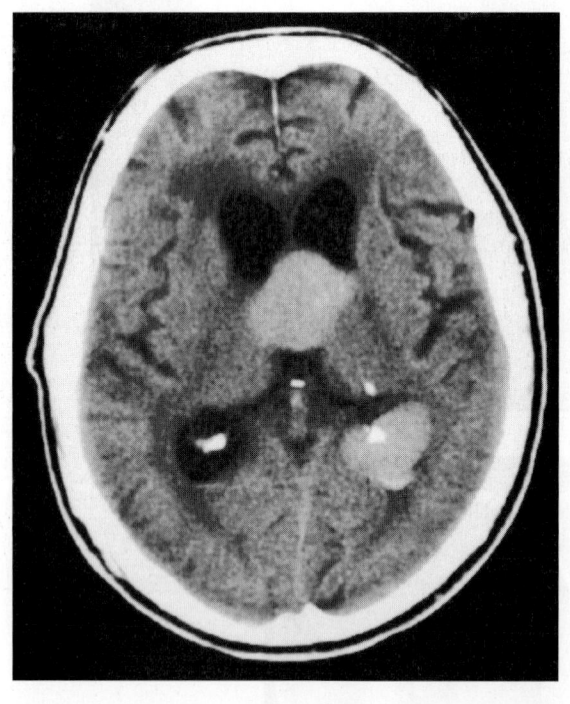

Figure 3.13. *Axial post-contrast CT scan. Ventricular lymphoma. There are homogeneously enhancing masses at the foramen of Monro and in the left trigone, the latter surrounding but not destroying calcification at the glomus of the choroid plexus. The ventricles are dilated with periventricular white matter low density. The fleck of high density in the left thalamus represents the lowermost end of a ventricular shunt tube.*

(a)

(b)

(c)

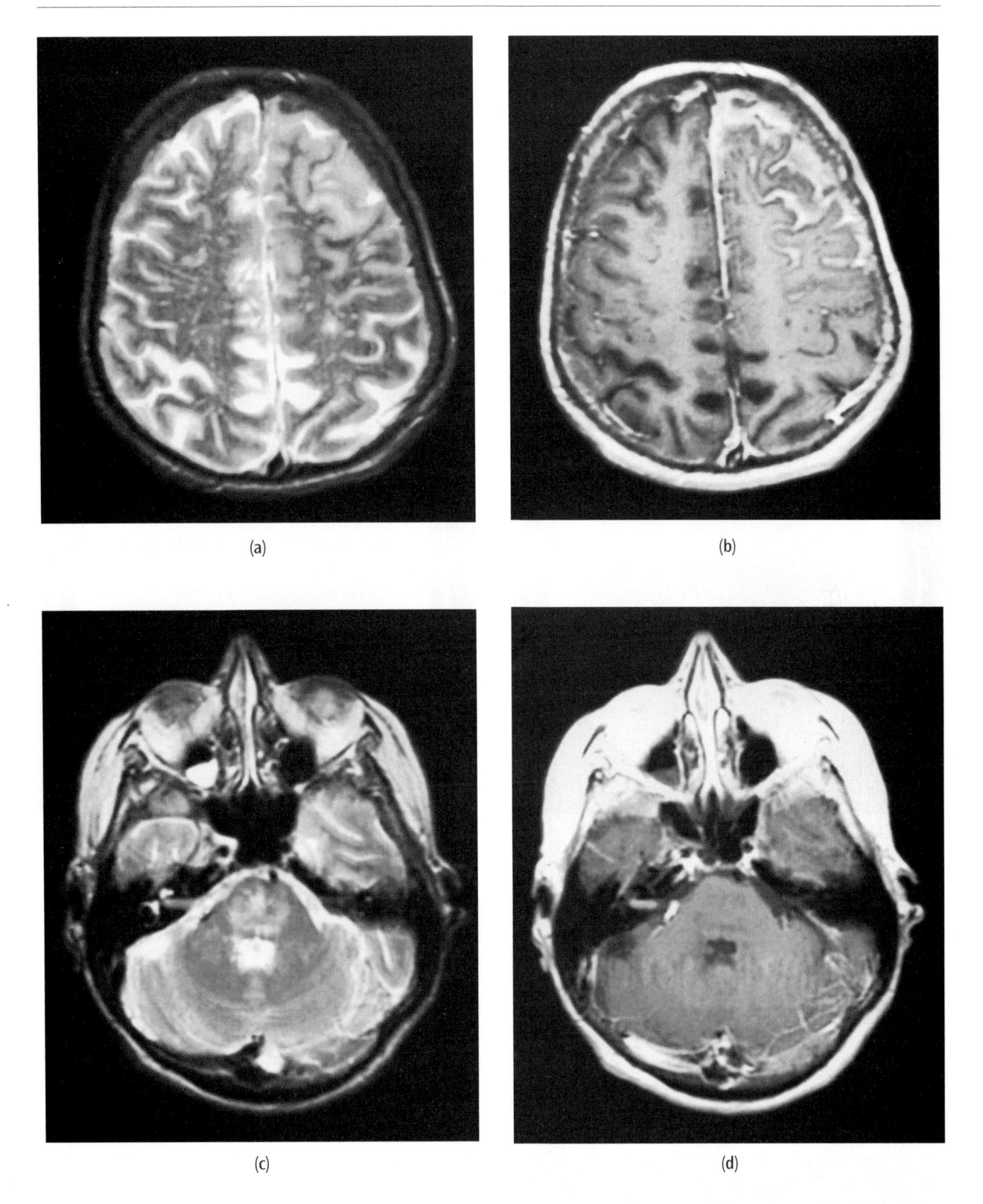

(d)

Figure 3.14. *Axial T2 (a) and post-contrast T1WI (b) show gyral thickening in the left frontal lobe and extensive associated leptomeningeal enhancement over most of this hemisphere. Further T2 (c) and post-contrast T1 (d) images through the pons shows signal change within the neural axis and an enhancing mass within the internal auditory meatus, again representing meningeal spread of lymphoma.*

detect more lesions than uncontrasted ones and that enhanced MRI is more sensitive than enhanced CT.[13] However, not every enhancing lesion is a metastatic deposit, and so post-contrast scans have to be read with caution. It is clinically important to identify those patients with a solitary metastasis (most commonly seen in carcinoma of the lung or breast, or melanoma) since there may be a surgical option and in this case contrast-enhanced MR is advisable to pick up other undetected deposits (Fig. 3.15). Similarly, in the staging of cancer, particularly those with a predilection for spread to the brain, contrast-enhanced MRI is indicated because the patient's treatment and prognosis may be substantially altered by finding a clinically silent metastasis. However, in the presence of numerous lesions typical of metastases on plain scans, the value of contrast enhancement is doubtful.

Some lesions may be particularly difficult to detect on plain scans and these include deposits within the cerebral cortex which tend not to excite oedema, and small

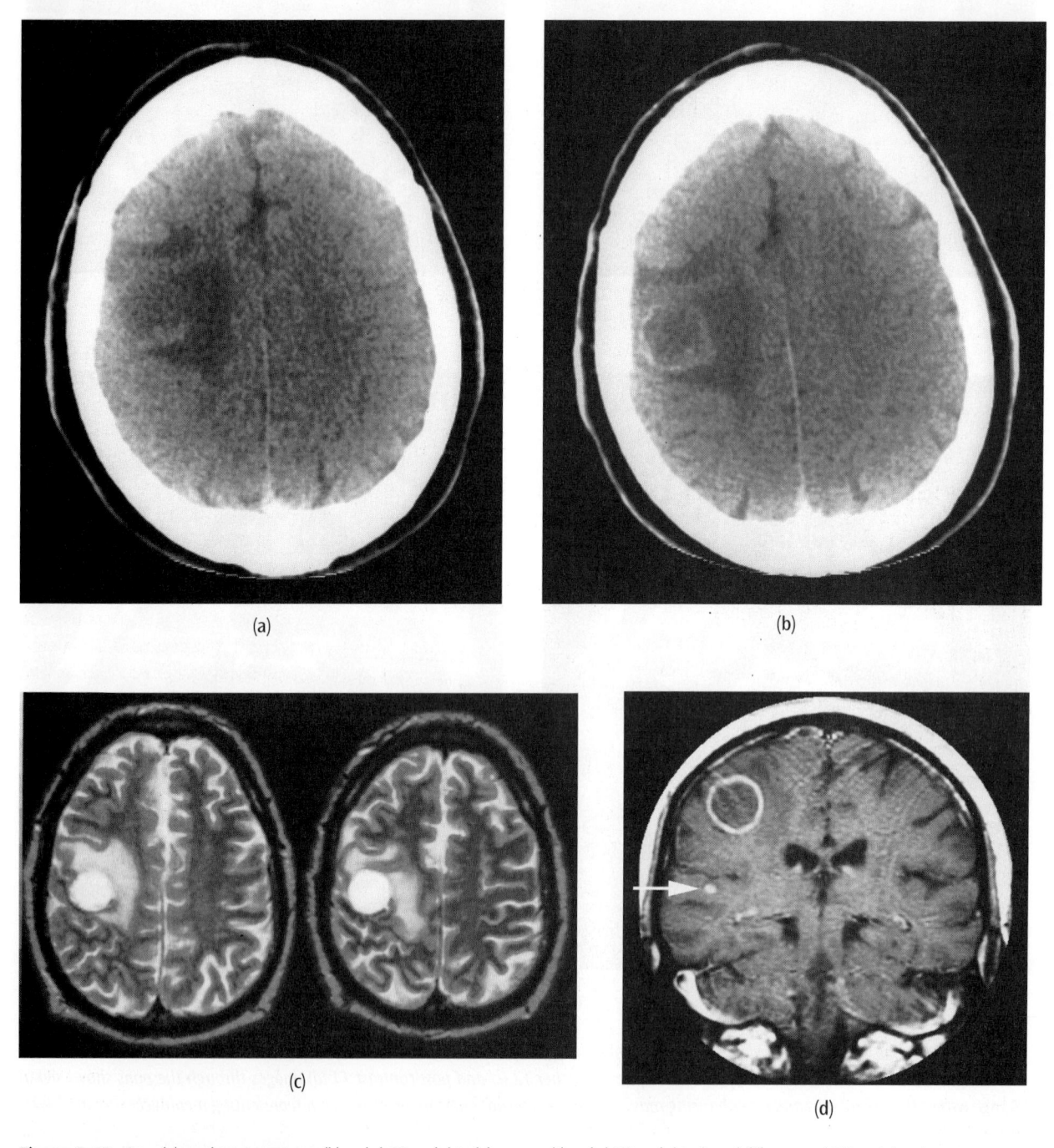

Figure 3.15. *Pre- (a) and post-contrast (b) axial CT weighted images; (c) axial T2-weighted and (d) coronal T1-weighted post-contrast MRI. There is a ring density at the grey/white matter junction of the posterior right frontal lobe which shows the typical mural enhancement of a metastasis. There is extensive localized vasogenic oedema. No other lesion was evident on CT but MRI demonstrated this lesion (c) and a second (arrow) in the superior temporal gyrus (d).*

lesions against a brain/CSF interface, which may be hidden on T2WI. Posterior fossa and anterior temporal lesions are commonly obscured on CT by beam-hardening artifact.

Most metastases are found at the grey/white interface, due to the small size of penetrating arteries at this site – metastatic abscesses occur here for the same reason. They are most common in the larger cerebral lobes. Typically they are associated with copious and almost disproportionate amounts of white matter oedema (Fig. 3.16), which tends not to spread across the corpus callosum, in contradistinction to that surrounding a glioma. Calcification is rare, but can be seen from a bony primary or some adenocarcinomas. Haemorrhagic metastases may appear hyperdense to grey matter on CT and this should not be mistaken for calcification. Some lesions, notably melanoma metastases, have short T1 times; in the case of melanoma this is said to be a direct effect of the short T1 of melanin, but amelanotic melanomas may have a similar appearance. Some metastases are micro-haemorrhagic, particularly those from breast, kidney, melanoma, and gestational trophoblastic disease, including choriocarcinoma: these may also have short T1 (and also T2) times. In some cases tumoral necrosis has been shown to shorten rather than prolong relaxation times.

Contrast-enhancement is to be expected but is not invariable. Small lesions usually demonstrate solid or nodular enhancement but as the metastasis grows it may outstrip its blood supply causing central necrosis. Such a lesion will then have a thick-walled irregular enhancing rim, with a lower density centre which approaches CSF density/intensity and does not enhance. Some studies have demonstrated that within an individual patient, some enhancing lesions (and therefore presumed metastases) may only be apparent on a delayed post-contrast scan, while others are apparent on immediate and delayed scans. However, most centres do not routinely perform delayed scans in the search for a cerebral metastasis. Double or even triple dose MR contrast-enhancement regimes have been described to increase the sensitivity of the detection of brain metastases, but this is at the expense of an increased number of false-positive results.[14]

Frank haemorrhage occurs in up to 20% of metastases. The resulting haematoma may obscure the underlying tumour and camouflage its enhancement, becoming apparent only on follow-up scans.

The differential diagnosis of a solitary large ring-enhancing mass lies between an abscess, which will usually have a smooth thin wall sometimes with short T1 and T2 times and a glioma, which may have less oedema, or oedema which passes across the corpus callosum. The former diagnosis should always be borne in mind, since it represents a lesion which is potentially both fatal and curable. It is a good rule to assess potential sources of infection such as the middle ear and paranasal sinuses when faced with such a lesion; if the scan shows for example extensive frontal sinusitis, then consider the possibility of abscess even if the imaging findings are not typical. Often, malignant glioma cannot be reliably distinguished from a solitary metastasis and these lesions are usually biopsied for a definitive diagnosis.

Multiple enhancing lesions can be seen on a variety of inflammatory conditions including multiple sclerosis, acute disseminated encephalomyelitis (ADEM), sarcoid, Whipple's disease, systemic lupus erythematosus (SLE), Behçet's disease and so on, but in these conditions perilesional oedema is absent or at least not a prominent feature. Multiple lesions associated with oedema raise the possibility of multifocal glioma or radiation necrosis. The first of these can be indistinguishable from metastases, except that the enhancing lesions of multifocal glioma are usually close to one another. Radiation necrosis can often be inferred from the history and typical clinical time course and will show evidence of decreased perfusion on single photon emission computed tomography (SPECT) or positron emission tomography (PET) scans. Microhaemorrhagic metastases can be indistinguishable from cerebral tuberculosis as both can produce multiple lesions which are of short T1 and T2 compared with normal brain.

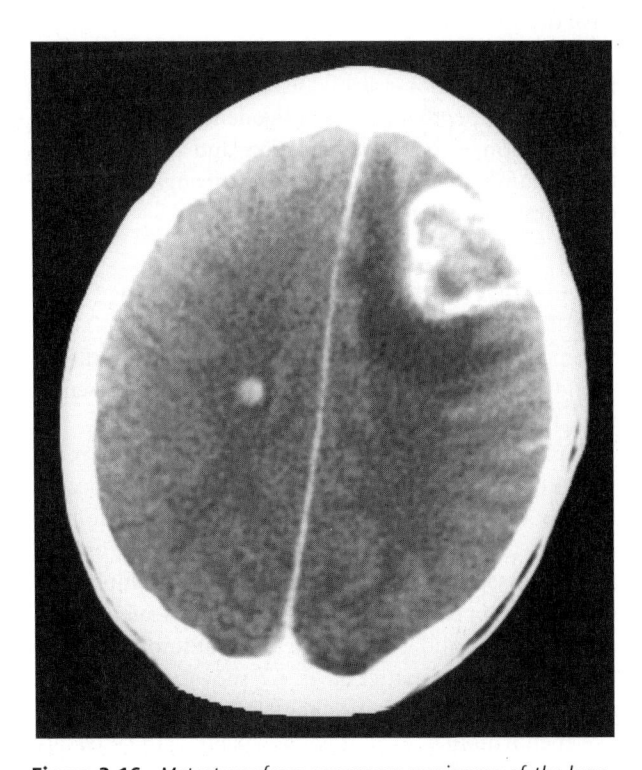

Figure 3.16. *Metastases from squamous carcinoma of the lung. Two types of metastasis are evident on this post-contrast CT scan. In the left frontal lobe there is a typical irregular thick-walled rim-enhancing lesion with copious surrounding vasogenic oedema but there is a second solid, homogeneously enhancing lesion in the medial white matter of the right frontal lobe.*

INTRAVENTRICULAR TUMOURS

Ventricular tumours can arise from any cell line of tissue normally found in the ventricular system. In addition, tumours such as glioma and meningioma can occur in a ventricle and are said to arise from embryonic cellular rests. Ventricular tumours usually present with hydrocephalus due to obstruction of CSF flow or to overproduction of CSF. They may spread locally, sometimes invading normal brain, or seed throughout the ventricles and subarachnoid space. Contrast-enhancement is usually required to detect the latter and consideration should be given to imaging the spine by MRI to detect drop metastases when a cerebral ventricular tumour is detected.

Ependymoma

In adults, ependymoma most commonly arises in the lateral ventricles, or spinal cord, but in childhood, it is most frequent in the fourth ventricle. It is characteristically irregular, with cysts, haemorrhage and calcification in about half of all cases and is inhomogeneous in density, signal intensity and contrast-enhancement (Fig. 3.17),[15] reflecting its heterogeneous matrix. Typically, when arising in the lateral ventricles of an adult, it extends locally to invade brain tissue. Seeding of tumour cells throughout the CSF, most commonly to the lumbosacral spinal canal, is common and should be routinely sought with enhanced MRI.

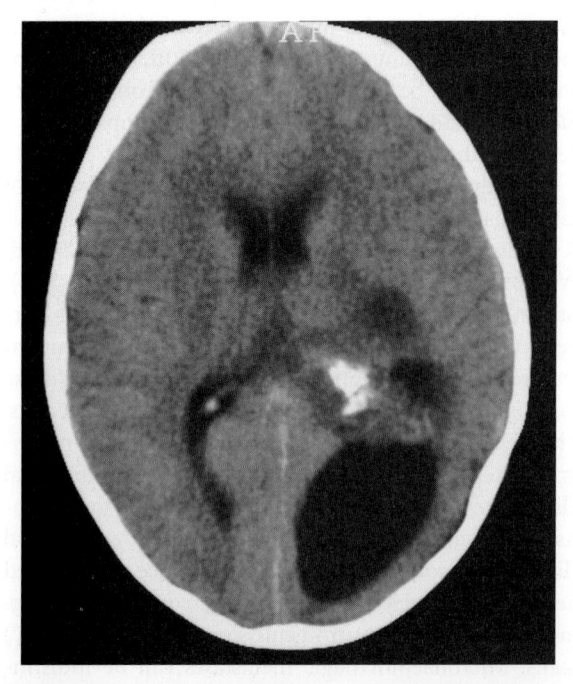

Figure 3.17. *Axial uncontrasted CT scan showing a partly calcified mass in the left trigone, trapping the occipital horn. It is irregular in outline and density and is typical of ependymoma.*

Ependymoma can usually be separated from meningioma by the characteristic appearance of the latter but can be indistinguishable from intraventricular glioma and central neurocytoma by imaging.[16] Generally, PNET appears as a homogeneously enhancing, less irregular mass. Occasionally ependymoma will arise *de novo* within brain substance, allegedly from cell rests and in this position is indistinguishable from cerebral glioma.

Central neurocytoma

Central neurocytoma was first recognized in 1982, when a histological reclassification of ependymomas and intraventricular gliomas showed many of them to have neuronal markers. They occur in young adults who present with signs of raised intracranial pressure. The typical lesion arises from the septum pellucidum or lateral ventricular wall (Fig. 3.18). Nearly all are found in the lateral ventricles, although large lesions can extend into the third and fourth ventricles. Approximately half show multiple small calcifications, and most are well circumscribed. Local spread into brain tissue and large calcified masses are recorded, but unusual. The MRI signal intensity resembles that of grey matter and there is moderate, usually inhomogeneous, contrast-enhancement.[17] Although originally described as a benign tumour which can be completely resected, more malignant varieties have been recognized.[18]

The imaging findings, like traditional light microscopy, cannot reliably separate central neurocytoma from ependymoma or oligodendroglioma, but a combination of good demarcation and attachment to the septum pellucidum are features strongly suggestive of central neurocytoma.

Subependymoma

Subependymoma is usually considered a variant of ependymoma but it has very different clinical presentation, appearance and outcome.

Typically, it arises in a middle-aged or elderly man, most commonly in the fourth ventricle but also occurring in the lateral and third ventricles where it may obstruct CSF flow. In the lateral ventricles, it usually abuts the septum pellucidum. It can be multiple and sometimes appears in the spinal cord. Small subependymomas are solid, homogeneous tumours, usually brighter than grey matter on T2WI, showing either no or moderate contrast-enhancement.[19] Larger lesions may, like ependymomas, exhibit heterogeneity with cysts, calcification and haemorrhage and tend to demonstrate more intense contrast-enhancement. Generally, however, they are indolent tumours which do not invade brain tissue, and are commonly discovered as incidental findings at autopsy.

When small, the lesions can be confused with

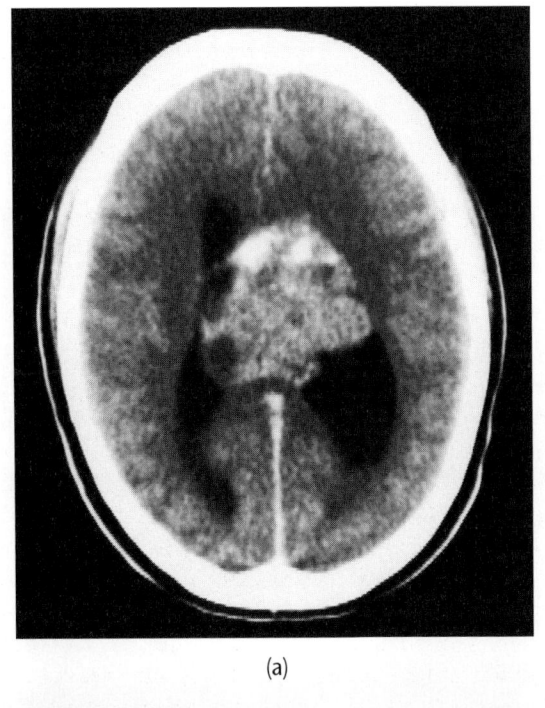

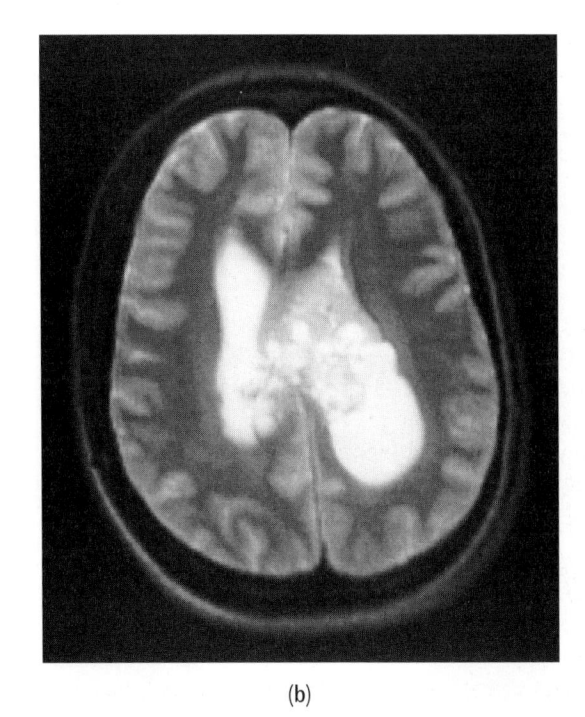

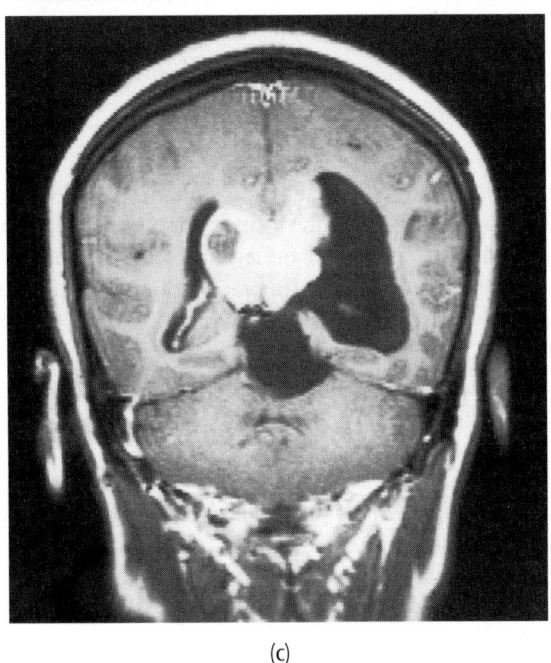

Figure 3.18. *Central neurocytoma. Axial post-contrast CT (a); T2-weighted (b); and post-contrast coronal T1-weighted MRI (c). Irregular but well-defined tumour with attachment to the septum pellucidum which shows calcification on CT and small intratumoral cysts.*

subependymal hamartoma or giant cell astrocytoma but evidence of tuberous sclerosis is almost invariably present in these. Heterotopic grey matter is always of grey matter density and intensity on all sequences but sometimes meningioma or ventricular glioma may mimic the lesion. Larger lesions are often indistinguishable from ependymoma, glioma and central neurocytoma. In particular, the diagnosis of subependymoma should be considered in the presence of a complete intraventricular lesion with little or no contrast-enhancement or surrounding oedema.

Meningioma

Intraventricular meningiomas are common intraventricular tumours, which nearly always appear as meningiomas do elsewhere. On CT they are well circumscribed, hyperdense, uniformly enhancing lesions which show calcification in a minority. On MRI they mimic grey matter on T2 and spin-density weighted images. Often they grow to a large size, particularly when arising in the trigone, the most common site, where obstruction of CSF flow results in focal enlargement or

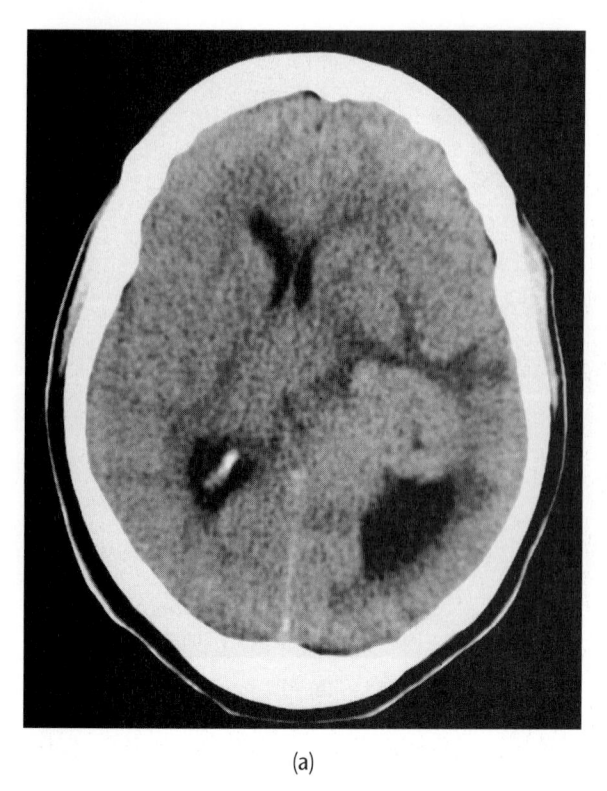

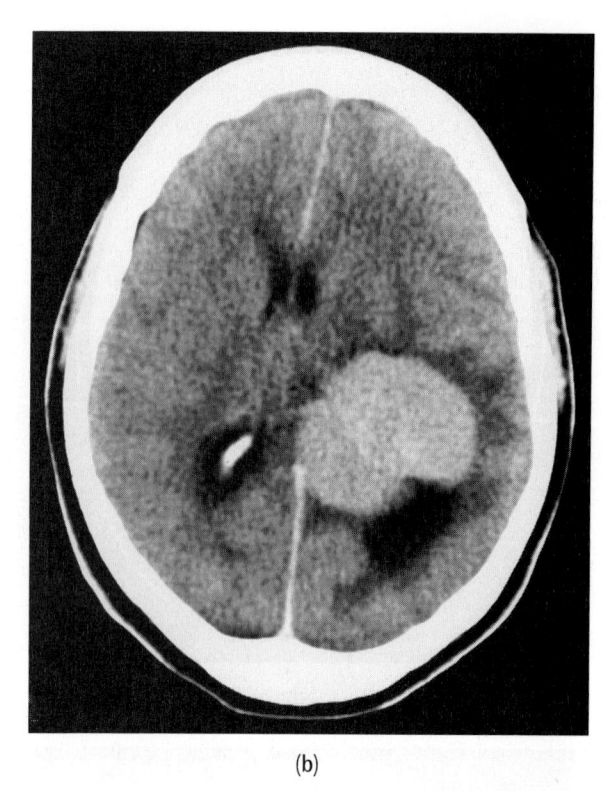

Figure 3.19. *Ventricular meningioma. Axial pre- (a) and post-contrast (b) scans. This slightly hyperdense homogeneous enhancing tumour is typical of meningioma elsewhere.*

'trapping' of the temporal horn (Fig. 3.19). Aggressive lesions may invade brain tissue.

The major differential diagnosis is lymphoma which can commonly appear in the immune-competent patient as a hyperdense uniformly enhancing intraventricular mass (Fig. 3.13). The frond-like outline of choroid plexus papilloma which frequently causes generalized ventriculomegaly is usually sufficient to differentiate it from meningioma.

Choroid plexus papilloma

In adults, the majority of choroid plexus papillomas occur in the fourth or lateral ventricles, while in children, 80% arise in a lateral ventricle and 15% in the fourth ventricle.[20] Third ventricular origin is relatively uncommon in both groups, while multifocal lesions are seen in around 5% of patients. Although they can be confused with meningioma or ependymoma, the typical choroid plexus papilloma is easy to recognize in that its papillary nature is revealed in its frond-like outline; it often looks simply like a large piece of choroid plexus (Fig. 3.20). Calcification is common, but variable in extent and evidence of large feeding vessels is frequently found on CT and MRI reflecting the marked vascularity of the tumour. Haemorrhage and cystic areas are frequently demonstrated. Contrast-enhancement is always intense, but often inhomogeneous due to cysts, calcification and flow voids from the feeding vessels. Even the calcified areas have been shown to enhance on MRI.

Hydrocephalus is almost invariable, either due to obstruction of ventricular outlets, or to overproduction of CSF; it may therefore appear as communicating or obstructive in pattern. Generally the ventricle is locally expanded next to a large lesion. Small papillomas may extend without tissue invasion along the CSF pathways, most commonly into and through the foramina of Magendie and Luschka.

Choroid plexus carcinoma is a rare malignant variety which may be indistinguishable from other aggressive ventricular lesions. It often demonstrates local, extraventricular invasion and distant metastases have been described.

Ventricular glioma

Most of these lesions are oligodendrogliomas but the literature of this tumour is marred by the fact that many lesions previously labelled as ventricular oligodendroglioma would now be classified as central neurocytoma. It comes as no surprise therefore that ventricular gliomas are said to be indistinguishable from central neurocytoma on imaging studies. Most arise in the lateral ventricles. They exhibit a range of appearances according to their aggressiveness. Invasion of surrounding brain is relatively common. Calcification, intratumoral cysts, and haemorrhage can be seen and there is usually moderate-to-marked contrast-enhancement

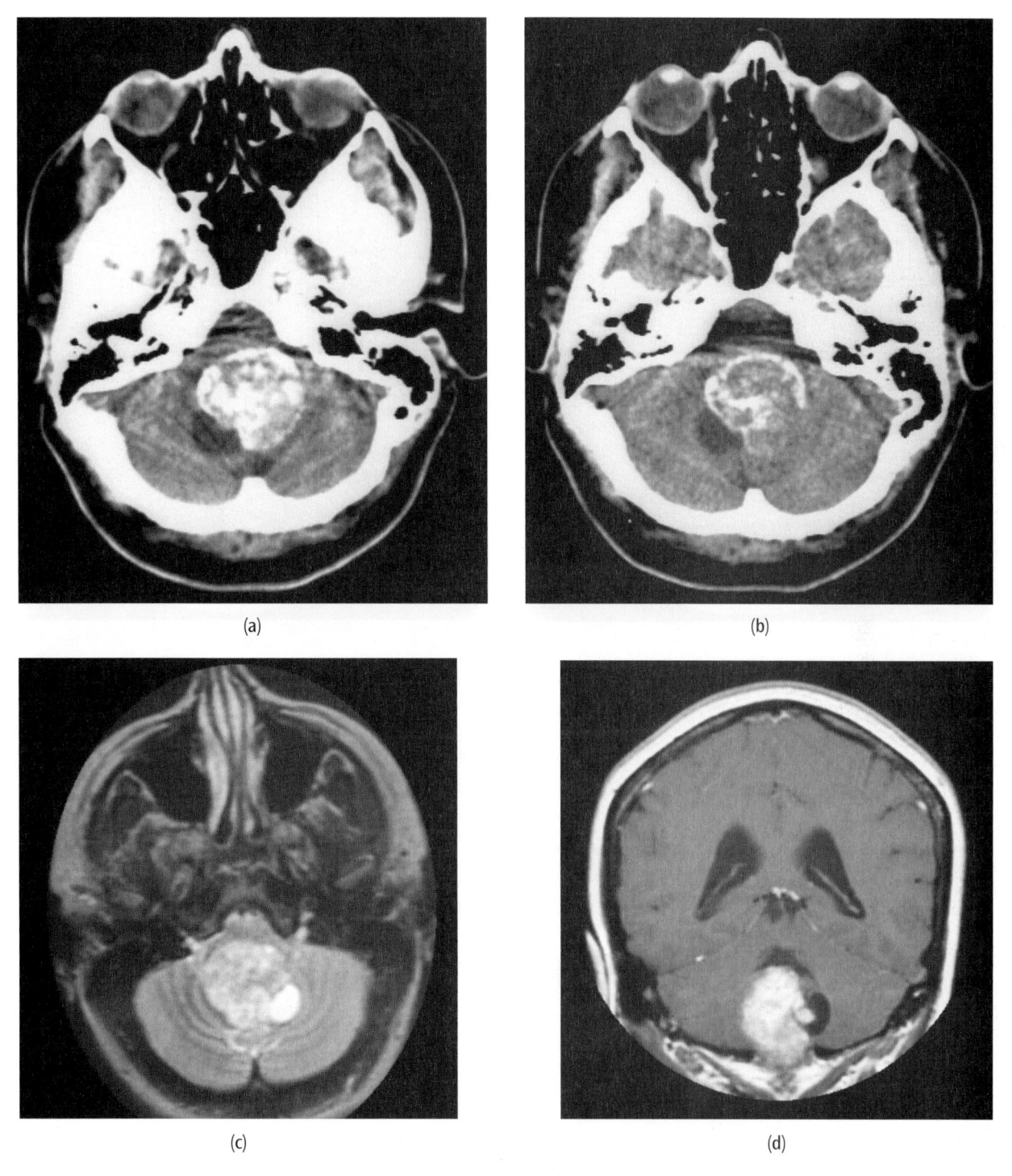

Figure 3.20. *Choroid plexus papilloma. Axial pre- (a) and post-contrast (b) scans. Axial T2-weighted (c) and post-contrast coronal T1-weighted (d) MR images. The 'frond-like' outline of the tumour reveals its nature. There is patchy calcification, inhomogeneous signal on MRI and contrast enhancement. Note how on the T2-weighted images the tumour extends into the foramina of Lushka.*

(Fig. 3.21). There are no pathognomic appearances which would indicate the true histology.

Ventricular cysts

The most common intraventricular cyst is the colloid cyst, which arises at the upper anterior third ventricle. It can easily obstruct the foramen of Monro causing hydrocephalus and sudden death is said to occur when a colloid cyst lodges in the foramen of Monro causing a catastrophic rise in intracranial pressure. Typically, colloid cysts are smooth, round, well defined lesions which are hyperdense on CT, although isodense and occasionally hypodense varieties may occur (Fig. 3.22).

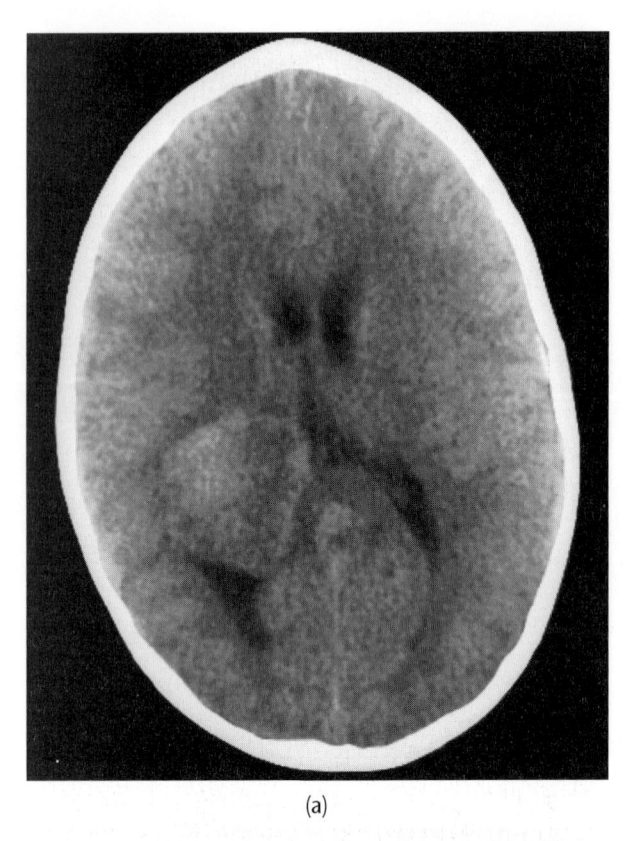

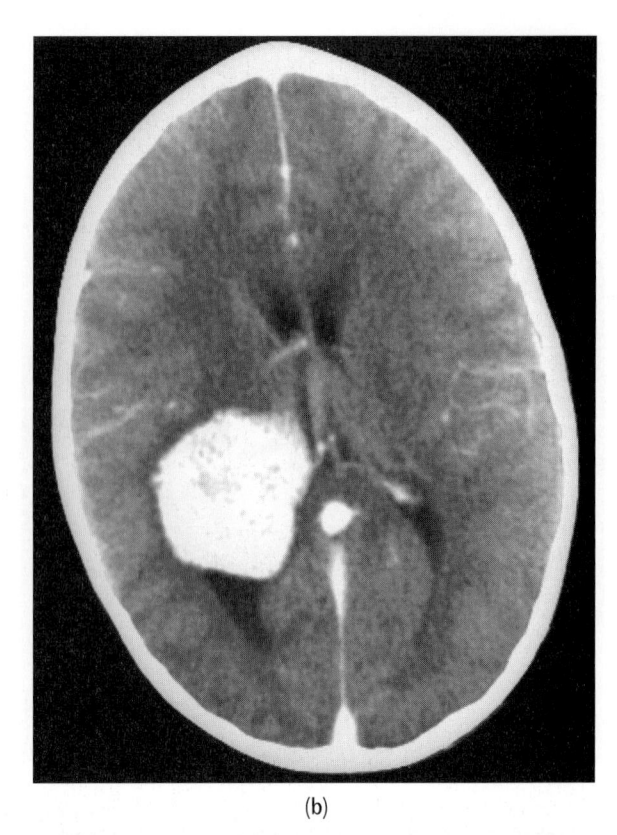

Figure 3.21. *Ventricular oligodendroglioma. Axial pre- (a) and post-contrast (b) CT scans show an essentially isodense brightly enhancing mass in the right trigone. There is no calcification and there are no pathognomic features.*

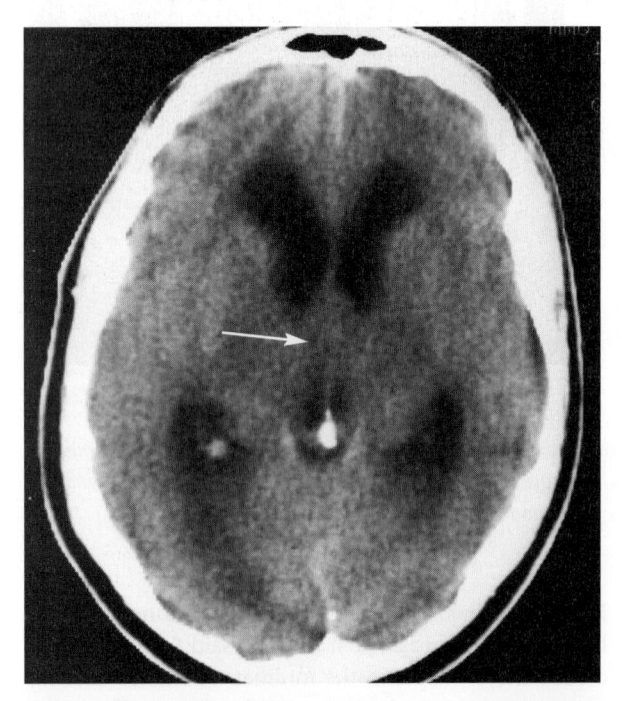

Figure 3.22. *Isodense colloid cyst on an axial CT scan through the third ventricle. There is a rounded isodense mass at the foramen of Monro (arrow) distorting its leaves and causing lateral ventricular enlargement.*

The lateral ventricles may not be enlarged at the time of scanning but hydrocephalus is usually apparent with larger lesions. Although some texts state that they can exhibit contrast-enhancement, this is not our experience and strong contrast-enhancement in a suspected colloid cyst is evidence against the diagnosis. The signal intensity also varies on MRI (Fig. 3.23). Some lesions are bright on T1WI, similar to white matter intensity; many of these will also be of low intensity on T2WI. Some approach the intensity of normal brain on all sequences and are therefore harder to see. Others are similar to CSF intensity, but this is unusual.[21]

Ependymal and choroidal cysts are CSF isodense/intense cysts which arise in the ventricle or choroidal fissure. They can be partly inside and partly outside the ventricle. They may cause hydrocephalus, perhaps localized to one temporal horn, by interrupting CSF flow. They do not show contrast-enhancement (Fig. 3.24).[22]

Intraventricular cysts may be seen in cysticercosis and cryptococcosis, where they may reach large size. Imaging cannot separate them from true cysts of neuroepithelial or endothelial origin unless there are associated features of cerebral infection.

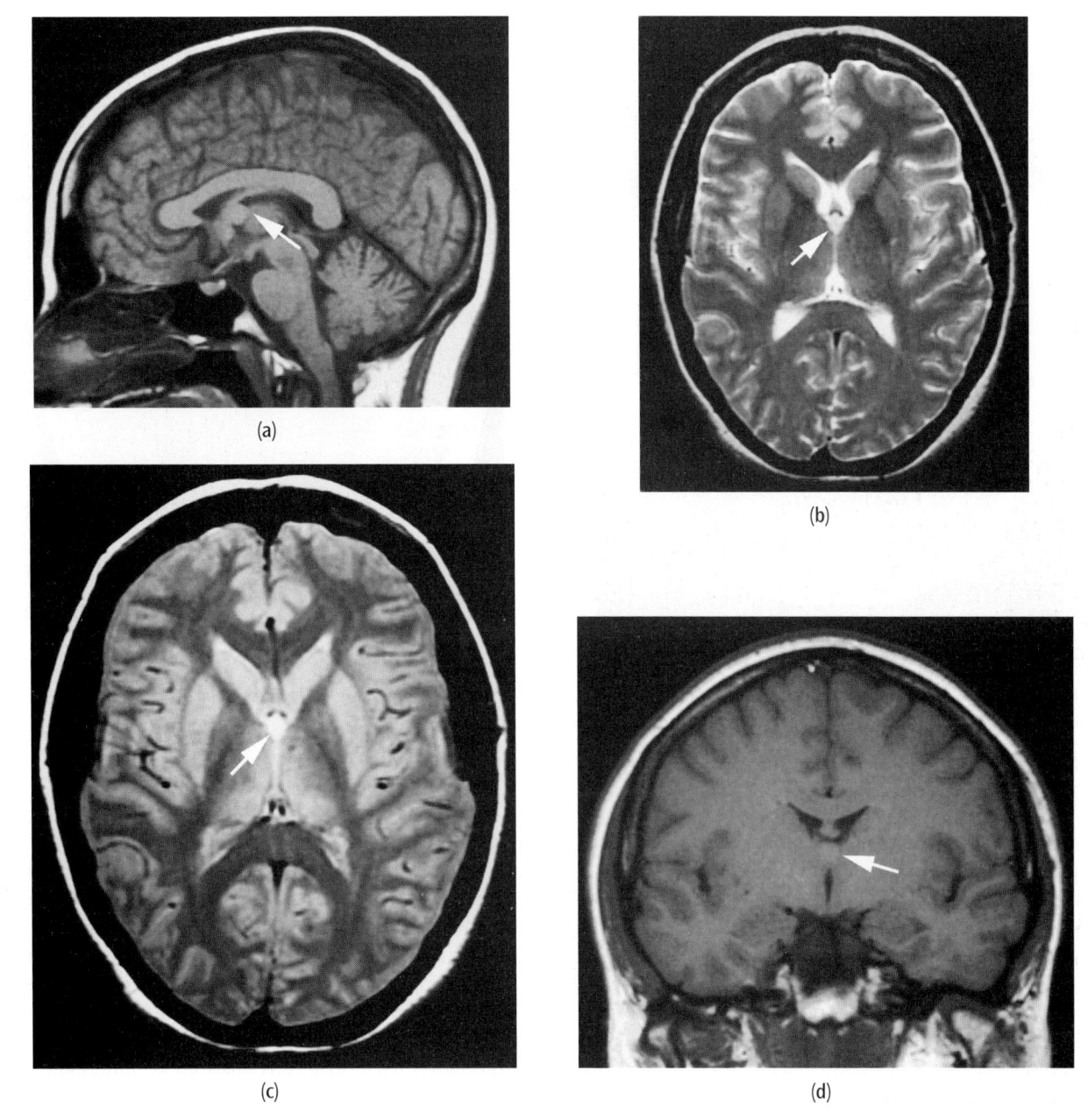

Figure 3.23. *Colloid cyst (arrows). Sagittal T1- (a), axial T2- (b), axial spin-density (c), and coronal T1- (d) weighted images show small lesion exactly in the position of the foramen of Monro. Note its position relative to the anterior commisure in image (a). In this patient the cyst fluid is isointense with white matter on T1WI but others may be even brighter and a few approach CSF signal intensity.*

Other lesions

Craniopharyngioma is described below. Rarely, metastases from non-CNS tumours may be seen lining the ventricular walls, particularly from breast, lung and melanoma. Ventricular spread may occur from any CNS tumour and is more common in children than adults. Arteriovenous malformations may be located completely inside a ventricle but can usually be recognized by their prominent feeding and draining vessels (Fig. 3.25).

PINEAL REGION TUMOURS

There can be no doubt that the nomenclature of tumours in this region is confusing and has led to considerable misunderstanding. The term 'pineal region' applies to that area bounded by the third ventricle anteriorly, the tectal plate of the midbrain and upper vermis inferiorly, the corpus callosum superiorly and the tentorium cerebelli posterolaterally (see Part 1, pp. 1–21). Tissue of several cell types exists in this region in addition to the pineal gland itself. 'Pineal region tumour'

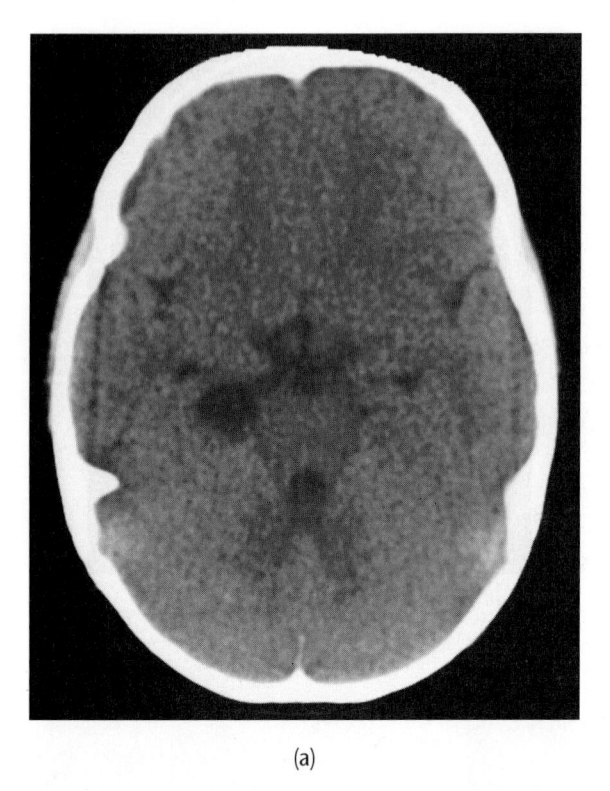

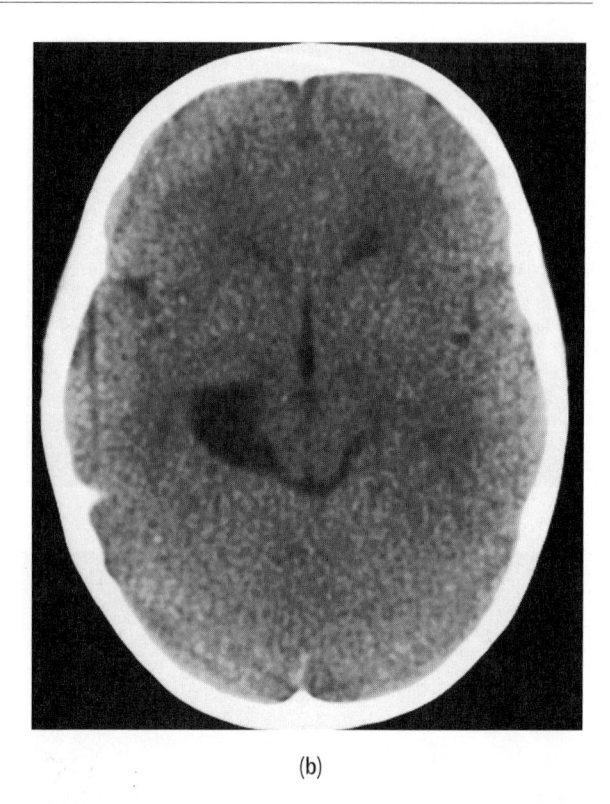

Figure 3.24. *Axial contiguous CT scans (a),(b). There is a choroidal cyst within the choroidal fissure and ambient cistern on the right side. Although such cysts may exert mass effect they never show contrast-enhancement and are almost invariably clinically irrelevant.*

encompasses many tumour types including glioma, meningioma, ependymoma and metastases, as well as tumours primarily of the pineal body itself. The pineal gland can be invaded by any surrounding tumour, for example by a glioma arising from the tectal plate.[23]

The commonest lesions found within the pineal region are tumours of the pineal itself, either primary or secondary, glioma of the tectal plate, and arachnoid cyst. Tumours of the pineal body itself can be divided into germ cell tumours and tumours of pineal cell origin. The term 'pinealoma' includes all pineal body tumours of germ cell or pineal cell origin and should not be used.

Germ cell tumours

These comprise a spectrum of tumours, ranging from mature teratoma, epidermoid and dermoid 'cysts' at the most benign end of the spectrum, to endodermal sinus tumours, embryonal cell tumours and choriocarcinoma at the malignant end, with germinoma and immature teratoma in the middle. Although germinoma and teratoma are by far the most common, a tumour can arise from any germ cell line, regardless of sex, and mixed histology is relatively common. There is a strong male predominance.

Germinoma tends to arise in the second decade and is the commonest pineal tumour (Fig. 3.26). Although it is a relatively aggressive tumour, which commonly invades surrounding tissue and seeds within the CNS, it is very radiosensitive and carries a favourable prognosis. Calcification may be seen in the tumour, and calcification of the pineal body itself is said to be commoner if there is a co-existent germinoma. When present, calcification may be surrounded and engulfed by germinoma. The tumour tends to be isodense/intense to grey matter on T2WI and enhances strongly and homogeneously. Intratumoral haemorrhage is relatively common and if present will alter the imaging appearance before and after contrast-enhancement. Local invasion of brain tissue may give rise to vasogenic oedema. Three-ventricular hydrocephalus is almost invariable with this lesion (and all pineal tumours) due to compression of the tectal plate and aqueduct.[24]

Pineal teratoma tends to arise in the first decade and carries a worse prognosis than germinoma. It is made up of tissue from all three germinal layers and may contain hair, teeth, or fat. It is therefore characterized by its heterogeneous appearance and variable contrast-enhancement as well as an unpredictable clinical course. Calcification, haemorrhage and CT or MRI evidence of fat are common findings (Fig. 3.27). Local invasion may occur with vasogenic oedema when present. A midline lipoma is composed entirely of fat, and so can be distinguished from teratoma by its homogeneity, chemical shift artifact and density/intensity of pure fat.

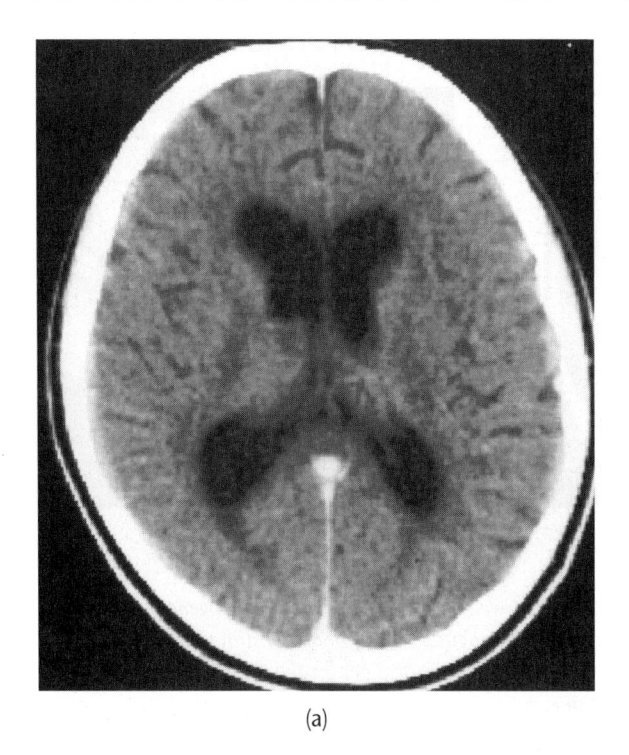

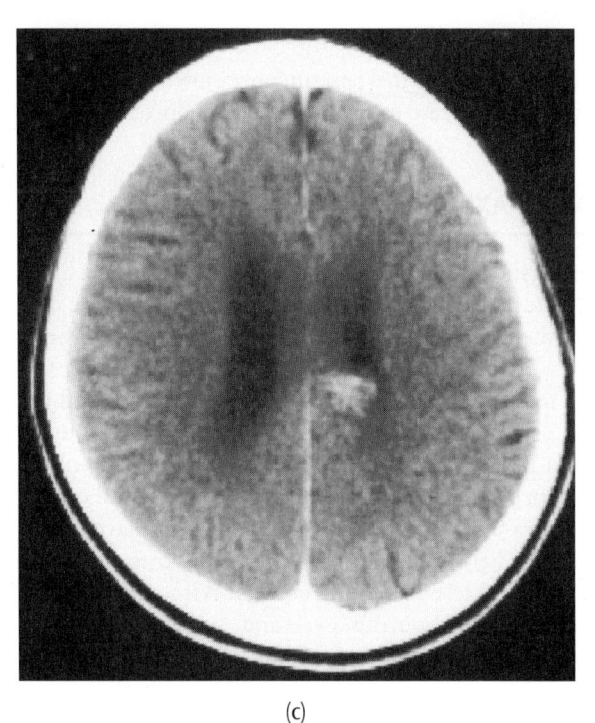

Figure 3.25. Ventricular vascular malformation. Post-contrast CT (a)–(c). The small brightly enhancing nodule (c) is non-specific except that an enhancing vein can be traced running from it (b) to a prominent vein of Galen (a).

Pineal cell tumours

These comprise pinealoblastoma and pinealocytoma but both cell lines often co-exist within an individual tumour. Pinealoblastoma occurs more often in children than adults and is sometimes grouped with PNET and medulloblastoma by neuropathologists. Imaging studies show it to have very similar characteristics to pineal germinoma, except perhaps that tumoral calcification is more common with pinealoblastoma.

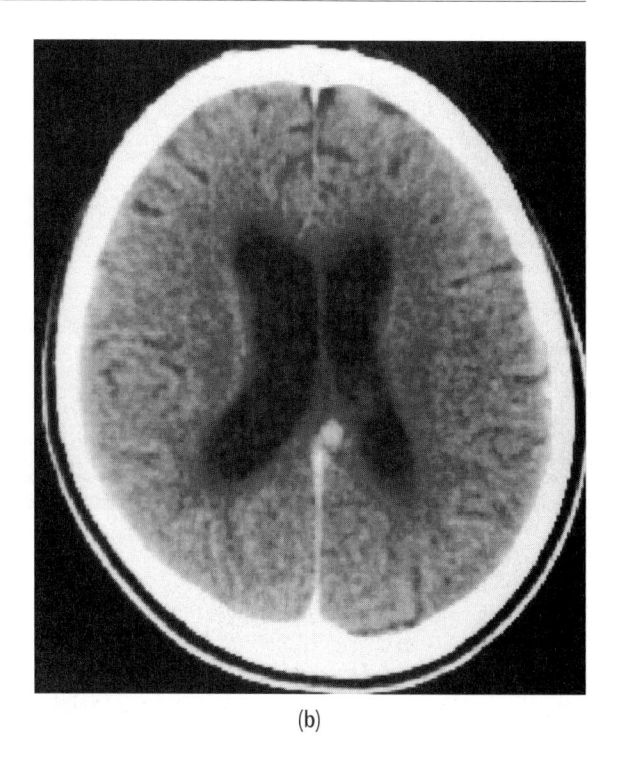

Haemorrhage and CNS seeding are relatively common, and often found at presentation.

Pinealocytoma tends to occur in adults (Fig. 3.28). It is usually well defined with smooth lobulated contours and local invasion is uncommon. Haemorrhage and calcification are common, resulting in inhomogeneous density and intensity. Contrast-enhancement is usually pronounced. The imaging appearances are variable, in part reflecting the variable biological behaviour of the tumour which can be at either end of the benign-to-malignant spectrum.[25]

Pineal glioma

Pineal glioma is yet another confusing label. The pineal gland is composed of lobules containing pinealocytes, which are specialized neuronal cells, and surrounding astrocytes. Pinealocytomas may exhibit neuronal or astrocytic differentiation but it is not clear whether this represents the basically pluripotential nature of pinealocytes or simultaneous change in the adjacent neurons or astrocytes. A glioma arising from the pineal gland itself can, therefore, be considered a variant of pinealocytoma and has similar imaging findings. Many pineal gliomas, however, result from a parapineal glioma which invades locally into the pineal gland and behave and appear as gliomas do elsewhere. The distinction between these is often difficult or impossible and so the term 'pineal region glioma' is preferred.

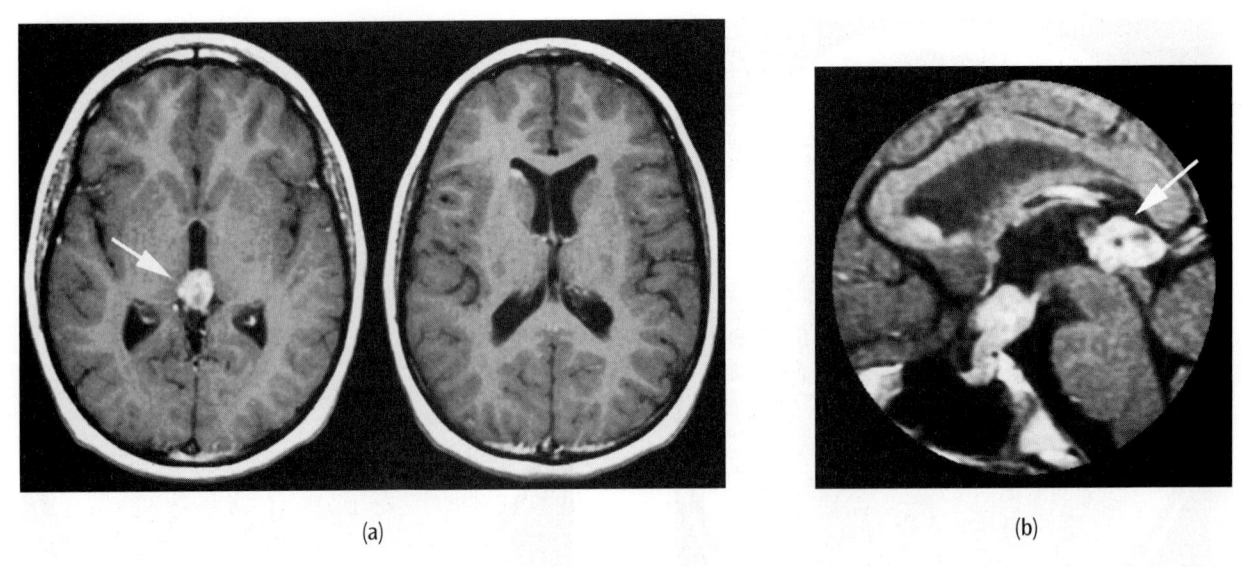

Figure 3.26. *Pineal germinoma. Contrast-enhanced MRI (a),(b). The pineal mass is well-defined (arrows) but inhomogenous in contrast-enhancement. The axial images show a second lesion in the right frontal horn. The sagittal image (b) demonstrates narrowing of the upper part of the aqueduct and other lesions present in the floor of the anterior third ventricle and in the hypothalamus, extending along the pituitary stalk. This is a common pattern of spread of germinoma.*

A glioma arising in the tectal plate will often present in an identical way to a pinealocytoma and may invade the pineal itself; such a lesion will often be indistinguishable from a pineal tumour invading the midbrain. A more indolent tectal plate tumour, however, most often presents with hydrocephalus. It can best be identified by sagittal MRI where the two humps of the quadrigeminal plate appear either as three, or as one, large mass; T2-weighted MRI can miss the lesion, as it can be hidden against bright CSF but it is more reliably shown on spin-density images (Fig. 3.29).

Pineal cyst

Pineal cysts are common incidental findings, particularly since the advent of MRI scanning. They have characteristic features which allow a confident radiological diagnosis, avoiding the need for biopsy. They tend to be small, usually less than 1.5cm in diameter. They are either CSF isointense on all sequences or demonstrate homogeneous high signal on spin-density images (and in this case often slightly higher signal than CSF on T1WI). They do not cause hydrocephalus or hormonal imbalance (except that some are found in the routine investigation of an endocrine disorder), and do not enhance after contrast medium administration. However, the surrounding normal pineal gland, as well as the leash of veins draining towards the vein of Galen, will show contrast-enhancement; this distinction is usually clear. Haemorrhage into the cyst, sometimes resulting in hydrocephalus, has been described but should be viewed with suspicion. Since they are more commonly seen in children, they presumably slowly regress; certainly any increase in size would be of concern.

EXTRA-AXIAL TUMOURS

The first decision a radiologist must make in assessing a CNS tumour is whether the lesion arises inside or outside the brain. The decision is often clear but in difficult cases the origin is usually clearer on MRI than on CT, due to its multiplanar capabilities and improved soft tissue contrast resolution. An extra-axial lesion pushes brain tissue away from itself. On one side of it will be dura or bone, while on the other will be cerebral cortex. An intra-axial tumour, however, will either have a layer of cortex between it and the dura, or the cortex itself will be clearly thickened and abnormal. With an extra-axial tumour, neighbouring gyri and sulci often appear squashed together like the folds of a concertina (Fig. 3.30), a feature seldom seen with a cerebral tumour. Hyperostosis only occurs with extra-axial lesions, although bone thinning can be seen with both.

Meningioma

This is by far and away the most common extra-axial CNS tumour. It has a predilection for certain sites, notably the parasagittal region, the olfactory groove, sphenoid wings, tuberculum sellae and parasellar region. Intraventricular and pial origin of the tumour, presumably from cellular rests, are also seen. Although commonest in the later stages of life, they do occur in

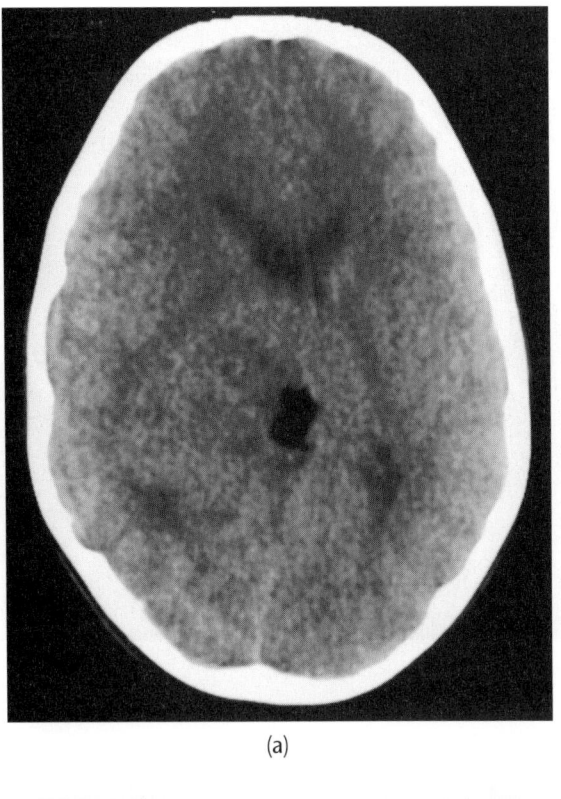

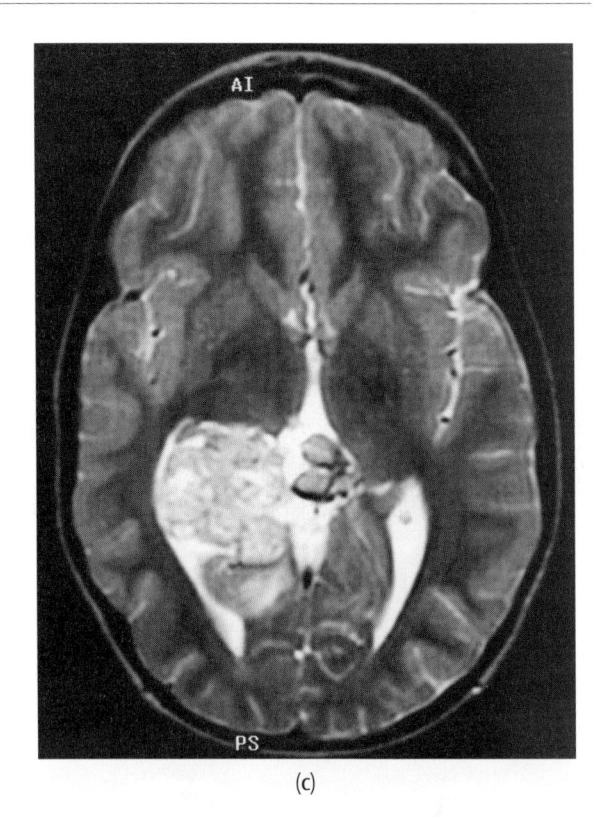

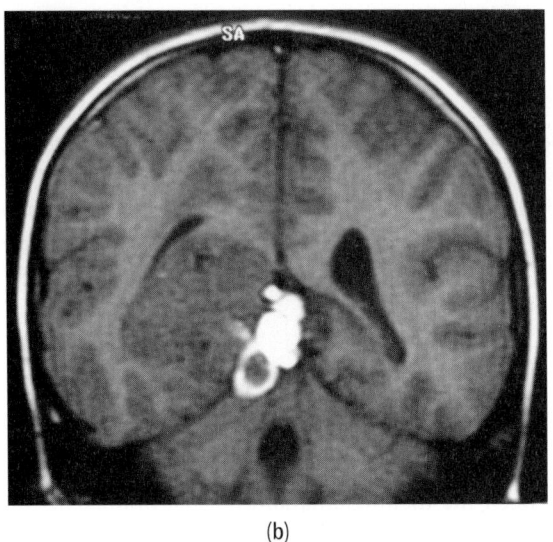

Figure 3.27. *Pineal teratoma. Axial post-contrast CT (a). Coronal T1WI (b) and axial T2WI (c). This complex irregular non-enhancing lesion contains fat medially within the pineal bed (note the chemical shift artefact on the T2WI). Not all teratomas will have calcification but most will show fat density/intensity.*

children and there is some evidence that meningioma in childhood is likely to carry an unfavourable outcome. In adults, there is a clear female predominance. Meningiomas may carry hormonal receptors and an association of meningioma with carcinoma of the breast has been reported. Multiple tumours are commonly seen, particulary in neurofibromatosis, a variant of which is termed by some as 'meningiomatosis'. Meningioma is also a common incidental finding at autopsy and heavily calcified psammomatous meningiomas are a frequent finding in CT scans of the elderly.

On CT, meningiomas typically are hyperdense, homogeneous, uniformly and brightly enhancing tumours (Fig. 3.30). Around 15% are calcified and a few are so heavily calcified that contrast-enhancement is not apparent. In the most indolent meningiomas surrounding vasogenic oedema may be absent but in most it is a prominent feature. Apical or 'capping' cysts are frequently seen in larger tumours and intratumoral haemorrhage may occur. Thickening of overlying bone is apparent in a minority of cases and is most commonly seen in meningiomas arising from the sphenoid bone. Hyperostotic bone is not necessarily invaded by tumour, however. Bone invasion or erosion are also occasionally seen. Convexity, sphenoid and parasellar meningiomas are often best seen using direct coronal scans and this

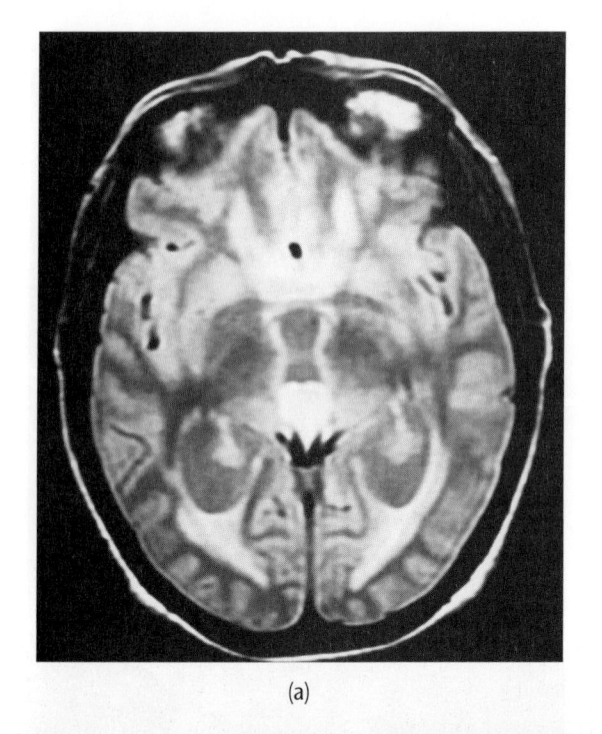

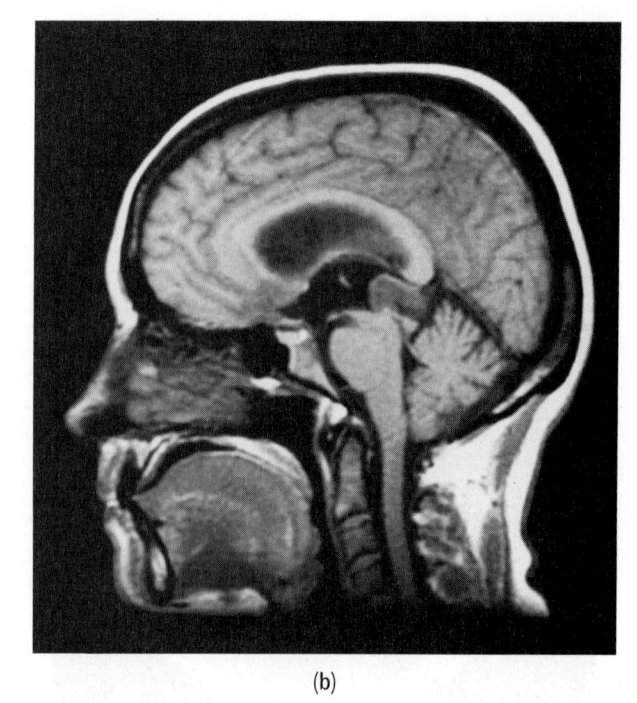

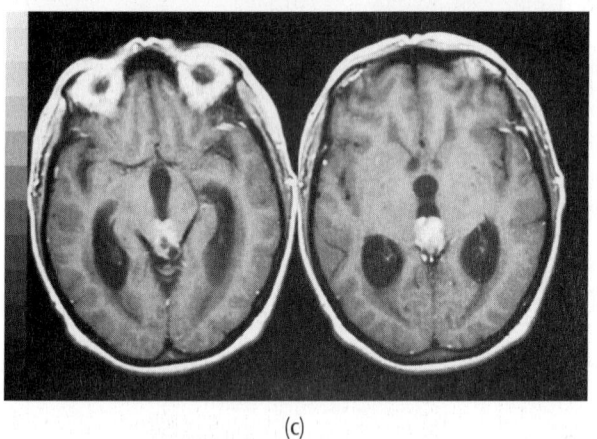

Figure 3.28. *Pinealocytoma. Axial spin-density (a) sagittal T1WI (b). Axial post-contrast T1WI (c). Spin-density images usually best demonstrate a pineal region tumour by providing contrast between tumour and low intensity CSF. This lesion has flattened the aqueduct causing three ventricular hydrocephalus and periventricular signal change.*

plane will demonstrate downward displacement of the ventricles as evidence of mass effect from a high convexity or parasagittal tumour better than axial scans.

On conventional or fast-spin echo MRI, using long and short echoes, meningioma is notorious for having very similar signal characteristics to grey matter and can easily be overlooked. Strong T1-weighting such as given by short TE inversion recovery images will, however, usually provide excellent tissue contrast, allowing the tumour to be separated from brain tissue. Some meningiomas will be relatively bright on T2WI and a correlation has been reported between T2 relaxation time and histological subtype.[26] However, T2-weighted signal patterns are commonly heterogeneous, reflecting intratumoral haemorrhage, calcification, cyst formation and/or cellular variety (Fig. 3.31).

A CSF isointense cleft is commonly seen on MRI between the meningioma and normal brain. This may represent one or a combination of compressed vessels, dura, or a true CSF collection (Fig. 3.32). Enlarged veins are often seen over the surface of a meningioma most commonly between the tumour and normal brain draining blood from both. Identification of such veins is of importance to the neurosurgeon in planning the surgical approach since patent veins cannot normally be sacrificed. A parasagittal tumour will often invade the superior sagittal sinus. If the sinus is occluded, then it can be sacrificed when resecting tumour but the sinus must be preserved if it is invaded but patent. Coronal T2-weighted scans, and magnetic resonance venography are very helpful in this situation, and a single slab two-dimensional phase-contrast technique, with velocity encoding set at 20cm/s or less, can be used to assess flow in the sinus.

Contrast-enhancement is invariable in meningioma

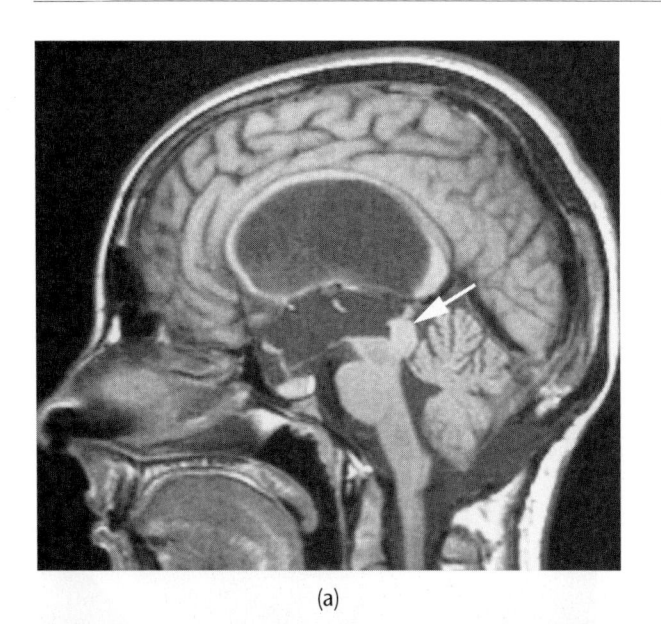

Figure 3.29. Sagittal T1WI (a) (TR/TE = 500/30) at 0.5T. Axial T2 (b) (TR/TE = 2200/90) and axial spin-density (c) (TR/TE = 2025/20). Tectal plate glioma. The tectal plate is bulky and appears as one mass (arrow) rather than two distinct humps formed by the quadrigeminal bodies. The lesion is easy to miss on T2WI (b) but is clearly shown on the spin-density scans(c).

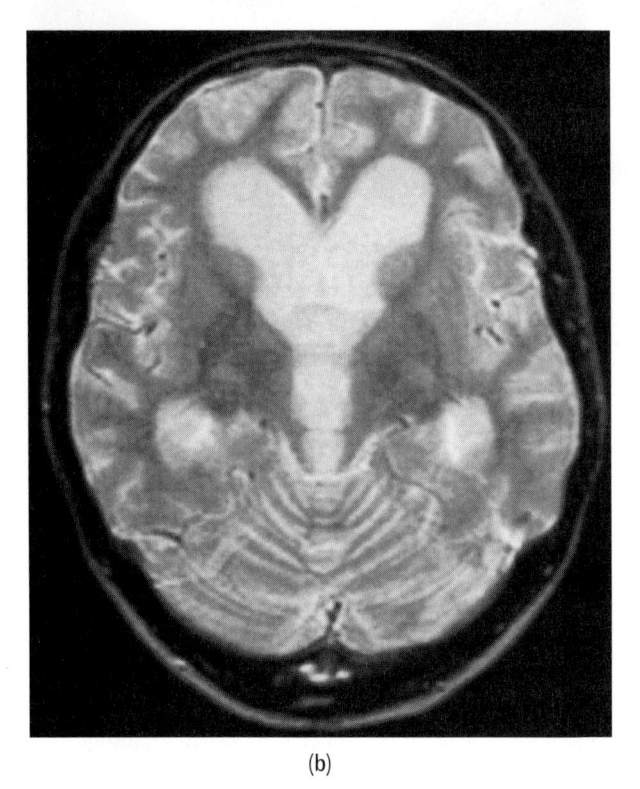

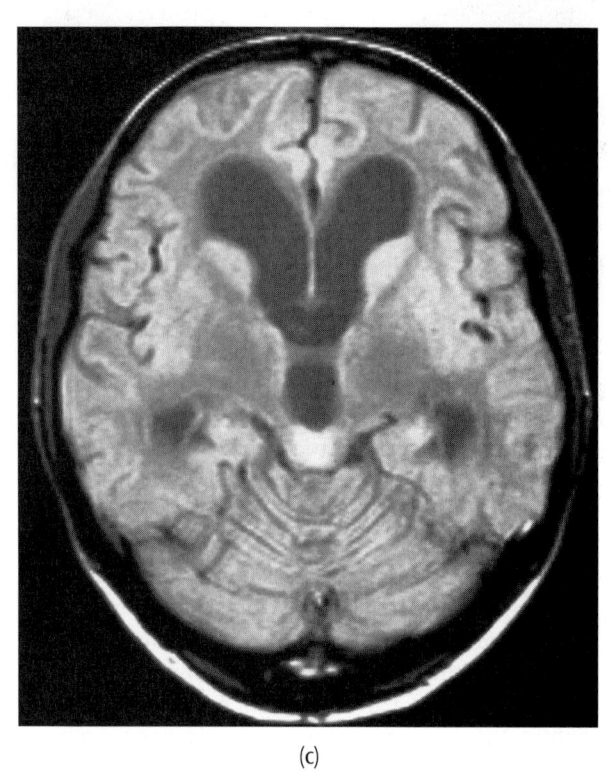

and is usually intense and homogeneous. Commonly, a dural 'tail' of enhancement is seen around a meningioma. This may or may not indicate *en plaque* spread of tumour, as some histologically examined cases have shown tumour in the thickened dura and some just reactive change. This dural tail sign has also more recently been reported in other lesions, including neuroma.[27]

The differential diagnosis of meningioma depends on its location and appearance but the following generalizations apply. Peripheral glioma may sometimes be confused as an extra-axial lesion, or an atypical meningioma which is perhaps inhomogeneous in density, intensity and enhancement can be thought to be intra-axial. Sarcoid and lymphoma can both produce dural masses which, if isolated, can be identical to meningioma but fortunately evidence of disease elsewhere is usually apparent. Metastases, particularly from carcinoma of the breast or lung, or melanoma can also give rise to dural masses which are usually, but not always, multiple. In the parasellar region inflammatory masses can mimic meningioma but the clinical picture is usually clear. Sometimes primary or secondary bone tumours will spread deeply to involve the dura and could be taken for meningioma with hyperostosis.

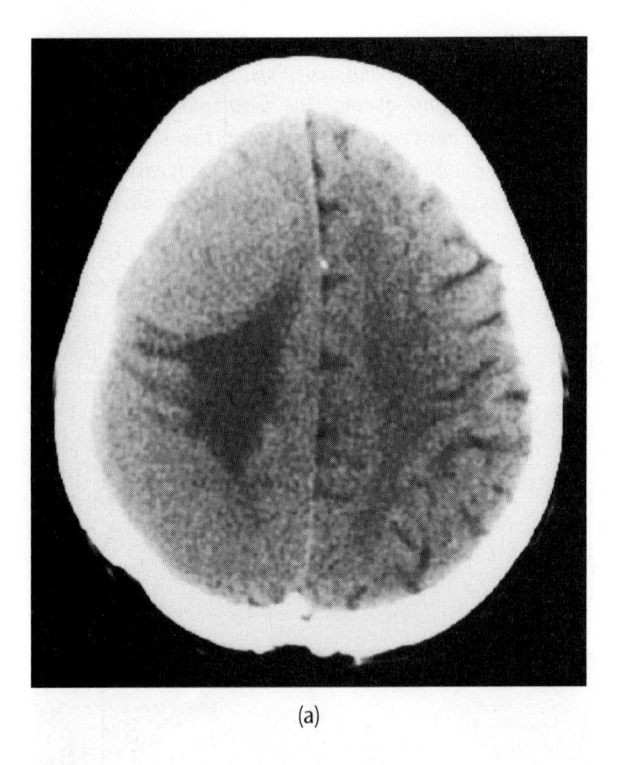

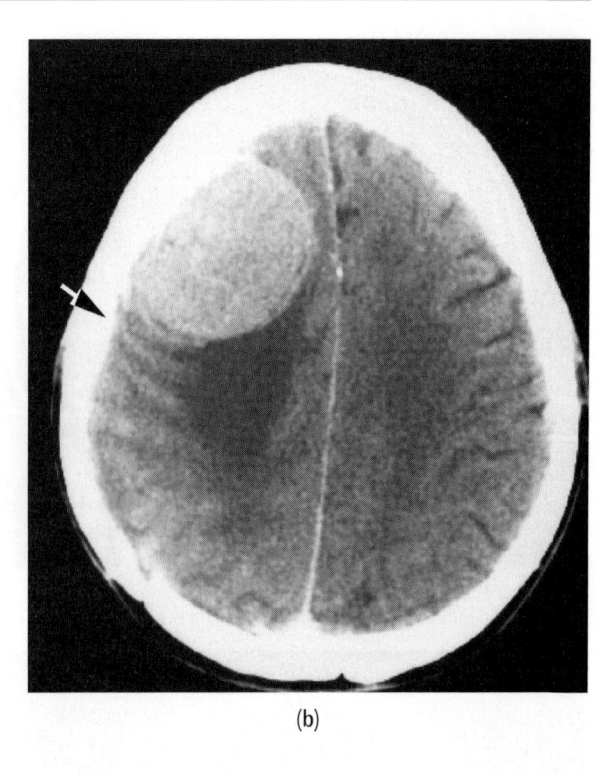

Figure 3.30. Pre- (a) and post-contrast (b) CT scan of a convexity meningioma. Note the compression of the right frontal gyri as evidence of an extra-axial lesion (arrow).

Congenital cysts

By far the most common of these is the arachnoid cyst. In the commonest location, the anterior part of the middle cranial fossa, they are almost always incidental findings even though they can be of impressive size. They are of identical signal intensity to CSF on all imaging sequences and all superficial cysts are associated with overlying bony thinning as evidence of their longstanding and benign nature. In other locations they can cause pressure effects, particularly if situated deep; for example in the quadrigeminal cistern they can sometimes compress the aqueduct. The temporal lobe adjacent to a large middle cranial fossa arachnoid cyst may seem small and slightly distorted and this again should not be considered as of pathological significance (Fig. 3.33).

Interhemispheric arachnoid cysts are a common accompaniment of congenital brain damage and are often seen in association with such diverse lesions as holoprosencephaly and Chiari malformation. Rarely, haemorrhage may occur into an arachnoid cyst which may then present as a subarachnoid or subdural haemorrhage. These should not be confused with epidermoid cysts which do not exactly match the density or intensity of CSF (Fig. 3.33b).

Neurenteric cysts are called by many synonyms, but the term is applied to any cyst lined by respiratory epithelium, although electron microscopy is often needed to separate endothelial from epithelial cysts histologically. These cysts occur in the midline, at the foramen magnum, or above the tentorium. Some, like colloid cysts, may contain fluid rich in protein or lipid, giving a high T1 signal. Like arachnoid cysts they are otherwise CSF isodense/intense. They may cause symptoms by pressure effects on local structures as they slowly grow.[28]

TUMOURS OF THE SELLAR AND PARASELLAR REGION

Pituitary adenoma

These are arbitrarily divided into microadenoma and macroadenoma according to their size; microadenomas are less than 10mm in diameter, while macroadenomas are larger. About 75% of pituitary adenomas secrete hormones; prolactin-producing tumours are by far the most common, followed by adrenocorticotropic hormone (ACTH) and growth hormone producing tumours. Because these tumours cause endocrine disturbance, they tend to present early, so that most prolactin and ACTH producing tumours are microadenomas, while non-functioning adenomas tend to present later, often with evidence of optic chiasmal compression.

In the search for a microadenoma, MRI is preferable to coronal CT which is often marred by beam-hardening artifact from the floor of the sella. Nevertheless thin coronal sections, using 100ml iodinated contrast

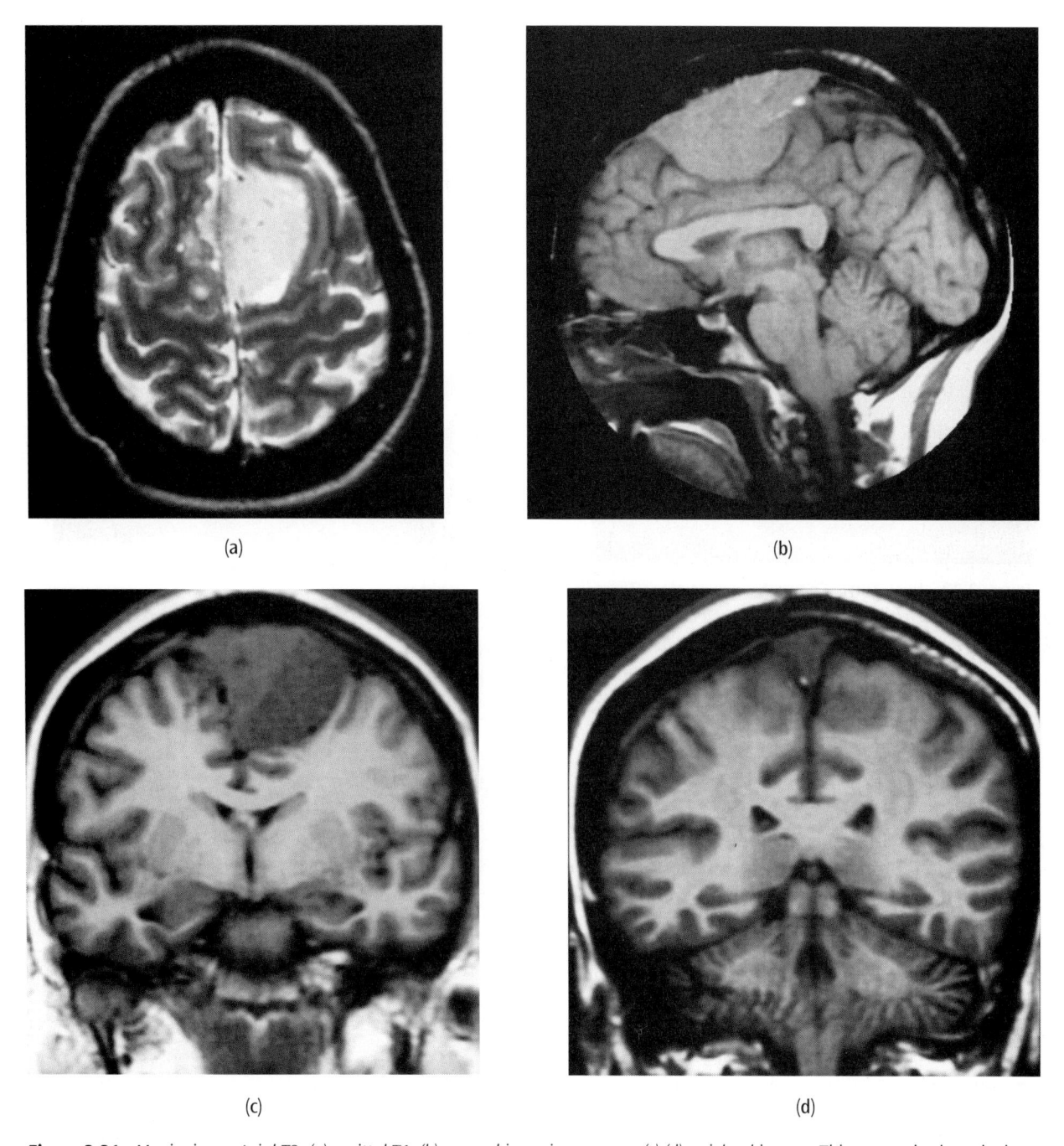

Figure 3.31. Meningioma. Axial T2- (a) sagittal T1- (b) coronal inversion recovery (c),(d) weighted images. This parasagittal meningioma is well-demonstrated with conventional images and the contrast resolution on the inversion recovery images is particularly good. Image (d) shows the tumour has grown into and expanded the sagittal sinus. On the sagittal image a tail of abnormal tissue can be seen extending anteriorly and posteriorly along the sagittal sinus. On the lateral surface of the tumour seen on coronal and axial images there is a thin band of grey matter with compression of local sulci again demonstrating the extra-axial position of the tumour.

medium and/or a contrast infusion for CT (Fig. 3.34), or T1-weighted spin echo MR (the gradient echo (GRE) technique suffers from susceptibility artifact produced at the pituitary/sella interface) will detect the majority of lesions as low density/intensity round tumours.[29] Displacement of the pituitary stalk, and depression of the floor of the sella are supportive features but of limited use by themselves. Contrast medium is not usually needed in MRI but if the lesion is not apparent on uncontrasted scans then further scans, after a standard dose of gadolinium chelate, increase sensitivity (Fig. 3.35). 'Standard' image settings on hard copy may, however, not best demonstrate the tumour; often a very narrow window width is preferable.

If a tumour is not visible on hard copy, examining the pre- and post-contrast scans on the MRI console while adjusting the window width and level will sometimes detect the lesion (Fig. 3.36). Dynamic scans during rapid

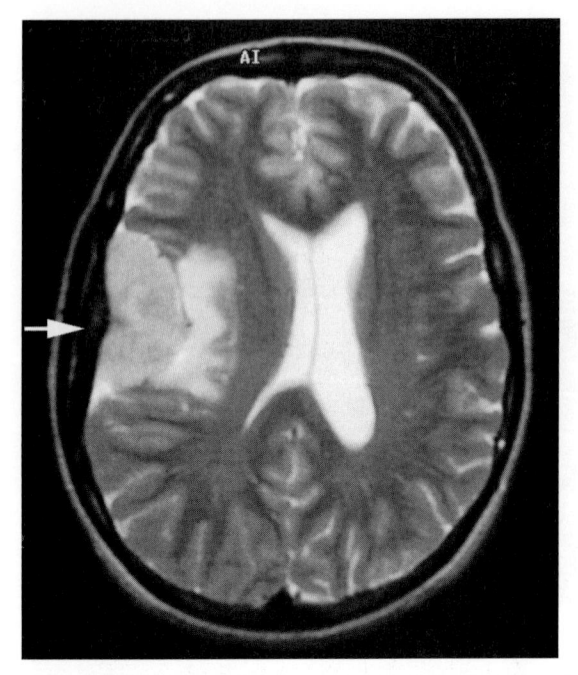

Figure 3.32. Axial T2WI. Convexity meningioma. There is a mixed intensity cleft between the tumour and brain tissue. This is composed partly of CSF and partly of flow-voids from blood vessels. Centrally in the dural surface of the tumour there is a 'hilum', said to represent the entry of feeding vessels (arrow). This is another common feature of meningioma.

contrast medium infusions will sometimes best display a small Cushing tumour, but this technique is time consuming and of limited benefit. Of course, not all microadenomas are low density/intensity. Some are isointense to normal pituitary and some are hyperintense. The former are particularly hard to find and probably account for the majority of false negative scans. Haemorrhage into a tumour can cause it to be hyperintense on T1WI. If such a lesion is seen, then contrast-medium is not needed (Fig. 3.37). Microadenomas have a variable appearance on T2-weighted FSE images but are usually hyperintense; occasionally lesions may be identified on T2WI which are not visible on T1WI.

There are a few confounding issues in the search for a microadenoma. First, pituitary adenomas are a common incidental finding at autopsy and rates of up to 27% have been quoted. Second, small cysts are commonly seen in the pars intermedia – that part of the pituitary gland at the interface between anterior and posterior lobes – and these should not be confused with microadenomas. Third, the portal vessels enter the pituitary from the stalk in the midline of the gland and then spread out. This results in the central portion of the gland enhancing more brightly than on either side.[30] Coupled with the normal slight inhomogeneity of pituitary enhancement, this can sometimes mimic a microadenoma (Fig. 3.38).

If a surgeon is to remove a microadenoma via the

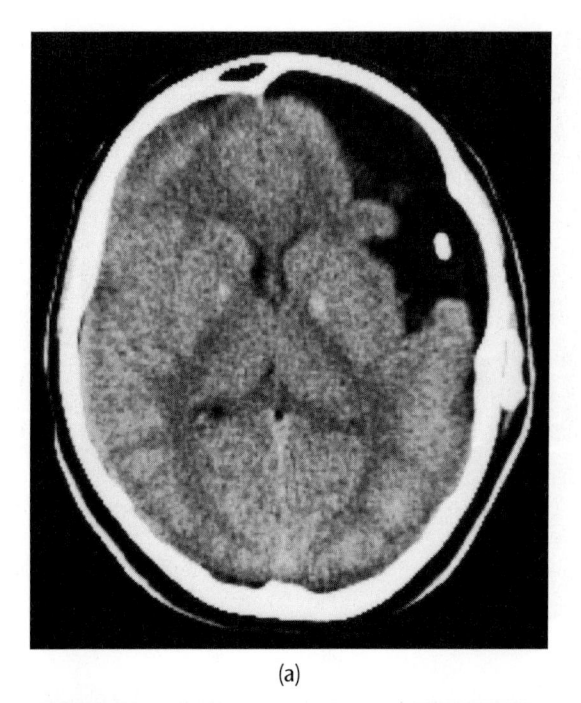

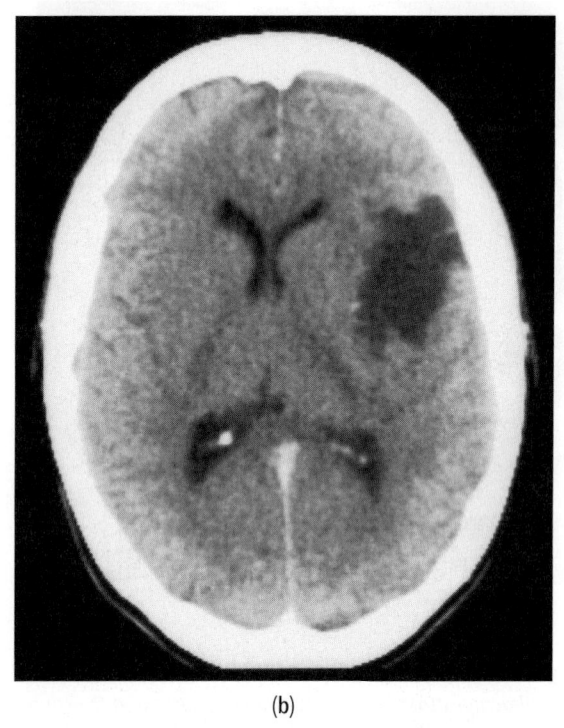

Figure 3.33. Axial CT scans of an arachnoid cyst (a) and epidermoid (b). Although unusually large, resulting in a surgical shunt tube being inserted, the arachnoid cyst is CSF isodense and tends to widen sulci. By contrast the epidermoid tumour although of low density is not CSF isodense.

trans-sphenoidal route, it is helpful to document the degree of aeration of the sphenoid sinus and to identify sagittal bony septa within it, since these may influence the approach. Although these septa can be seen on MRI, undoubtedly CT demonstrates them better.

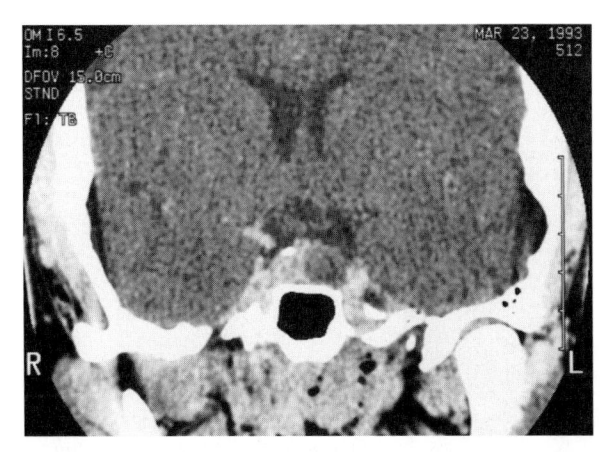

Tumours of the sellar and parasellar region 129

Figure 3.34. *Pituitary microadenoma. Coronal CT. Using a bolus and infusion technique, high vascular and pituitary gland contrast-enhancement is obtained allowing the non-enhancing microadenoma to be clearly defined. Although the lesion bulges into the chiasmatic cistern, the chiasm is not compressed.*

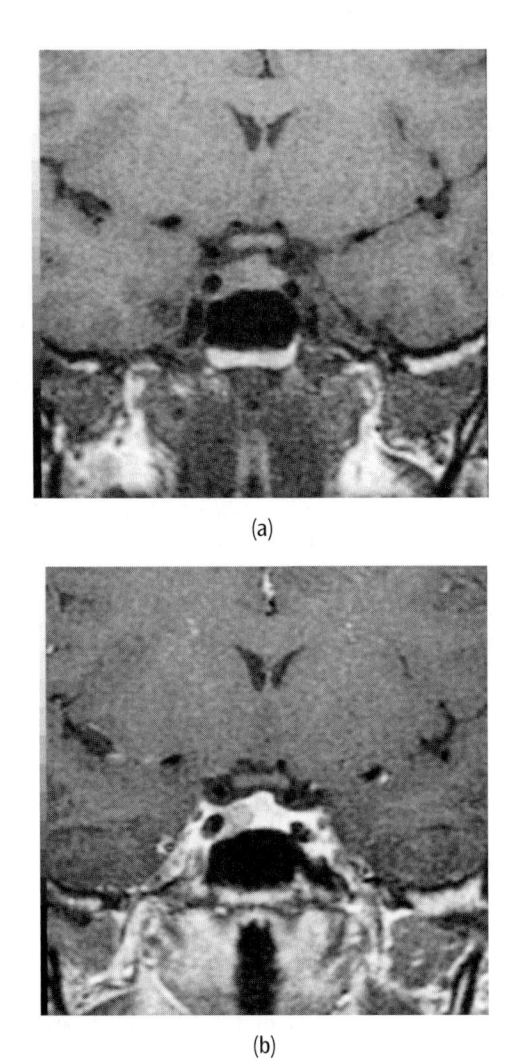

Figure 3.35. *Coronal pre- (a) and post-contrast (b) T1WI. The right-sided prolactin producing microadenoma is visible on the plain scans but is much more obvious on the post-contrast scan.*

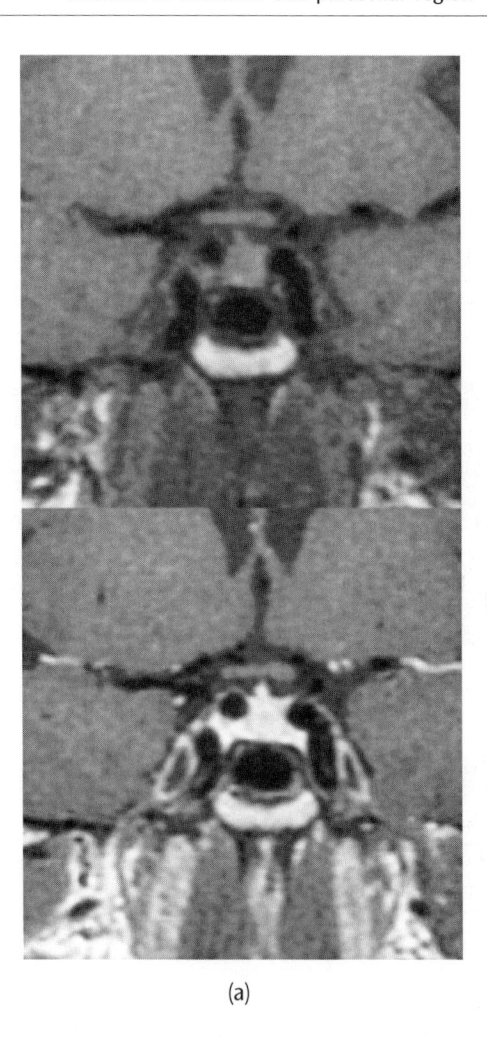

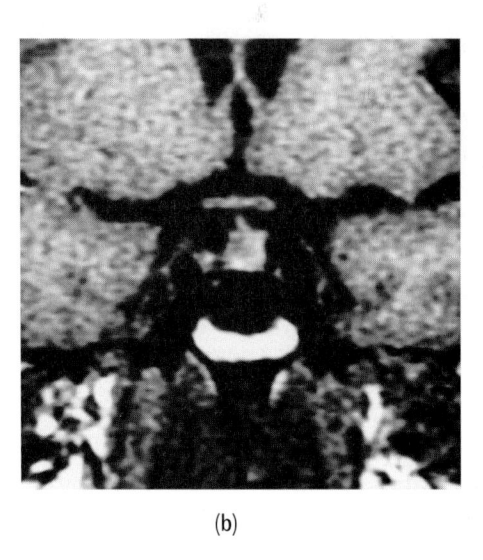

Figure 3.36. *Pituitary microadenoma. T1WI. The lesion is better displayed on non-contrast scans with a narrow window width (b) even though the overall image is less pleasing to the eye than in 'routine' image settings on the pre- and post-contrast scans (a). Note the deviation of the pituitary stalk to the left.*

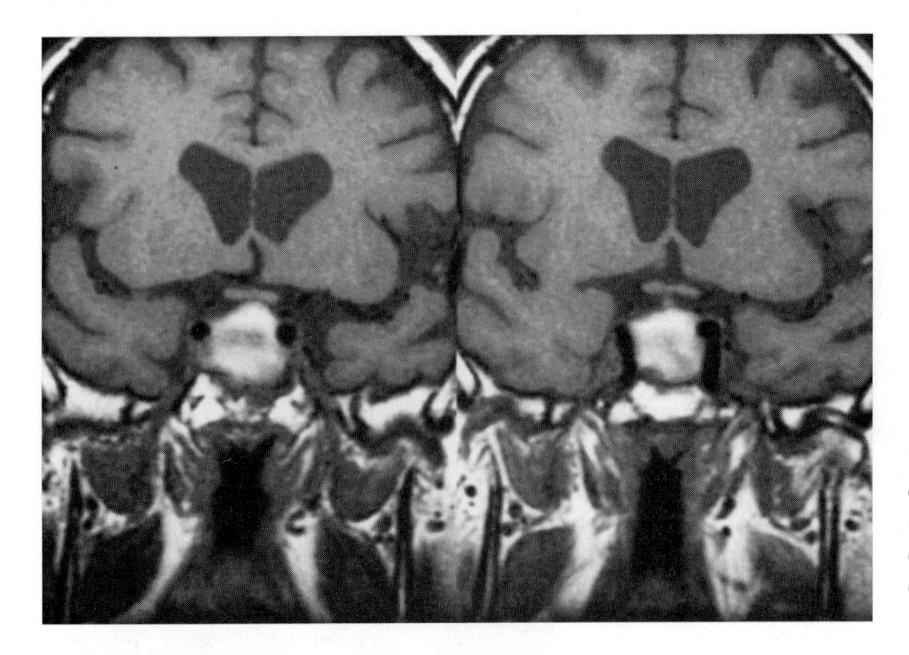

Figure 3.37. *Haemorrhagic pituitary adenoma. Uncontrasted coronal T1WI through the pituitary gland show deviation of the stalk and a short T1 mass consistent with recent haemorrhage.*

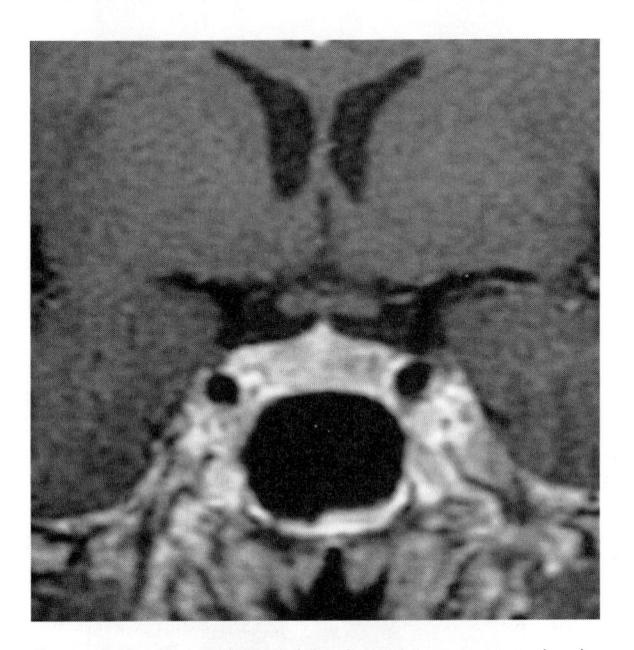

Figure 3.38. *Coronal T1-weighted MRI post-contrast showing slight but normal pituitary gland heterogeneity.*

When examining a macroadenoma, it is important to define the position and extent of optic nerve/chiasm/tract compression, to define the tumour boundaries, and to assess the cavernous sinuses for tumour invasion. To this end, images both before and after gadolinium are necessary on MRI, in at least coronal and sagittal planes. Uncontrasted scans, surprisingly, better demonstrate the compressed chiasm, while contrasted scans are better able to demonstrate the normal dural boundary between the sella and the cavernous sinus (Fig. 3.39).

Unfortunately the medial dural wall of the sinus is extremely thin and often cannot be seen. Asymmetry of size of the cavernous sinuses is strongly suggestive of tumour invasion and tumour which spreads more laterally may interpose between the cavernous segment of the carotid artery and the lateral wall of the sinus, usually without significantly narrowing the artery. Sometimes the unenhanced scans are more helpful than those after contrast-enhancement in this regard. Again more than one window setting may be necessary, particularly in assessing the cavernous sinus.

Large pituitary adenomas may have a capping cyst, and haemorrhage is common. The largest tumours usually have a very heterogeneous density/intensity. Haemorrhage into a pituitary tumour may result from pituitary apoplexy when a tumour suddenly infarcts (Fig. 3.37). Invasion of the floor of the sella is common with larger tumours and is well demonstrated with CT and MRI.

The differential diagnosis of a pituitary lesion is wide. The pituitary gland can be physiologically enlarged in puberty and around pregnancy or when stimulated by lack of end-organ response, such as is sometimes seen in hypothyroidism. Compression of the chiasm has been described in this situation with regression of the changes after appropriate hormone replacement.

It is vital not to confuse an aneurysm, which can flop down into an empty sella, with an adenoma. This can be avoided by maintaining high intravascular contrast medium concentration with CT, perhaps by using a bolus and infusion technique. We routinely give 100ml of 300mgI$_2$/ml contrast-medium plus an infusion of 150mgI$_2$/ml for a pituitary CT scan. The presence of flow void on MRI is adequate to exclude an aneurysm (Fig. 3.40).

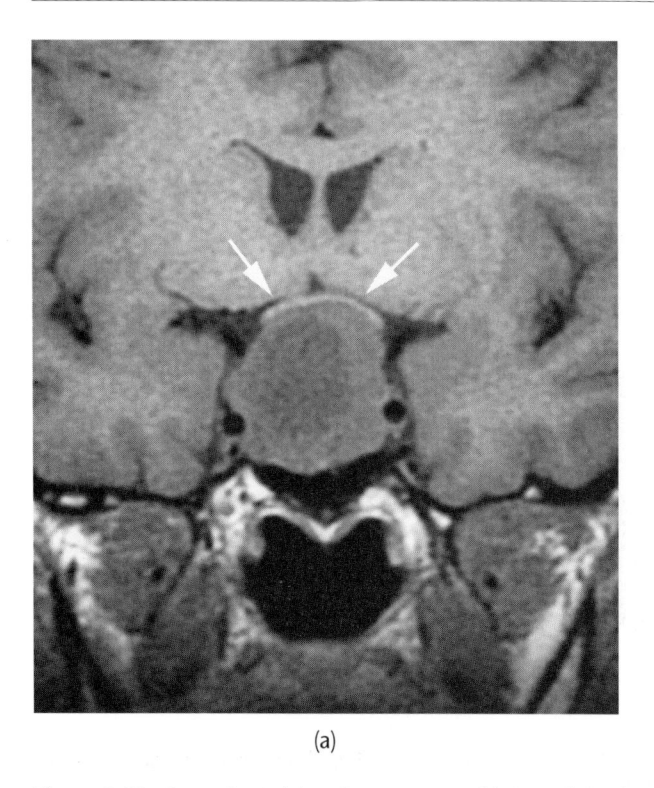

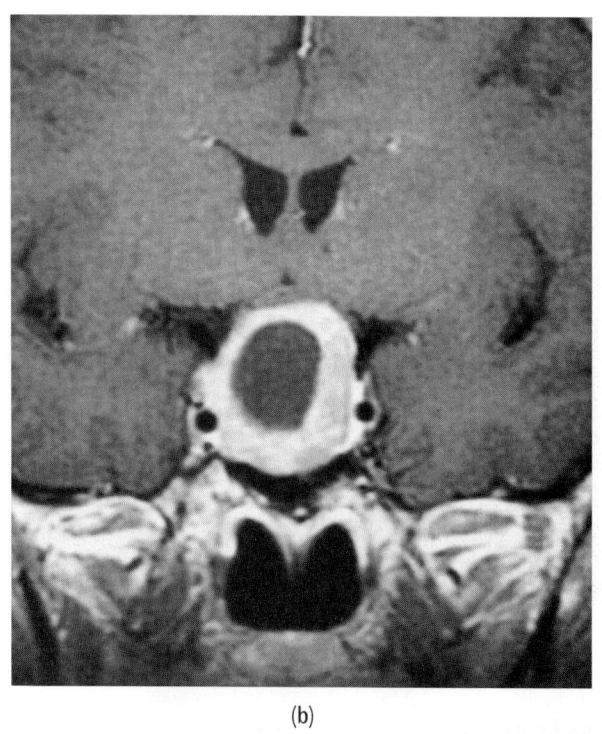

Figure 3.39. Coronal pre- (a) and post-contrast (b) T1WI through a pituitary microadenoma. The uncontrasted scan better shows the chiasm which is stretched over the dome of the tumour (arrows) while the contrasted scans better demonstrate the signal intensity difference between the cavernous sinus and the adenoma.

Suprasellar meningioma can appear similar to a pituitary tumour, except it is centred usually on the planum sphenoidale, and the sella is normal in size or minimally enlarged. The sphenoid sinus is characteristically ballooned upwards towards a meningioma (Fig. 3.41) but this feature is not always seen. Sagittal MRI is the best technique for separating the two lesions and contrast enhancement may demonstrate a dural tail with meningioma.

Lymphocytic adenohypophysitis is an autoimmune inflammatory condition which can exactly mimic an adenoma, causing compression of the chiasm. The presentation is usually different, characteristically occurring in young women, often late in pregnancy or in the post-partum period. Many of these patients have a history of recurrent aseptic meningitis due to the pituitary inflammation. Pituitary abscess is rare but can also appear similar to an adenoma except that abnormal enhancement may extend to meninges beyond the sella (Fig. 3.42).

Craniopharyngioma

This tumour arises from remnants of Rathke's pouch. It has a bimodal age distribution with the largest peak at around 5 years and a second peak in the sixth decade. Most frequently, it is centred on the pituitary stalk but may extend into the sella as well as up into the hypothalamus. The sella is usually not as enlarged with craniopharyngioma as it would be with a pituitary adenoma of the same size. The majority of childhood craniopharyngiomas are heavily calcified, and indeed they may only be visible as a discrete lump of calcification in or above the sella (Fig. 3.43). Most adult lesions are also calcified but calcification is not as prominent or as common a feature as in children.[31]

Larger tumours are almost invariably cystic to a lesser or greater extent. The cysts contain fluid described by surgeons as 'engine oil' due to its lipid component and are often very bright on T1-weighted MRI. They are commonly septated. Even if the cysts dominate the appearance, there is always a solid nodule of active tumour at their base which is best detected by contrast-enhanced scans (Fig. 3.44). In children, a post-surgical remnant of dense calcification may be present and then CT may be preferable in follow-up. Craniopharyngioma typically grows along the line of the pituitary stalk, whereas pituitary adenomas extend in all directions. Rarely, craniopharyngioma may be found entirely within the third ventricle, usually as a bright round cyst on T1-weighted MRI (Fig. 3.45).

132 Supratentorial tumours

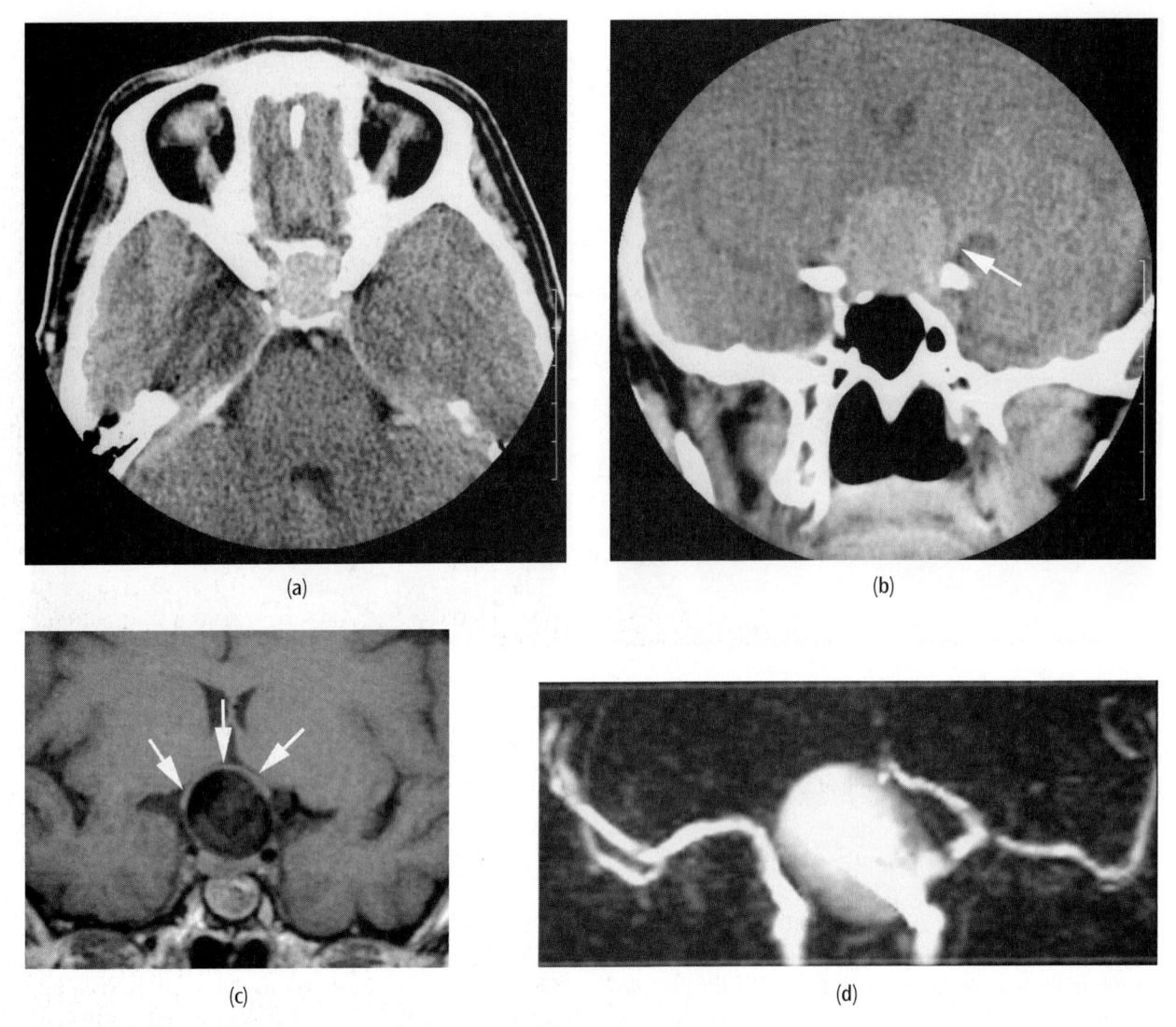

Figure 3.40. Axial (a) coronal (b) post-contrast CT scans with coronal uncontrasted T1-weighted MR (c) and maximum intensity protection reconstruction of three-dimensional time-of-flight MR angiogram. This large carotid/ophthalmic artery aneurysm appears very similar to a pituitary adenoma. Note the density of the lesion is identical to that of the terminal carotid artery (arrow in image b). Using a dynamic contrast enhancement technique would have emphasized in this patient the vascular nature of the lesion. Areas of flow-void and vortex signal within the aneurysm are clear on MRI. Note the compression of the chiasm (arrows image c). The diagnosis is confirmed by the magnetic resonance angiogram.

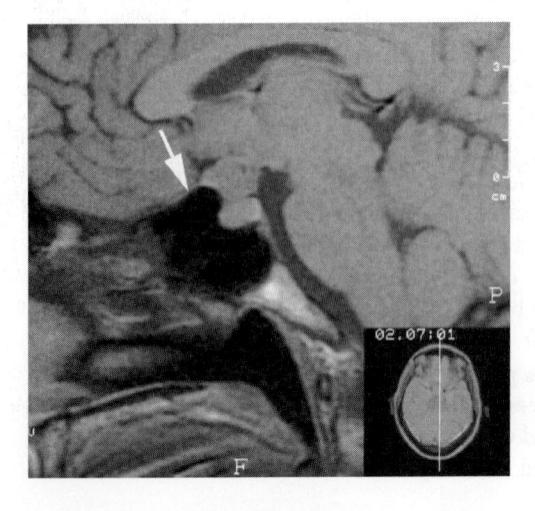

Figure 3.41. Suprasellar meningioma. Unenhanced sagittal T1-weighted MR image. The sphenoid sinus is 'blistered' upwards (pneumosinus dilatans, arrow). The tumour mass reaches up to compress the chiasm. It has a broad dural base and passes a little way into the sella but differs in intensity from the pituitary gland itself.

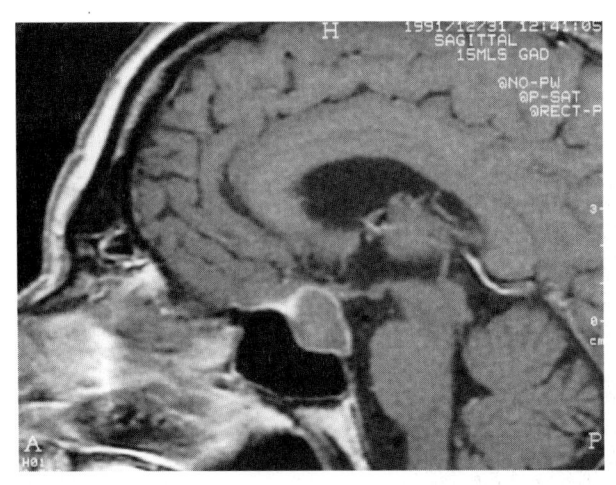

Figure 3.42. Pituitary abscess. Sagittal T1-weighted MR image after gadolinium enhancement. The pituitary gland is replaced by a low intensity rim-enhancing mass with enhancement passing anteriorly onto the planum sphenoidale. This appearance is quite distinct from pituitary adenoma.

(a)

(b)

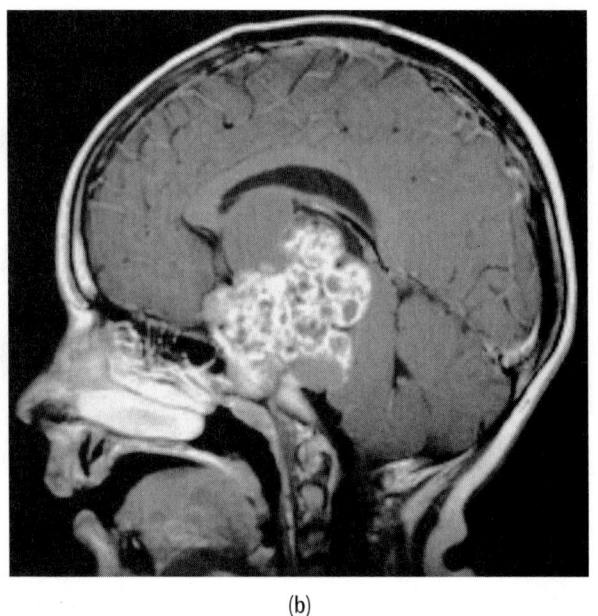

Figure 3.44. Sagittal pre- (a) and post-enhanced (b) MRI images of a young child with craniopharyngioma. Note different components to the mass. 'Engine oil' cysts are seen superiorly and inferiorly. Some are of iso- or slight hyperintensity to white matter (long arrows) while others are of very short T1 (arrow heads). The non-cystic portions of the tumour show extensive irregular enhancement (b).

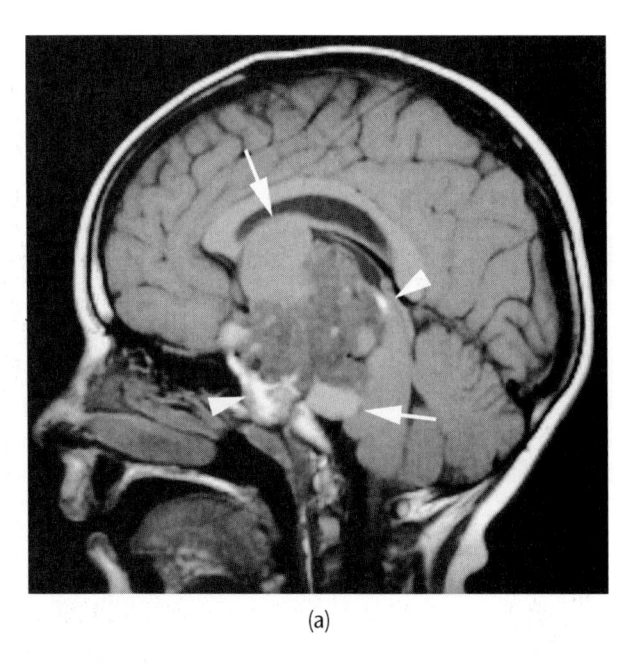

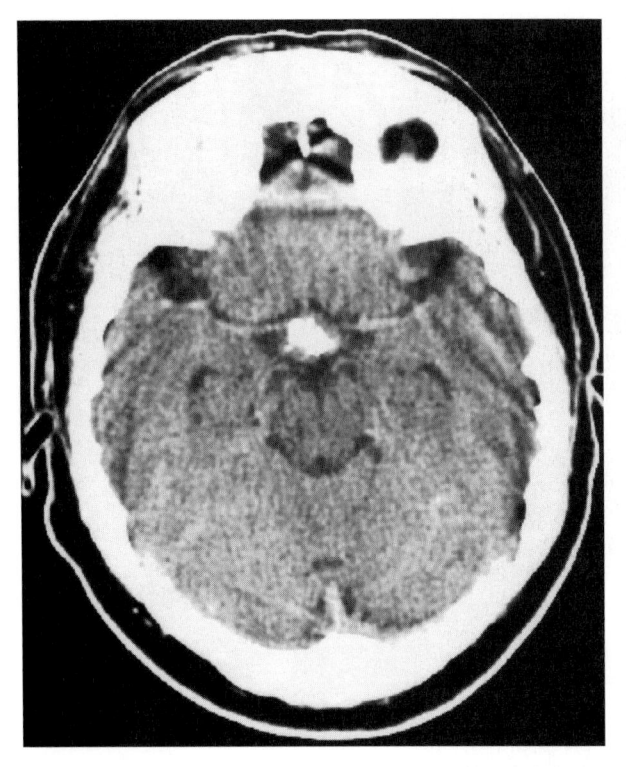

Figure 3.43. Craniopharyngioma. Axial post-contrast CT scan. There is a densely calcified sellar and suprasellar mass which is intimately related to the chiasm. This is a typical appearance of a craniopharyngioma particularly in a young person.

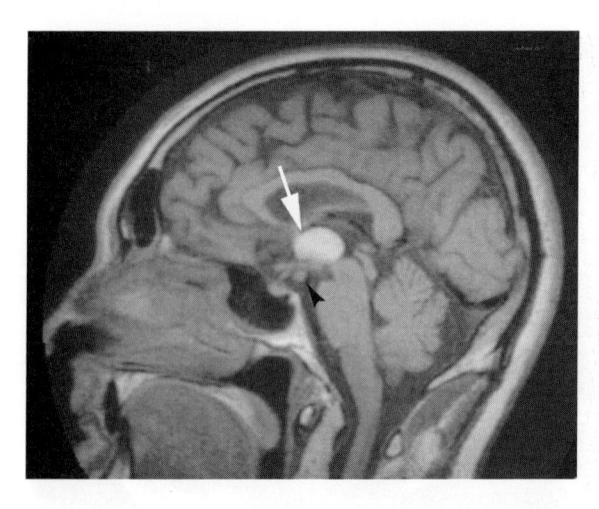

Figure 3.45. *Intraventricular craniopharyngioma. Sagittal T1WI. This short T1 mass (arrow) contained fluid typical of that seen in the craniopharyngioma. The normal pituitary stalk is seen but there is a small nodule of soft tissue intensity immediately below the chiasm (arrowhead).*

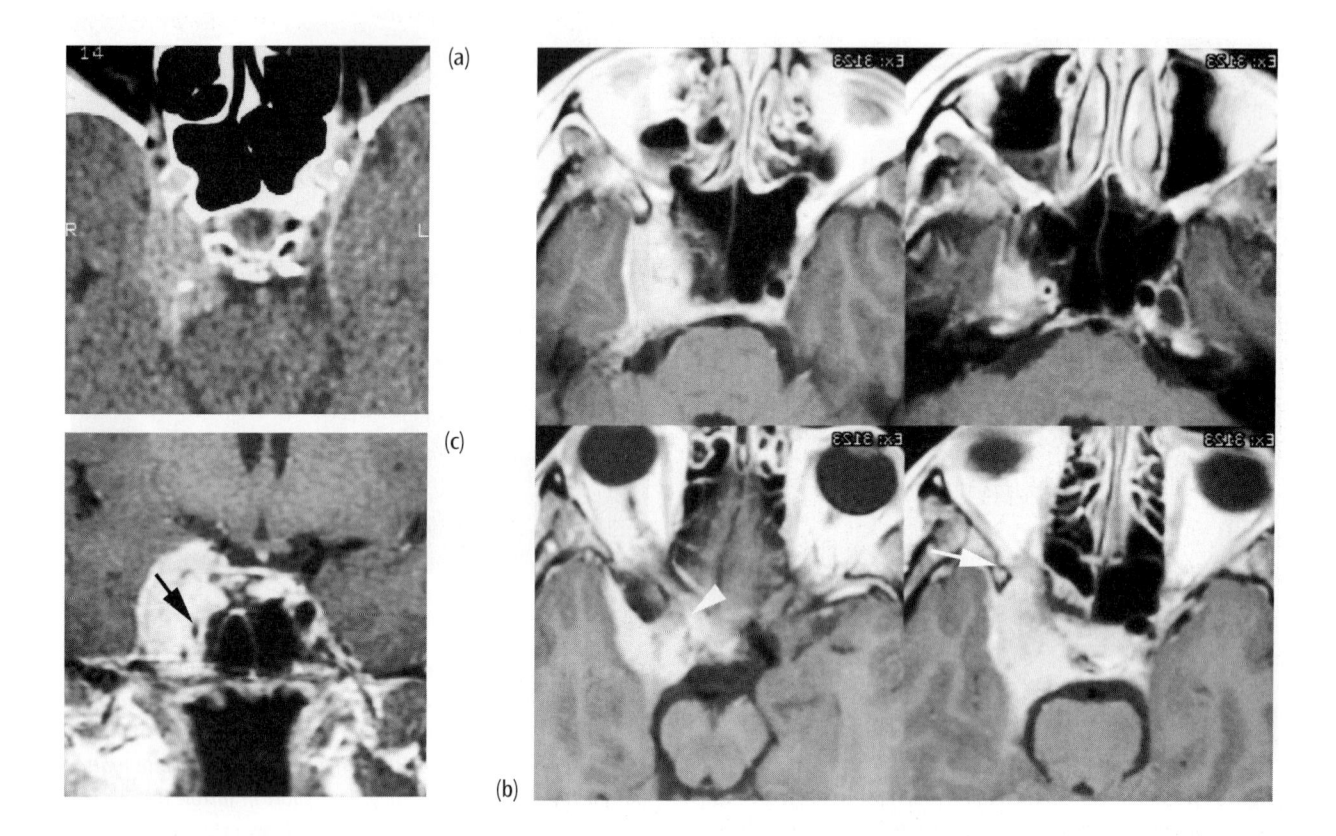

Figure 3.46. *Parasellar meningioma. Axial post-contrast CT scan (a), post-contrast axial MR (b) and post-contrast coronal MR (c). There is an irregular bulky mass within the right cavernous sinus which bulges underneath the free edge of the tentorium to abut the pons (a). The MR images (of a different patient) demonstrate that the tumour abuts and expands the superior ophthalmic fissure (arrow) and reaches the cranial end of the optic foramen (arrowhead in (b)). Distortion and narrowing of the cavernous carotid artery are demonstrated by reduction in diameter of the flow-voids in (b) and arrowed in (c).*

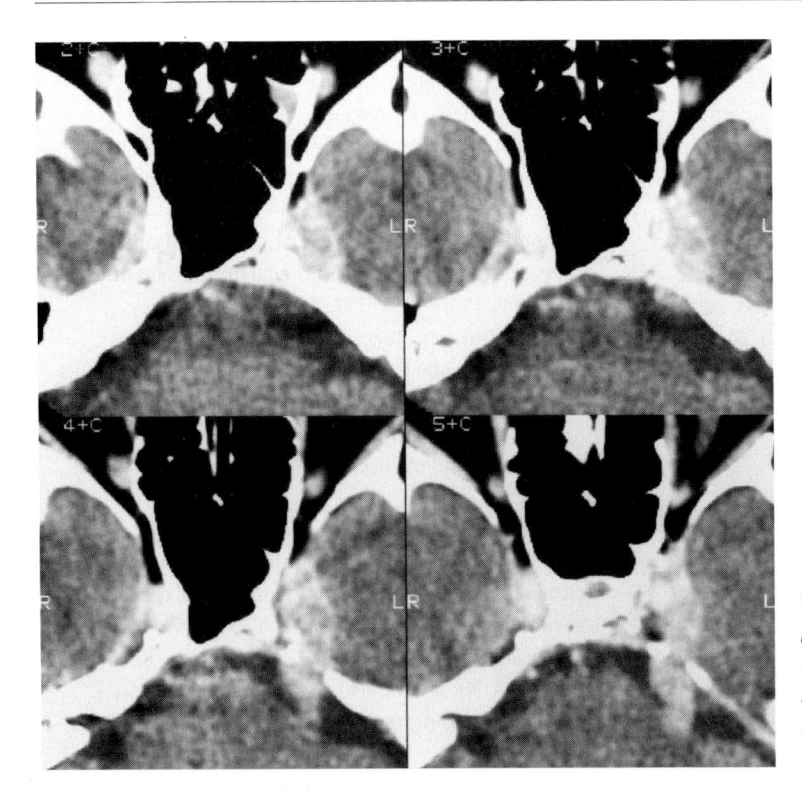

Tumours of the sellar and parasellar region 135

Figure 3.47. Axial post-contrast CT scan. This patient presented with pain and numbness in the left trigeminal nerve distribution. The cavernous sinus is bulky and an enhancing mass extends along the intracranial portion of the left Vth nerve. These features are typical of neurinoma.

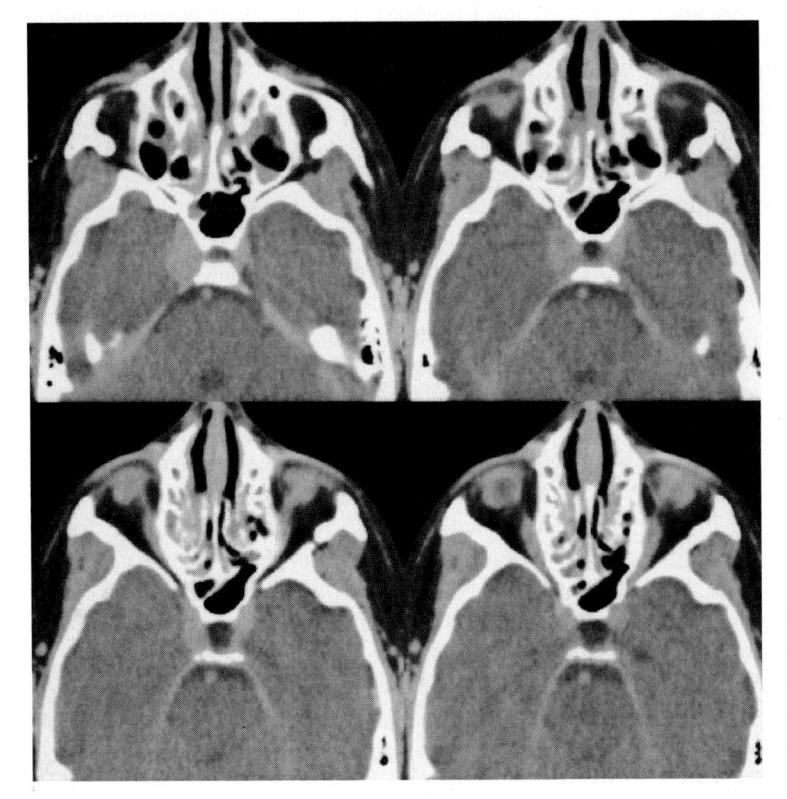

Figure 3.48. Inflammatory parasellar mass. Axial post-contrast CT scans show inflammatory changes in the paranasal sinuses and a smooth regular mass in the right cavernous sinus. With a typical history as in this patient, the diagnosis is usually clear.

Rathke pouch cysts can be considered a benign variant of craniopharyngioma, having the same embryological origin. They can be seen in the midline in the upper nasopharynx, the sella, or in the pituitary stalk. Many but not all are bright on T1WI. They do not show contrast-enhancement.

Sometimes the posterior pituitary fails to migrate from the tuber cinereum and remains lodged in the hypothalamus. This entity has been associated with breech delivery and is easily separated from a Rathke cleft cyst because the stalk is absent, and the high T1 signal of the posterior lobe is not seen in the sella.

Parasellar lesions

Tumours such as meningioma and neurinoma can grow in the cavernous sinuses, or can spread to this site from the orbital apex, brainstem or planum sphenoidale. The region can be examined with thin coronal sections, before and after contrast-enhancement. Meningioma within the cavernous sinus tends to distort and narrow the carotid artery (Fig. 3.46) and a soft tissue mass may be more apparent before rather than after enhancement, because the cavernous sinus invariably enhances strongly. Often, dural enhancement will extend onto the planum sphenoidale, or along the tentorium. Neurinomas tend to be 'softer', often distorting the carotid artery less. They follow the anatomical course of the nerve from which they arise (Fig. 3.47), and so particular care needs to be taken to look at the relevant skull base and orbital foramena and fissures. They appear as brightly enhancing lesions which approximate to grey matter density/intensity. They grow slowly and so tend to remodel bone around them, rather than eroding or invading it. Both neurinoma and meningioma can be limited to a small non-specific cavernous sinus mass and are usually indistinguishable in this context. Inflammatory lesions can also appear in this manner but present with a very different clinical picture, most often a painful ophthalmoplegia (Fig. 3.48).

REFERENCES

1 *WHO International Histological Classsification of Brain Tumours*. Kleihaus P, Burger PC, Scheithaeur BW (Eds). Berlin: Springer Verlag, 1993.
2 Dean BL, Drayer BP, Bird CR, Flom RA, Hodak JA *et al*. Gliomas: classification with MR imaging. *Radiology* 1990; **174**: 411–15.
3 Lee YY, Van Tassel P. Intracranial oligodendrogliomas: imaging findings in 35 untreated cases. *Am J Neuroradiol* 1989; **10**: 119–27.
4 Rippe DJ, Boyko OB, Radi M, Worth R, Fuller GN. MRI of temporal lobe pleomorphic xanthoastrocytoma. *J Comput Assist Tomogr* 1992; **16**: 856–9.
5 Felsberg GJ, Silver SA, Brown MT, Tien RD. Radiologic-pathologic correlation. Gliomatosis cerebri. *Am J Neuroradiol* 1994; **15**:1745–53.
6 Fulham MJ, Melisi JW, Nishimiya J, Dwyer AJ, Di Chiro G. Neuroimaging of juvenile pilocytic astrocytomas: an enigma. *Radiology* 1993; **189**: 221–5.
7 Raymond AA, Fish D, Halpin SFS, Scaravilli F, Alsanjari A *et al*. Dysembryoplastic neuroepithelial tumour: features in 16 patients. *Brain* 1994; **117**: 461–75.
8 Castillo M, Davis PC, Takei Y, Hoffman JC. Intracranial ganglioglioma: MR, CT, and clinical findings in 18 patients. *Am J Neuroradiol* 1990; **11**: 109–14.
9 Altman NR. MR and CT characteristics of gangliocytoma: a rare cause of epilepsy in children. *Am J Neuroradiol* 1988; **9**: 917–21.
10 Robles HA, Smirniotopoulos JG, Figueroa RE. Understanding the radiology of intracranial primitive neuroectodermal tumors from a pathological perspective: a review. *Semin US CT MR* 1992; **13**: 170–81.
11 Roman-Goldstein SM, Goldman DL, Howieson J, Belkin R, Neuwelt EA. MR of primary CNS lymphoma in immunologically normal patients. *Am J Neuroradiol* 1992; **13**: 1207–13.
12 Li C, Yousem DM, Hayden RE, Doty RL. Olfactory neuroblastoma: MR evaluation. *Am J Neuroradiol* 1993; **14**: 1167–71.
13 Sze G, Shin J, Johnson C, Liu D, Deck MDF. Intraparenchymal brain metastases: MR Imaging versus contrast enhanced CT. *Radiology* 1998; **168**: 1013–20.
14 Sze G, Johnson C, Kawamura Y, Goldberg N, Lange R *et al*. Comparison of single and triple dose contrast material in the MR screening of brain metastases. *Am J Neuroradiol* 1998; **19**: 821–8.
15 Spoto GP, Press GA, Hesselink JR, Solomon M. Intracranial ependymoma and subependymoma: MR manifestations. *Am J Neuroradiol* 1990; **11**: 83–91.
16 Jelinek J, Smirniotopoulos JG, Parisi JE, Kanzer M. Lateral ventricular neoplasms of the brain: differential diagnosis based on clinical, CT and MR findings. *Am J Neuroradiol* 1990; **11**: 567–74.
17 Goergen SK, Gonzales MF, McLean CA. Intraventricular neurocytoma: radiologic features and review of the literature. *Radiology* 1992; **182**: 787–92.
18 Wichmann W, Schubiger O, Deimling A, Schenker C, Valavanis A. Neuroradiology of central neurocytoma. *Neuroradiology* 1991; **33**: 143–8.
19 Hoeffel C, Boukobza M, Polivka M, Lot G, Guichard JP, Lafitte F, Reizine D, Merland JJ. MR manifestations of subependymomas. *Am J Neuroradial* 1995; **16**: 2121–9.
20 Coates TL, Hinshaw DB, Peckman N, Thompson JR, Hasso AN *et al*. Pediatric choroid plexus neoplasms: MR, CT and pathologic correlation. *Radiology* 1989; **173**: 81–8.
21 Maeder P, HoltOes SL, Basibüyük LN, Salford LG, Tapper UAS, Brun A. Colloid cysts of the third ventricle: correlation of MR and CT findings with histology and chemical analysis. *Am J Neuroradiol* 1990; **11**: 575–81.
22 Numaguchi Y, Foster RW, Gum GK. Large asymptomatic

noncolloid neuroepithelial cysts in the lateral ventricle: CT and MR features. *Neuroradiology* 1989; **31**: 98–101.

23 Tien RD, Barkovitch AJ, Edwards MSB, MR imaging of pineal tumours *Am J Neuroradiol* 1990; **11**: 557–65.

24 Hoffman HJ, Otsubo H, Hendrick EB *et al*. Intracranial germ cell tumours in children. *J Neurosurg* 1991; **74**: 545–51.

25 Makagawa H, Iwasaki S, Kichikawa K *et al*. MR imaging of pineocytoma: report of two cases. *Am J Neuroradiol* 1990; **11**: 195–8.

26 Elster AD, Challa VR, Gilbert TH, Richardson DN, Contento JC. Meningiomas: MR and histopathological features. *Radiology* 1989; **170**: 857–62.

27 Bourekas EC, Wildenhain P, Lewin JS, Tarr RW, Dastur KJ *et al*. The dural tail sign revisited. *Am J Neuroradiol* 1995; **16**: 1514–6.

28 Sherman JL, Camponovo E, Citrin CM. MR imaging of CSF-like choroidal fissure and parenchymal cysts of the brain. *Am J Neuroradiol* 1990; **11**: 939–45.

29 Elster AD. Modern imaging of the pituitary *Radiology* 1993; **1987**: 1–14.

30 Tien RD. Sequence of enhancement of various portions of the pituitary gland on gadolinium enhanced MR images: correlation with regional blood supply *Am J Radiol* 1992; **158**: 651–4.

31 Zimmerman RA Imaging of intrasellar, suprasellar, and suprasellar tumors. *Semin Roentgenol* 1990; **25**: 174–97.

FURTHER READING

1 Kaye AH, Laws ER (Eds). *Brain Tumors: an encyclopedic approach*. New York: Churchill Livingstone, 1995.
2 Russel DS, Rubenstein LJ. *Pathology of Tumors of the Nervous System*. Baltimore: Williams and Wilkins, 1989.
3 Atlas SW. Intra- and extra-axial brain tumors. In: *Magnetic Resonance Imaging of the Brain and Spine*. New York: Raven Press, 1991

APPENDIX

SUGGESTED SCAN PROTOCOLS FOR COMMON CLINICAL PRESENTATIONS

Protocol 1 *Symptoms/signs of raised intracranial pressure/suspicious headaches*

	MRI	CT
Essential	Axial T2	Axial routine scan
Additional scans and notes	Axial PD or FLAIR. Coronal T2 or IR. Contrast-enhancement not necessary for 'normal' scan	Contrast-enhancement not necessary for 'normal' scan

Protocol 2 *Generalized tonic–clonic epilepsy*

	MRI	CT
Essential	Axial T2 + PD + Coronal IR or T1-weighted volume	Axial routine scan
Additional scans and notes	High resolution coronal T2WI through area of EEG abnormality. Contrast-enhancement not necessary for 'normal' scan	Contrast-enhancement not necessary for 'normal' scan

Protocol 3 *Headache or epilepsy with focal symptoms or signs*

	MRI	CT
Essential	Axial T2 + PD or FLAIR + Coronal IR or T1-weighted volume	Axial routine scan before and after contrast-enhancement
Additional scans and notes	High resolution coronal T2WI through area of EEG abnormality. Contrast-enhancement not necessary for 'normal' scan	Consider coronal scans or altered axial scan plane for temporal lobe

Protocol 4 *Partial seizures/temporal lobe epilepsy*

	MRI	CT
Essential	Axial T2 + Coronal IR or high resolution T2WI, ideally orthogonal to the plane of the temporal lobe	Axial routine scan
Additional scans and notes	Post-contrast images in 2 planes if tumour present. If not consider T1-weighted volume acquisition, and thin reformatted images.	Consider altered axial scan plane. Enhanced scans if suspicious or if tumour seen. Contrast medium is usually otherwise unhelpful.

Protocol 5 *Lesion affecting orbital apex or cavernous sinus (i.e. any combination of palsies of the IInd to VIth cranial nerves)*

	MRI	CT
Essential	Axial T2 + PD. Coronal T1-weighted thin sections from globe to clivus before and after contrast	Coronal thin sections from globe to clivus with rapid infusion of contrast
Additional scans and notes	T1-weighted fat sat post-contrast T2-weighted fat sat before contrast	Axial post-contrast scans through the head. Thin axial sections through the orbit, particularly if reformatting capability not good

Protocol 6 *Lesion at the cerebellopontine angle i.e. affecting the VIIth and VIIIth nerves*

	MRI	CT
Essential	Either high resolution axial T2WI or post-contrast axial and coronal T1WI	Routine whole head scan, before and after contrast medium
Additional scans and notes	Unenhanced T1WI are recommended in at least one plane before any contrast medium injection. Axial whole head T2WI ideal	Thin sections through the skull base and petrous bones strongly recommended with soft tissue and bone windows.

Protocol 7 *Trigeminal neuralgia or other Vth nerve lesion*

	MRI	CT
Essential	Axial T2WI, starting low (C2 level). Coronal T1WI from globe to pons before and after gadolinium	Routine whole head, starting at C2, with additional thin sections through skull base and petrous before and after high dose contrast medium
Additional scans and notes	High resolution T2WI from CP angle to midbrain. Possibly MR angiography	Coronal post-contrast images from globe to pons

Protocol 8 *Lesion of the lower cranial nerves*

	MRI	CT
Essential	Axial T2 and PDWI. Contrast medium if suspicious areas	Routine whole head scan, before and after contrast medium
Additional scans and notes	Plain and enhanced T1WI in axial and/or coronal planes	Thin sections through the skull base and foramen magnum with soft tissue and bone windows

4

Infratentorial tumours

MARGARET D HOURIHAN

Introduction	140	Extra-axial tumours	152
Intra-axial tumours in children	140	Uncommon extra-axial tumours	155
Intra-axial tumours in adults	146	References	161
Uncommon intra-axial tumours	150		

INTRODUCTION

The general principles of imaging and diagnosis of brain tumours discussed in the introduction of the previous chapter also apply to the infratentorial region. The sensitivity of computed tomography (CT) to detect lesions in the posterior fossa is increased with thin slice thickness e.g. 2–5 mm, and intravenous contrast medium. Magnetic resonance imaging (MRI), however, is the investigation of choice in patients suspected of having a posterior fossa tumour because of its greater resolution, increased sensitivity and virtually artefact-free imaging; MRI better defines the extent and the site of tumour origin i.e. intra-axial or extra-axial, an important feature when trying to predict tumour type and when making a preoperative assessment.

Infratentorial tumours account for 25% of all brain tumours in adults and 15–20% of intra-axial brain tumours. Metastases are the most common intra-axial posterior fossa tumour in an adult, with haemangioblastoma the second most common accounting for 7–10% of posterior fossa tumours. The common extra-axial tumours seen within the posterior fossa in adults are schwannoma, meningioma and epidermoid.

Central nervous system (CNS) tumours are the second most common childhood neoplasm after leukaemia, accounting for 15% of all paediatric neoplasms. The posterior fossa, either cerebellum or brainstem, is the most common site of primary CNS tumours in children older than 1 year. Whilst metastases to the CNS are rare in children, CNS spread of primary intracerebral neoplasms is more common and in this age-group the preoperative assessment of any posterior fossa tumour should include enhanced MRI of the whole neuroaxis to look for seeding.

The clinical presentation of posterior fossa tumours is essentially the same for all age groups. The symptoms result from either obstruction to cerebrospinal fluid (CSF) flow and hydrocephalus, or focal neurological deficits which will depend on the structures involved e.g. vermis or cerebellar hemisphere. The clinical presentation is therefore of little help when trying to differentiate between posterior fossa tumours. The most helpful features are the age of the patient (adult or child), the location of the tumour (intra-axial or extra-axial), and certain morphological features determined on imaging. Specific features of the common posterior fossa tumours are summarized in Table 4.1.

INTRA-AXIAL TUMOURS IN CHILDREN

Cerebellar astrocytoma

Cerebellar astrocytoma and medulloblastoma are the most common paediatric posterior fossa tumours. (Studies differ as to which is the more common.) Cerebellar astrocytomas differ from astrocytomas elsewhere in the brain, as they occur in early life, within the first two decades with a peak at 10 years. There are two histological types of astrocytoma – pilocytic and fibrillary.

Pilocytic astrocytomas are most common (85%) and have a good prognosis with the highest survival rate of all primary brain tumours (80–90%: 10 years survival). With total resection the cure rate approaches 100%, although late recurrences, after 20 years, have been reported. Both CT and MRI demonstrate a well defined

Table 4.1 Differential diagnosis of the common infratentorial tumours

Tumour type	Age group (peak in years)	Location	Imaging features (CT/MRI)
Cerebellar astrocytoma	Child (10)	Intra-axial Hemisphere, vermis	Large, cystic tumour with mural nodule which enhances. Minimal oedema. Displaces fourth ventricle. Hydrocephalus (50%) on presentation.
Medulloblastoma	Child (5–9) Adult (25–30)	Intra-axial Midline, roof of fourth ventricle	Well defined, homogeneous. Hyperdense on unenhanced CT scan. Hypo/isointense T1WI, hyperintense T2WI, but may be hypointense to grey matter. Homogeneous enhancement. Subarachnoid spread common. Displaces fourth ventricle anteriorly. Hydrocephalus (95%).
Brainstem glioma	Child – 2nd decade (10–20)	Intra-axial Midline, brainstem	Enlarges brainstem (pons). Displaces fourth ventricle posteriorly. Hydrocephalus relatively uncommon except when tectal plate involved
Ependymoma	Child (10–15) Adult (mid 30s)	Intraventricular – fourth ventricle (90% of infratentorial ependymomas)	Lobulated heterogeneous mass which fills fourth ventricle and extends through foramina into subarachnoid cisterns. Calcification common (50%). Heterogeneous enhancement. Subarachnoid spread occurs (10–30%). Associated hydrocephalus
Metastasis	Adult (> 40)	Intra-axial (but maybe extra-axial/calvarial)	Variable appearance depending on primary tumour. Discrete mass often marked associated oedema. Moderate-to-marked enhancement. Hydrocephalus at presentation
Haemangioblastoma	Adult sporadic (50–60) VHL (30s)	Intra-axial Hemisphere (80–85%), medulla (2%), spinal cord (5–15%)	Well defined cystic tumour with mural nodule that strongly enhances. May be multiple in von Hippel-Lindau (VHL)
Choroid plexus papilloma	Adult Child	Intraventricular – fourth ventricle – adult lateral, third ventricle – child	Well defined lobulated often pedunculated, heterogeneous mass. Strongly enhancing. Hydrocephalus due to obstruction of fourth and/or overproduction of CSF.

partly cystic mass with a solid mural nodule of vascular tissue, arising in the vermis or cerebellar hemisphere, with minimal surrounding oedema (Fig. 4.1). Calcification is uncommon (less than 10%), but if present is better shown on CT. On CT there is marked but variable enhancement of the solid portion. The cyst wall, which consists of compressed cerebellum, may occasionally show some faint enhancement. The fourth ventricle is displaced and compressed by tumour and obstructive hydrocephalus may be present particularly if the tumour arises from the vermis.

The diagnosis of a pilocytic astrocytoma can be made on MRI by identifying a large, mainly cystic tumour arising in the cerebellar hemisphere or vermis. The cystic portion is iso- or hyperintense to CSF on T2-weighted imaging (T2WI), due to a high protein content. The smaller solid portion is hypo- or isointense to grey matter on T1WI and moderately hyperintense on T2WI and enhances homogeneously (Fig. 4.2). The fibrillary type (15%) is frequently anaplastic and infiltrative and carries a worse prognosis. These tumours are more likely to occur in the older age-group (early adulthood). More solid tumours may be associated with necrosis and haemorrhage. Astrocytomas displace and compress the fourth ventricle rather than fill it, important features when differentiating from ependymoma. Calcification is also more frequent in ependymomas. Medulloblastoma, the other common posterior fossa tumour in the paediatric age-group is usually a homogeneous midline mass, which is hyperdense on CT and homogeneously enhances. In adults an atypical medulloblastoma may be indistinguishable from an astrocytoma. The age of onset may help differentiate haemangioblastoma which is rarely seen before the age of 20 years.

Medulloblastoma

Medulloblastoma is a primitive neuroepithelial tumour (PNET) which originates from primitive, undifferentiated cells capable of differentiating along glial or neuronal lines. Cerebellar PNETs can be associated with other tumours and several syndromes e.g. basal cell naevus (Gorlin) syndrome; 75% present before the age of 10 years, with 40% within the first 5 years. There is a slight male predominance and 15% present in adults with a second peak between 25 and 30 years. Overall 5-year survival rates of greater than 50% are reported.

A total of 75% of medulloblastomas are midline tumours arising from the roof of the fourth ventricle, which they fill and obstruct. Not infrequently these tumours may arise laterally (25%); this is more common in the adult group. These lateral tumours may extend through the foramina of Luschka or Magendie, and can

(a)

(b)

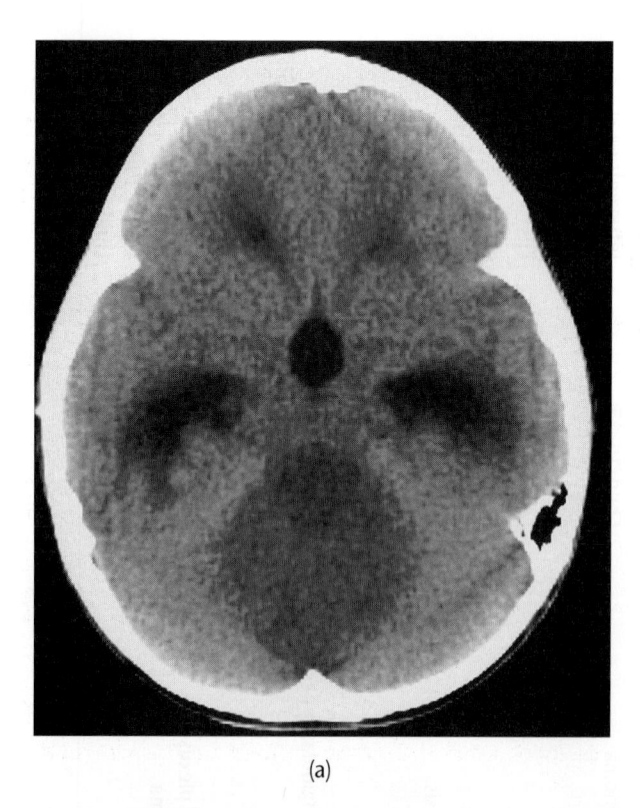

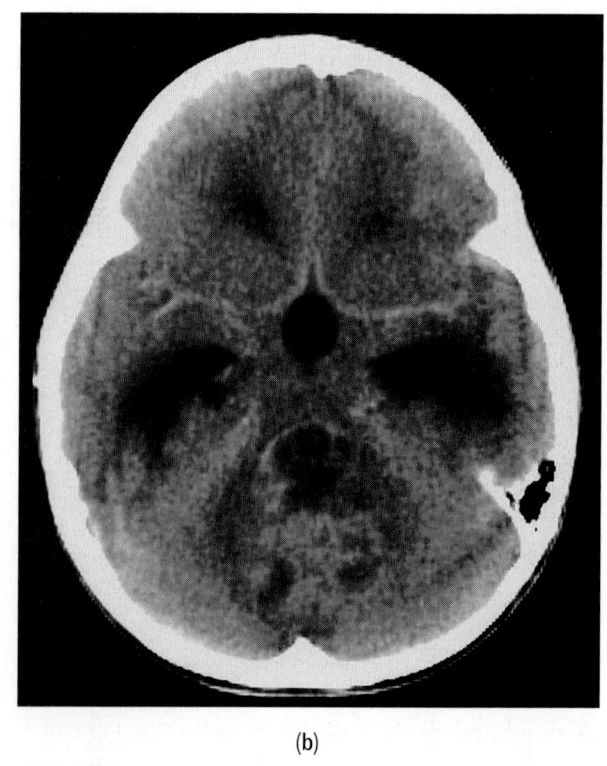

Figure 4.1 *Astrocytoma. (a) Axial CT scan. A hypodense vermian mass is demonstrated, it compresses and displaces the fourth ventricle anteriorly. There is associated obstructive hydrocephalus. (b) Enhanced axial CT scan. Note the irregular enhancement of this partly cystic, partly solid tumour.*

Intra-axial tumours in children 143

(a)

(b)

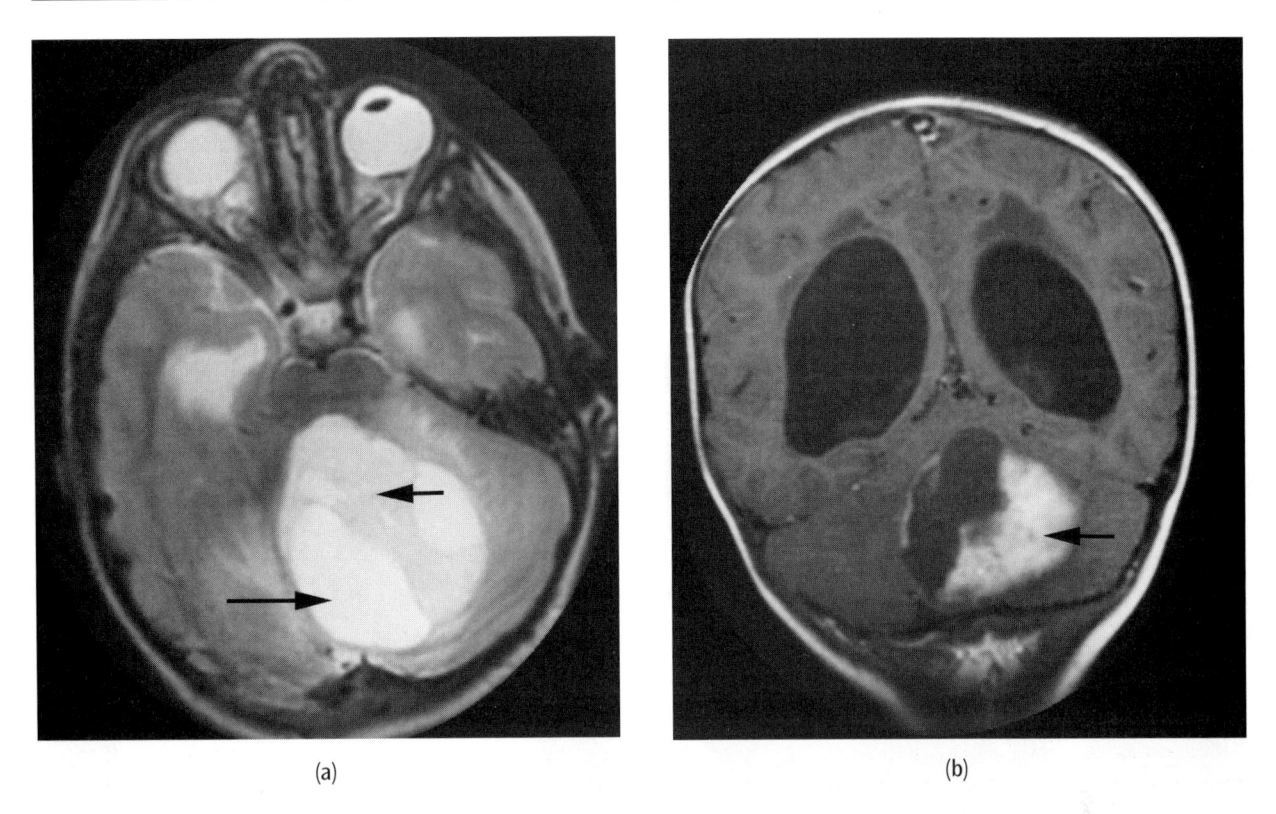

Figure 4.2 *Astrocytoma. (a) T2-weighted axial MR scan. A hyperintense, partly cystic (long arrow), partly solid (short arrow) mass is seen arising in the vermis. This displaces and compresses the fourth ventricle. (b) T1-weighted post-contrast axial MR scan. The solid component of this pilocytic astrocytoma enhances intensely and inhomogeneously (arrow).*

(a)

(b)

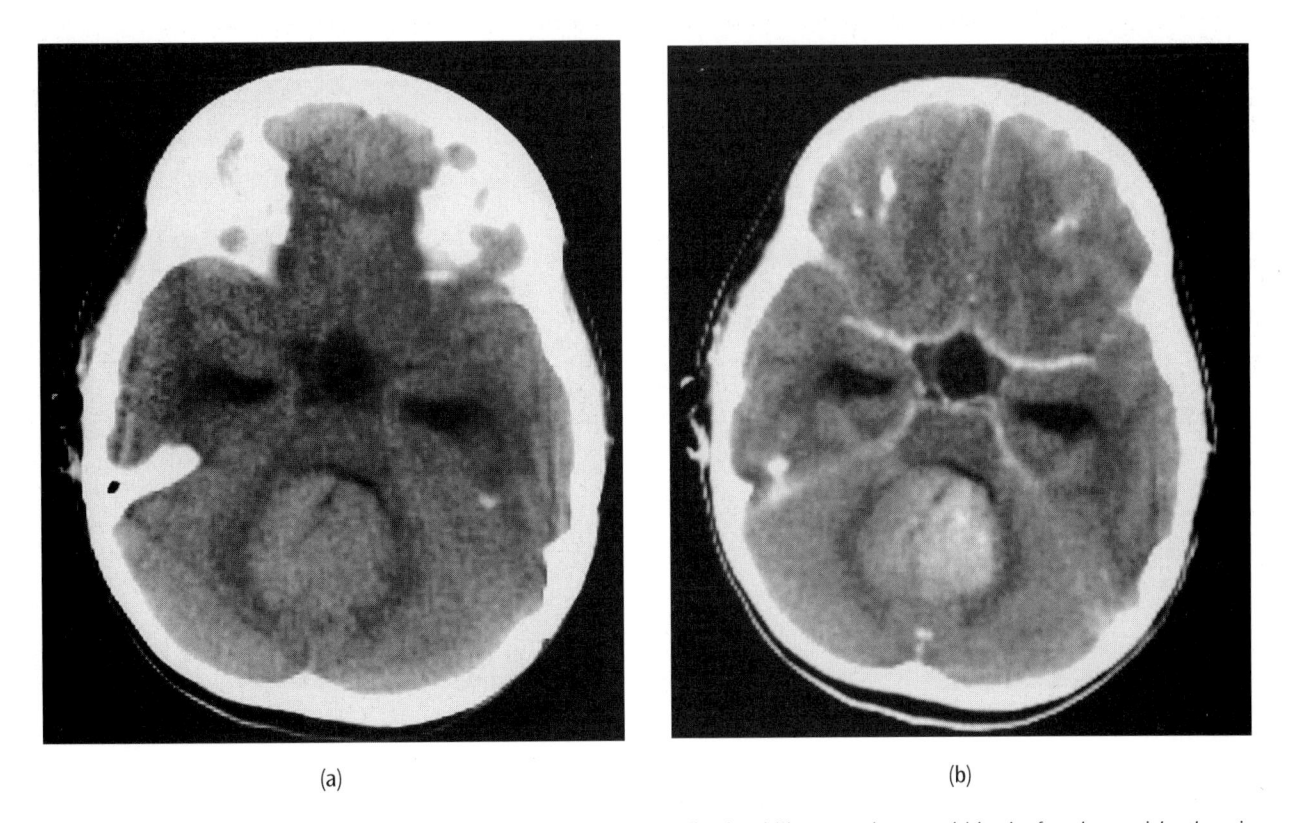

Figure 4.3 *Medulloblastoma. (a) Axial CT scan. A hyperdense, well defined, midline mass is seen within the fourth ventricle, there is associated obstructive hydrocephalus. (b) Enhanced axial CT scan. Marked enhancement of this tumour is seen.*

rarely be seen at the cerebellopontine angle and may invade the leptomeninges. Typically on CT, medulloblastomas are rounded or lobulated, well-defined midline posterior fossa mass lesions which are homogeneously hyperdense and enhance (Fig. 4.3). Obstructive hydrocephalus is present in 95% of cases. Calcification is seen uncommonly (15–50%). Heterogeneity with cystic areas or necrosis occurs (65%) and is more prominent in lateral tumours. The presence of necrosis carries a worse prognosis. The midline intraventricular mass on MRI has a relatively homogeneous signal intensity which is hypo- to isointense on T1WI and iso- or slightly hyper-

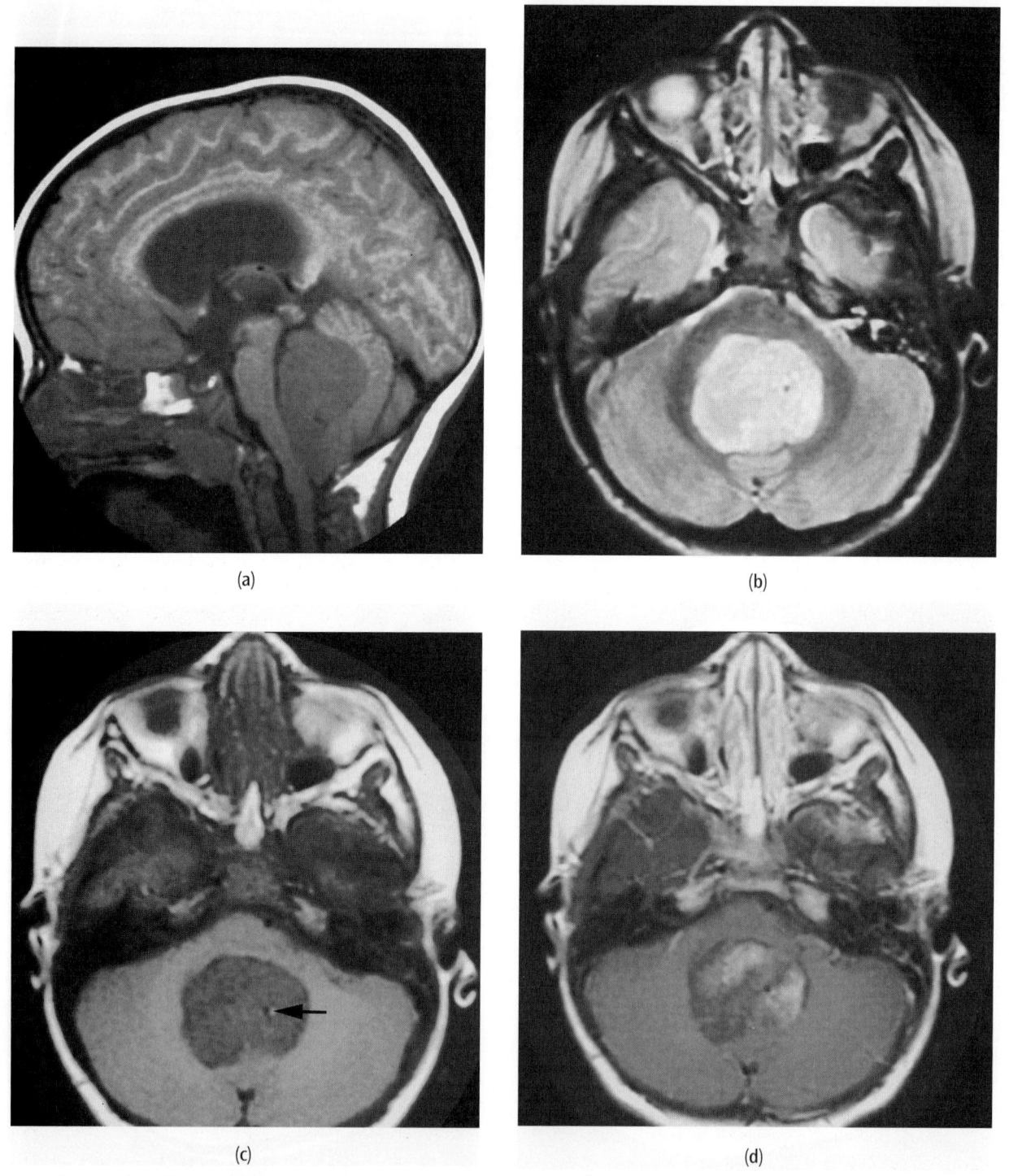

Figure 4.4 *Medulloblastoma. (Same patient as in Fig. 4.3.) (a) T1-weighted sagittal MR scan. The fourth ventricle is filled with a large homogeneous mass which is isointense to grey matter. (b) T2-weighted axial MR scan. The tumour is hyperintense to grey matter and displaces the brainstem anteriorly. (c), (d) T1-weighted pre- and post-contrast axial MR scans. Heterogeneous enhancement after contrast is seen in this tumour. Note the signal void from a dilated feeding vessel (arrow).*

intense on T2WI and may even be hypointense to grey matter (Fig. 4.4). They are therefore not typically hyperintense, and this may be an important distinguishing feature. Tumours enhance homogeneously but it is not unusual to find areas of signal heterogeneity due to haemorrhage (rare), cysts or necrosis, features better seen on MRI. Dissemination through the CNS is common (50–60%) and it is important at the time of diagnosis to image the whole neuroaxis, by enhanced MRI, to look for subarachnoid spread. Medulloblastomas are the most common CNS tumour to metastasize outside the CNS although this occurs rarely (6%). Secondaries are most common in bone but occasionally lymph nodes, abdominal viscera or lung are affected.

Atypical features are common in these tumours i.e. lack of enhancement, calcification, cystic or necrotic areas, and lateral location, and these should be considered when making a radiological diagnosis. The main differential diagnoses for midline tumours, usually in the paediatric age group, are ependymoma and vermian pilocytic astrocytoma and for the laterally based tumours usually seen in adults, pilocytic astrocytoma, ependymoma, haemangioblastoma, choroid plexus papilloma and metastases.

Brainstem glioma

Brainstem glioma is usually a slow growing astrocytoma of the fibrillary, infiltrating type. It is the third most common posterior fossa tumour (15–25%) and accounts for 10% of all childhood and adolescent brain tumours. The pons is most commonly involved either unilaterally or bilaterally and extension into the medulla, midbrain and cerebellar hemispheres occurs. The tumour diffusely infiltrates the brainstem and children present with either cranial nerve deficit, long tract signs, and/or gait disturbance. Hydrocephalus is relatively uncommon except if the tumour involves the tectal plate. Posterior displacement of the fourth ventricle may be a helpful sign in differentiating brainstem glioma from the other intraventricular or vermian tumours of childhood. Because of its anatomic location and its infiltrative nature, this tumour is not surgically resectable. The prognosis is poor with an overall 5-year survival of 20%.

Pilocytic astrocytomas of low grade also occur in the brainstem, mainly in the medulla or at the cervicomedullary junction. Usually focal in nature, these tumours carry a slightly better prognosis. Without MRI the diagnosis of brainstem glioma is difficult to make and suspicion of the diagnosis is made when secondary signs of localized or diffuse enlargement of the brainstem, which is slightly lower in density than normal, is seen on CT, in a child with progressive cranial nerve palsies. The investigation of choice to confirm this diagnosis is MRI. Ill-defined abnormal signal is seen within the involved brainstem, usually within the pons and this may extend throughout the brainstem, into the cerebellum and, in an exophytic tumour, may be seen in the cerebellopontine angle. The tumour is hypo- or isointense to grey matter on T1WI and hyperintense on T2WI (Fig. 4.5). On T1WI, heterogeneity may be present due to cysts, microcalcification (15–25%), or haemorrhage, which are more common in high grade tumours. These tumours may not enhance but, if present, enhancement is often irregular. Rarely CSF dissemination may occur. The differential diagnosis of abnormal signal within the brainstem of a child includes encephalitis, infarction, demyelination, arteriovenous or occult vascular malformations. Each of these should be excluded by the clinical presentation, in particular the pattern of onset of symptoms and their progression. Stereotactic biopsy may be performed to confirm the clinical and radiological diagnosis.

Ependymoma

Ependymoma is the fourth most common (15%) posterior fossa tumour in children. There is an association with neurofibromatosis type 2 (NF2). Their peak incidence is between 10 and 15 years but there is a small second peak in the mid-30s. Most ependymomas occur infratentorally (60%) and of these the majority can be found filling the fourth ventricle where they have arisen from the ependymal lining of the floor. Ependymomas characteristically extend into the lateral recesses and through the foramen of Luschka to the cerebellopontine cisterns and through the foramen of Magendie into the cisterna magna. These relatively slow growing tumours are moderately radiosensitive and have a variable prognosis with an overall 5-year survival of 45%. Frequently CNS dissemination occurs (10–30%) but less often than in primitive neuroectodermal tumour (PNET). It is important to screen the whole neuroaxis by enhanced MRI preoperatively and on postoperative follow-up scans, to look for subarachnoid seeding. Extracranial metastases are fortunately rare. Characteristically ependymomas are partly cystic, with punctate calcification (50%), but they may be haemorrhagic and therefore have a heterogeneous appearance. Typically there is a lobulated mass, isodense on CT with heterogeneous enhancement, which fills and dilates the fourth ventricle and is associated with obstructive hydrocephalus (Fig. 4.6). Extension through the foramina into the subarachnoid cisterns occurs and tumour can extend through the foramen magnum into the upper cervical canal compressing the posterior aspect of the upper cervical cord. This appearance is diagnostic of ependymoma and is best seen on sagittal MRI (Fig. 4.7). On MRI the tumour mass has a heterogeneous mixed signal with the solid portion hypo- or isointense to grey matter on T1WI and hyperintense on T2WI (Fig. 4.8). The cyst fluid has sim-

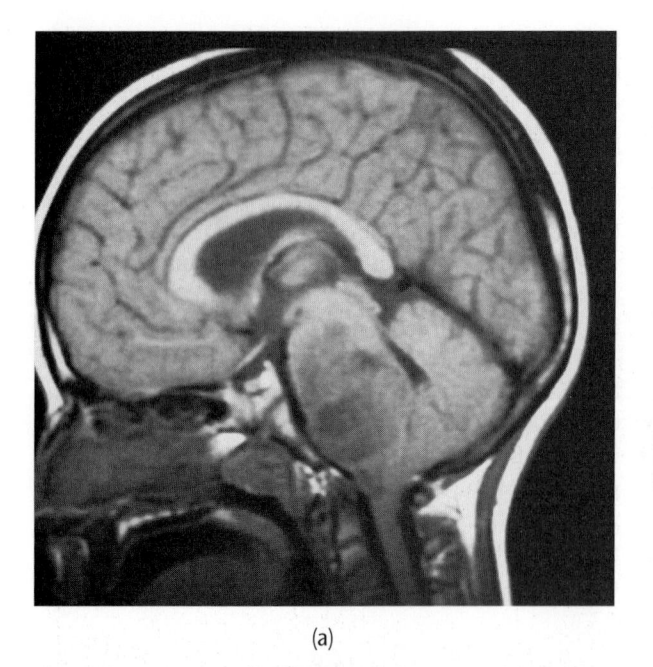

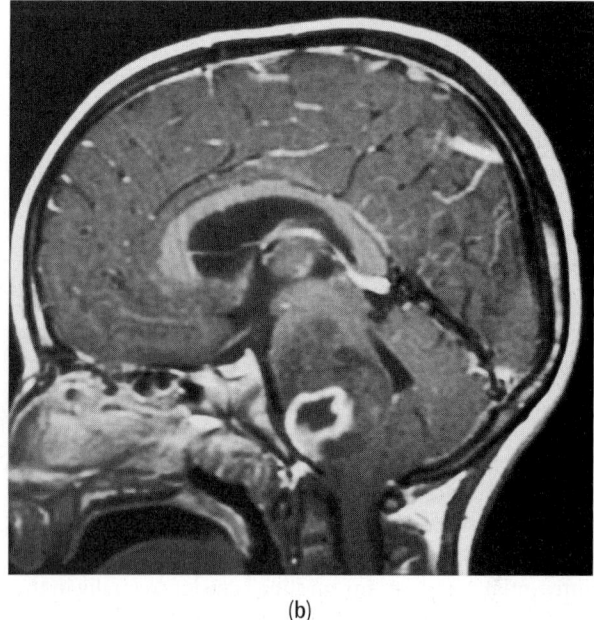

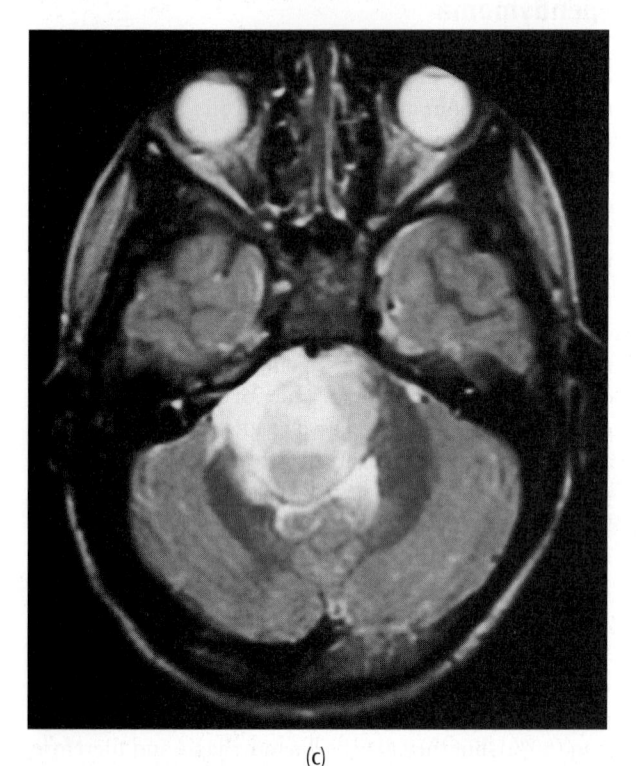

Figure 4.5 Brainstem glioma. (a), (b) T1-weighted pre- and post-contrast sagittal MR scans. An unhomogeneous ill-defined mass expands the pons. Irregular enhancement is present. (c) T2-weighted axial MR scan. The hyperintense mass (to grey matter) is compressing the fourth ventricle and displacing it posteriorly.

ilar signal characteristics to CSF. This tumour may be difficult to differentiate from a midline, homogeneously enhancing, medulloblastoma but not from a vermian pilocytic astrocytoma with its large cyst and mural nodule. Brainstem glioma (pontine astrocytoma) causes diffuse brainstem infiltration and displacement of the fourth ventricle posteriorly and choroid plexus papilloma rarely occurs in the fourth ventricle unless in adults and are seen to enhance more homogeneously.

INTRA-AXIAL TUMOURS IN ADULTS

Metastases

A metastasis is the commonest cause of a intra-axial posterior fossa tumour in adulthood and although occurring at all ages, the highest incidence is between the fourth and sixth decades. The presenting symptoms may be related to the anatomic location of the lesion or, more often, secondary to obstructive hydrocephalus caused by the tumour mass and its surrounding oedema. Patients with solitary lesions may benefit from urgent surgical removal of the solitary lesion or shunting, to relieve hydrocephalus. A preoperative enhanced MR scan should be performed to exclude other 'silent' secondary lesions. Metastatic disease in the posterior fossa may come from lung (45–50%), breast (15%), melanoma (10–15%), the gastrointestinal and genitourinary tracts (10–15% each). The primary site will remain unknown in 10–15% of cases. Parenchymal metastases from the above may involve both the supratentorial and infratentorial regions, although metastases from a renal cell carcinoma tend to be solitary and involve the infratentorial region. In many (45%) the finding of intracranial metastatic disease precedes the diagnosis of primary cancer. Secondary involvement of the cerebellum may also occur by direct spread from secondaries in the calvarial bone or dura. Contrast-enhanced MRI is more sensitive than CT for detection of brain metastases. The

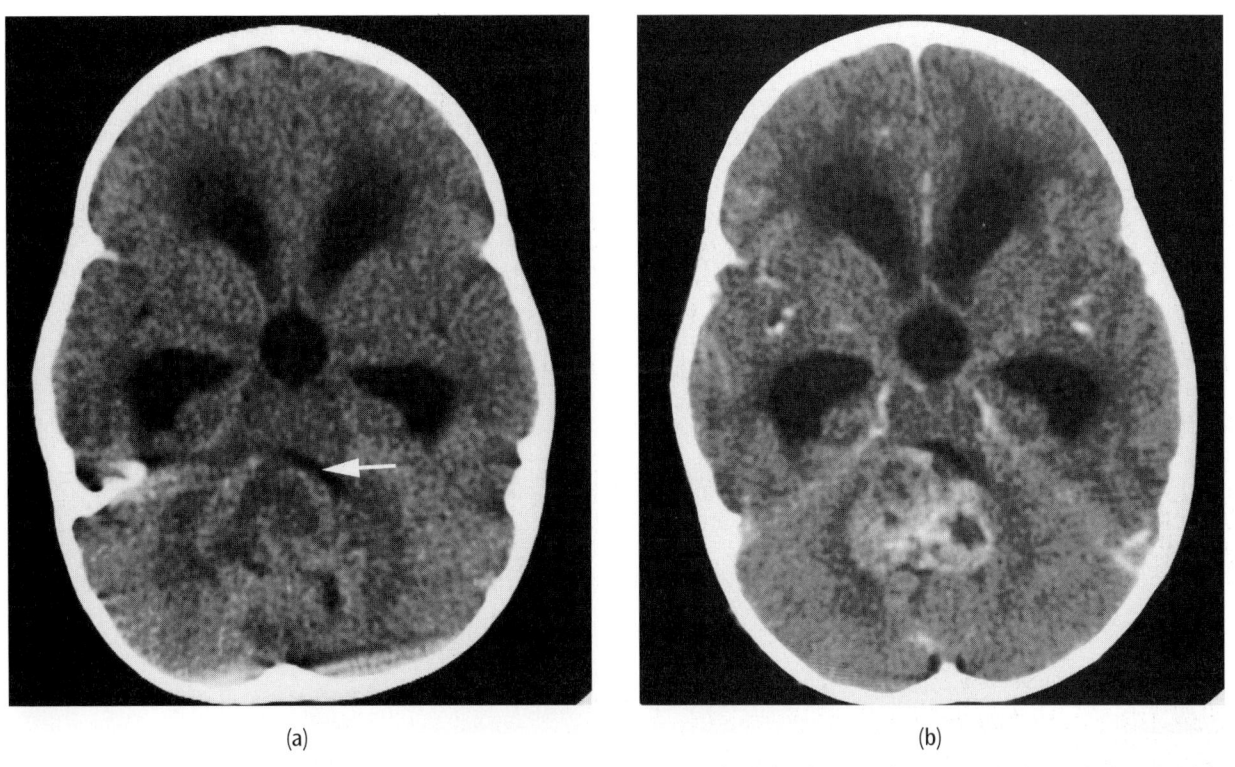

Figure 4.6 *Ependymoma. (a), (b) Axial CT scans pre- and post-contrast. A mixed density mass is present within the fourth ventricle (arrow) with irregular enhancement. There is associated obstructive hydrocephalus.*

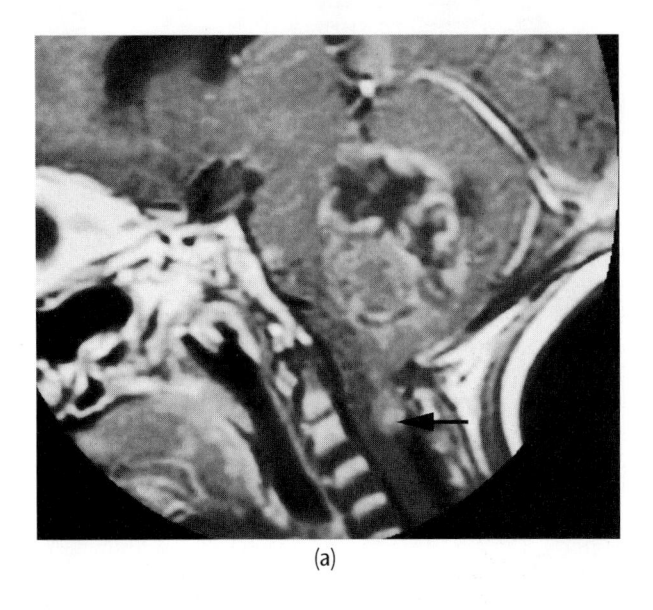

Figure 4.7 *Ependymoma. (a) T1-weighted post-contrast sagittal MR scan. The ependymoma extends into the upper cervical canal (arrow). (b) T1-weighted axial post-contrast MR scan. Tumour also extends into the left cerebellopontine angle (arrow).*

CT and MRI features of metastases and their differential diagnoses have been covered in the preceding chapter. The differential diagnosis of a solitary posterior fossa tumour in an adult should include haemangioblastoma and lymphoma. The former is typically a cystic mass with a peripheral strongly enhancing mural nodule. Multiple haemangioblastomas, in von Hippel–Lindau syndrome (VHL), should also be considered in the differential of multiple metastases. Primary cerebral lymphoma rarely involves the posterior fossa unless the

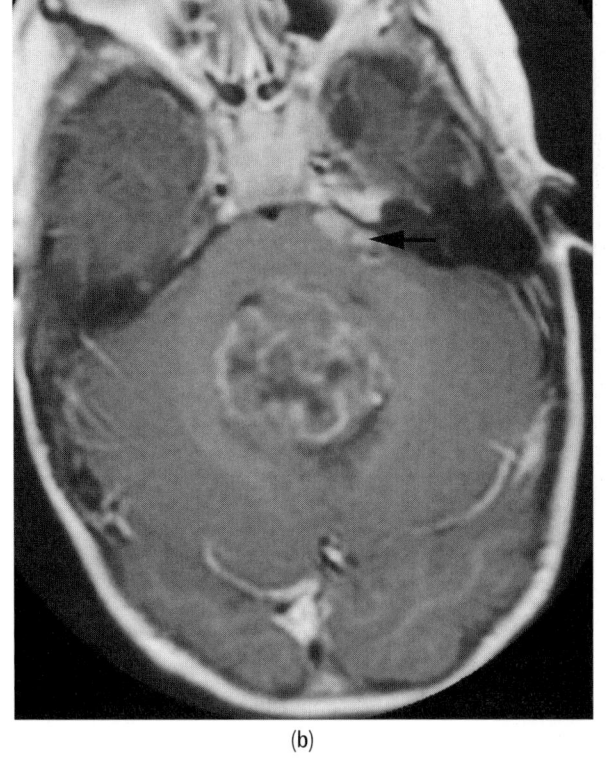

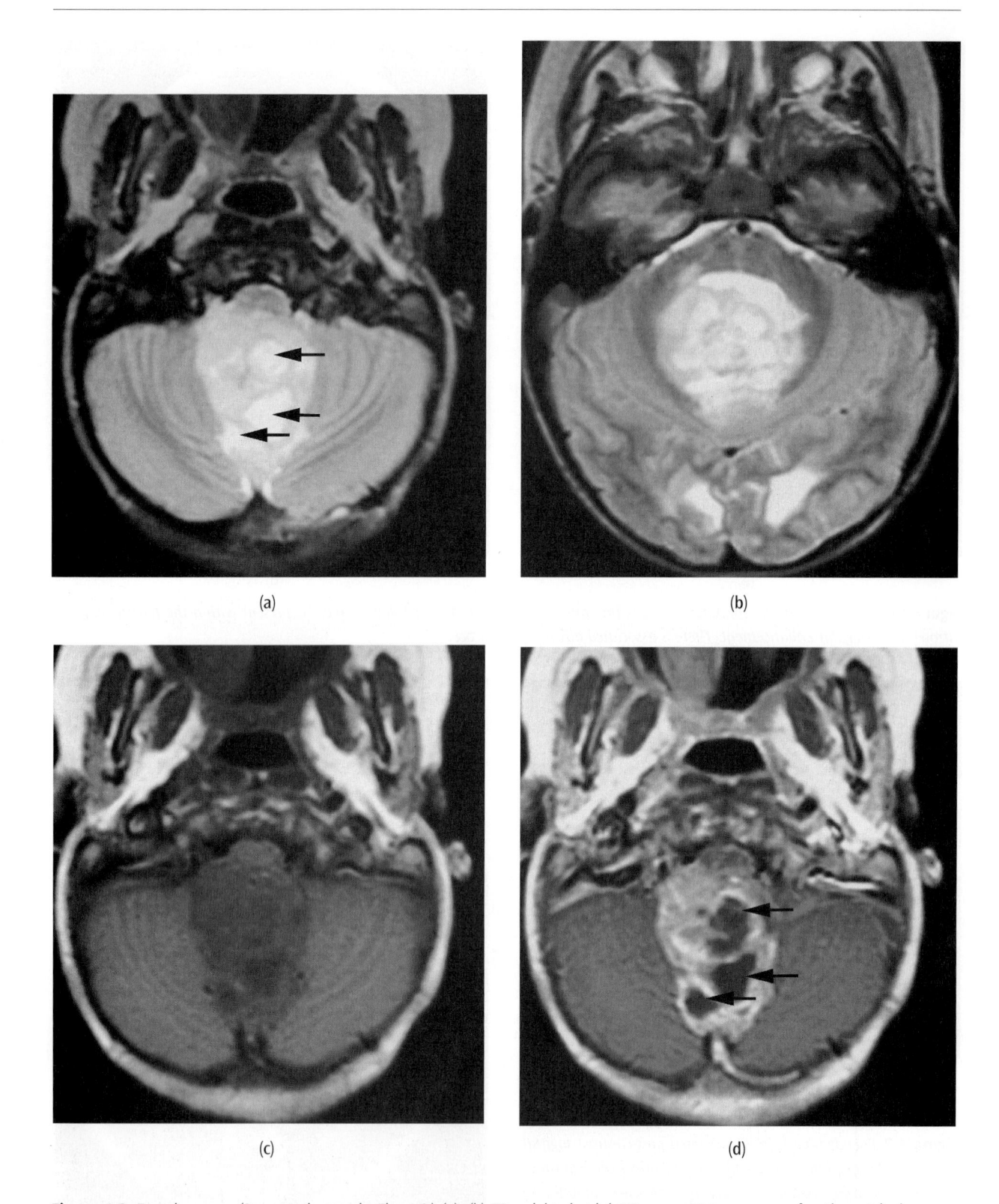

Figure 4.8 *Ependymoma. (Same patient as in Fig. 4.6.) (a), (b) T2-weighted axial MR scans. Heterogeneous fourth ventricular mass extending through the foramen of Magendie. (c), (d) T1-weighted pre- and post-contrast axial MR scans (at the same level as (a)). Heterogeneous enhancement of the solid portion of the tumour is present. Cystic areas within the tumour are noted (arrows).*

patient is immunocompromised, in which case the imaging features are atypical and toxoplasmosis should be considered in the differential diagnosis. The imaging features of lymphoma have been discussed in the preceding chapter.

Cerebellar haemangioblastoma

This tumour only accounts for 1–2% of primary intracranial tumours, 10% being located within the posterior fossa making it the most common intra-axial tumour in adults after metastases. There is a well documented association with the inherited (autosomal dominant) VHL. It is important to genetically screen all patients once the diagnosis of haemangioblastoma is made to ensure patients with VHL are identified and family screening programmes set up. These tumours are seen in sporadic cases during the 5th and 6th decade, and in young adults when associated with VHL. Tumours are usually solitary, but multiple lesions occur in 10% of sporadic cases and up to 40% in VHL. Tumours are occasionally seen in the medulla and rarely in the spinal cord and supratentorial locations.

Haemangioblastomas are large, well defined tumours which usually (80–85%) involve the cerebellar hemispheres. They are usually cystic (60%) and have a solid, strongly enhancing vascular mural nodule which tends to abut the pial surface (Fig. 4.9). Entirely solid tumours (40%) are more commonly seen in the supratentorial region. These are benign tumours and patients present with symptoms dependent on the location of the tumour. Polycythemia may be present as 10–40% of these tumours secrete erythropoietin. If completely removed they carry a very good prognosis. Preoperative assessment must include localization of the vascular nodule and identification of any other lesions. In this respect MRI is superior to CT and the MRI appearances are virtually pathognomonic. The solid portion of the tumour is isointense to grey matter on T1WI and slightly hyperintense on T2WI and strongly enhances. The sharply demarcated cystic portion often has a slightly higher signal than CSF on T1WI and T2WI due to its increased protein content (Fig. 4.10). The wall of the cyst typically does not enhance. Heterogeneity of signal may be present if haemorrhage has occurred. Signal flow voids may be present within or at the periphery of the tumour due to large feeding and draining vessels. Depending on the location of the tumour and the planned operative approach, preoperative angiography may be helpful in some cases to further delineate these vessels. Lesions in the medulla and spinal cord may be associated with a tumour syrinx. The identification of a syrinx, in the absence of a Chiari malformation, should raise the possibility of a tumour and the need for an enhanced MR scan.

The differential diagnosis should include a pilocytic astrocytoma, but this tumour usually occurs in childhood and a cystic metastasis, the most common intra-axial posterior fossa tumour in adults. Usually, the entire wall of a cystic metastasis enhances.

(a)

(b)

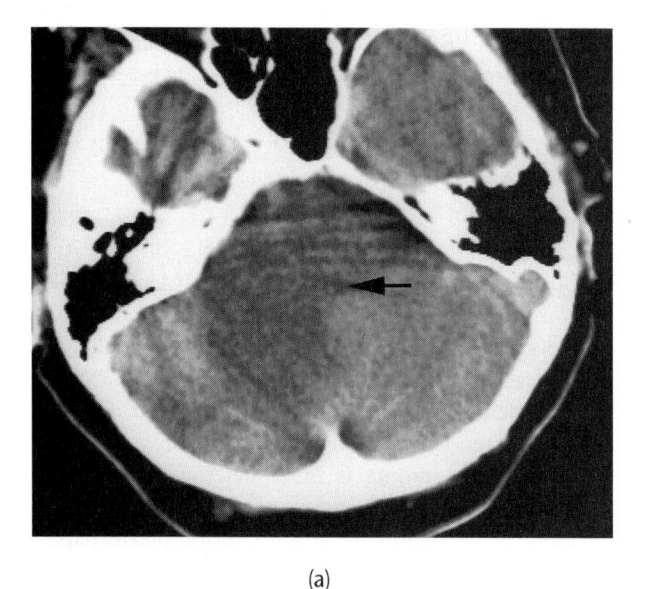

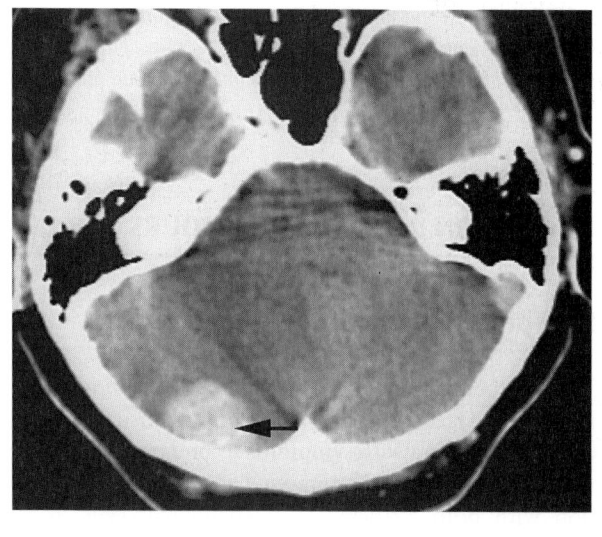

Figure 4.9 *Haemangioblastoma. (a) Axial CT scan. An ill-defined hypodense right cerebellar mass displaces the fourth ventricle (arrow). (b) Enhanced axial CT scan. Strongly enhancing mural nodule (arrow) is demonstrated after contrast.*

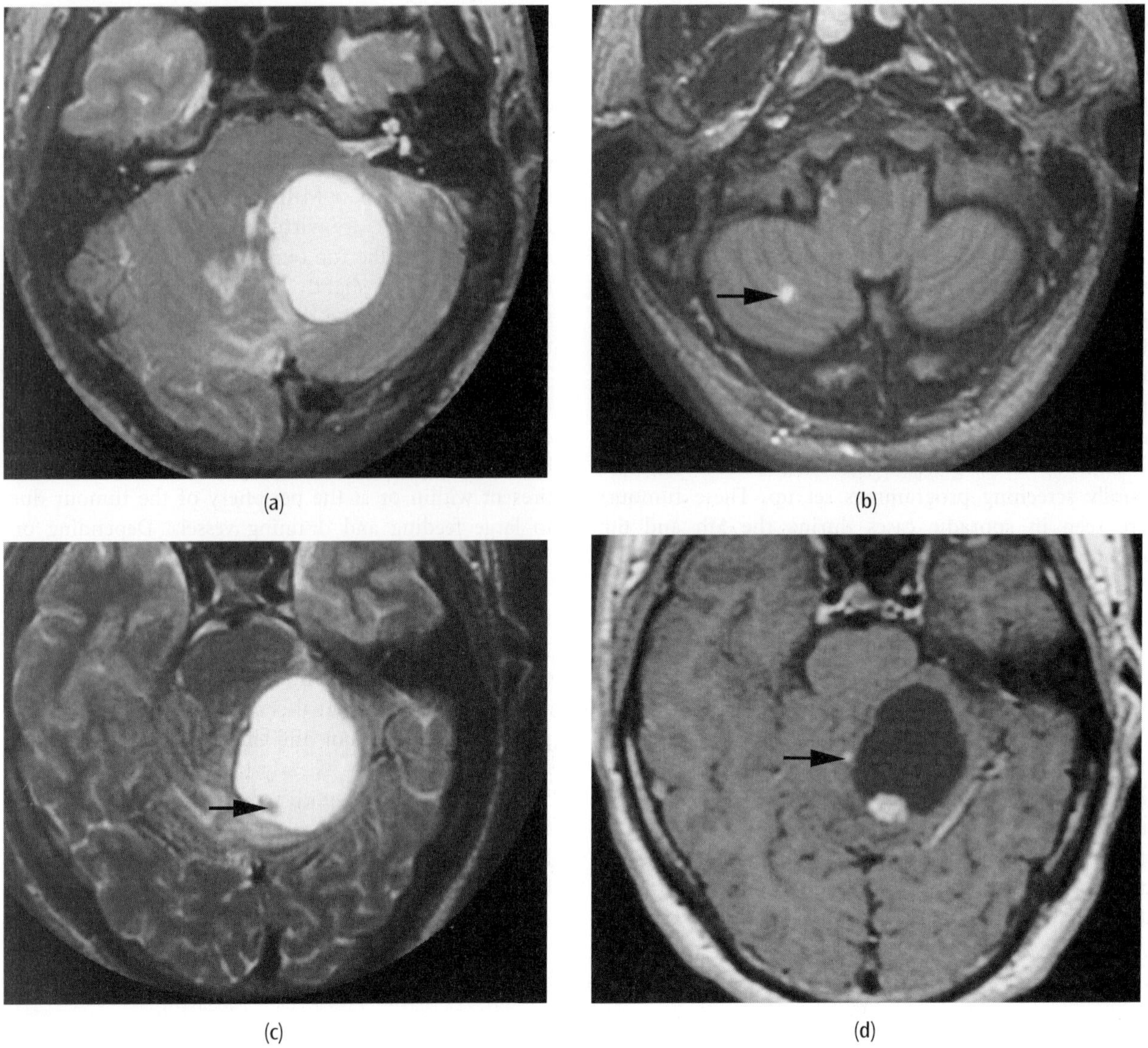

Figure 4.10 *Haemangioblastoma. (a), (b) T2-weighted axial MR scans. A large left cerebellar mass which is mainly cystic is demonstrated, as is a second smaller right cerebellar lesion in a patient with VHL. (c) PD axial MR scan at a higher level demonstrates the small solid nodule within the large cyst (arrow). (d) T1-weighted post-contrast axial MR scan. The mural nodule strongly enhances after contrast. Note third small enhancing haemangioblastoma (arrow).*

UNCOMMON INTRA-AXIAL TUMOURS

Subependymoma

This rare benign tumour is often an incidental finding in the middle-aged or elderly. Patients are usually male adults and present with symptoms secondary to obstructive hydrocephalus. The tumour has a mixed composition with both astrocytes and ependymal cells. It is usually located along a ventricular wall, especially beneath the floor of the inferior fourth ventricle (75%) and septum pellucidum. In the fourth ventricle the tumour is imaged as a well defined subependymal or intraventricular mass hypo- or isodense on CT. It is hypo- or isointense to grey matter on T1-weighted MRI and mildly hyperintense on T2-weighted MRI. Heterogeneity may occur as a result of cystic change, subclinical haemorrhage or (infrequently) calcification. Enhancement is variable from none to marked. The differential diagnosis includes other fourth ventricular tumours. Ependymoma is more heterogeneous, more frequently calcified and enhances moderately. Intraventricular meningioma and choroid plexus papilloma can be differentiated as they both strongly enhance. Differentiation from a metastasis can be difficult and, after all, this is the most common posterior fossa tumours in adults.

Choroid plexus papilloma

Choroid plexus papilloma is a rare tumour and accounts for 0.5% of adult primary intracranial tumours and 2–5% of paediatric intracranial tumours. In adults this tumour usually occurs within the fourth ventricle or its lateral recess. In children it is more commonly found in the trigone of the lateral ventricle or third ventricle. Choroid plexus carcinomas are uncommon and usually occur in the lateral ventricles.

Choroid plexus papilloma has a good prognosis even though recurrence after resection is common. They arise from secretory epithelial cells and patients can present with symptoms secondary to hydrocephalus, or due to overproduction of CSF and/or impaired resorption due to blockage in the subarachnoid cisterns. Well defined, lobulated, often pedunculated, homogeneously iso- or hyperdense, markedly enhancing intraventricular masses are seen on CT. Calcification may occur (Fig. 4.11). The papilloma is hypo- or isointense to grey matter on T1WI and isointense or slightly hyperintense on T2WI (Fig. 4.12). It appears more heterogeneous on MRI than CT with a 'mottled' appearance due to trapped CSF, haemorrhage, calcification and vascular flow voids and if present there is heterogeneous enhancement.

Preoperative angiography may be helpful to identify the position of the enlarged choroidal arteries and early draining veins prior to planning surgical access. The tumour is highly vascular and a prolonged tumour blush is noted. The differential diagnosis of this fourth ventricular mass, most commonly seen in adults, includes medulloblastoma which is a rare adult tumour, ependymoma which usually enhances less, haemangioblastoma which is typically a cystic mass with a solid enhancing mural nodule, and a solitary metastasis from which it may be indistinguishable.

Oligodendroglioma

Oligodendroglioma is a relatively uncommon glial tumour and accounts for 5–10% of gliomas. Usually located in the supratentorial region they may invade the ventricles. Posterior fossa oligodendrogliomas are uncommon and are more likely to occur in children. Their imaging characteristics have been discussed in the previous chapter.

Dysplastic gangliocytoma of the cerebellum (Lhermitte–duclos disease)

This rare lesion is probably a hamartoma or cortical dysplasia which causes focal progressive expansion of the cerebellar folia, and disorganization of hypertrophic neurons within the cerebellar cortex. It presents in adults with symptoms of raised intracranial pressure, due to displacement and compression of the fourth ventricle which results in hydrocephalus in 50% of cases. Cerebellar dysfunction is uncommon. There is an association with other congenital abnormalities i.e. megalencephaly, heterotopia, polydactyly and Cowden syndrome. On CT the focally enlarged cerebellar folia are seen as a hypodense non-enhancing cerebellar mass and on MRI as a slightly hyperintense mass which has a typically striated appearance caused by the thickened ribbon like folia.

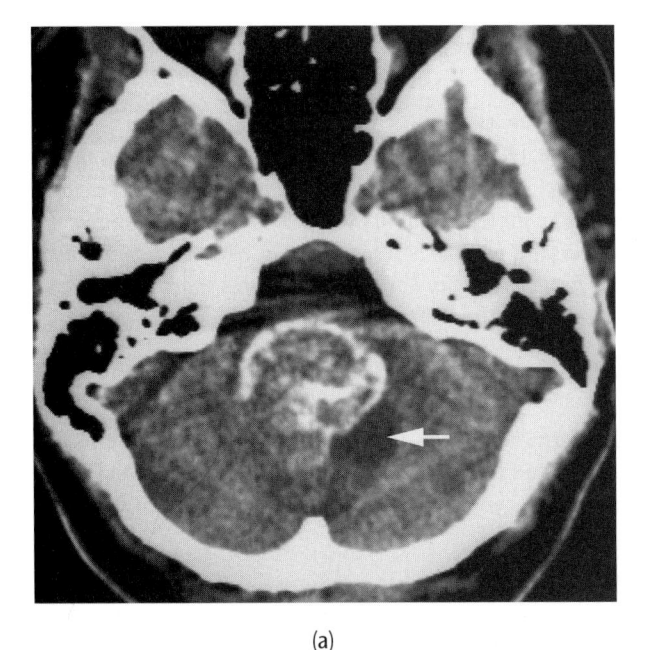

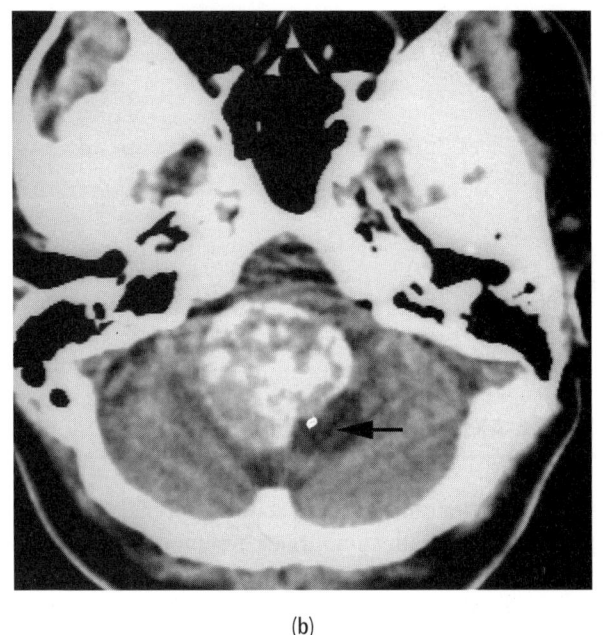

(a) (b)

Figure 4.11 *Choroid plexus papilloma. (a) Axial CT scan. A lobulated, calcified mass expands the fourth ventricle. (b) Enhanced axial CT scan. This mass enhances after contrast. Note lateral cyst (arrow).*

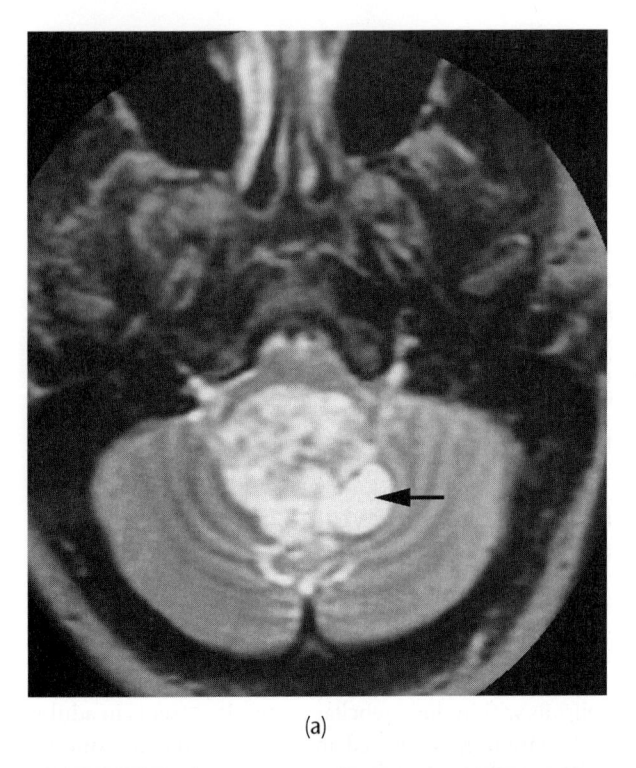

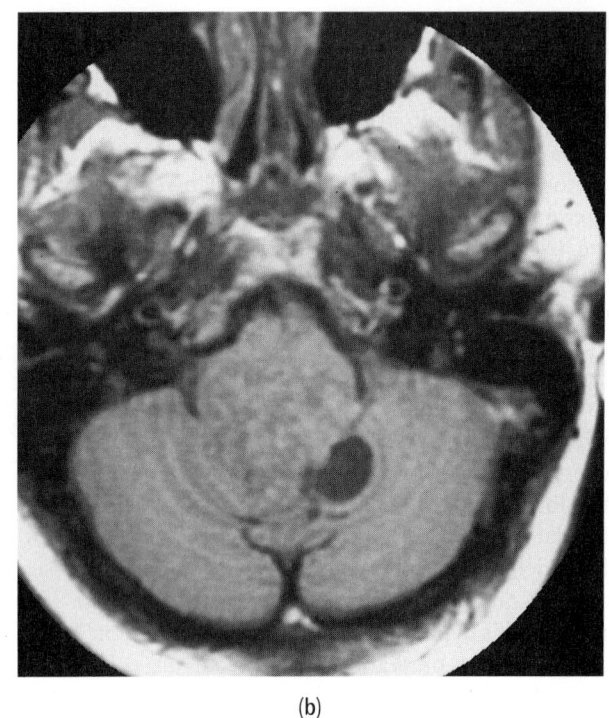

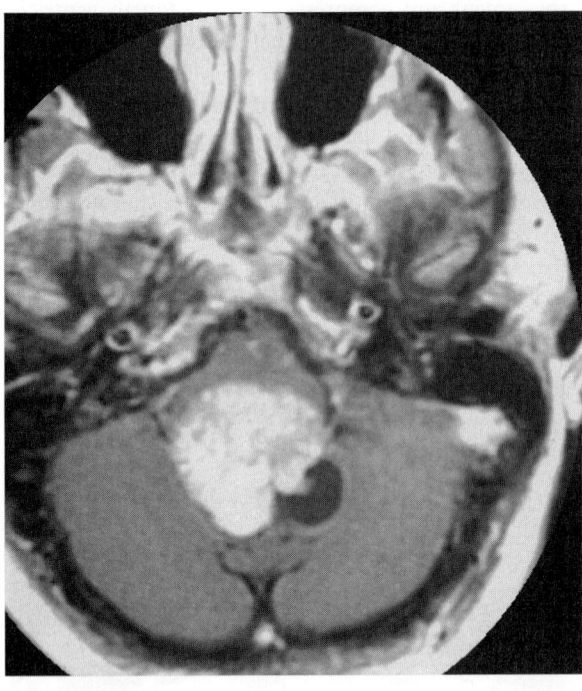

Figure 4.12 *Choroid plexus papilloma. (Same patient as in Fig. 4.11.) (a) T2-weighted axial MR scan demonstrating a heterogeneous fourth ventricular mass with a lateral cyst (arrow). (b), (c) T1-weighted pre- and post-contrast axial MR scans demonstrating the papilloma, which has a heterogeneous signal due to the calcification. The mass intensely enhances.*

EXTRA-AXIAL TUMOURS

Extra-axial tumours are more common in the adult age-group: nerve sheath tumours (schwannoma, neurilemmoma or acoustic neurinoma), meningioma, chordoma and paraganglioma. Congenital dermoid and epidermoid cysts are rare tumour-like lesions and account for only 1% of primary brain tumours. They occur at any age but are usually seen between 20 and 60 years. Epidermoids are 5–10 times more common than dermoids and have to be considered in the differential diagnosis of a cerebellopontine angle mass (Table 4.2).

Schwannoma

Schwannoma (neurilemmoma or neurinoma) is a benign tumour which arises from schwann cells of nerve sheaths. Schwannomas commonly involve the cranial

Table 4.2 *Differential diagnosis of common cerebellopontine angle (CPA) masses*

Lesion	Frequency	Age range (years)	Imaging features (CT/MR)
Schwannoma (neurinoma) Cranial nerves – 8 Cranial nerves 5 & 7	75% 2–5%	40–60	Sharply delineated. Small lesions – homogeneous. Large lesions – heterogeneous. May be cystic. Hyperintense to brain parenchyma on T2-weighted MRI. Enhances markedly. Acoustic schwannoma resembles an 'ice-cream cone' protruding from an enlarged IAM into CPA.
Meningioma	8–10%	40–60	Well-defined. Homogeneous but can be partly cyst. Calcification Isointense to brain parenchyma on T2-weighted MRI. Enhances markedly. Broad dural base with dural tail. Unusual to extend into IAM.
Epidermoid	5%	20–60	Isointense to CSF on T1-weighted, iso/hyperintense on T2-weighted MRI. Difficult to see tumour margins. Rarely enhances and calcification uncommon. Spreads along CSF cisterns and may extend into supratentorial region.
Metastasis	8–10%	> 40	Isointense to brain parenchyma on T1-weighted and T2-weighted MRI. Enhances moderately. Usually associated with multiple parenchymal metastases (75%) and meningeal lesions.
Paraganglioma	1–2%	40–60	Well-defined. Isodense/isointense enhancing mass which erodes bone and extends into CPA from jugular fossa.

Ependymoma and exophytic cerebellar and brainstem astrocytomas, arachnoid cyst, lipoma, vascular ectasia and aneurysms uncommonly occur in the CPA but should be considered in the differential diagnosis of a CPA mass.

nerves, most frequently the VIIIth cranial nerve (acoustic schwannoma). This presents as a cerebellopontine angle mass usually arising from the vestibular division of the nerve. These account for 6–8% of primary intracranial neoplasms and 75–80% of cerebellopontine angle tumours. There is an association with neurofibromatosis, and in NF2, bilateral acoustic schwannomas are more common. Usually occurring in older adults (40–60 years) acoustic schwannomas present at a younger age (20–30, years) in NF2. There is a predilection for females (2:1). The onset of symptoms is usually gradual and, while dependent on the location of the tumour, high frequency sensorineuronal deafness and tinnitus are the presenting features when the VIIIth cranial nerve is involved. Vestibular symptoms occur uncommonly. When the VIIth cranial nerve is involved gradual facial paralysis and occasionally hemifacial spasm is seen. When the Vth cranial nerve is involved facial pain, numbness and weakness of mastication are presenting symptoms. Large tumours in the cerebellopontine angle may involve multiple cranial nerves and symptoms of brainstem compression and/or hydrocephalus may be present. These slow growing tumours are unlikely to undergo malignant change.

Other imaging modalities have been replaced by MRI for the investigation of patients suspected of having an acoustic schwannoma. With the newer MR sequences, a single heavily T2-weighted scan (fast spin echo or turbo fast) can show the neurovascular bundles in the internal auditory meatus (IAM) (Fig. 4.13) although very small lesions may require T1WI post-contrast for confident detection. These tumours generally involve most of the intracanalicular portion of the vestibular division of the VIIIth nerve, and protrusion of a well defined rounded mass into the cerebellopontine angle at the level of the enlarged IAM is seen well on MRI and appears as an 'ice-cream cone' (Fig. 4.14). Smaller tumours are homogeneous but larger tumours may be heterogeneous if haemorrhage, necrosis or tumour cysts are present. Solid tumours enhance markedly after contrast and if the above sequences are not available pre- and post-contrast axial scans will exclude this clinical diagnosis. The differential diagnosis includes other cerebellopontine angle tumours. When MRI is not available, CT should be performed with enhancement so that isodense tumours are not missed. Images taken on 'bone' window settings will demonstrate the enlarged IAM and this will help differentiate a meningioma, which rarely extends into the IAM, usually has a broad base on the petrous ridge and may have a dural tail of enhancement. Metastasis, paraganglioma (typically heterogeneous signal due to vascular flow voids), ependymoma and choroid plexus papilloma, which are rarely isolated in the cerebellopontine angle, should be considered in the differential diagnosis. Enhancement of slightly enlarged nerves can be seen in cases of neuritis e.g. Ramsey–Hunt syndrome. This enhancement can be seen for some time (at least 1 year after the onset of symptoms). A follow-up scan is necessary to confirm this diagnosis and exclude a schwannoma.

Trigeminal nerve schwannoma (neurinoma)

The trigeminal nerve is the second most common site for schwannomas to occur. They are seen along its course and may involve the cisternal segment and/or extend into Meckel's cave at the petrous apex (Fig. 4.15). The imaging characteristics are similar to those described above for acoustic schwannoma and the key to the diagnosis is the anatomical location of the tumour.

Meningioma

Meningioma is the second most common intracranial neoplasm and 10% occur within the posterior fossa. They commonly arise from the dura of the clivus, petroclival or sinodural angle, the posterior surface of the petrous bone or the foramen magnum, especially its anterior margin. Others arise from the tentorium or rarely within the fourth ventricle. Meningiomas and their imaging features have been discussed in the previous chapter. When they occur in the cerebellopontine angle (10%) they have to be differentiated from acoustic schwannomas. Their broad dural base, frequent calcification, marked enhancement with a 'dural tail', lack of extension into the IAM and occasional hyperostosis, all aid differentiation (Fig. 4.16). Cystic change does occur but is rare. Meningiomas usually present between the 4th and 6th decade, but when they occur in childhood may

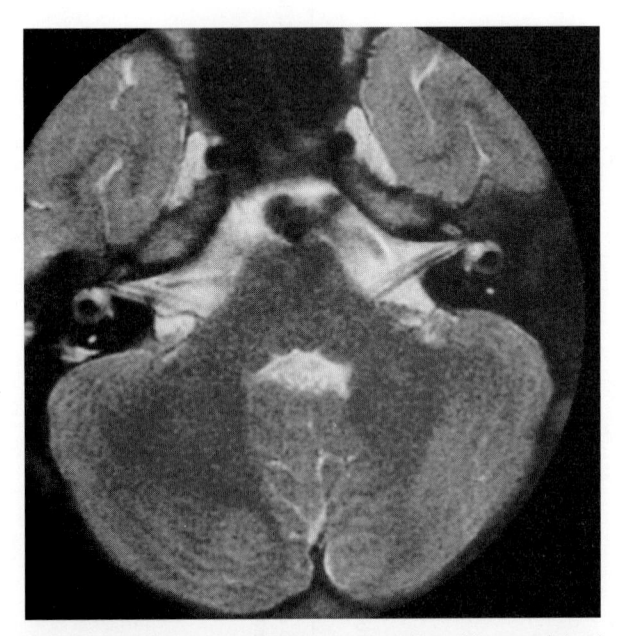

Figure 4.13 Normal neurovascular bundles. (a) T2-weighted axial MR scan (TR3300; TE100). Normal VIIth (anterior) and VIIIth (posterior) cranial nerves are seen crossing the cerebellopontine angle into the IAM.

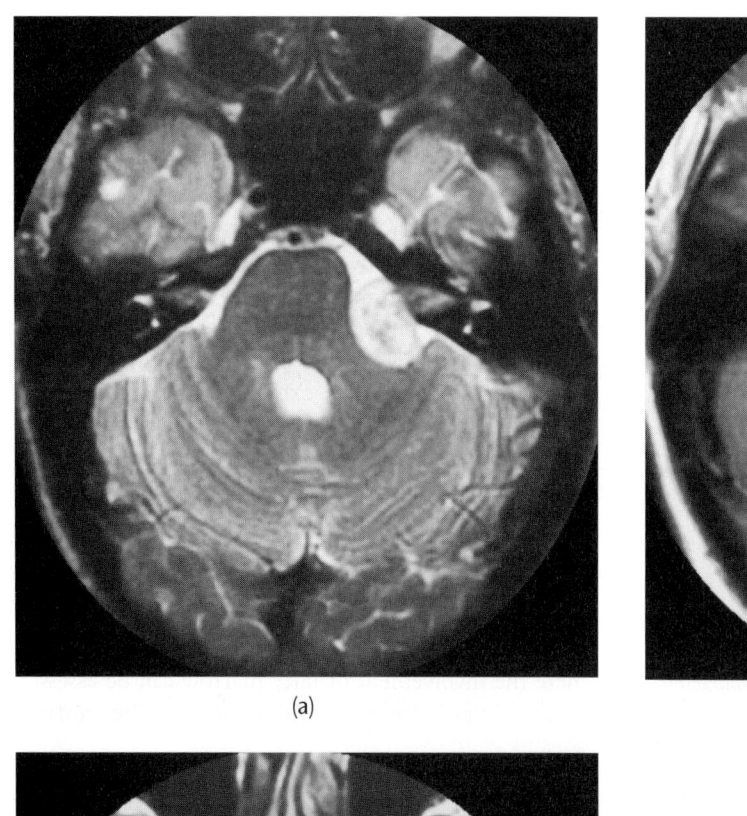

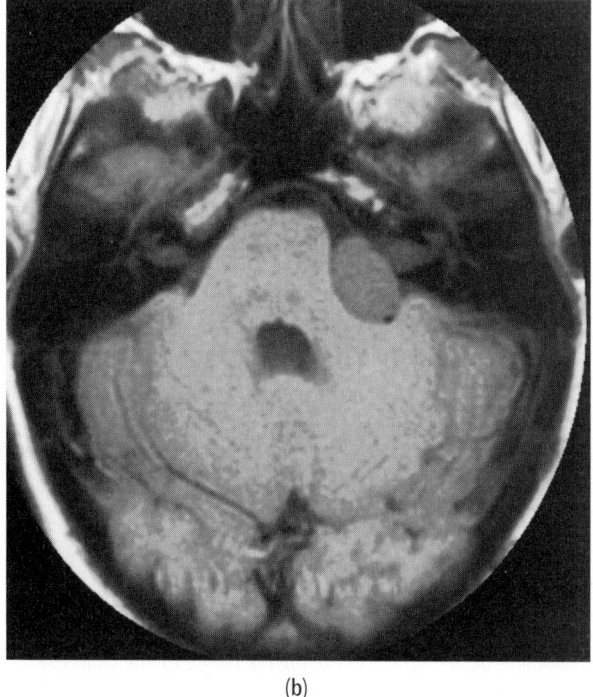

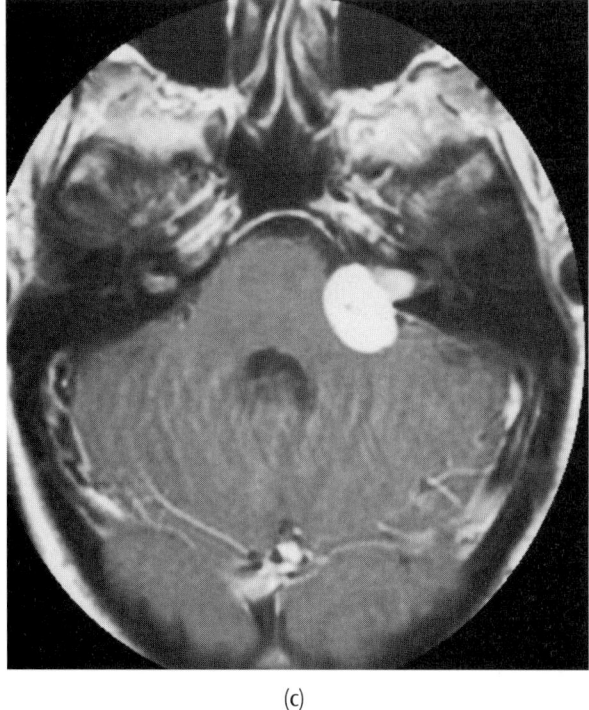

Figure 4.14 *Acoustic schwannoma. (a) T2-weighted axial MR scan. A slightly heterogeneous cerebellopontine angle mass is demonstrated. The right VIIth and VIIIth nerves are not identified in the IAM. (b), (c) T1-weighted pre- and post-contrast axial MR scans. The cerebellopontine angle mass is isointense to grey matter and markedly enhances and extends into the IAM. Note enhancement of the smaller right-sided acoustic schwannoma in this patient with NF2.*

be located in an atypical location, such as the posterior fossa.

UNCOMMON EXTRA-AXIAL TUMOURS

Haemangiopericytoma

Haemangiopericytoma is a rare meningeal-based tumour which arises from mesenchymal pericytes around capillaries rather than meningothelial cells. They are no longer considered as a subtype of meningioma in the World Health Organization classification but, as they occur at similar locations as meningioma, they need to be considered in the differential diagnosis. Occurring in a similar age group, but with a slight male rather than female predilection, they are distinguished from a meningioma by their heterogeneous signal pattern and their more aggressive nature, invading the adjacent calvarial bone and extending into the soft tissues of the scalp. These features

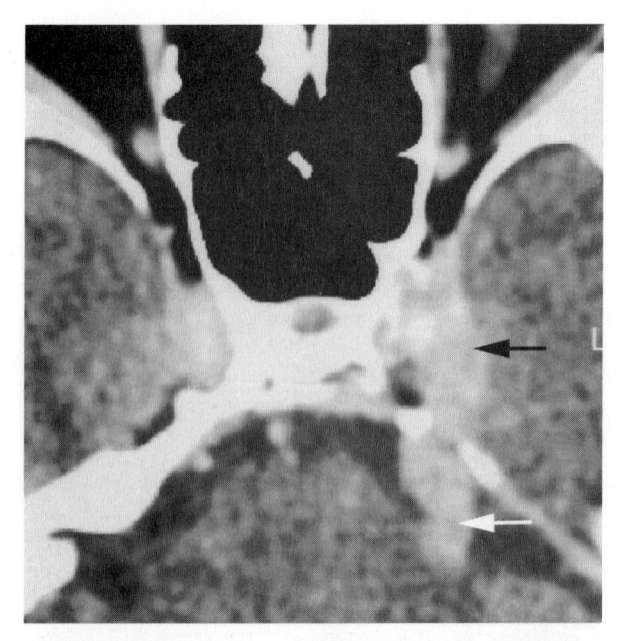

Figure 4.15 *Trigeminal schwannoma. Enhanced axial CT scan. Homogeneous enhancement along the course of the enlarged left Vth cranial nerve (arrows).*

are better demonstrated on MRI. After removal they more commonly recur (75–80% of cases), and they can metastasize (10–15%), usually to bone and lung.

Chordoma

The chordoma is an uncommon primary bone tumour (1–5%) which arises from notochordal remnants in the skull base, and commonly involves the clivus or the sacrum. Usually presenting between the ages of 30–70 years, there is a slight male predilection. A destructive mass involving the clivus, extending intracranially and extradurally to involve both the middle and posterior cranial fossa is seen. It usually occurs in the midline but can occasionally be off-centre and extend predominantly into the cerebellopontine cistern. Symptoms are caused by local invasion of cranial nerves or brainstem, brain compression, or anterior extension into the nasopharynx. These tumours have a variable appearance on MRI. The extent is best demonstrated on T1-weighted scans where the involvement of fatty marrow can be assessed by the hypointense lesion replacing the normal

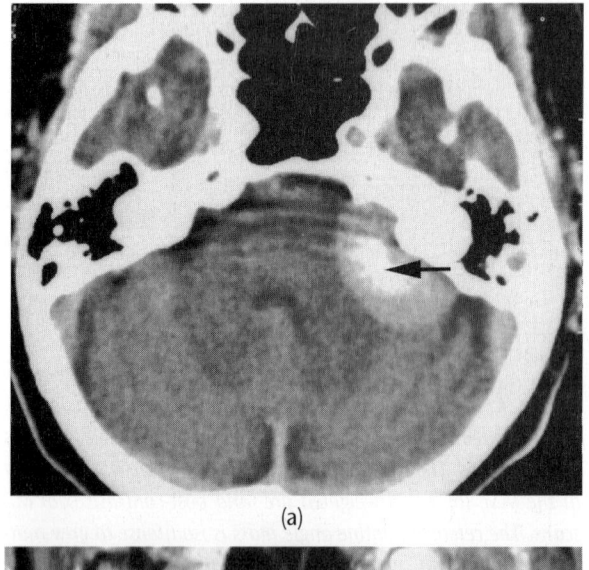

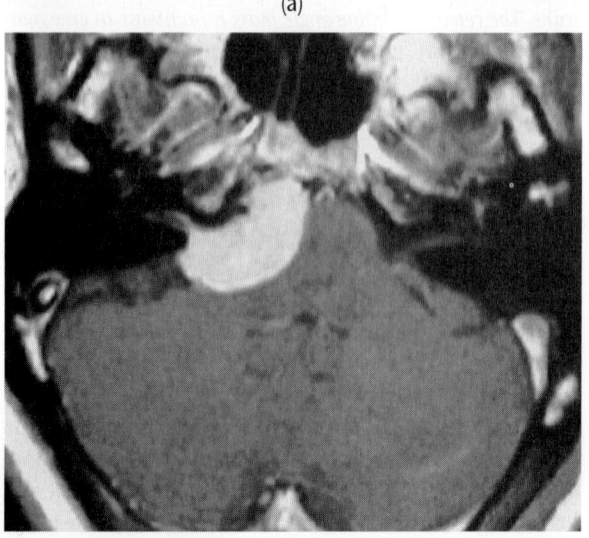

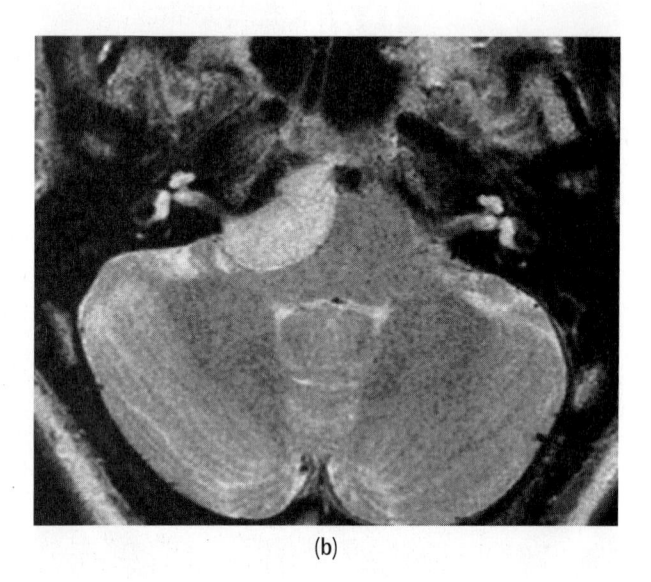

Figure 4.16 *Meningioma. (a) Enhanced axial CT scan. Enhancing, partly calcified (arrow), broad based left cerebellopontine angle mass. (b) T2-weighted axial MR scan. (Different patient to Fig. 4.16a). Broad-based homogeneous right cerebellopontine angle mass lesion, which is isointense to grey matter. The IAM is normal in size. (c) T1-weighted post-contrast axial MR scan. Homogeneous enhancement of the mass with a 'tail' of enhancement in the IAM.*

(a) (b)
(c) (d)

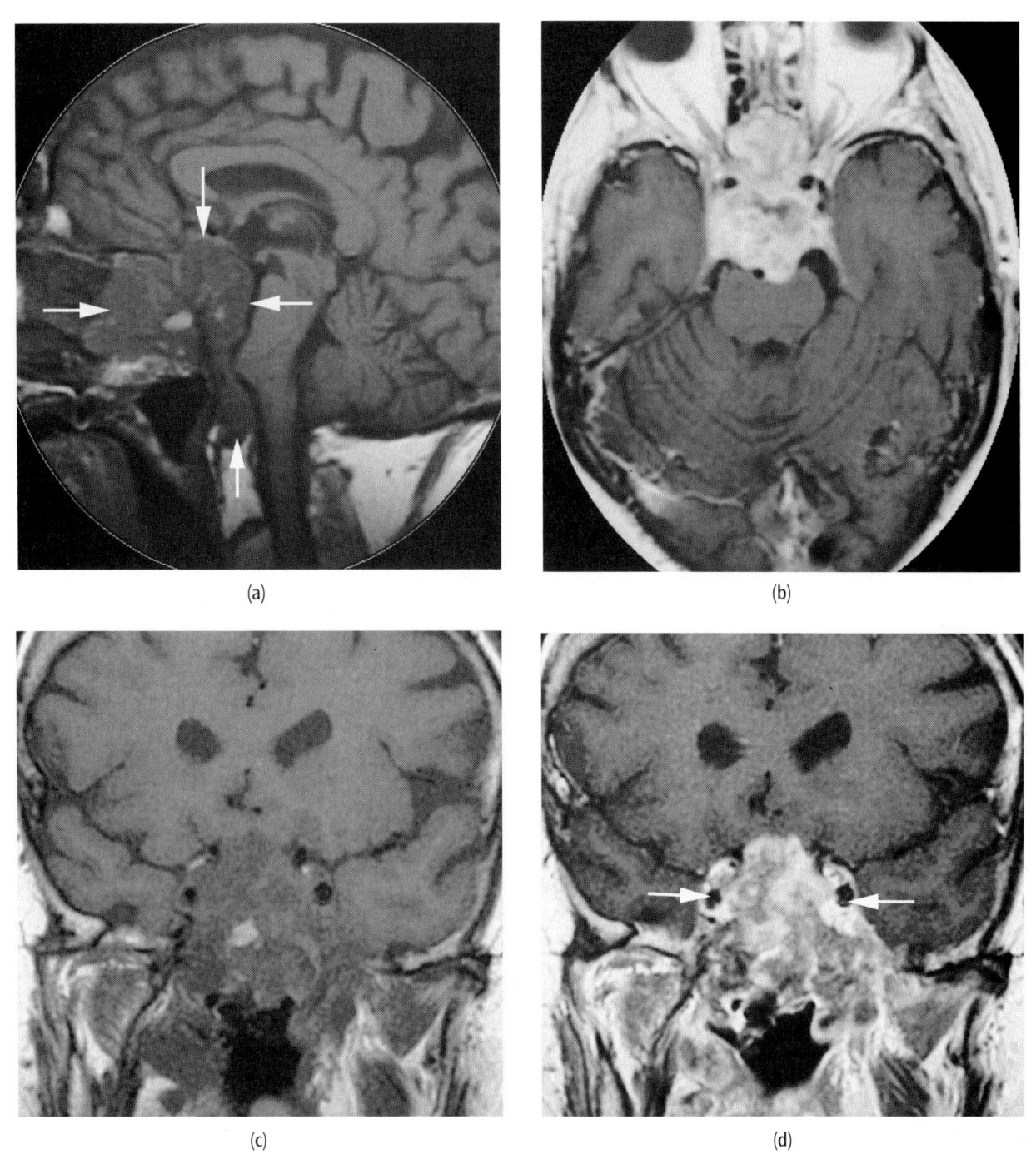

Figure 4.17 Chordoma. (a) T1-weighted sagittal MR. The normal high signal from the bone marrow of the clivus has been replaced by tumour which extends upwards into the suprasellar region, anteriorly into the nasopharynx, inferiorly eroding the odontoid peg and posteriorly into the prepontine cistern (arrows). (b) T1-weighted post-contrast axial MR scan. The tumour extends into the nasopharynx anteriorly and into the prepontine cistern posteriorly and compresses the brainstem. (c), (d) T1-weighted pre- and post-contrast coronal MR scans. This inhomogeneously enhancing tumour is encasing the cavernous carotid arteries (arrows).

hyperintense fatty marrow (Fig. 4.17). A hyperintense destructive mass is seen on T2WI with heterogeneity caused by focal areas of calcification, signal void areas due to vascularity, bony sequestration or tumoral haemorrhage, all of which are variable findings (20–70%).

Treatment includes resection and radiotherapy, but this tumour is prone to recur locally and occasionally metastasizes. Chondrosarcomas may have a similar appearance to chordoma. Bone metastases should be considered in the differential diagnosis.

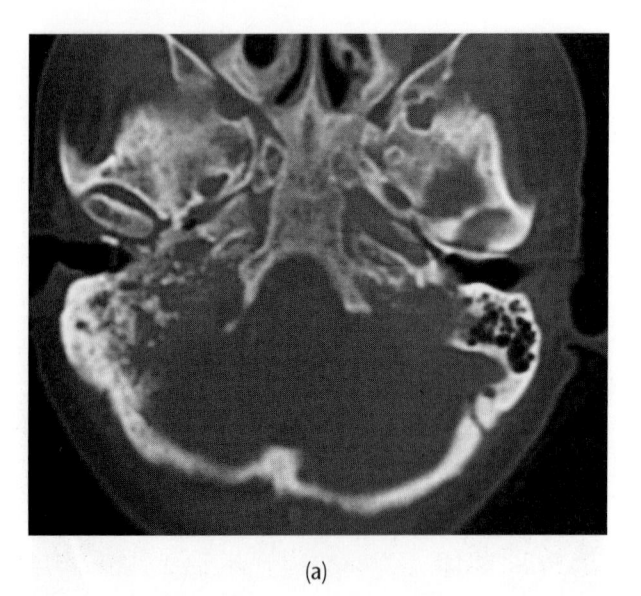

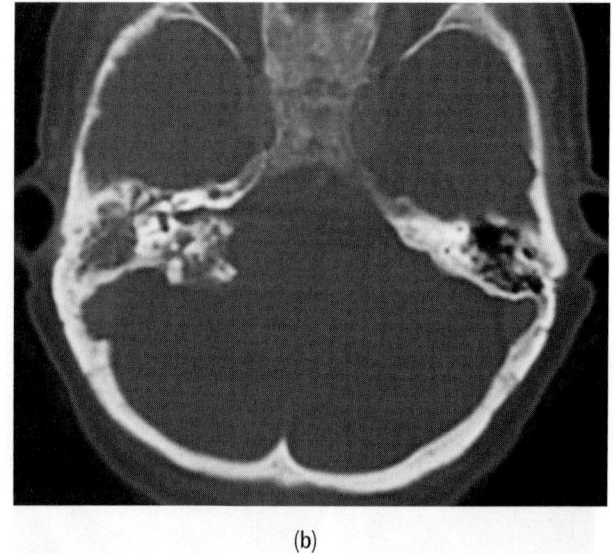

Figure 4.18 *Paraganglioma. (a) Axial CT scan (on bone windows) demonstrating the bony destruction associated with bilateral glomus jugulare tumours. (b) Axial CT scan at a slightly higher level than (a). On the right the tumour has extended extradurally into the cerebellopontine angle and into the right middle ear. The tumour is calcified as a result of previous radiotherapy.*

Paraganglioma

The paraganglioma (chemodectoma or glomus tumour) is a neuroendocrine tumour which arises in paraganglionic tissue and is commonly found originating in the middle ear (glomus tympanicum) or lateral aspect of the jugular foramen (glomus jugulare). The jugulotympanic paraganglioma extends from the jugular foramen into the middle ear where it may erode the bone and extend into the CPA. Tumours usually present between 40 and 60 years and have a female predilection. Symptoms are location-dependent, but lower cranial nerve palsies and pulsatile tinnitus are common for temporal bone tumours. A vascular retrotympanic mass may be visible if a glomus tympanicum is present. Although the bony changes, loss of the bony margin and erosion of the jugular foramen are best seen on CT (Fig. 4.18), MRI in axial and coronal planes with T1-weighted fat suppressed sequences pre- and post-gadolinium and if available fat suppressed T2-weighted sequences, optimally demonstrate the extent of these tumours (Fig. 4.19). Hypo- or isointense to grey matter on T1WI and hyperintense on T2WI, the signal is typically heterogeneous due to vascular flow voids giving a speckled 'salt and pepper' appearance. Marked heterogeneous enhancement is seen in this vascular mass, the nature of which can be confirmed by angiography. A well delineated dense tumour blush with possible arteriovenous shunting, supplied by the ascending pharyngeal branch and often other branches of the external carotid artery is seen. Embolization of these tumours is frequently performed preoperatively to reduce surgical blood loss. Local recurrence is frequent after operation (50% for glomus jugulare).

Lipoma

Subarachnoid lipomas arise from a congenital abnormality of the leptomeningeal membranes and are most frequently found in the pericallosal cistern but may rarely be found in the cerebellopontine angle and perimesencephalic cistern. These are often incidental findings, but may cause brain compression and hydrocephalus when large, or cranial nerve deficits. The CT and MRI characteristics are of a discrete non-enhancing fatty mass. On MRI the signal may be heterogeneous due to elements of non-lipomatous tissue within the mass and chemical shift artefact may be evident. Calcification is common. Vascular flow voids may be seen in the variant angiolipoma.

Congenital cysts

EPIDERMOID AND DERMOID

These are not tumours but are congenital inclusion cysts from ectodermal elements during neural tube closure. This inclusion occurs at different gestational times and this may explain the differing histology and the more midline and varied location of the dermoid. Although rare, epidermoids (1%) are 5–10 times more common than dermoids (<0.5%). Epidermoids may arise in the parasellar region, the middle cranial fossa or in an intraventricular location, but most (40–50%) occur in the cerebellopontine angle. The tumour may insinuate along CSF spaces and may be shown to be involving both infra- and supratentorial regions and if present this is pathognomonic of epidermoid. There is no sex predilec-

Uncommon extra-axial tumours 159

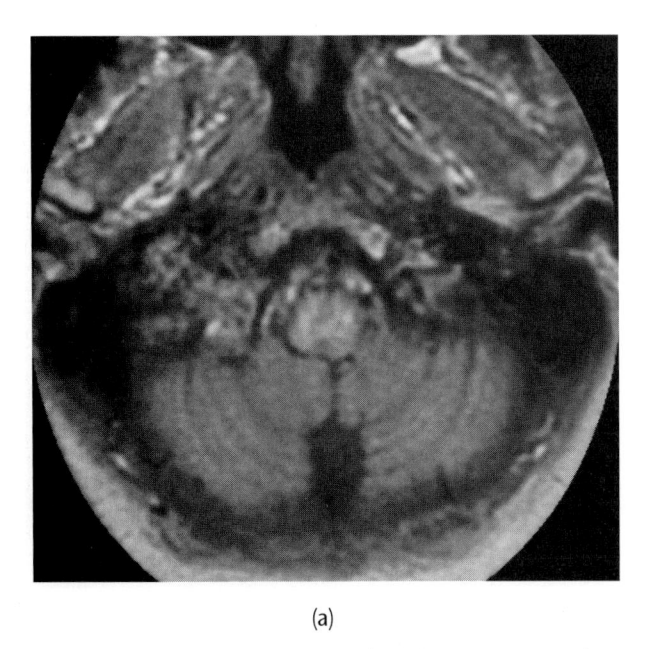

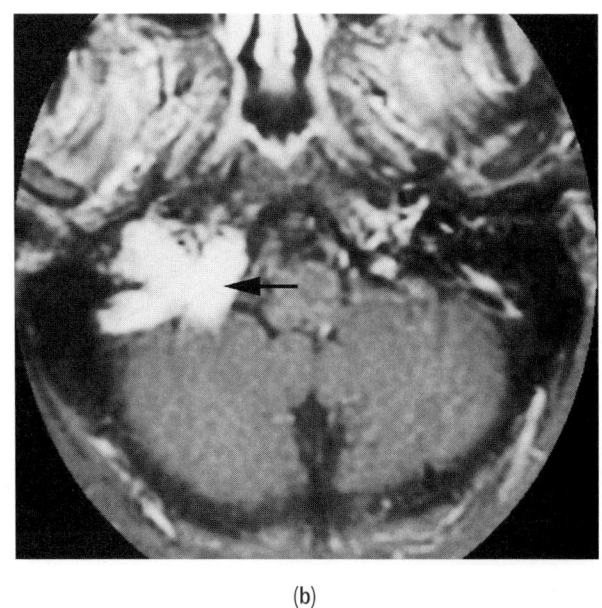

(a) (b)

Figure 4.19 *Paraganglioma. T1-weighted FAT SAT pre- and post-contrast MR scans. An enhancing irregular mass extending is seen extending extradurally (arrow) from the right jugular foramen (glomus jugulare tumour).*

tion and although they can occur at any age they are most commonly diagnosed between the ages of 20 and 60 years. These are slow growing tumours and symptoms are non-specific, depending on their location. When incompletely resected, or if a cyst ruptures, persistent tumour may produce devastating results and a recurrent chemical meningitis. The epidermoid contains solid crystaline cholesterol and no dermal appendages, so it appears as a lobulated, fairly discrete, homogeneous CSF density mass. On CT, the CSF cistern appears widened. The actual margin of the cyst is difficult to perceive unless calcified, and this is uncommon (Fig. 4.20). Enhancement is rarely seen. The signal is usually similar to CSF on T1-weighted MRI but is usually heterogeneous and slightly hyperintense to CSF on T2WI, due to an increased protein content in the form of keratin and cellular debris (Fig. 4.21). If the cyst contains a high fatty content the MRI appearance is similar to that of a dermoid. Heavily T1-weighted or spin density weighted images may be helpful to define the margins of this lesion preoperatively. The differential diagnosis is as for acoustic schwannoma and also includes cystic meningioma, arachnoid cyst and exophytic pilocytic astrocytoma. Cholesterol granulomas, which originate within the petrous temporal bone and secondarily invade the IAM, are hyperintense on T1WI due to their fatty content and can therefore be differentiated.

The rarer dermoid cyst may be found in the posterior fossa within the fourth ventricle and vermis. There may be a persistent skin defect overlying a sinus tract which extends to the intracranial portion. They are seen in a similar age-group (30–50 years) and there is a slight male

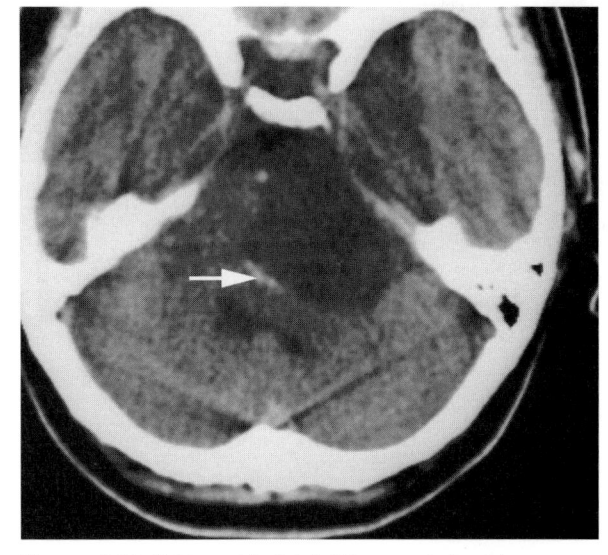

Figure 4.20 *Epidermoid. Axial CT scan. A hypodense mass enlarging the left cerebellopontine angle cistern with calcification within its wall medially (arrow). Note the mass effect on the brainstem.*

predominance. Because of the presence of liquid cholesterol and lipid metabolites the CT and MR signal characteristics are of fat (CT – hypodense, MRI – hyperintense T1WI). Calcification is more common, as is rupture of the cyst with subarachnoid spread of its contents which may result in a chemical meningitis or ventriculitis.

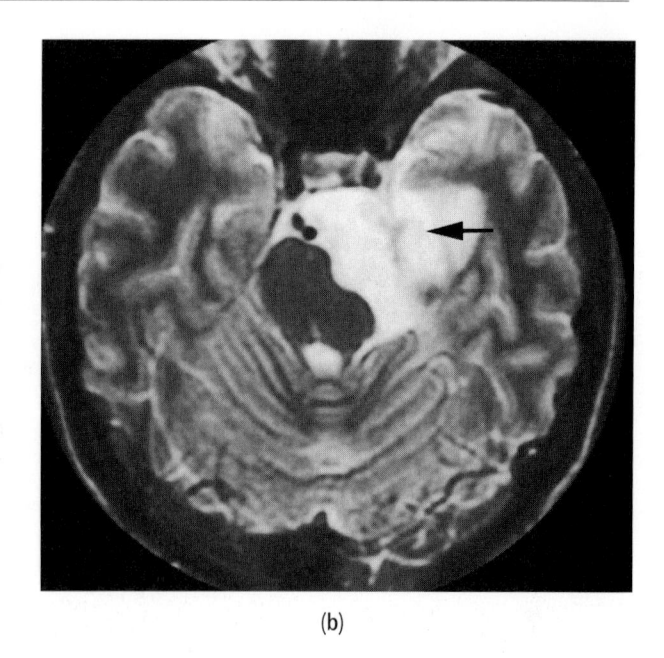

Figure 4.21 Epidermoid. (a), (b) T2-weighted MR scans. The left cerebropontine angle cistern is enlarged and there is mass effect on the brainstem. The margins of the epidermoid are ill-defined. The boundaries of this mass cannot be defined because of the similar signal characteristics to CSF on this sequence. There is extension of the mass into the medial aspect of the left middle cranial fossa (arrow). (c) T1-weighted coronal MR scans. The epidermoid is slightly hyperintense compared with CSF. This aids in identifying the extent of the epidermoid.

ARACHNOID CYST

Congenital arachnoid cysts (Fig. 4.22) probably occur secondary to an abnormal development of the arachnoid membrane. They account for about 1% of intracranial masses and 50–65% of these occur in the middle cranial fossa where they are associated with partial agenesis of the temporal lobe. About 5–10% are seen in the posterior fossa, commonly in the CPA or cisterna magna. They are often asymptomatic but with progressive, albeit slow, increase in size may become symptomatic when they compress the brain or obstruct the CSF pathway and cause hydrocephalus. They may present at any age but presentation is most common in childhood (75%). Expansion and erosion of the inner table of the vault may be appreciated on plain films and CT. Typically there is a well defined extra-axial, non-enhancing, smooth-walled homogeneous mass which has the signal characteristics of CSF. Occasionally, pulsation artefacts may cause hypointensity on the T2WI. Arachnoid cysts may be associated with subdural collections.

Acquired arachnoid cysts also occur, most often secondary to trauma, meningitis or subarachnoid haemorrhage.

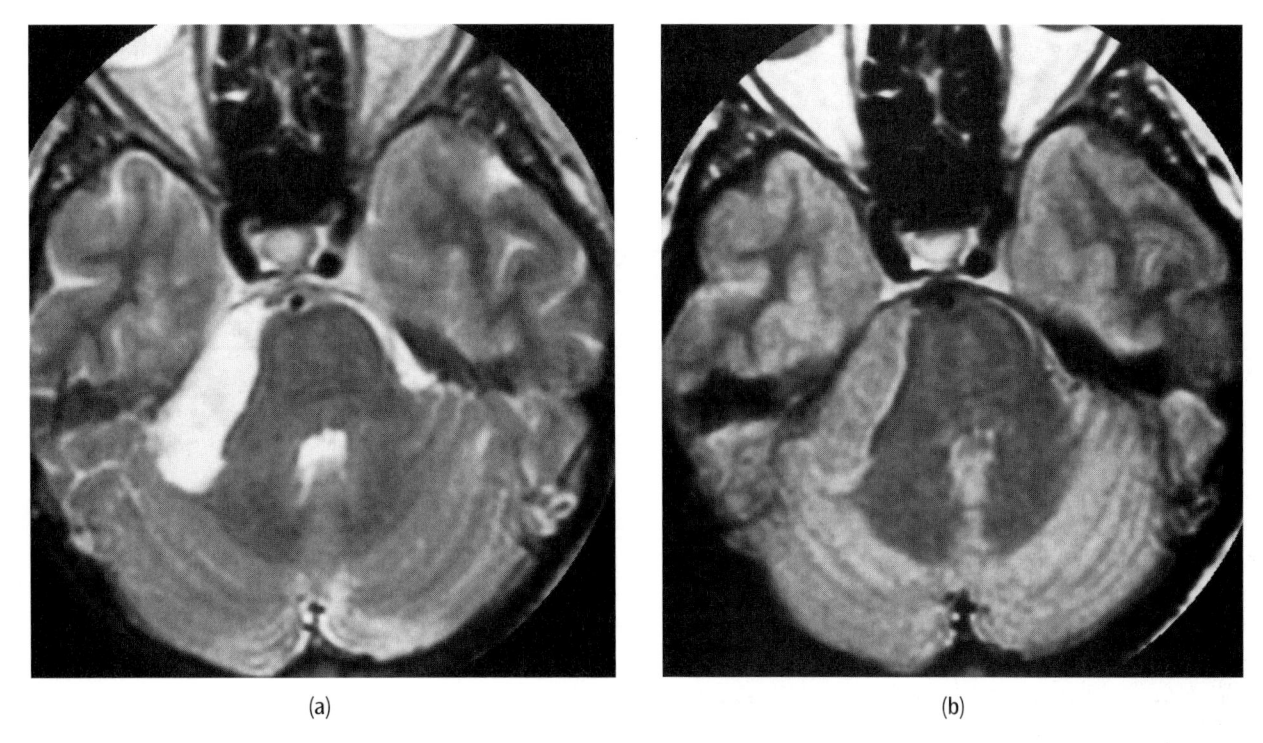

Figure 4.22 *Arachnoid cyst. (a), (b) T2-weighted and PD axial MR scan demonstrating a well-defined mass in the right cerebellopontine angle cistern with signal characteristics similar to CSF on both sequences. Note slight mass effect on the brainstem and cerebellar hemisphere.*

REFERENCES

1. Osbourne AG, Tong KA. *Handbook of Neuroradiology: Brain and Skull* 2nd edn. St Louis: Mosby, 1996.
2. Russell DS, Rubinstein LG. *Pathology of Tumours of the Nervous System* 5th edn. London: Arnold, 1989.
3. Altas SW. Intra and extra-axial brain tumors. In: *Magnetic Resonance Imaging of the Brain and Spine*. pp. 223–378. New York: Raven Press, 1991.
4. Barkovich AJ. Brian tumors of childhood. pp. 321–437. In: *Pediatric Neuroimaging* 2nd edn. New York: Raven Press, 1995.

5

Haemorrhagic vascular disease

PAUL D GRIFFITHS, ANIL GHOLKAR

Introduction	162
Anatomical sites of intracranial haemorrhage	162
Pathophysiological basis of imaging	165
Rationale for imaging protocols for intracranial haemorrhage	167
Specific conditions producing intracranial haemorrhage	170
Intracranial haemorrhage in children	179
Recent advances in interventional neuroradiology	182
References	185

INTRODUCTION

Intracranial haemorrhage describes bleeding into one or more of the intracranial compartments. There are many causes of intracranial haemorrhage, the commonest being trauma which is discussed fully in Chapter 3. This chapter deals with the imaging findings of non-traumatic intracranial haemorrhage. It is useful to describe intracranial haemorrhage by the compartment(s) involved. The meninges permit division into extradural, subdural and subarachnoid haemorrhage while haemorrhage into the brain substance is termed intraparenchymal. The fifth compartment is intraventricular which is usually found in conjunction with bleeds into other compartments. These terms are purely descriptive of anatomy and in no way implicate a particular pathology. For example, there are many causes of subarachnoid haemorrhage although ruptured aneurysm is the commonest non-traumatic cause. However, ruptured aneurysms may also produce intraparenchymal, intraventricular or subdural haemorrhage alone, or in combination. After describing these anatomical points we discuss the rationale for investigating patients with intracranial haemorrhage in terms of the pathophysiology and imaging techniques available. This is followed by a more detailed discussion of some of the commoner causes of non-traumatic intracranial haemorrhage. The chapter is concluded by a discussion of intracranial haemorrhage in children and an introduction to the recent advances in interventional neuroradiology particularly in relation to the treatment of aneurysms.

ANATOMICAL SITES OF INTRACRANIAL HAEMORRHAGE

Haemorrhage affecting the brain itself is referred to as intraparenchymal haemorrhage/haematoma in this chapter. Those related to the meninges and ventricular system are grouped as extra-axial haemorrhages. They usually have distinctive appearances which allow classification into extradural, subdural, subarachnoid or intraventricular haemorrhage. Knowledge of the anatomy of the meninges makes the radiological appearances understandable.

Extra-axial haemorrhage

EXTRADURAL HAEMORRHAGE

Haemorrhage at this site occurs between the periosteal and meningeal layers of the dura mater. The majority of cases of extradural haemorrhage are caused by trauma, very often by tearing of the middle meningeal artery. The acute extradural haematoma is usually biconvex in shape and because the dura is firmly attached at the skull sutures, the haematoma does not cross these structures (Fig. 5.1). Other causes are unusual; however, extradural metastases extending from the adjacent skull may mimic haemorrhage (Fig. 5.2).

SUBDURAL HAEMORRHAGE

Subdural haemorrhage occurs in the potential space between the arachnoid mater and the dura mater.

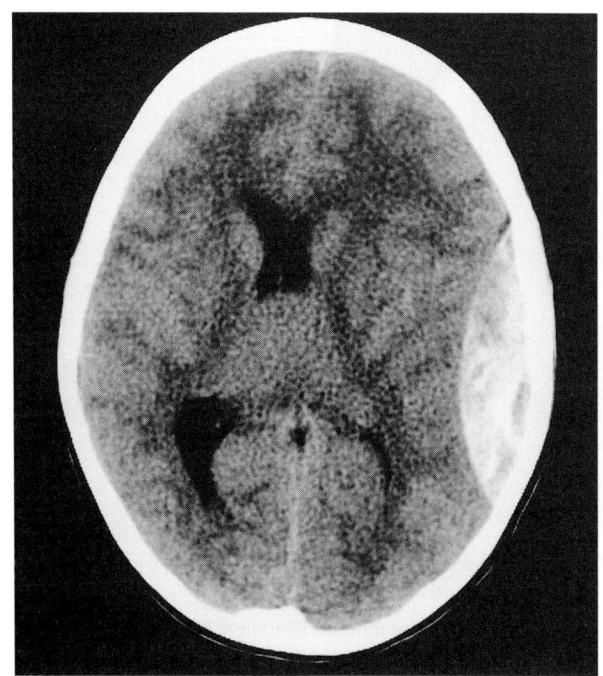

Figure 5.1. *CT of a typical acute extradural haematoma showing a high attenuation, biconvex collection which is confined by the sutures. There are isodense regions within this extradural haematoma indicating continuing haemorrhage (i.e. hyperacute).*

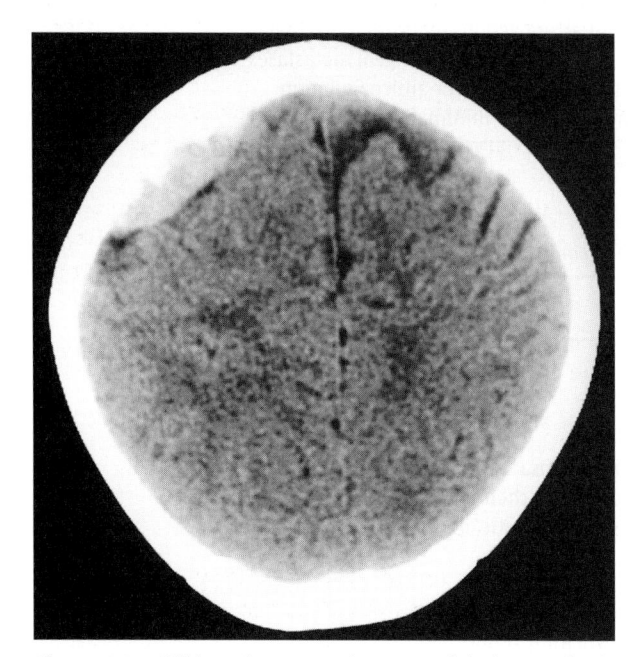

Figure 5.2. *Child aged 6 years. The extra-axial abnormality in the right frontal region looks like an acute extradural haematoma. However, there is also bone destruction. Two similar abnormalities were present at the vertex and were vault metastases with extradural extensions from neuroblastoma primary.*

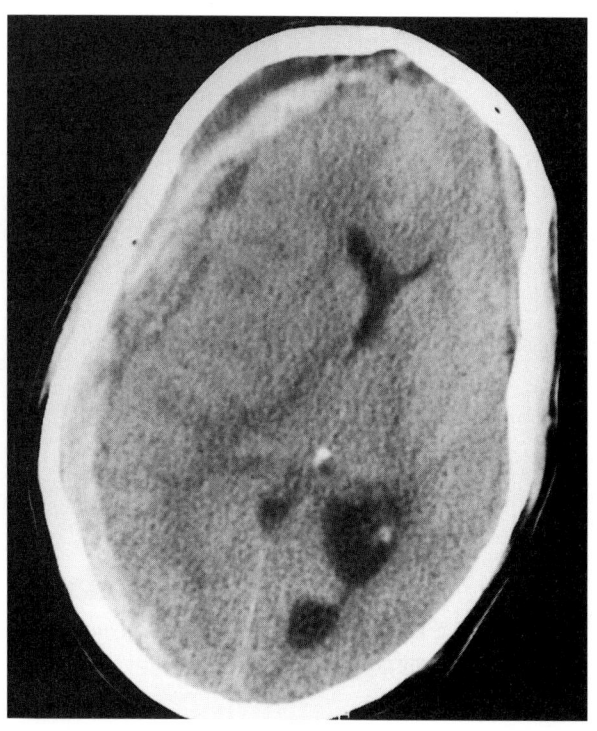

Figure 5.3. *Acute on chronic haematoma. A 63-year-old with known acute myeloid leukaemia and coagulopathy. There is a large mixed high and low attenuation collection overlying all the right hemisphere with midline shift. Obstruction of the left lateral ventricle at the foramen of Monro has produced contralateral hydrocephalus.*

Because haemorrhage in this space is not confined by the sutures they tend to spread out over the surface of the cerebral hemisphere to produce a convex/concave shaped haematoma (Fig. 5.3). Subdurals may extend into the interhemispheric fissure; however, because it is confined by the arachnoid on the deep surface it does not extend into the cortical sulci. Causes of non-traumatic subdural haemorrhage are outlined in Table 5.1.

SUBARACHNOID HAEMORRHAGE

Subarachnoid haemorrhage occurs between the arachnoid mater and pia mater, that is the space occupied by cerebrospinal fluid (CSF). Therefore subarachnoid haemorrhage in the cranium can usually be diagnosed by examination of CSF taken by lumbar puncture. On computed tomography (CT) subarachnoid blood can be shown in any CSF space but common regions include interhemispheric fissure, suprasellar cistern, sylvian fissures and the perimesencephalic cisterns (Fig. 5.4). Because of the anatomical predisposition of the subarachnoid space, blood tracks into the cortical sulci unlike subdural haemorrhage. Subarachnoid haemorrhage has a high prevalence and is a common referral for catheter angiography and is usually due to ruptured berry aneurysms. Vascular abnormalities of the spinal cord and meninges can also produce subarachnoid haemorrhage. This is important to bear in mind when dealing with patients with xanthochromic CSF and normal cerebral angiograms. Other causes are given in Table 5.2.

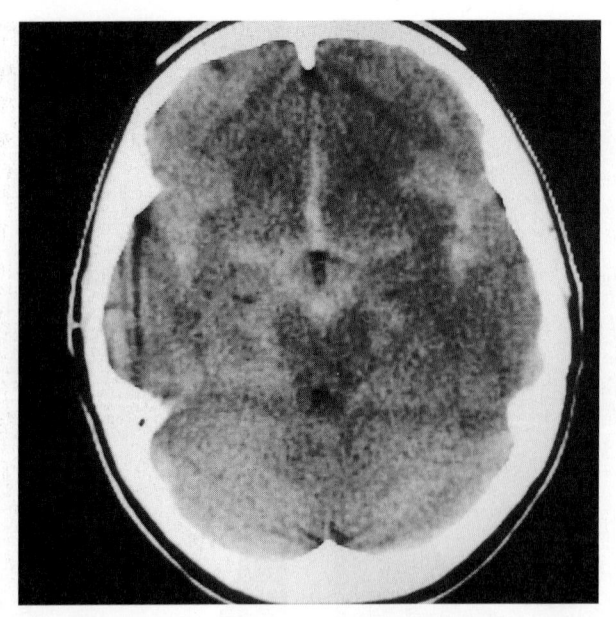

Figure 5.4. *Diffuse subarachnoid haemorrhage in a patient with ruptured anterior communicating artery aneurysm.*

Table 5.1 *Causes of non-traumatic subdural haemorrhage*

Uncommon	
Superficial vascular abnormalities	Aneurysm or arteriovenous malformations (AVM)
Tumours	Particularly haemorrhagic meningeal metastases
Coagulopathies	Mainly iatrogenic due to over-anticoagulation
	May be precipitated by minimal trauma

Table 5.2 *Causes of non-traumatic subarachnoid haemorrhage*

Common	
Ruptured aneurysm	Berry, (rare – myotic or malignant)
Ruptured vascular malformation	Pial AVM, (rare – cavernous angioma, dural AVM)
Uncommon	
Vasculitis	Polyarteritis nodosa, SLE, Wegener's granulomatosis, rheumatoid arthritis
Coagulopathy	Iatrogenic, neoplastic, inherited
Benign perimesencephalic haemorrhage	
Haemorrhage in superficial tumours	
Illicit drug use	Cocaine, amphetamine; may also have a structural abnormality
Arterial dissection	With re-entry haemorrhage
Others	Moyamoya, vein thrombosis, septicaemia, meningitis

SLE: systemic lupus erythematosus

INTRAVENTRICULAR HAEMORRHAGE

Intraventricular haemorrhage without blood in other intracranial compartments is unusual (Fig. 5.5). Intraventricular haemorrhage usually occurs as an extension from intraparenchymal haemorrhage or subarachnoid haemorrhage. There is a constant relationship between the presence of intraventricular haemorrhage and the development of hydrocephalus.

Intraparenchymal haemorrhage

Intraparenchymal haemorrhage has many, diverse causes. The major ones are listed in Table 5.3. The appearance of the haemorrhage is exceptionally variable on CT and magnetic resonance imaging (MRI) and depends on the timing of the scan after the bleed. Anatomically, haemorrhages can be described as infratentorial or supratentorial. Infratentorial haemorrhages can be divided into cerebellar or brainstem. In the supratentorial compartment the major distinction is between lobar (frontal, temporal, parietal or occipital) and those affecting the subcortical structures: basal ganglionic, thalamic, corpus callosum or central deep white matter. The site of 100 non-traumatic haematomas from our recent study is shown in Table 5.4.[1] Intraparenchymal haematomas are frequently accompanied by surrounding oedema which contributes to the overall mass effect (Fig. 5.6). Large haematomas may produce compartmental herniations, the commonest being subfalcine (Figs 5.6, 5.7) and supra to infratentorial (Fig. 5.7).

PATHOPHYSIOLOGICAL BASIS OF IMAGING OF INTRACRANIAL HAEMORRHAGE

Computed tomography

Computed tomography utilizes X-rays to produce cross-sectional images, usually in the axial plane. Contrast between different tissue results from differing densities, particularly electron densities, of the constituents. In a normal, non-enhanced CT examination of the brain the vascular structures are isointense to the brain because flowing blood has an electron density comparable with brain. This is also the case as blood leaves the vessel in a hyperacute timescale. Therefore it is very difficult to see haemorrhage as it occurs on CT. However as resorption of the fluid component of haemorrhage proceeds the haematocrit and protein concentration increases. Protein

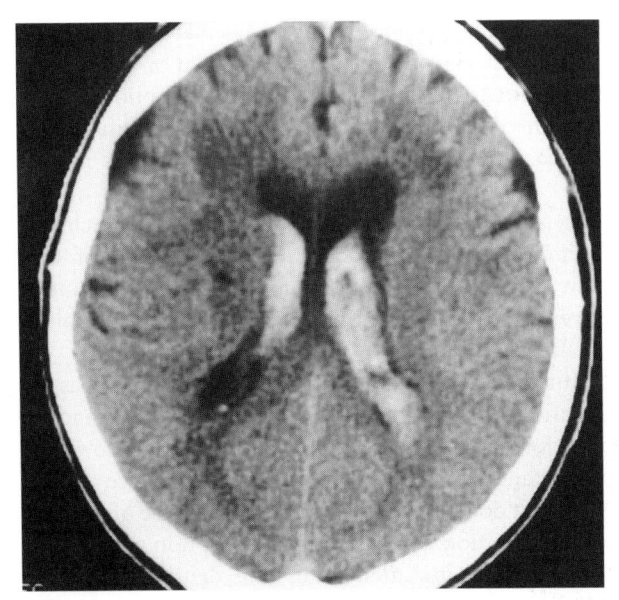

Figure 5.5. *Acute intraventricular haemorrhage in a patient with bilateral carotid and left vertebral artery occlusion. Angiography did not demonstrate the site of haemorrhage.*

Table 5.3 *Causes of non-traumatic intraparenchymal haemorrhage*

Common	
Hypertension	
Amyloid angiopathy	
Haemorrhagic stroke	Embolic>> thrombotic
Ruptured vascular malformation	Pial AVM, cavernous angioma, (rare dural AVM, capillary telangiectases)
Ruptured aneurysm	
Coagulopathy	Iatrogenic, neoplastic, inherited
Tumours	metastases, pituitary adenoma, glioma

Uncommon	
Venous infarction	Sinus or venous thrombosis
Vasculitis	
Encephalitis	Common in herpes encephalitis
Abscess	

Table 5.4 *Anatomical distribution of 100 intracerebral haematomas and the findings of immediate angiography*

SITE	Number	Aneurysm	AVM	Normal
Supratentorial	91	22	25	44
Lobar	75	22	21	32
Frontal	16	4	6	6
Temporal	37	18	7	12
Parietal	10	0	4	6
Occipital	12	0	4	8
Ganglionic/thalamus	14	0	3	11
Corpus callosum	2	0	1	1
Infratentorial	9	0	2	7
Brainstem	3	0	0	3
Cerebellum	6	0	2	4

seen within an established acute haematoma (Fig. 5.1). This indicates continuing haemorrhage or rebleed. As the haematoma organizes there is resorption of the protein component which decreases the attenuation of the haematoma. The rate at which this occurs is variable and depends primarily upon the age of the patient and the site of haemorrhage. Subarachnoid haemorrhage tends to clear quicker because of CSF flow as well as resorption of protein, whereas intraparenchymal bleeds tend to remain high attenuation for longer.

It is frequently quoted that subdural haematomas are iso attenuating to brain 7–21 days after the bleed and are therefore difficult to see on CT. Narrow CT windowing is important in this situation in order to visualize cortical sulci that do not reach the calvarium because of the subdural collection. Further protein resorption will eventually produce a low attenuation (CSF density) collection. Mixed-age subdural collections are sometimes seen (Fig. 5.3). In the presence of chronic subdural haematoma, the small veins that bridge the subdural space are stretched and are prone to rupture, even with minor trauma.

Magnetic resonance imaging

The appearance of intracranial haemorrhage on MRI depends on many factors, including the age of the haemorrhage, the site of the haemorrhage, pulse sequence and field strength of the scanner. The signal changes during the evolution of a haematoma are mainly due to the iron and haemoglobin, particularly in the change from oxyhaemoglobin to deoxyyhaemoglobin, to methaemoglobin (intracellular and extracellular) to the long-term iron storage compounds of ferritin and haemosiderin. Many exhaustive texts are available concerning these changes and for an excellent overview the interested reader should consult Ref. 2. Table 5.5 presents the expected sequence of signal change in intracranial haemorrhage (see Part 2, pp. 22–44).

Catheter angiography

Most patients with non-traumatic intracranial haemorrhage will need diagnostic angiography to identify the source of haemorrhage. Magnetic resonance, CT and X-ray angiography are all able to demonstrate intracranial vessels; CT and magnetic resonance angiography (MRA) are both relatively less invasive but their resolution when compared with X-ray angiography is poor (Fig. 5.8) and very small aneurysms may be missed. Therefore X-ray angiography is still the method of choice for investigating patients with intracranial haemorrhage. In selected cases MRA may be useful as an adjunct to catheter angiography in assessing aneurysm configuration prior to endovascular occlusion and in post-coiling follow-up.

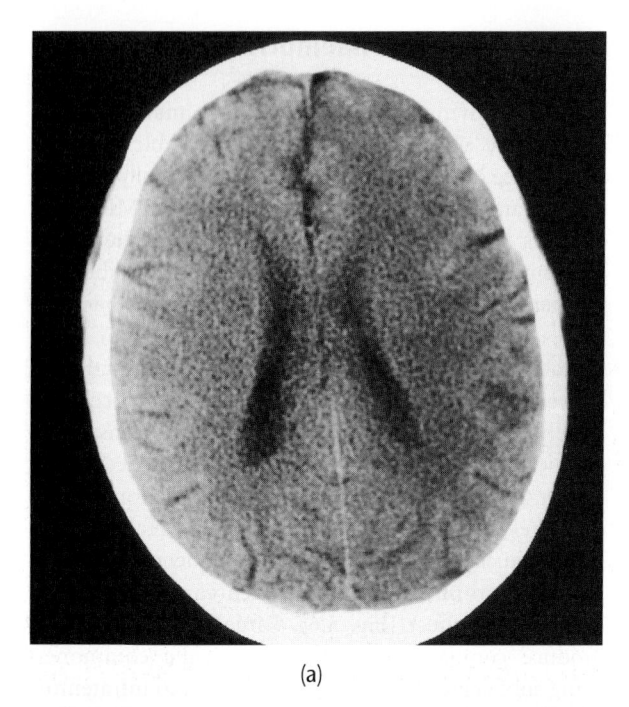

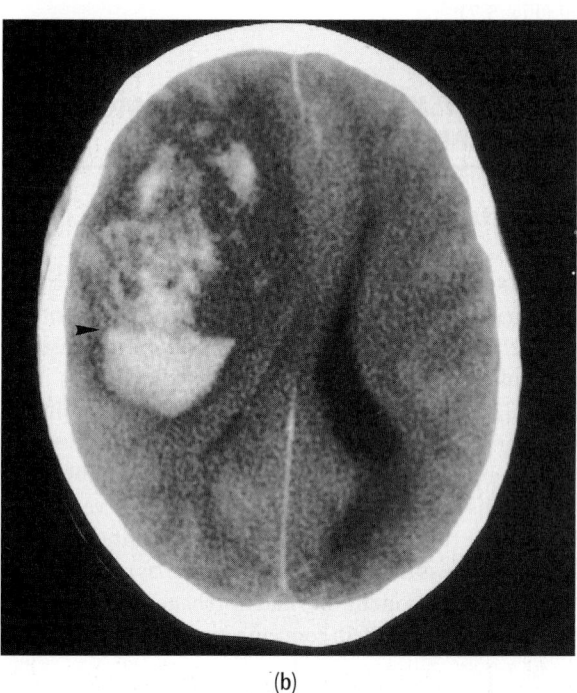

Figure 5.6. *A 64-year-old with a known coagulopathy due to chronic liver disease presented with confusion. The initial CT is normal (a). The following day she became comatose and the repeat CT (b) now shows a large acute haematoma in the right frontal and parietal lobes with a blood fluid level (arrowhead). Note the midline shift anteriorly suggesting anterior, subfalcine herniation.*

has high electron density and therefore an evolving, acute haematoma becomes high attenuation on CT which greatly facilitates detection. This is true for all of the intracranial compartments.

Occasionally active bleeding (isointense) may be

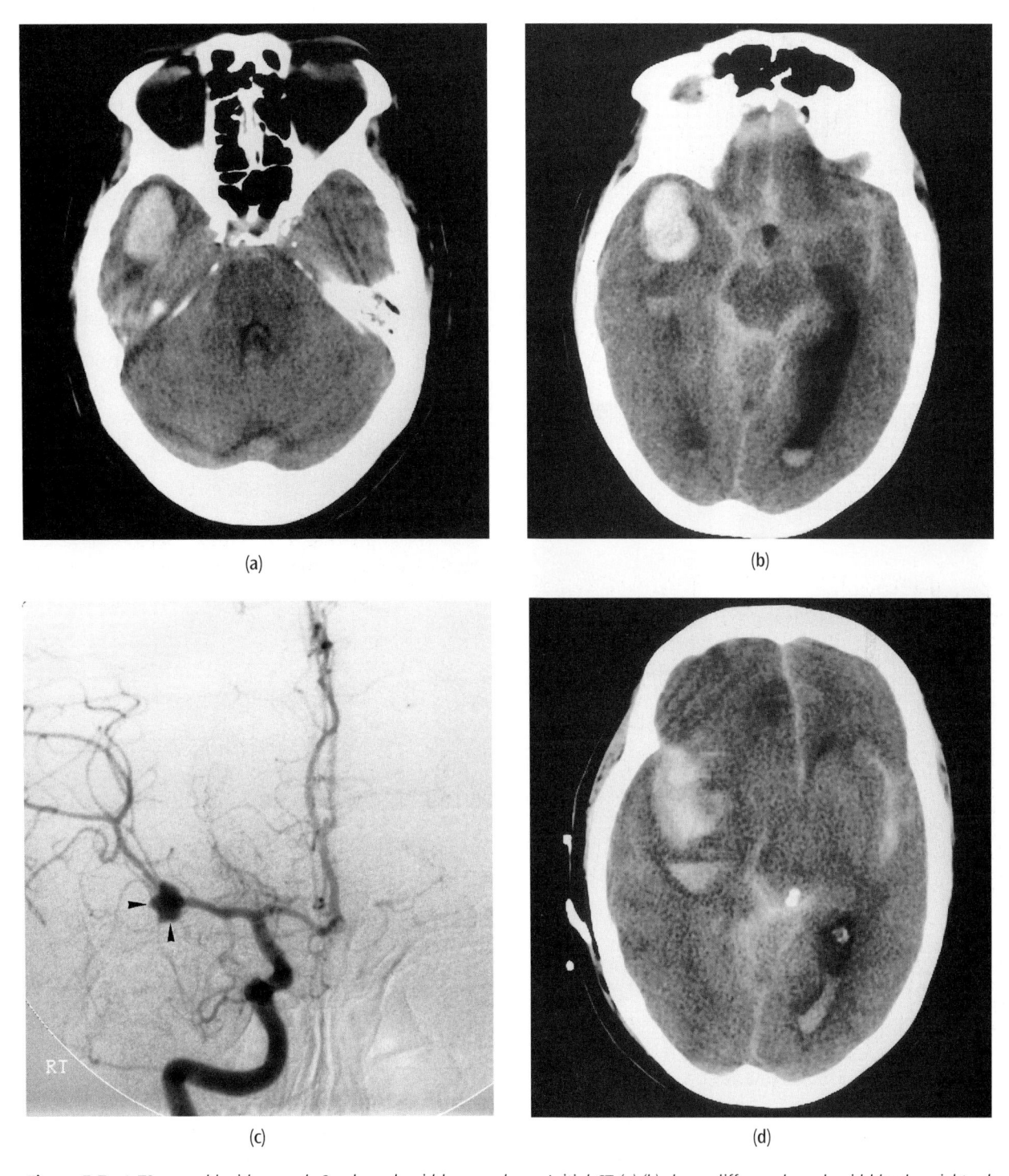

Figure 5.7. *A 73-year-old with a grade 3 subarachnoid haemorrhage. Initial CT (a),(b) shows diffuse subarachnoid blood, a right sylvian fissure haematoma and a temporal lobe haematoma. This combination is very suggestive of ruptured middle cerebral artery aneurysm (confirmed in (c): arrowheads). The fluid level in the haematoma is unusual in this situation. Three days later (d) there is widespread hemisphere oedema with subfalcine herniation and asymmetry of the perimesencephalic cistern suggesting tentorial herniation.*

RATIONALE OF IMAGING PROTOCOLS FOR INTRACRANIAL HAEMORRHAGE

The imaging method of choice for acute intracranial haemorrhage is CT. This is because of the inherent sensitivity of CT to acute haemorrhage; CT scan times are short and acutely unwell patients are managed easily in CT scanners. As described previously the morphology of acute extra/axial haemorrhage is characteristic and there is usually no difficulty with diagnosis by CT. However, small subacute subdurals may be difficult to see on CT and in this context MRI may be useful. This is particu-

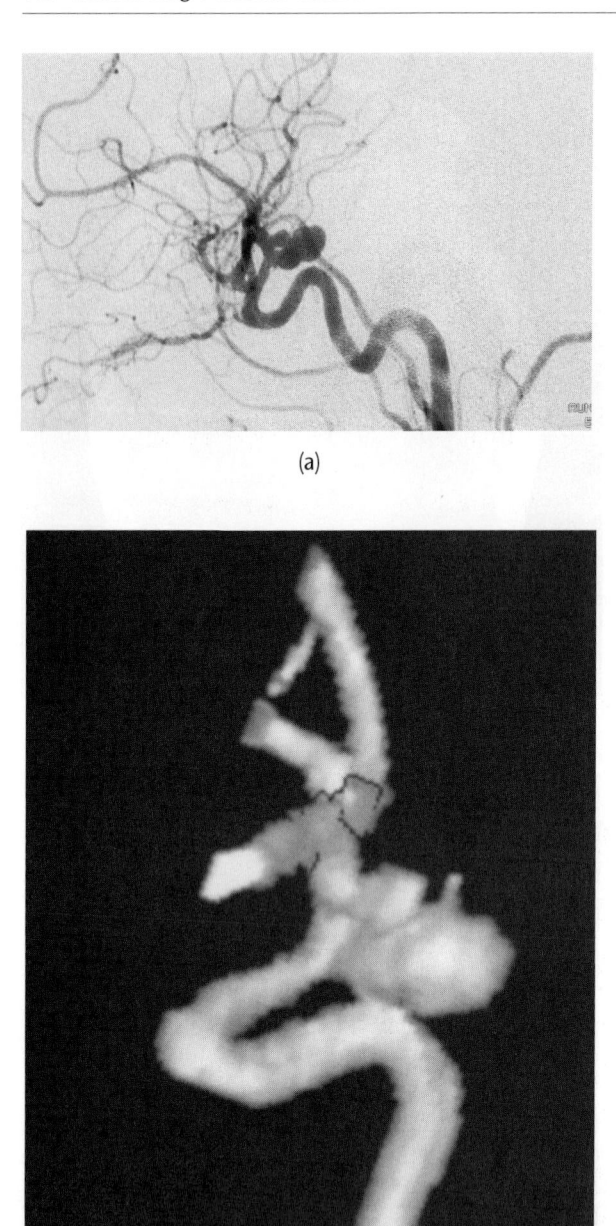

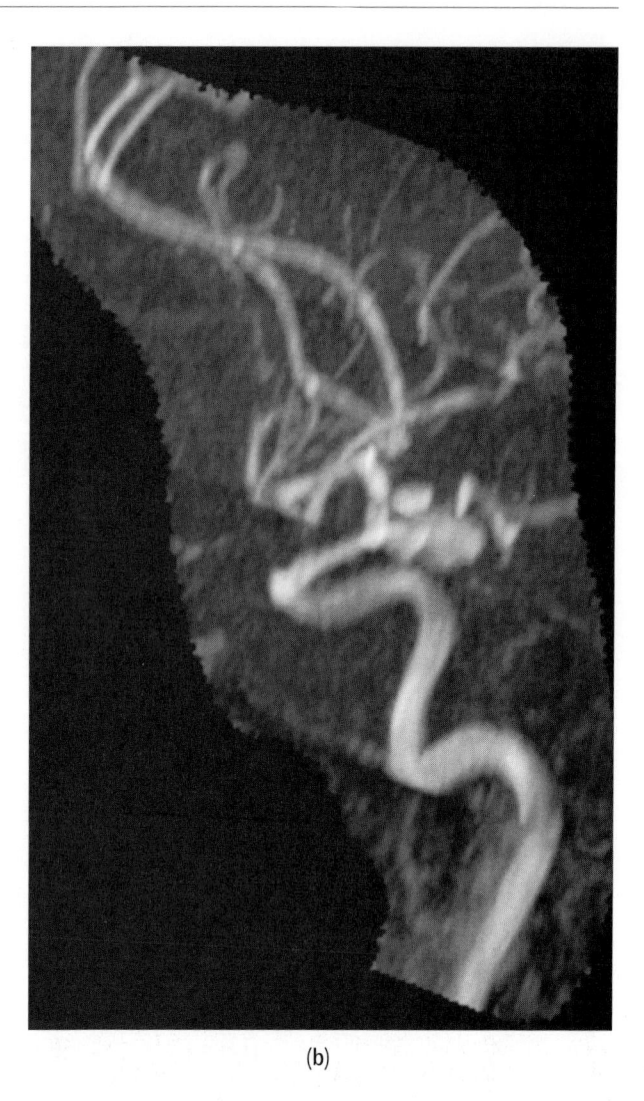

Figure 5.8. *Left posterior communicating and anterior choroidal aneurysms shown on conventional angiography (a), and time-of-flight MRA presented as a maximum intensity projection (b) and 3-D surface reconstruction (c). Spatial detail is superior in the lateral angiogram image (a) and is still the technique of choice. However, the MRA images (also presented as lateral views in (b) and (c) can be rotated and interrogated in near-real time on a work-station when aneurysm configuration is complex.*

larly so in the investigation of possible non-accidental injury in children. The radiological investigation of patients with suspected subarachnoid haemorrhage should ideally start with non-enhanced CT after history-taking and resuscitation if necessary. As well as confirming the diagnosis of subarachnoid haemorrhage, the scan may show features that will affect immediate management. Hydrocephalus may be shunted as an emergency measure, or other pathology may be shown that makes lumbar puncture unsafe, e.g. a large intraparenchymal haematoma.

In addition, CT is useful in planning angiography. Subarachnoid haemorrhage patients may be confused and agitated which can make angiography difficult and it may not be possible to complete a full, four-vessel study on the first examination. Therefore the vessel studied first should be the one with the highest suspicion of abnormality and the distribution of subarachnoid and/or intraparenchymal haemorrhage may be useful in this respect. Cranial CT may be interpreted as normal in cases of true subarachnoid haemorrhage. The commonest cause for this is a delay in performing the scan. In

Table 5.5 *A summary of the expected changes in MR signal on T1- and T2-weighted sequences with the evolution of intracranial haemorrhage*

	Haemoglobin state	T1-weighted images	T2-weighted images
Hyperacute (4–6 hours)	Oxyhaemoglobin, intracellular	Isointense	Hyperintense
Acute (6 hours–3 days)	Deoxyhaemoglobin, intracellular	Isointense	Hypointense
Early subacute (4–7 days)	Methaemoglobin, intracellular	Hyperintense	Hypointense
Late subacute (1–4 weeks)	Methaemoglobin, extracellular	Hyperintense	Hyperintense
Chronic (months–years)	Haemosiderin and ferritin	Hypointense	Hypointense

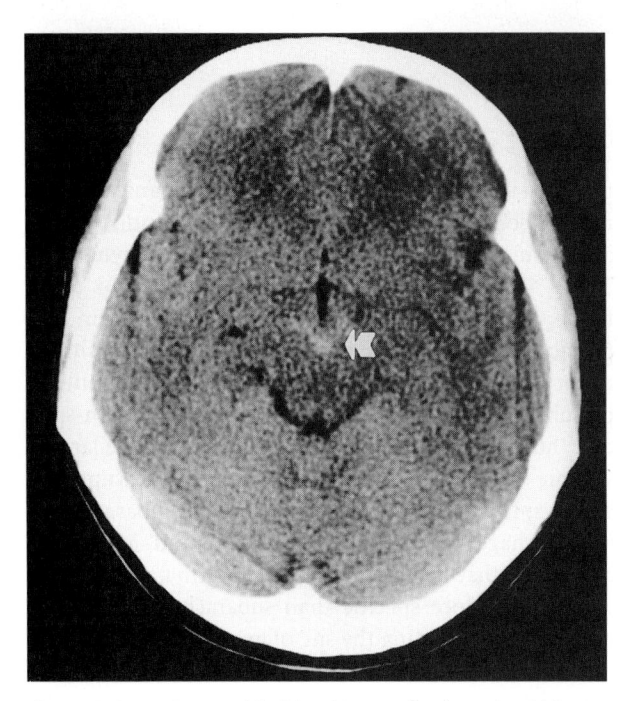

Figure 5.9. *A 40-year-old with a history of subarachnoid haemorrhage. The only abnormality seen was blood within the interpeduncular cistern (arrow). This is a subtle finding but this region is an important review area. Angiography and MRI was normal giving a presumptive diagnosis of benign perimesencephalic haemorrhage.*

cases of proven subarachnoid haemorrhage the CT will be positive in 90% of cases 1 day after the ictus but only 50% after 7 days. This is due to resorption of the blood form the subarachnoid space. Another possible cause of a scan being reported as normal in cases of true subarachnoid haemorrhage is observer error. This is also linked to the timing of the scan after ictus because blood becomes increasingly difficult to detect. It is important to examine carefully the potential 'pitfall' areas such as the interpenduncular cistern (Fig. 5.9), the dependent portions of the ventricular system, the anterior interhemispheric fissure and the sylvian fissures. A commonly quoted but rarely seen cause of CT-negative subarachnoid haemorrhage is a vascular abnormality that bleeds into the spinal CSF system rather than the intracranial compartment. Possible causes include: posterior inferior cerebellar artery aneurysms and spinal artery aneurysms/arteriovenous malformations. It is essential that a patient with a history suggestive of subarachnoid haemorrhage should have CSF examination by lumbar puncture if the CT is normal.

In cases of traumatic contamination of the sample, centrifugation and colorimetric examination are useful to detect subtle xanthochromia. If CT and lumbar puncture are negative it may still be necessary to perform angiography if the history is highly suggestive of subarachnoid haemorrhage.

Table 5.6 *Epidemiological findings of non-traumatic subarachnoid cases over a 3-year period from Newcatle General Hospital*

Number of angiograms for subarachnoid haemorrhage	140 per year
Prevalence of patients receiving angiography for subarachnoid haemorrhage	5.6 per 100 000 per year
Angiograms positive for ruptured aneurysm	81%
Angiographic negative examinations	11%
Multiple aneurysms	30%

170 Haemorrhagic vascular disease

(a)

(b)

(c)

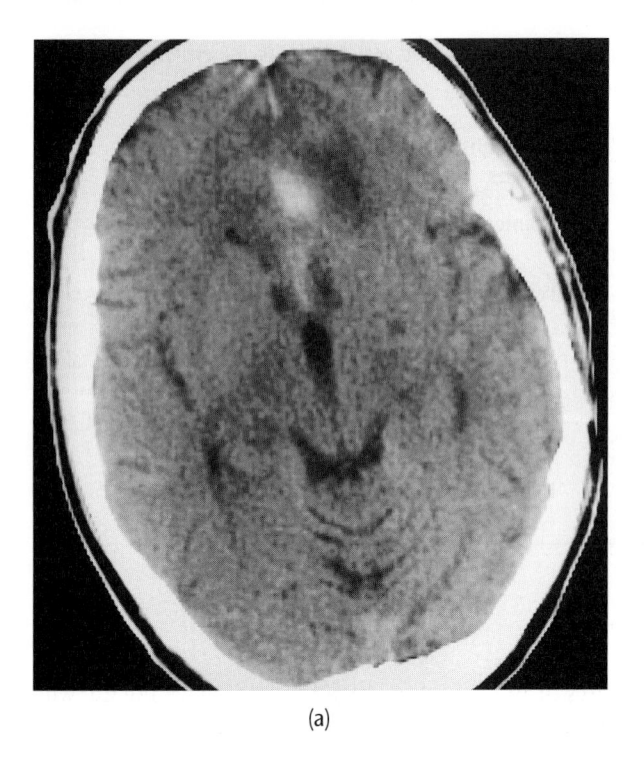

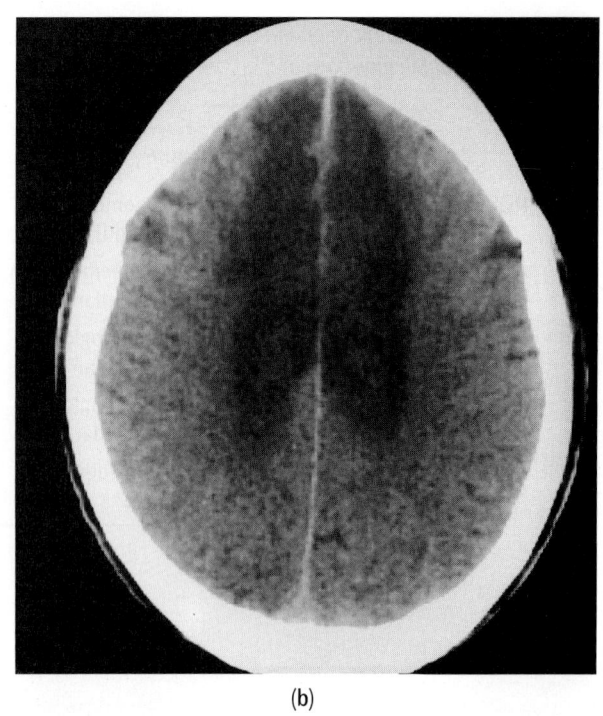

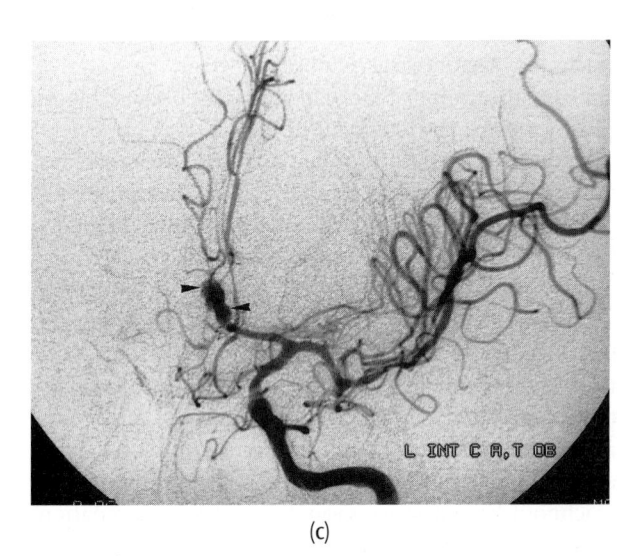

Figure 5.10. *A 52-year-old with a history suggestive of subarachnoid haemorrhage 6 days previously but who had not sought medical advice. He presented with seizures and decreased level of consciousness. The CT shows blood in the anterior interhemispheric fissure and a septum pellucidum haematoma (a). There is also bilateral infarction in the anterior cerebral territory (b). The first angiogram showed vascular spasm. Repeat angiography 2 weeks later showed a bilobed anterior communicating artery aneurysm (c) (arrowheads).*

Occasionally it is possible to predict the site of a ruptured aneurysm with confidence from the distribution of the intracranial haemorrhage (see above). Even in this situation it will be necessary to perform angiography prior to surgery in order to gain more anatomical information concerning the projection of the fundus of the aneurysm, size of the neck and local flow dynamics. These will influence the surgical approach and technique. Angiography will also provide information not possible by CT, such as the presence of multiple aneurysms or vasospasm. In many cases the distribution of subarachnoid haemorrhage is diffuse and non-specific, however the location of the cistern with the largest volume of blood is likely to be close to the ruptured aneurysm. Although the distribution of subarachnoid haemorrhage maybe useful Sengupta and McAllister concluded that haematomas, paraenchymal or within a cistern, are more specific than subarachnoid haemorrhage when predicting the site of aneurysm rupture.[3]

SPECIFIC CONDITIONS PRODUCING INTRACRANIAL HAEMORRHAGE

Subarachnoid haemorrhage

Aneurysms may present by mass effect, seizures or cranial nerve palsy, but the most frequent presentation is by rupture. This may produce subarachnoid, intraventricular or intraparencymal haemorrhage alone or in combination. A superficial aneurysm may occasionally produce subdural haematoma. Of these combinations pure subarachnoid haemorrhage is the commonest in our experience. The results of an angiographic audit from Newcastle General Hospital over a 3-year period of patients with non-traumatic subarachnoid haemorrhage are shown in Table 5.6. These figures are comparable with those quoted in the general literature and highlight the need to perform four-vessel angiography wherever possible. In cases of acute subarachnoid haemorrhage not related to trauma, conventional catheter angiography is indicated as soon as patients condition permits and operative procedures can be arranged.

Ruptured aneurysms at specific sites[3]

ANTERIOR COMMUNICATING ARTERY ANEURYSM

This is the commonest site for a ruptured aneurysm (32%) and produces interhemispheric subarachnoid haemorrhage in nearly 70% of cases. When the subarachnoid haemorrhage from an anterior communicating artery aneurysm is more extensive it involves the sylvian fissures and suprasellar cistern. Anterior communicating aneurysms are associated with haematoma in 45% of cases and are most common in the septum pellucidum (Fig. 5.10) and frontal lobe.

It is often not possible to predict by CT which side of the anterior circulation the aneurysm will fill from on angiography. It is also important to assess anatomical variations of the circle of Willis which may influence surgery.

POSTERIOR COMMUNICATING ARTERY ANEURYSM

Posterior communicating aneurysms account for approximately 22% of ruptured aneurysms and frequently produce subarachnoid haemorrhage in the suprasellar, perimesencephalic cisterns with extension into one or both sylvian fissures and the interhemispheric fissure. They produce a haematoma in a minority of cases (10%) and these are usually in the adjacent temporal lobe. Sometimes CT may show asymmetric intracranial haemorrhage within the suprasellar cistern or a small collection next to the cavernous sinus which will localize the side of the aneurysm.

MIDDLE CEREBRAL ARTERY ANEURYSM

Middle cerebral artery aneurysms account for about 20% of ruptured aneurysms. Most of the aneurysms on this vessel occur at its bi/trifurcation, therefore unilateral subarachnoid haemorrhage in the sylvian fissure is the commonest finding (over 65%). Haematomas are common (44%) and a localized haematoma in the sylvian fissure with a temporal haematoma extending to the inferior pole is highly characteristic of ruptured middle cerebral artery aneurysm (Fig. 5.7). In our experience, on the rare occasions when a subdural haematoma is caused by an aneurysm, ruptured middle cerebral artery or posterior communicating aneurysms are found in most cases.

INTERNAL CAROTID ARTERY BIFURCATION ANEURYSM

Intracranial carotid bifurcation aneurysms are more likely to produce intraparenchymal haematoma or intraventricular haemorrhage rather than pure subarachnoid haemorrhage (only 6/20[3]). The commonest site for intraparenchymal haematoma is in the basal ganglia/thalamus although lobar frontal and temporal haematomas may occur. This is the commonest site of ruptured aneurysm in the second decade of life and accounts for about 6% of all ruptured aneurysms overall.

BASILAR TIP ANEURYSM

Approximately 3% of ruptured aneurysms occur at the basilar tip. The majority of the subarachnoid haemorrhage is usually sited in the perimesencephalic (interpeduncular, ambient, quadrigeminal) and pontine cisterns. Intraventricular haemorrhage is also common.

POSTERIOR INFERIOR CEREBELLAR ARTERY ANEURYSM (PICA)

These make up around 2% of ruptured aneurysms. Subarachnoid haemorrhage in the cisterns of the posterior fossa may be present but PICA aneurysms may not produce CT-detected subarachnoid haemorrhage or haematoma. This may in part be due to problems in imaging the posterior fossa by CT, due to beam hardening and streak artifact, or PICA aneurysms may only produce spinal subarachnoid blood because of the anatomical site of the vessel.

PERICALLOSAL ARTERY ANEURYSM

Although these are rare aneurysms (2%), the pattern of interhemispheric and pericallosal cistern subarachnoid haemorrhage and haematoma in the genu of the corpus callosum are characteristic (Fig. 5.11).

Complications of subarachnoid haemorrhage include hydrocephalus, arterial spasm leading to cerebral ischaemia and rebleed. Ventricular dilatation is common in the acute stage of subarachnoid haemorrhage and in cases where the blood is difficult to see on CT, ventricular dilatation must alert the radiologist. This is likely to be due to decreased absorption of CSF across the arachnoid villi due to obstruction by red blood cells and fibrin. Some patients show a gradual clinical decline after the ictus with signs of cerebral ischaemia/infarction. This is thought to be due to arterial spasm and is maximal 5–7 days after the initial haemorrhage. The precise cause of arterial spasm is unknown but blood products and/or endothelial agents are likely causes. Ischaemia is brought about by vasoconstriction and there appears to

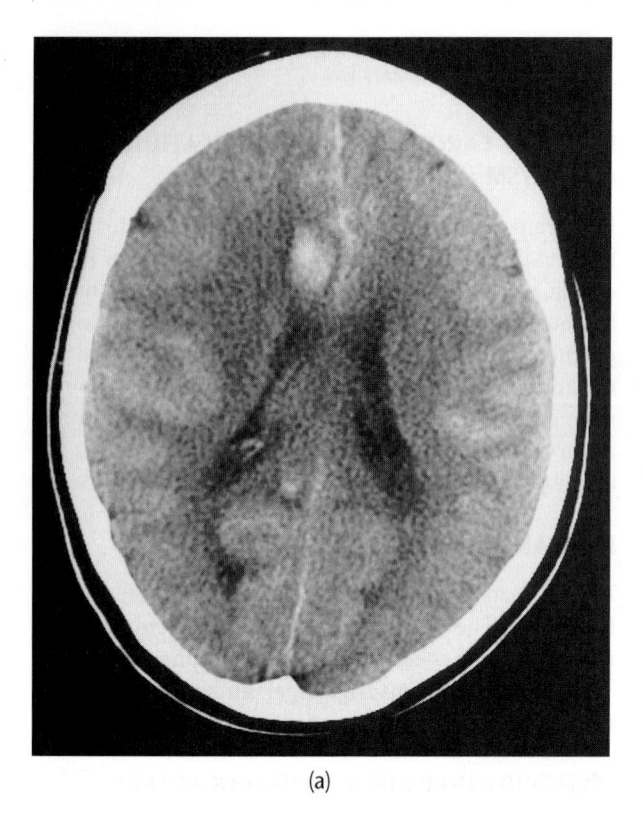

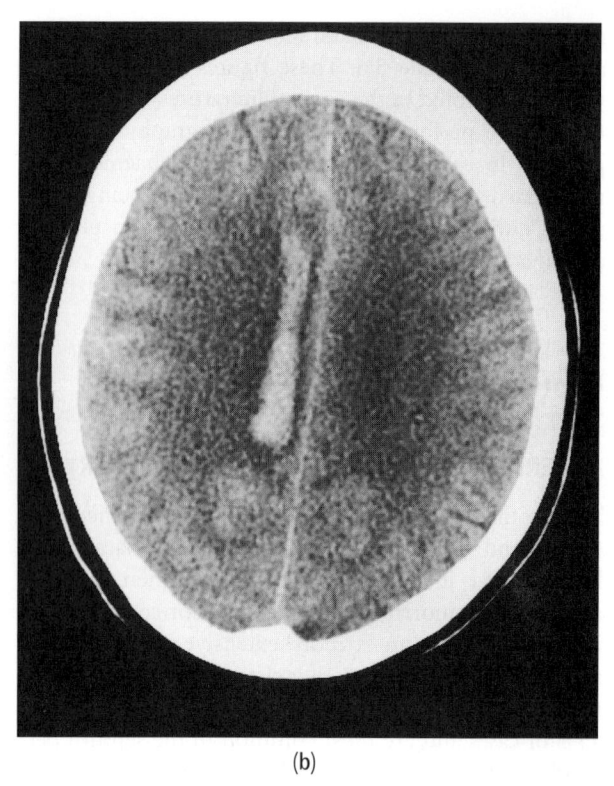

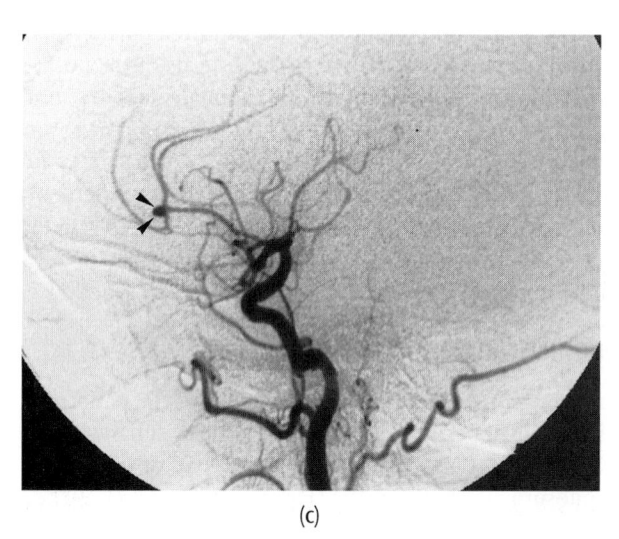

Figure 5.11. *A 42-year-old with a history of subarachnoid haemorrhage. CT (a), (b) shows interhemispheric subarachnoid blood. There is also a haematoma in the genu and body of the corpus callosum. These features are typical of a ruptured pericallosall aneurysm which was confirmed by angiography (c) (arrowheads).*

be a disorder of cerebral pressure autoregulation. A severe case of infarction due to vasospasm is demonstrated in Fig. 5.10.

Rebleed from an untreated ruptured aneurysm is a significant risk. In this situation over one-third die within the first week. The rebleed rate is 10% in the first week after the ictus, 7% per week in the third week and 1.8% per week at 3 months. In the first 6 months 50% of patients will rebleed if the aneurysm is not treated.[3]

Intraparenchymal haemorrhage

The anatomical features of intraparenchymal haemorrhage/haematoma have already been described and a list of causes is given in Table 5.3.

In this section we will discuss in some detail three of the commoner causes, which are AVM, hypertensive haemorrhage and haemorrhagic infarction. In addition, we also comment upon a relatively recently recognized cause in older patients, amyloid angiopathy and also an increasingly common cause in younger patients, haemorrhage due to substance abuse. The usual method to investigate suspected intraparenchymal haemorrhage is CT. In the acute stage the CT will show the haemorrhage to be of high attenuation and may be accompanied by intraventricular or subarachnoid haemorrhage. Mass effect may also be a prominent feature. Large haematomas may produce intercompartmental herniations. Subfalcine herniation produces major midline shift with displacement of the ipsilateral anterior cerebral artery across the midline and contralateral hydrocephalus (Fig 5.3). Supra to infratentorial herniation is demonstrated in the axial plane by effacement or asymmetry of the perimesencephalic cisterns (Fig 5.7). The major challenge for CT in cases of intraparenchymal haematoma, is to distinguish cases with an underlying vascular abnormality (aneurysm or AVM etc), from haemorrhagic tumour, and cases where there is no macroscopic abnormality. We have found that it is impossible to exclude aneurysm or AVM by the distribution of the intraparenchymal haematoma. This is at variance with much of older CT literature.[1]

We have shown old patients with hypertension and basal ganglionic haemorrhage who have had underlying AVM (Fig. 5.13) or aneurysm (usually internal carotid bifurcation).

In all, 20% of hypertensive patients in our study had underlying aneurysm or AVM as a cause of the intraparenchymal haemorrhage. Conversely there are distributions of haemorrhage that are highly suggestive of underlying aneurysm or AVM. Temporal lobe haematomas were the commonest site of intraparenchymal haemorrhage and aneurysm/arteriovenous malformation were found in 67%. When the haematoma extended to the inferior pole of the temporal lobe, or was associated with subarachnoid haemorrhage, aneurysm/arteriovenous malformation were found in 95% of cases. As described previously there are distributions of haematoma that are reasonably specific for aneurysms at various sites.

It is often difficult to distinguish haemorrhagic tumour from a simple haematoma by CT. There are features suggestive of the presence of tumour. Occasionally a blood fluid level may be seen within the tumour (Fig. 5.12) although this is also seen in coagulopathies (Fig. 5.6). The high attenuation region in non-neoplastic

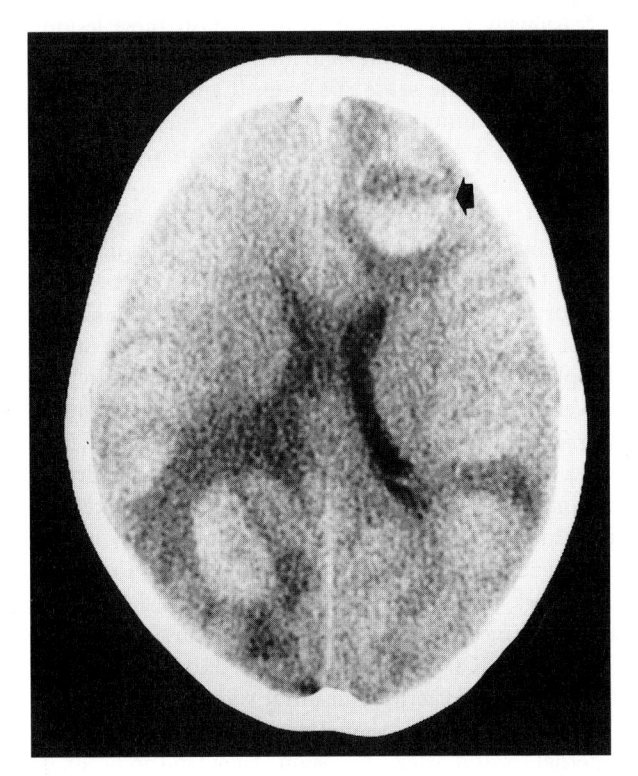

Figure 5.12. *Multiple metastases from a melanoma primary. Note the fluid level in the left frontal lobe (arrow) which confirms haemorrhage.*

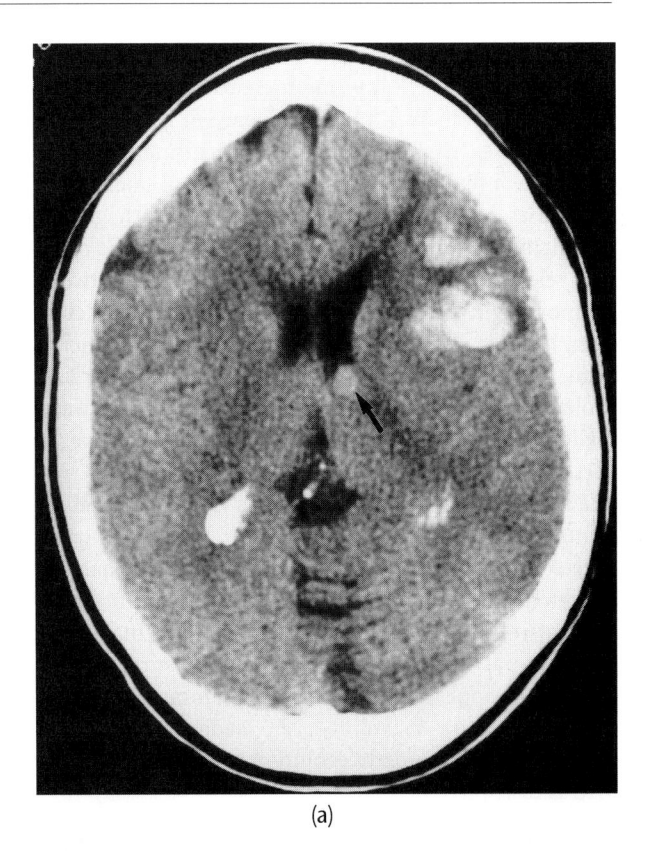

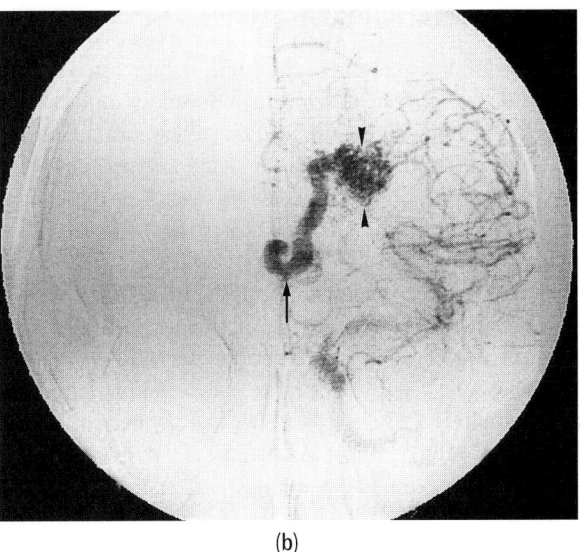

Figure 5.13. *There is an acute left frontal haematoma (a). In addition there is a rounded structure lateral to the left foramen of Monro suggestive of an enlarged vessel (arrow). The angiogram (b) demonstrates a frontal pial arteriovenous malformation (arrowheads) with an enlarged single draining vein (arrow). This was visualized on the CT.*

intraparenchymal haemorrhage tends to be homogenous whereas tumour often has non-haemorrhagic portions which may enhance after contrast. Multiple haemorrhages usually indicate a coagulopathy or possibly metastatic disease or multiple abscesses. Haemorrhage is common in metastases (around 15%)

most commonly seen from bronchogenic carcinoma (especially small cell), melanoma and renal carcinoma. Although rare, there is a high incidence of haemorrhage in metastases from choriocarcinoma primaries. Note that high attenuation deposits in cases of melanoma metastases do not necessarily indicate haemorrhage.

Melanin has an inate high attenuation because of its high electron density; MRI can distinguish between haemorrhagic and non-haemorrhagic melanoma metastases if clinically relevant and occasionally convincing signs of haemorrhage are present on CT (Fig. 5.12). Probably MR is more useful for distinguishing between malignant tumours and non-malignant haemorrhage. In particular the presence of a complete haemosiderin ring in a subacute or chronic haematoma is good indication of non-malignant pathology. However, there are no definite confirmatory signs on a single CT or MRI that will definitely rule out malignancy. In these circumstances interval re-investigation is very useful. Non-malignant haematomas tend to resolve and the surrounding oedema disappears. Neoplastic haematomas, however, tend to increase in volume, the oedema persists or increases and the orderly evolution of haemorrhage on MRI is disrupted.

VASCULAR MALFORMATIONS

Vascular malformations of the brain include: pial AVM, cavernous angioma, developmental venous anomalies, capillary telangiectasias and dural arteriovenous malformations. In children the vein of Galen aneurysmal malformation may also be added to this list. There is a very small risk of intracranial haemorrhage with developmental venous anomalies (although they are frequently associated with cavernous angioma), but all of the others significantly increase the risk of intracranial haemorrhage. The greatest risk occurs with pial AVM.

The annual risk of rupture in these malformations is approximately 2.5%. A pial AVM is a congenital lesion consisting of a compact collection of abnormal, thin-walled vessels connecting enlarged, arterialized draining veins with no interposed capillaries. Arterial, intranidal or venous aneurysms may be associated. These aneurysms and venous outflow obstruction may predispose the AVM to rupture. The estimated prevalence of pial AVM is 1–2/100 000. Most AVM are supratentorial (16:1, supratentorial: infratentorial) and most frequently involve the middle cerebral artery territory (Fig. 5.13). A commonly used grading system has been proposed by Spetzler[4] based upon size, venous drainage and the eloquence of the brain involved. This is used to predict outcome and to help decide between the treatment options which are surgical resection, endovascular obliteration, radiosurgery, any combination of these or no treatment. Intracranial haemorrhage is the commonest presentation of pial arteriovenous malformations (65% parenchymal, 50% subarachnoid, 5% intraventricular).

Non-haemorrhagic presentations include headache, seizures, stroke or transient ischaemic attacks, or focal neurological deficits.

Cavernous angiomas are irregular sinusoidal vascular spaces lined by endothelium and are well demarcated from the adjacent brain. Cavernous angioma are usually not shown by catheter angiography and along with the developmental venous anomalies and capillary telangiectasias are sometimes classified as 'angiographically occult vascular malformations'.

The imaging method of choice for these is MRI and the prevalence may be as high as 0.4% in unselected patients. Cavernous angioma are most frequently found in the supratentorial compartment but ones in the brainstem are most likely to produce a clinically significant haemorrhage. The MR features are characteristic. On spin echo T2-weighted images (T2WI) the abnormalities have a core of mixed signal. A surrounding low-intensity rim of haemosiderosis is usually present. High signal changes on T1WI indicated recent haemorrhage. Cavernous angioma are multiple in over 50% of cases and may show familial tendency. T2* gradient echo sequences are useful to show smaller cavernous angiomas because of the 'blooming' effect (Fig. 5.14) due to microcalcification, microhaemorrhage or haemosiderosis. The annual risk of clinically relevant intracranial haemorrhage is estimated as 0.5% although subclinical bleeds are common.

Capillary telangiectasia most frequently affect the brainstem capillaries with normal brain interposed. Occasionally it is difficult to distinguish these lesions from cavernous angiomas and many authorities consider them part of the same spectrum. Capillary telangiectasias are common and are frequently incidental findings. They are most frequently detected on MRI as small multiple low signal areas on T2-weighted sequences in the pons. Contrast enhanced T1WI show discrete focus of enhancement with irregular or brushlike border (Fig. 5.15). Lack of mass effect, benign clinical course, minimal or no T2 prolongation and characteristic enhancement on MR distinguishes these lesions from a neoplasm.

Venous angiomas represent the most common intracranial vascular malformation. They consist of a network of dilated medullary veins, surrounding and draining into a large central vein. The intervening parenchyma is normal suggesting that venous angiomas may in fact represent a developmental venous anomaly. Contrast-enhanced MRI beautifully demonstrates the characteristic appearance described as the 'caput medusa'.

Dural AVM and fistulae are acquired communications between dural arteries and dural veins and/or sinuses. They are sometimes sequelae of sinus thrombosis or internal carotid artery occlusion. They tend to occur in the older age range and may present with headache or bruit. They rarely produce intracranial haemorrhage but retrograde venous flow in the cortical veins and venous

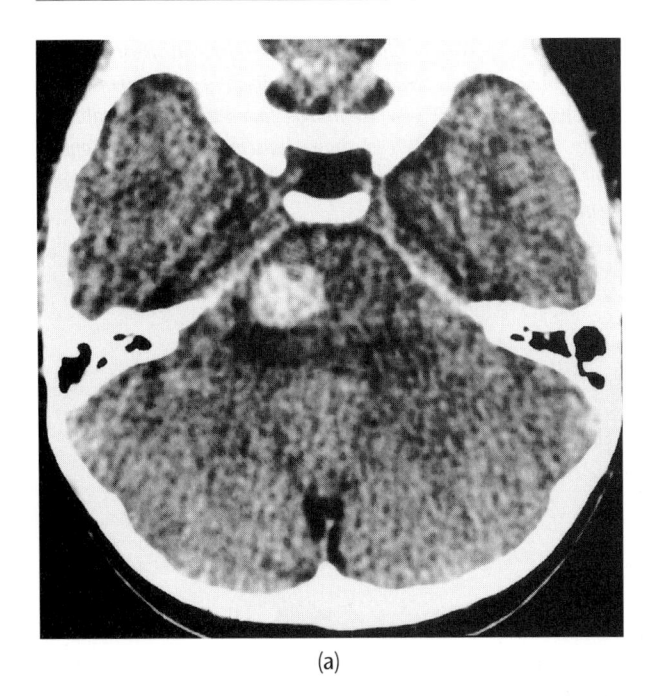

Figure 5.14. *A 2-year-old with a sudden onset of headache and hemiplegia. CT shows an acute 1 cm haematoma in the right side of the pons (a). Standard spin echo MRI showed no further abnormality but coronal gradient echo T2* sequences (b), (c) showed multiple areas of low signal 'blooming' in both cerebral hemispheres. This sequence is very sensitive for microcalcification and/or microhaemorrhage. A case of multiple cavernous angiomas.*

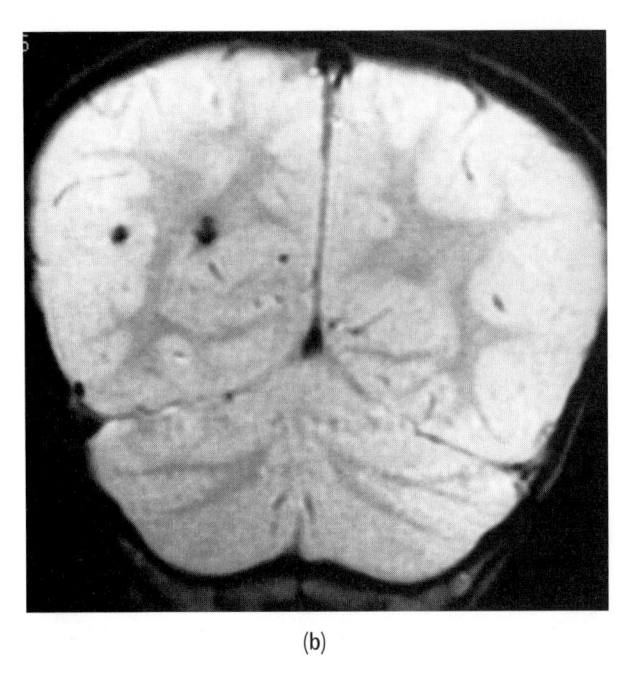

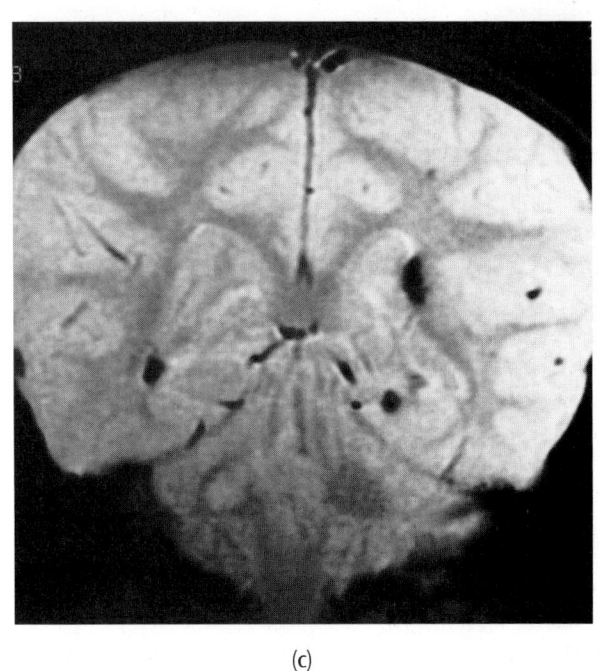

varices significantly increases the risk. Catheter angiography is the imaging method of choice to show the fistulae and endovascular techniques are frequently used to treat these lesions.

HYPERTENSIVE INTRACRANIAL HAEMORRHAGE

Hypertension frequently causes intraparenchymal haemorrhage with or without extension into other compartments. The commonest sites are basal ganglia, thalamus and brainstem which are regions supplied primarily by small perforator branches. One suggested aetiology of hypertensive parenchymal haemorrhage is rupture of microaneurysms on perforating branches (Charcot–Bouchard aneurysms). These are not visible on angiography. However, approximately 20% of hypertensive haemorrhage have a lobar distribution and intraventricular haemorrhage is also common. The early CT literature states that in a hypertensive patient with an intraparenchymal haematoma in a typical distribution, angiography is not indicated. Some authors suggested that is was 'ethically unacceptable' to perform angiography on hypertensive patients. We do not hold with this view and believe that the distribution of the haematoma cannot be used to exclude the presence of structural vascular abnormalities with certainty.

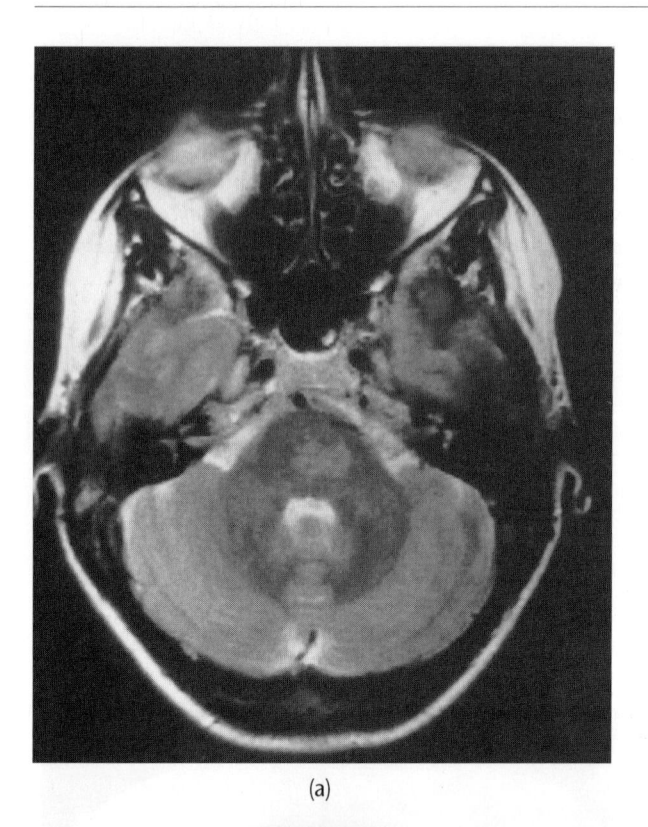

Figure 5.15. A 46-year-old patient presented with hearing loss. T2-weighted MRI (a) showed a lesion with mild hyperintensity in the pons. Pre-contrast T1WI (b) images failed to show any abnormality. Post-contrast T1WI (c) showed discreet focus of enhancement with irregular brush like borders typical of capillary haemangioma.

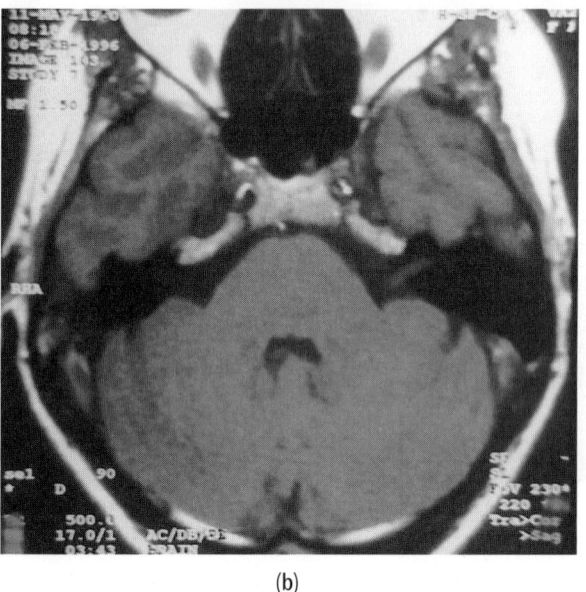

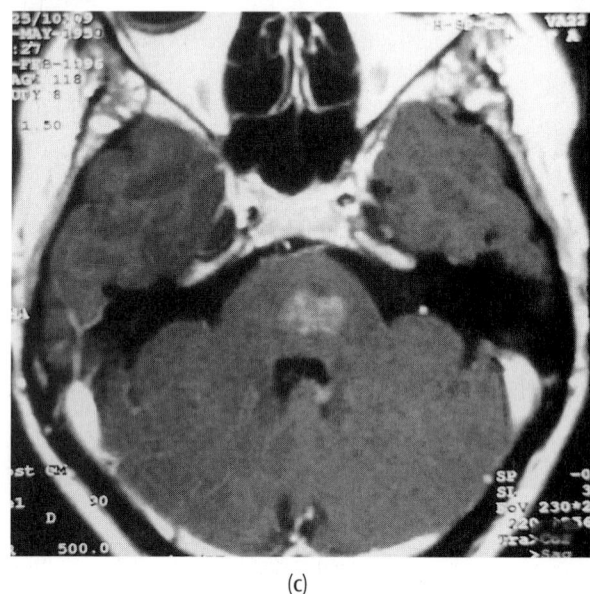

For example we have shown arteriovenous malformations in hypertensive patients with basal ganglia haematoma (Fig. 5.16). In a recent review of 100 consecutive intraparenchymal haematomas at Newcastle General Hospital, 25 patients were hypertensive and five (20%) had structural abnormalities (four aneurysms, one AVM).[1] The decision to perform angiography should be based on the individual clinical situation.

Most hypertensive bleeds will occur in the older age group. Occasionally a young patient will develop intracranial haemorrhage as a result of a known systemic disease producing hypertension e.g. chronic renal failure, or intracranial haemorrhage may be the presenting feature of a systemic disorder. Recreational substance abuse should also be considered in young patients with intracranial haemorrhage.

SUBSTANCE ABUSE

Many of the chemicals implicated in illegal substance abuse have pronounced effects on the cerebral vasculature as well as on the neurotransmitter/receptor system.

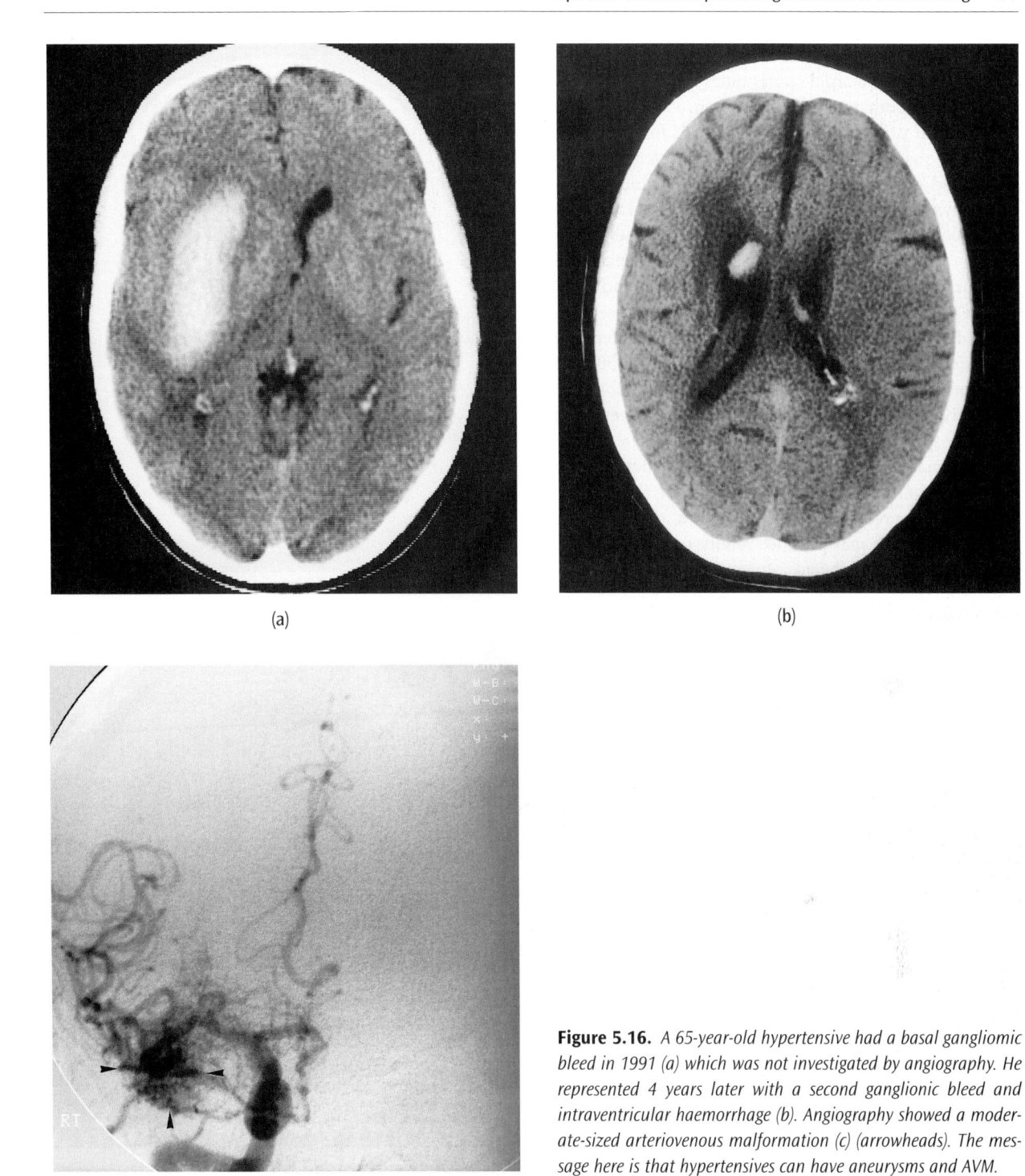

Specific conditions producing intracranial haemorrhage   177

Figure 5.16. *A 65-year-old hypertensive had a basal gangliomic bleed in 1991 (a) which was not investigated by angiography. He represented 4 years later with a second ganglionic bleed and intraventricular haemorrhage (b). Angiography showed a moderate-sized arteriovenous malformation (c) (arrowheads). The message here is that hypertensives can have aneurysms and AVM.*

Prominent amongst these are cocaine hydrochloride, free-base and 'crack' cocaine, amphetamine and methylene dioxymethylamphetamine (ecstasy). The range of CNS complications following the use of these substances include infarction, subarachnoid haemorrhage, vasculitis, arterial spasm, intraparenchymal haemorrhage, seizures and infective sequelae. Some complications are due to embolic, vasculitic or infective phenomenon of inert 'bulking agents' such as talc or sugar. These complications particularly, but not exclusively, occur when these substances are administered intravenously.

The pharmacology of these substances and their effects on the CNS vasculature are complicated and often dose-dependent and idiosyncratic. However, a frequent sequence of events is early cerebral vasoconstriction due to the effects on the vessels' (alpha)-adrenergic receptors and calcium channels. The common combination of cocaine and amphetamine potentiates these effects. This results in smooth muscle constriction, vascular spasm and cerebral ischaemia/infarction. This is followed by a period of vasodilation and systemic hypertension. It is postulated that this mechanism may produce intraparenchymal haemorrhage in cocaine users and the neuroradiological findings of this have been reviewed by Brown et al.[5] The distribution of intraparenchymal haemorrhage usually involves the basal ganglia and bears a close similarity to hypertensive haemorrhage seen in the older age group (Fig. 5.17). However, underlying structural vascular abnormalities are found in 50% of cases of intracranial haemorrhage related to substance abuse, most commonly aneurysm and AVM.[6] These may produce subarachnoid haemorrhage as well as intraparenchymal haemorrhage. Cocaine also increase the risk of thrombosis by increasing platelet thrombotic agents. This predisposes to sinus and cortical vein thrombosis which may produce venous infarction which is frequently haemorrhagic.

HAEMORRHAGIC INFARCTION

Haemorrhagic infarction can be due to occlusion of either the cerebral arteries or the draining veins and/or sinuses. Haemorrhagic infarction is more common in sinus or cortical vein thrombosis than arterial thrombosis and tends to involve the white matter rather than cor-

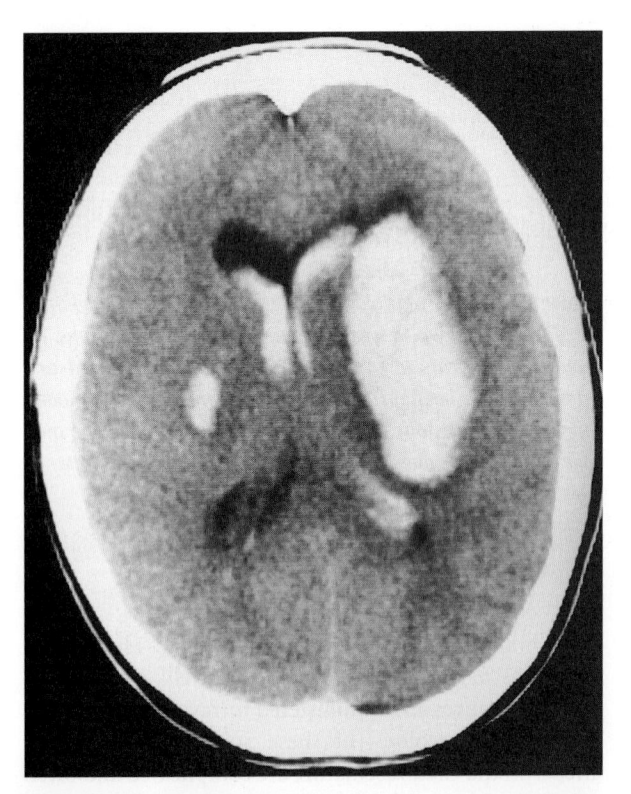

Figure 5.17. *Bilateral basal gangliomic haematoma with intraventricular extension in a 16-year-old following amphetamine use. Angiography was normal.*

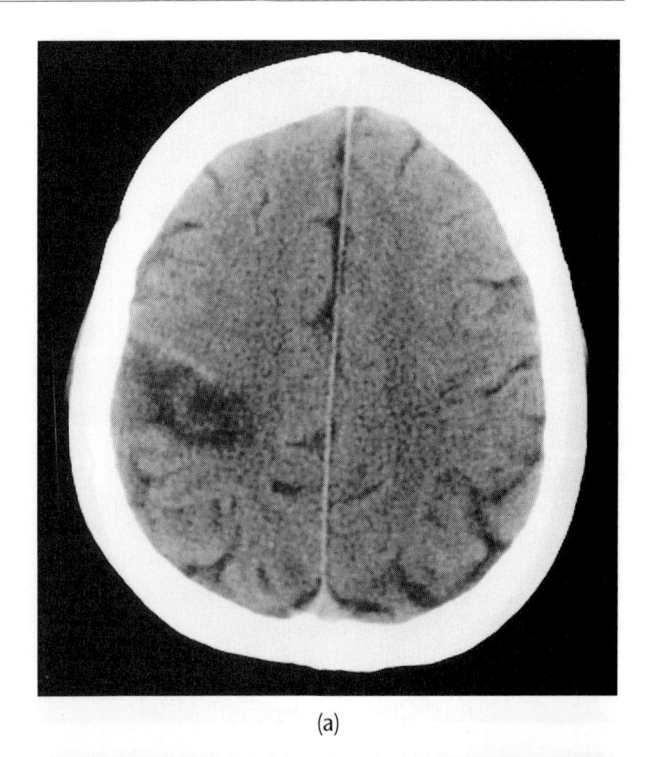

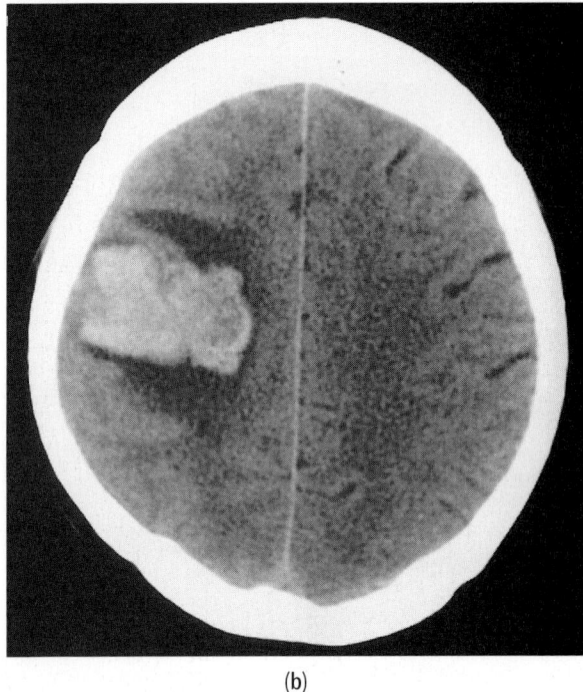

Figure 5.18. *Haemorrhagic change in a bland cerebral infarction. CT 36 hours after stroke (a) shows a wedge-shaped area of low attenuation in the right parietal lobe. A repeat scan at 4 days (b) shows haemorrhagic change within the region of infarction.*

tex. Bilateral involvement is common in sinus thrombosis, cerebral hemisphere in cases of superior sagittal thrombosis and basal ganglia or thalamus in cases of straight sinus thrombosis. Other CT features of sagittal sinus thrombosis are a triangular high attenuation region in the sinus on non-enhanced scans in the acute

Table 5.7 *Typical features of haemorrhagic infarction and intraparenchymal haematomas*

Haemorrhagic infarction	Parenchymal haematoma
1 Bland infarction in the first few hours	Haemorrrhagic at onset
2 Heterogenous, patchy high attenuation	Dense, homogenous high attenuation
3 No extra mass effect	Mass effect a major feature
4 May extend into the cortex	May extend into the ventricles
5 Gyral enhancement	Rim enhancement
6 No change in clinical condition at the time of haemorrhage	Often catastrophic clinical deterioration

stage or the empty sinus or 'delta' sign on contrast-enhanced scans when the thrombus has organized. Common causes of sinus/cortical vein thrombosis include pregnancy, oral contraception, infection, dehydration, trauma and tumour invasion.

Haemorrhagic infarction probably occurs in approximately 50% of all strokes due to arterial occlusion and is more frequent in strokes due to proximal emboli. A major radiological concern is distinguishing between parenchymal haematoma and haemorrhagic infarction following arterial occlusion. This may be difficult and the only way to be entirely sure is to have CT documentation of haemorrhage into a previously bland infarction (Fig. 5.18). However, many patients with stroke are not imaged early in their admission and features which may help to distinguish between the two are listed in Table 5.7.

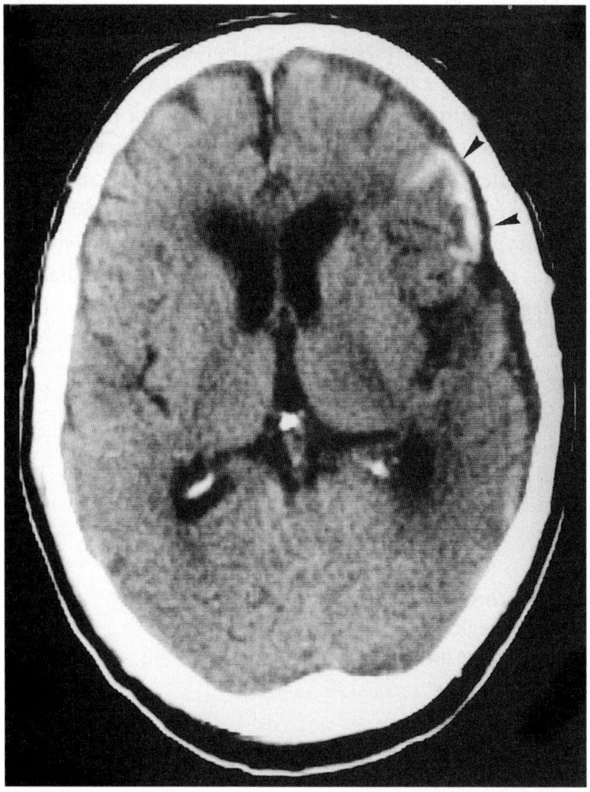

The significance of haemorrhage into infarction is not known with certainty but many authors consider that haemorrhagic infarction alone is not necessarily a serious complication with respect to outcome. The difficult choice arises in the decision to anticoagulate the patient or not. The concern is changing a previously bland infarction into a haemorrhagic one or possibly into a haematoma (Fig. 5.19). Factors which predispose to this are, over anticoagulation, large volume of infarction, hypertension and embolic stroke.

CEREBRAL AMYLOID ANGIOPATHY

This is a recently recognized cause of non-traumatic intracerebral haemorrhage in older patients that does not invoke a hypertensive aetiology (Fig. 5.20). It has been estimated that 20% of intraparenchymal haemorrhages in the over 70 age-group are due to cerebral amyloid angiopathy. Amyloid angiopathy may produce bland infarction as well as haemorrhage. The amyloid laid down in the vessel walls in this disorder is virtually identical to those in the plaques of Alzheimer's disease and the two disorders frequently co-exit (40–45%). There is a roughly equal sex distribution with a mean age of presentation between 70 and 74 years. It most frequently presents as recurrent haemorrhage, although 32% also have a clinical history of hypertension. The haemorrhages are most frequently lobar in the distribution frontal > parietal > occipital > temporal.

INTRACRANIAL HEAMORRHAGE IN CHILDREN

Neonatal period

Intracranial haemorrhage in the neonatal period is frequently caused by birth trauma which can affect both premature and term babies. The haemorrhage can affect any of the intracranial compartments and is more fre-

Figure 5.19. *Right hemiplegia in a 75-year-old who was taking warfarin. The CT scan, 1 day after the ictus, showed subtle low attenuation in the perisylvian frontal lobe indicating infarction and gyriform haemorrhage in the cortical mantle (arrowheads).*

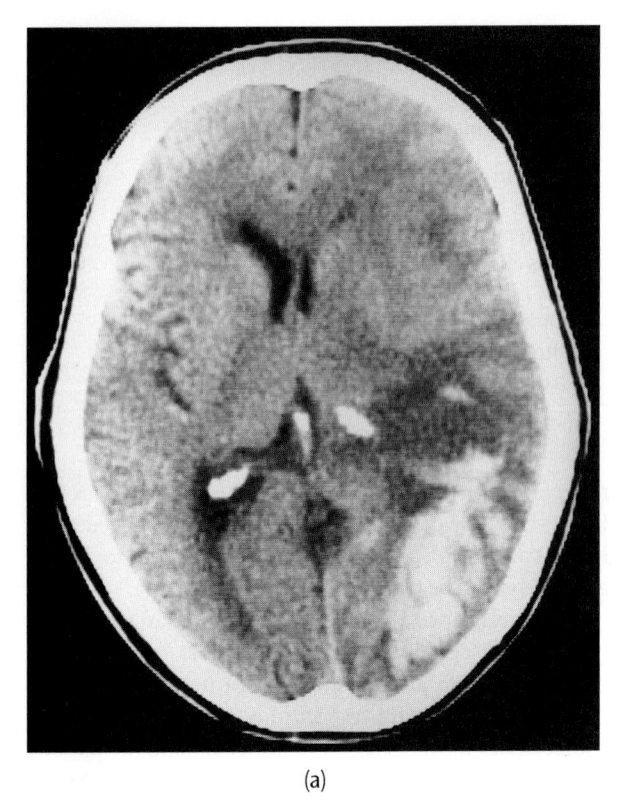

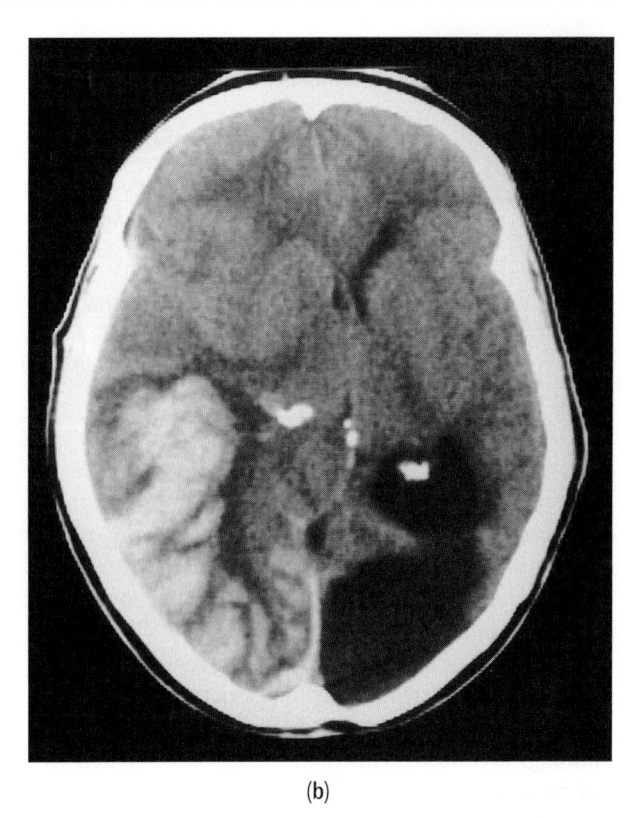

Figure 5.20. Left parietal and occipital lobe haematoma in a 70-year-old non-hypertensive (a). Angiography was normal. After 4 months the patient represented with right parietal and occipital haematoma (b). The diagnosis of cerebral amyloid angiography was confirmed on histology at the second presentation.

quent in interventional vaginal deliveries such as forceps or vacuum-assisted deliveries. For a full synopsis of this subject see Ref. 5.

THE TERM BABY

There are many causes of non-traumatic intracranial haemorrhage in the term baby. These are outlined in Table 5.8 but it is important to realise there may be multiple and/or interrelated causes. For example neonatal infection may cause intracranial haemorrhage by producing disseminated intravascular coagulation, infective vasculitis, embolism, sinus thrombosis or direct infection of the meninges or ependyma, alone or in combination. Two entities warrant brief discussion, the first being primary subarachnoid haemorrhages of the newborn. This is the commonest single cause of intracranial haemorrhage in the term newborn occurring in 37% of all

Table 5.8 Causes of non-traumatic intracranial haemorrhage in the term newborn

Common	
Asphyxia	
Primary subarachnoid haemorrhage of the newborn	
Uncommon	
Venous infarction	Dural sinus or cortical vein thrombosis
Arterial infarction	Often haemorrhagic
Coagulopathy	Particularily diffuse intravasular coagulopathy
Infection	Direct or systemic
Rare	
Polycythaemia	Especially in cyanotic heart disease
Vascular malformations	
Primary thalamoventricular haemorrhage	
Syndrome related	e.g. Sturge–Weber, Wyburn–Mason, Weber–Rendu–Osler syndromes

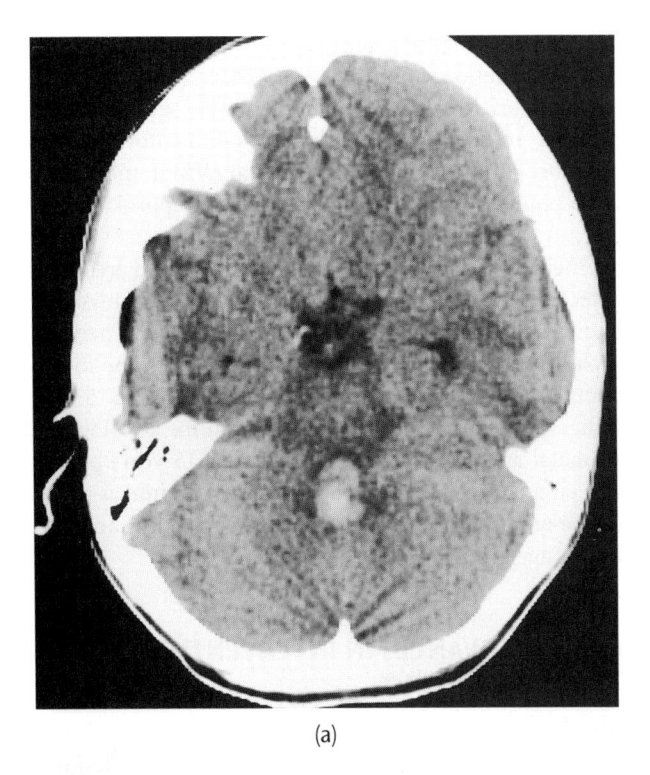

Figure 5.21. *A 12-year-old with an acute onset of headache and neck stiffness. CT at presentation shows an acute haematoma localized to the cerebellar vermis (a). Early arterial phase angiography shows a pial arteriovenous malformation fed by the right superior cerebellar artery (b) (arrowhead) and late arterial phase angiography shows an enlarged vein draining (arrowhead) to the straight sinus via the Galenic system (c).*

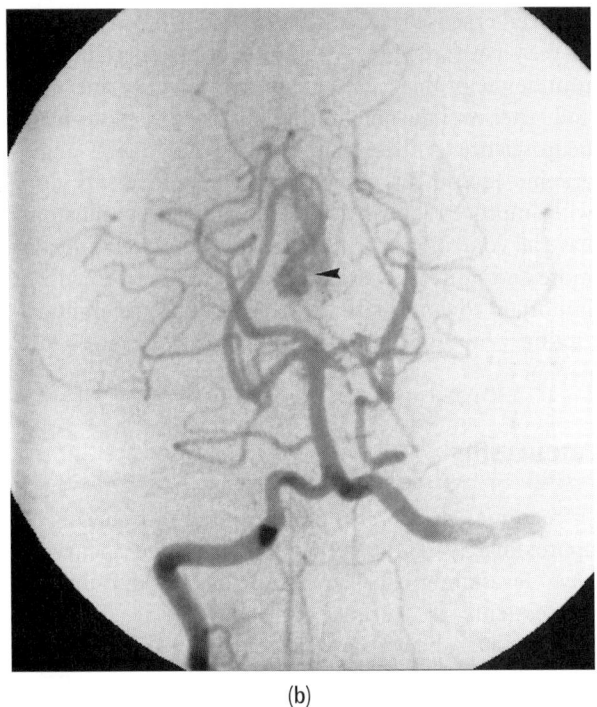

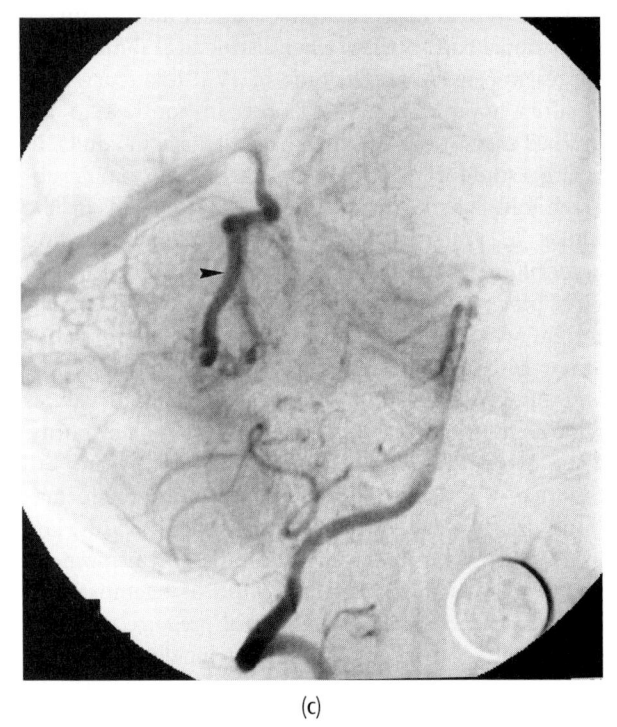

(a)

(b)

(c)

intracranial haemorrhage in one study. It has been observed in 20% of spontaneous vaginal deliveries and 40% of instrument-assisted deliveries. Many of these are due to the mechanical trauma of childbirth but other factors include asphyxia, venous congestion and focally raised intracranial pressure.

Primary thalamoventricular haemorrhage is unilateral thalamic haemorrhage in a term child. This usually presents between 3 and 21 days post-delivery. Seizures and irritability in a previously well baby is the commonest clinical setting. Most cases are thought to occur secondary to venous thrombosis, particularly at the internal cerebral vein. Outcome is usually poor, death in 3/29 and cerebral palsy is 13/29 in Govaert's series.[7]

THE PREMATURE BABY

Many of the previously described pathologies can affect the pre-term neonate; however, germinal matrix haemorrhage is common in these children. It is the result of hypoxic–ischaemic damage affecting the metabolically active germinal matrix in the periventricular region, particularly in the caudate/thalamic notch. This region is rendered hypoxic and on subsequent reperfusion the weakened blood vessels rupture. It is not the mechanism of haemorrhage that is peculiar to this age group but the site of the most susceptible area. Germinal matrix haemorrhage is unusual after 34 weeks of gestation. The anatomical four-point grading system proposed by Volpe is frequently used.[8] Children with the less severe (grade I–II) haemorrhage have a 23% mortality rate, while in children with grade III–IV haemorrhage the mortality is 74%. Serious long-term neurological sequelae are common in survivors. Ultrasound is the usual means of detection and follow-up of children with germinal matrix haemorrhage.

Intracranial haemorrhage in older children

Non-traumatic intracranial haemorrhage in children is uncommon because most of the causes listed in Tables 5.2 and 5.3 are rare in this age group. In persons under 15 years AVM is the commonest cause of non-traumatic intracranial haemorrhage when a structural abnormality is present (Fig. 5.21). The ratio of AVM to aneurysm in children approaches 3:1.[9] This is in contrast to the marked excess of aneurysmal haemorrhage in adults. In a large study of 6368 patients with aneurysmal subarachnoid haemorrhage only 0.6% occurred in the under 19 years group. Arteriovenous malformation account for 20% of all 'strokes' in children and 20% of all AVM have presented by the age of 20 years. Vascular malformations include pial AVM, developmental venous anomalies, cavernous angioma, capillary telangiectasia and dural AVM. Pial AVM are congenital abnormalities with an estimated prevalence of 1–2/1000 newborns. They occur sporadically although family clusters are reported. Cases of multiple arteriovenous malformations are unusual outside Osler–Weber–Rendu (Fig. 5.22) and Wyburn–Mason syndromes. Arteriovenous malformations may present because of haemorrhage, seizure, headache, raised intracranial pressure, progressive neurological deficits or may be an incidental finding. The non-haemorrhagic presentations may be due to many causes and can be multifactorial. Mass effect, venous hypertension and vascular steal have been implicated. Headache may result from hypertrophy of dural vessels.

There are significant differences between AVM in children and adults. In a large study from the Hospital for Sick Children, Toronto 132 children with brain AVM were reviewed over a 40-year period.[10] Presentation was by intracranial haemorrhage in 79% and seizures accounted for 12%.[8] This is in contrast to adults in whom intracranial haemorrhage is the mode of presentation in approximately 50% (65% parenchymal, 30% subarachnoid and 5% intraventricular). In reports from adult populations there is a marked preponderance of supratentorial AVM (approximately 94% supratentorial and 6% infratentorial). Although supratentorial AVM are more common than infratentorial AVM in the paediatric population the ratio is reduced to approximately 3:1.

Aneurysms are less common in children and are often infective in nature. The aetiology of non-mycotic aneurysms in children is open to debate. Theories include enlargement of vestigial stumps from the foetal circulation or large arterial media defects (Fig. 5.23). Others have implicated birth trauma in the aetiology of neonatal aneurysms. In children under 15 years posterior circulation aneurysms are twice as common as those of the anterior circulation. Multiple aneurysms are rare in this age group.

RECENT ADVANCES IN INTERVENTIONAL NEURORADIOLOGY

Endovascular treatment of intracranial vascular lesions has been practised since the late 1960s. However the past 10 years have seen great expansion of this speciality with routine use of this technique for treatment of aneurysm and arteriovenous malformations in the most major neuroscience centres. Improvements in digital angiographic equipment, catheter and embolic agents along with improved knowledge of functional neuroanatomy have all contributed to the success of this technique. As more and more of these procedures are performed it is important to emphasize the need for a proper multidisciplinary approach and commitment towards total patient care.

Aneurysms

Intracranial aneurysms are common, occurring in approximately 2% of population. Ruptured aneurysms have devastating consequences with only one-third of the patients recovering with mild or no disability. Endovascular therapy can treat aneurysms or the spasm associated with subarachnoid haemorrhage. Large proximal aneurysms are preferably treated with parent vessel occlusion, where the vessel bearing the aneurysm is blocked with detachable balloons at or below the neck of the aneurysm. Most aneurysms, however, are now treated by endosaccular occlusion using detachable coils. Guglielmi detachable coils (GDC) are platinum coils which are soldered on to a stainless steel delivery wire. Once positioned in the aneurysm they are detached with electrothrombosis. Immediate results of GDC treatment of aneurysms are comparable with surgical results; however the long-term security of treated aneurysm remains to be seen.

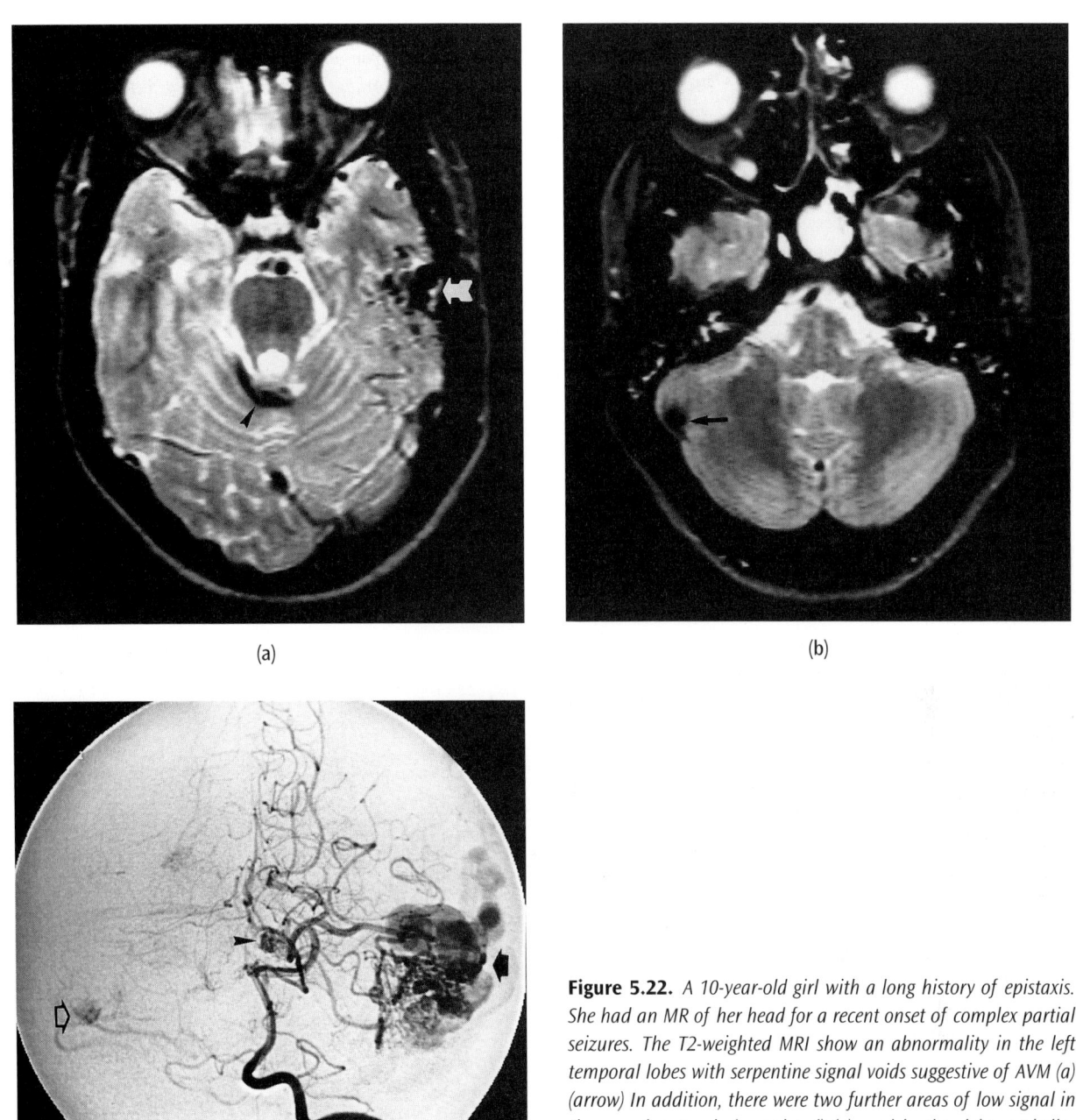

Figure 5.22. *A 10-year-old girl with a long history of epistaxis. She had an MR of her head for a recent onset of complex partial seizures. The T2-weighted MRI show an abnormality in the left temporal lobes with serpentine signal voids suggestive of AVM (a) (arrow) In addition, there were two further areas of low signal in the superior vermis (arrowhead) (a), and in the right cerebellar hemisphere (arrow) (b). Catheter angiography showed three AVM (c) (solid arrowhead), open arrow and solid arrow). The diagnosis of Osler–Weber–Rendu syndrome was made.*

Which patients should be treated by endovascular methods is at present uncertain. In most centres, patients with surgically difficult, for example basilar aneurysms, are now referred for endovascular treatment (Fig. 5.24). In our unit, we also treat patients who may be medically unfit for major intracranial surgery. A randomized study comparing surgery with endovascular treatments in ruptured intracranial aneurysms is now ongoing in many centres around Europe. Results of this study may give us guidelines for using this new and exciting technique.

Arteriovenous malformations

Arteriovenous malformations most often present with an intracranial haemorrhage although presentation with epileptic fits or neurological deficits are not uncommon. Many more incidental AVM are also being detected because of the increased use of CT and MRI. Once detected, an AVM has a 2–3% per year risk of rupture. With use of this knowledge of natural history, management of AVM is based on the age and existing neurological deficit of patient as well as Spetzler grade of the lesion.

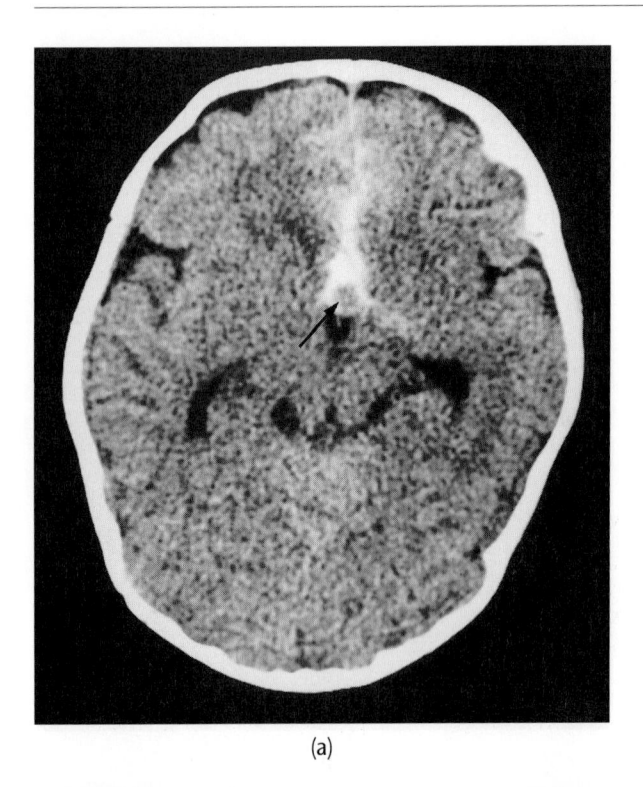

Figure 5.23. A 6-week infant presented with listlessness and a bulging anterior fontanelle. CT showed interhemispheric subarachnoid haemorrhage outlining a filling defect anterior to the third ventricle (arrowed) (a). T1-weighted MRI showed acute haemorrhage in the region of the anterior communicating artery (b) (arrowhead). Catheter angiography showed a complex aneurysm extending over the anterior communicating artery and the A1 and A2 segments of the anterior cerebral artery (c) (arrowhead).

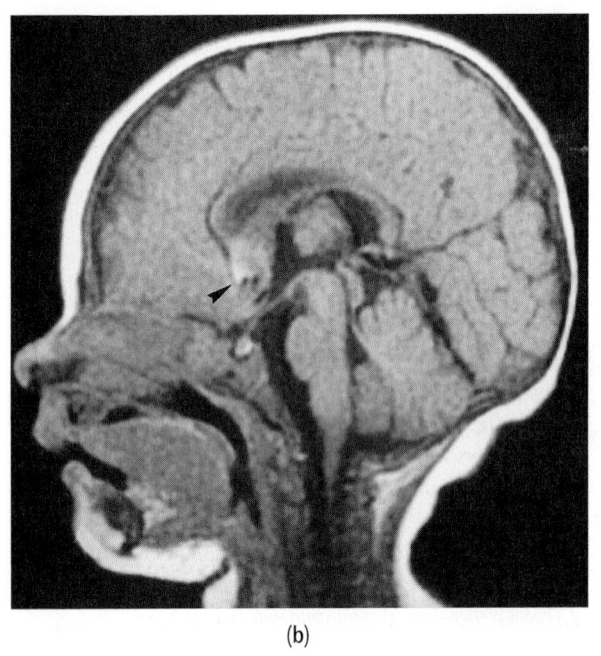

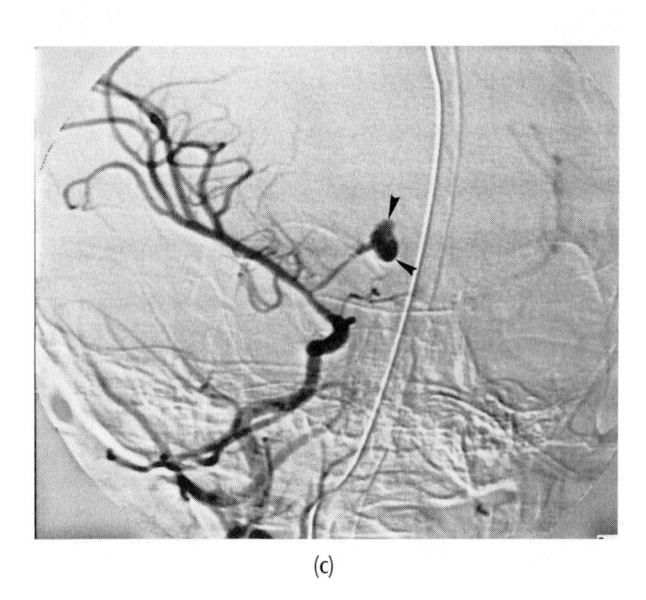

Treatment options include conservative management, surgery, radiosurgery and endovascular embolization. In the case of definitive treatment, the goal is to completely obliterate the lesion. This may be achieved by any one of the above treatments or in combination with others. The initial method of treatment is usually decided after multidisciplinary consultation.

Endovascular treatment involves catheterizing the nidus of the AVM using either flow-guided or wire-guided microcatheters. In most cases embolization is performed using a glue (Histoacryl blue) and Lipiodol mixture. Some operators prefer to use other embolic agents such as polyvinyl alcohol (PVA) particles, silk, microcoils, alcohol, Ival etc. A small number of malformations (approximately 15%) can be completely obliterated by embolization alone. The rest of the malformations will need either surgery and/or radiosurgery for complete obliteration (Fig. 5.25). Such multidisciplinary treatment has revolutionized the management and outcome of patients with AVM.

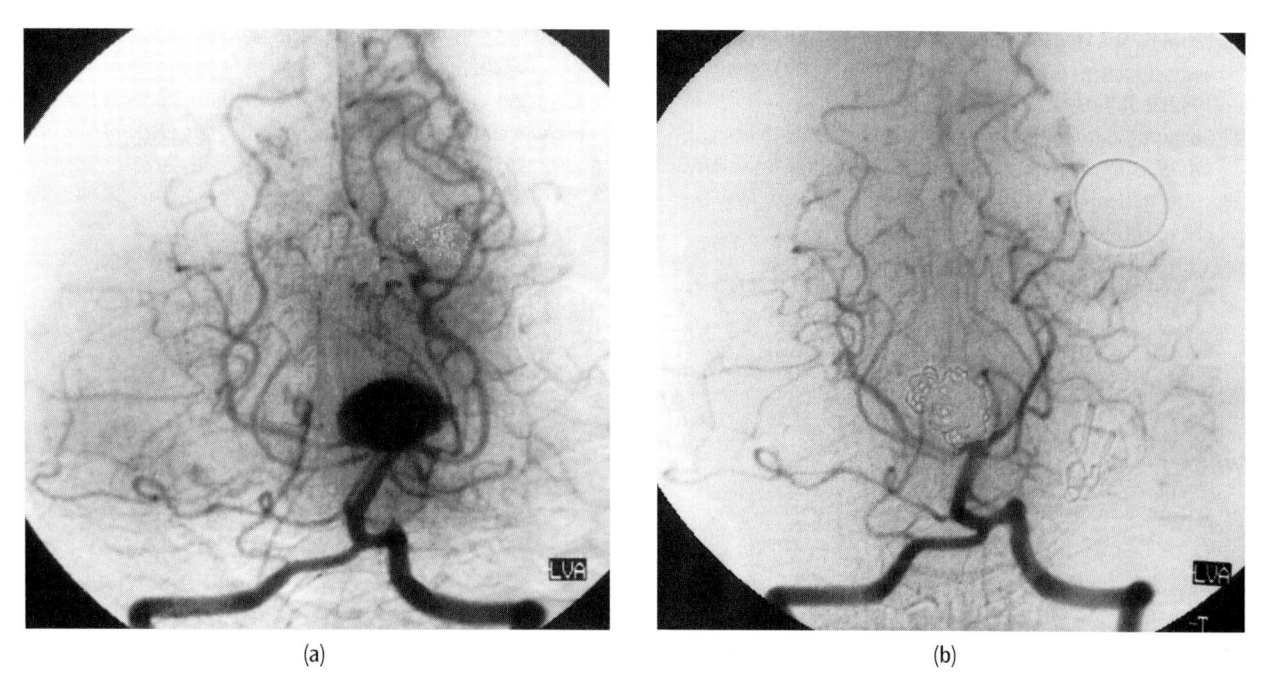

Figure 5.24. *(a) Endosaccular coil embolization of a large basilar tip aneurysm using GDC coils. Follow-up angiogram (b) performed 1 year after treatment shows persistent complete occlusion.*

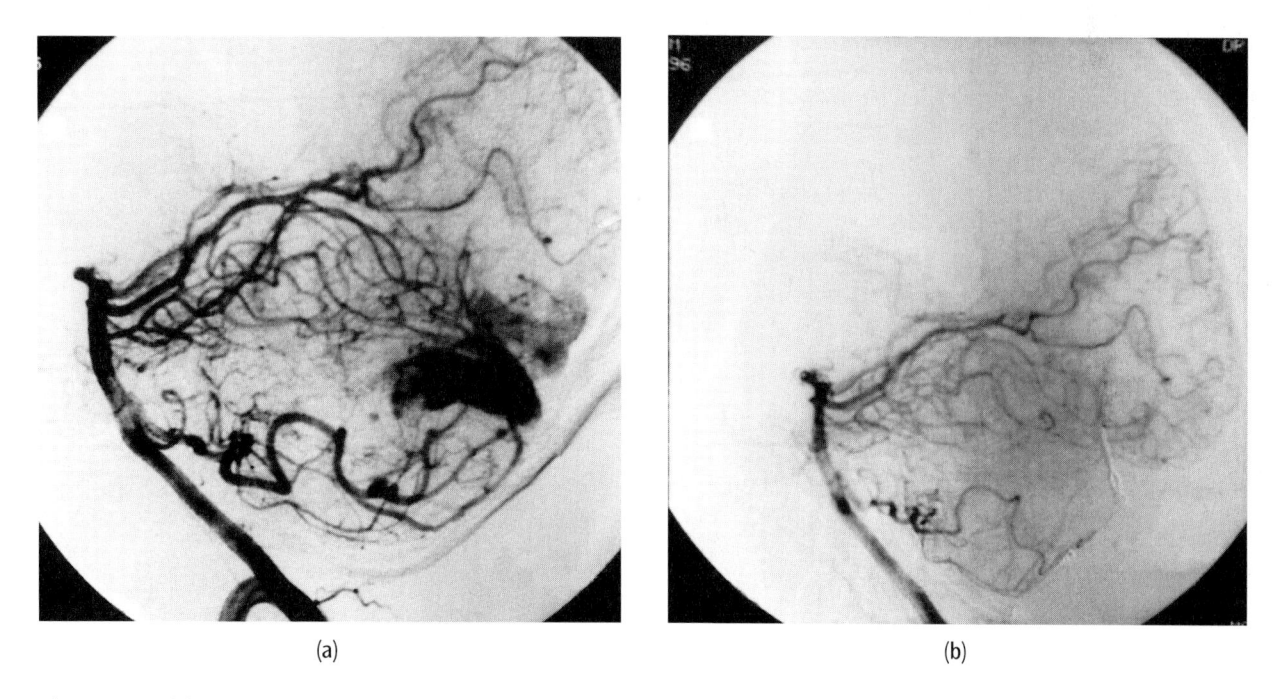

Figure 5.25. *(a) Cerebellar AVM treated by combination of embolization and surgery. The AVM was embolized with glue and the residual lesion was then completely excised by surgery (b).*

REFERENCES

1 Beveridge CJ, Griffiths PD, Gholkar A. *Cerebral angiography for non-traumatic intracerebral haematoma*: p. 28. Rontgen Centenary Congress. 1995.
2 Osborne AG. *Diagnostic Neuroradiology*. pp. 154–68. St Louis: Mosby, 1994.
3 Sengupta RP, McAllister VL. *Subarachnoid Haemorrhage* pp. 93–163. Berlin: Springer–Verlag, 1986.
4 Spetzler R. A proposed grading system for arteriovenous malformations. *J Neurosurg* 1986; **65**: 476–83.
5 Brown E, Prager J, Lee H-Y, Ramsey RG. CNS complications of cocaine abuse: prevalence, pathophysiology and neuroradiology. *Am J Roentgenol* 1991; **159**:137–47.

6 Landi JL, Spickler EM. Imaging of intracranial haemorrhage associated with drug abuse. *Neuroimaging Clin N Amer* 1992; **2**:187–94.
7 Govaert P. *Cranial Haemorrhage in the Term Newborn Infant*. Cambridge: MacKeith Press, Cambridge University.
8 Volpe JJ. Neonatal intraventricular haemorrhage. *New Engl J Med* 1981; **304**:886–91.
9 Humphreys RP Haemorrhage stroke in childhood. *J Pediatr Neurosci* 1986; **2**:1–10.
10 Kondziolka, D *et al*. Arteriovenous malformations of the brain in children. A 40 year experience. *Can J Neurol Sci* 1992; **19**:40–45.

6

Non-haemorrhagic vascular disease

PAUL BUTLER

Introduction	187	Imaging strategies in cerebral ischaemia	202
CT and MRI in cerebral infarction	188	Craniocervical arterial dissection	203
The evolution of cerebral infarction	189	Cerebral arterial ectasia	203
Haemorrhagic infarcts	194	Cerebral vasculitis and other angiopathies	204
Posterior circulation infarction	196	Cerebral venous infarction	205
Watershed infarction	196	Cerebrovascular disease in children	207
Lacunar infarcts	198	References	210
Magnetic resonance angiography	200	Further reading	211

INTRODUCTION

Stroke is a lay term defined clinically as the sudden onset of a focal neurological deficit lasting longer than 24 hours. Its commonest manifestation is as a hemiparesis. A transient ischaemic attack (TIA) is a focal neurological deficit resolving, by convention, within 24 hours. It may take the form of hemiparesis, dysphasia or amaurosis fugax (transient monocular blindness).

Eighty per cent of strokes result from cerebral infarction, most often in the territory of the middle cerebral artery. The remainder are due to haemorrhage and the distinction between the two on clinical grounds may not be possible. Most cerebral infarcts are caused by cerebral thromboembolism which may arise due to atherosclerosis in the craniocervical arteries or from emboli originating from the heart. Many conditions are associated with cerebral ischaemia (Table 6.1) but even after extensive investigation, including such techniques as transoesophageal echocardiography, no underlying cause is apparent in a proportion of cases.

Paroxysmal dysrhythmias are the principal cause of cardiogenic cerebral emboli. Valvar disease, cardiac ischaemia and endocarditis may also be responsible. Atrial myxomas are a rare cause. Strokes associated with coronary artery bypass graft surgery are usually embolic in origin.[1]

Although the precise pathogenesis is uncertain, there does appear to be association between ischaemic stroke and migraine, particularly in the territory of the poste-

Table 6.1 *Causes of cerebral ischaemia*

Atherosclerosis
Embolism
   cardiac
   cervical arterial
Hypotension
   e.g. following cardiac arrest
Trauma
   severe closed head injury
   penetrating injury
   dissection
   angiography
Arterial spasm
   subarachnoid haemorrhage
Angiopathies
   collagen diseases, SLE, PAN
   moyamoya disease
   sarcoidosis
   Takayasu's disease
   substance abuse
Blood dyscrasias
   sickle cell disease
   oral contraceptives
Migraine
Venous infarction

SLE: Systemic lupus erythematosus
PAN: Polyarteritis nodosa

rior cerebral artery.[2,3] Females taking oral contraception are at risk from both arterial infarction and, much less frequently, superior sagittal sinus thrombosis.[4] Systemic

188 Non-haemorrhagic vascular disease

lupus erythematosus may also give rise to both cerebral arterial and venous occlusion as well as to a fulminating vasculitis.

Computed tomography (CT) is the initial imaging investigation of choice in suspected stroke. It is simple, quick and straightforward for the patient. It is widely available and readily identifies the presence of haemorrhage.

Magnetic resonance imaging (MRI) has a number of advantages over CT including superior contrast resolution and the ability to image in multiple planes without altering the patient's position within the imaging facility. In purely practical terms, however, an MR examination takes longer than CT and the representation of haemorrhage on MRI is complex. In the acute stage and depending on the pulse sequence used, it may be indistinguishable from infarction.

CT AND MRI IN CEREBRAL INFARCTION

An established cerebral infarct is shown on CT or MRI as a region of parenchymal change conforming to a vascular territory. The vascular territories are illustrated on pp. 20, 21. When the entire vascular territory is affected, the change will involve both grey and white matter with a well defined margin (Fig. 6.1). The three major cerebral arteries which supply the cortical mantle and subcortical white matter have collateral pathways to re-establish perfusion after occlusion. Smaller arteries supplying the

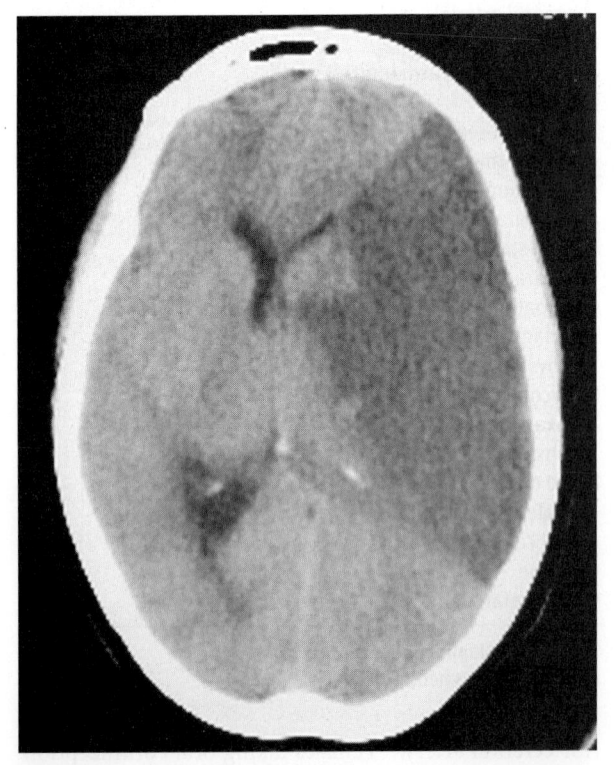

Figure 6.1 *Cranial CT. Acute left middle cerebral artery territory infarct.*

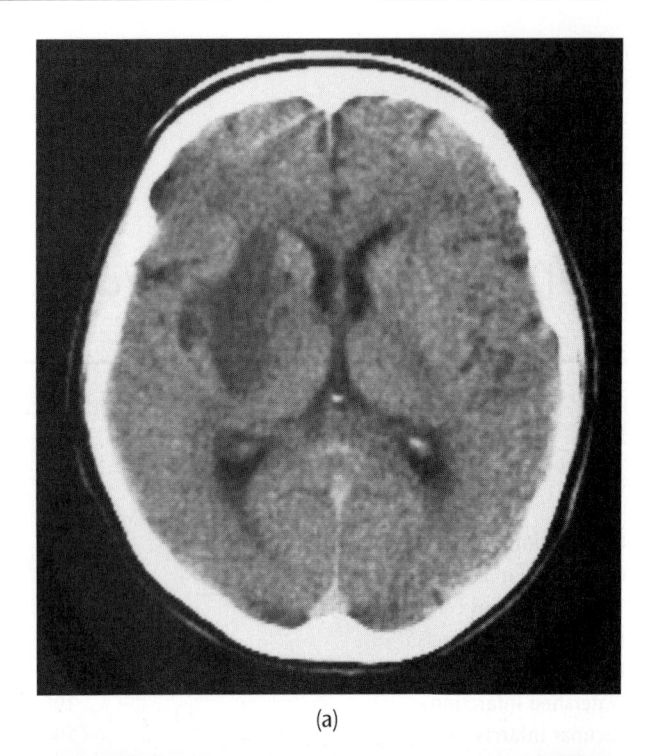

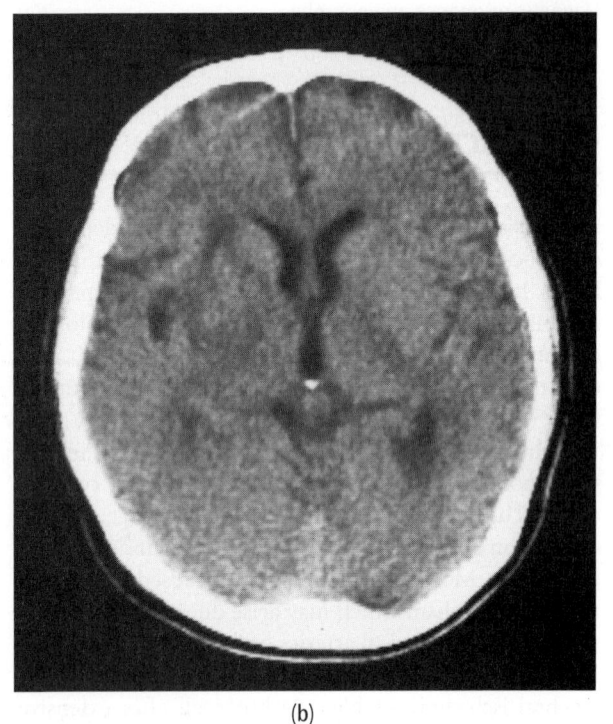

Figure 6.2 *Cranial CT. Right hemisphere infarction: (b) was obtained 7 days after (a). Note the resolution of the hypodensity.*

deep hemispheres may be end arteries. If a collateral circulation exists or if only a small branch is occluded the parenchymal change will be less extensive and the diagnosis more problematic. These appearances could also be due to an infiltrating neoplasm.

To assist in interpretation it is important to appreciate that an infarct evolves fairly rapidly through a series of

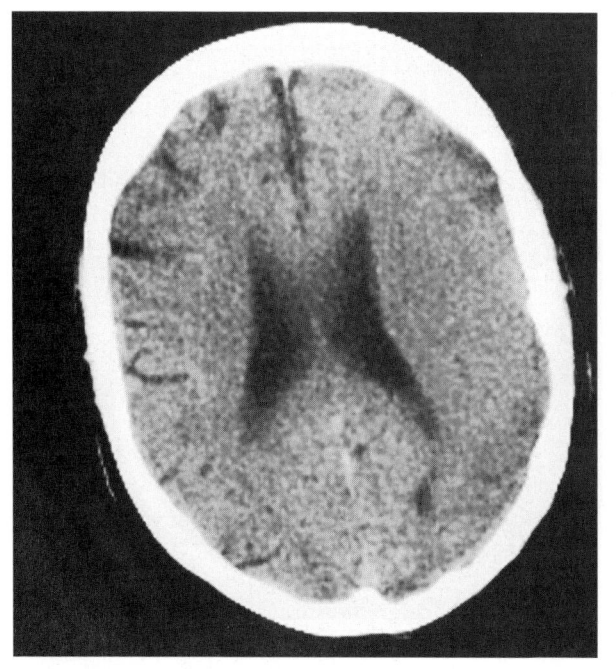

Figure 6.3 Cranial CT. Early left middle cerebral artery territory infarction. Sulcal effacement is evidence of mass effect.

stages towards maturity, reflecting the pathophysiology of ischaemia. Untreated neoplasms usually either increase in size or remain unchanged. Sequential scanning may therefore resolve the issue in cases of doubt (Fig. 6.2). Four helpful signs assist in distinguishing infarct from tumour within the supratentorial compartment on CT:[5]

- Enhancement of the grey matter following intravenous contrast medium and sparing of the thalamus favoured infarction
- Oedema and ring enhancement within the white matter indicating tumour

The importance of scanning in the acute stage of stroke is to exclude haemorrhage so that anticoagulant or thrombolytic therapy can be instituted as appropriate.

THE EVOLUTION OF CEREBRAL INFARCTION

Similar criteria to those used in CT are also employed in the MRI diagnosis of cerebral infarction. However, MRI is more sensitive in the detection of parenchymal change unimpeded by artefacts arising from bone. Smaller lesions can be identified and MRI is particularly valuable in the diagnosis of posterior fossa infarction. Enhancement of the ischaemic region with intravenous contrast agents is rather more complex than is found with the iodinated agents used with CT.

In the first 24 or 48 hours following infarction CT may

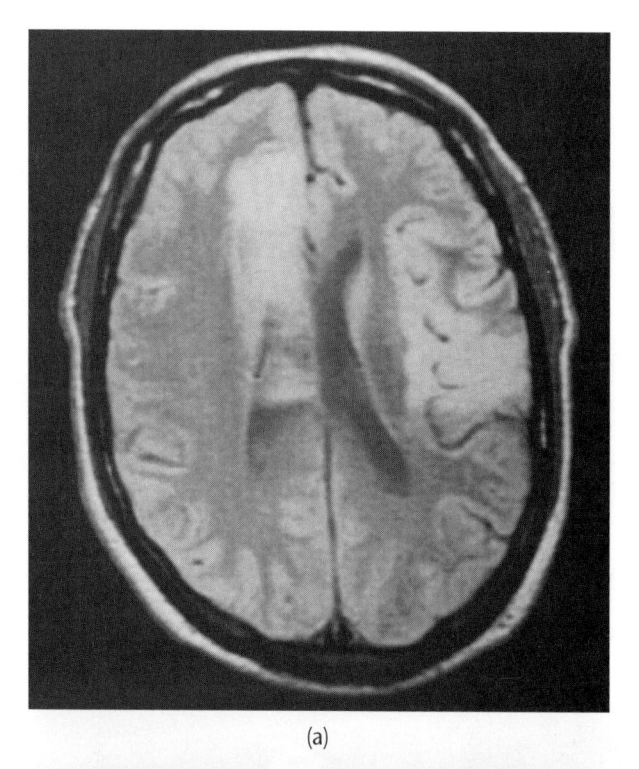

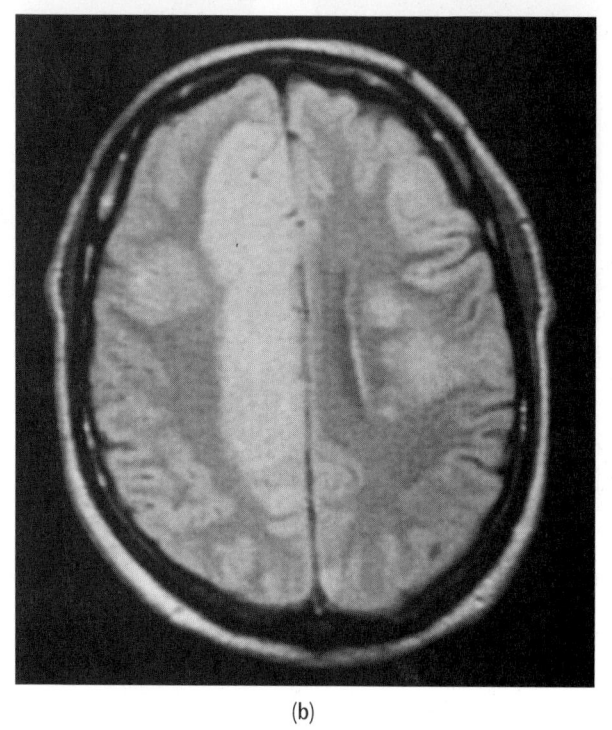

Figure 6.4 Cranial MRI: axial proton density images (a),(b). Right anterior and bilateral middle cerebral artery territory

be normal although, in the presence of hemiparesis, a normal scan is a valuable diagnostic clue.

The cessation of oxidative metabolism in infarction leads to cytotoxic oedema due to the accumulation of intracellular sodium and potassium. This affects grey matter, the site of cell bodies, and which is more active metabolically than white matter in the adult.

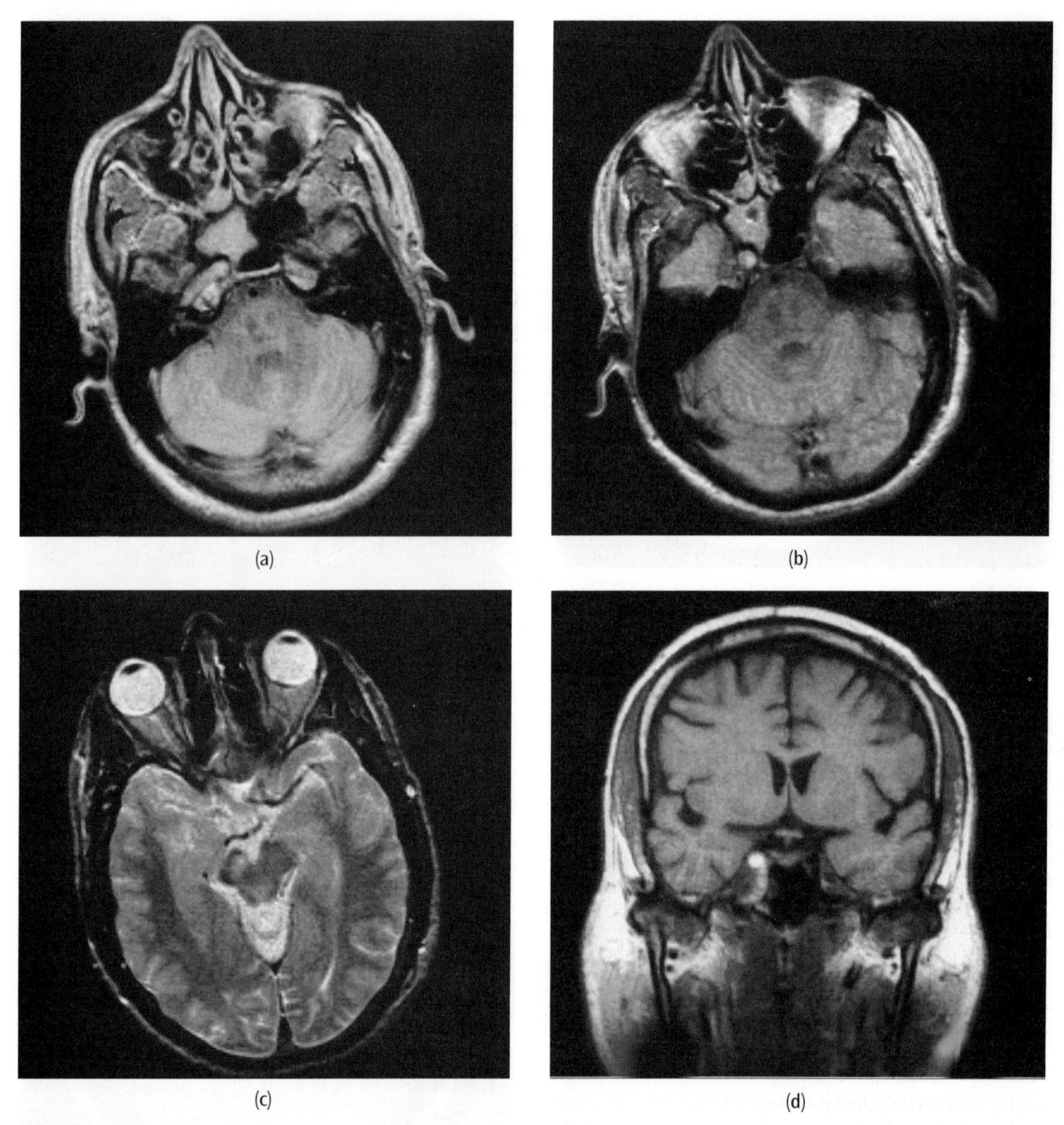

Figure 6.5 Cranial MRI: (a), (b) proton density; (c) T2-weighted axial images; (d) T1-weighted coronal image. Longstanding occlusion of the right internal carotid artery. The right carotid artery shows central high signal (a),(b),(d) on T1WI and lack of normal flow void on T2WI (c). Note the Wallerian degeneration of the right cerebral peduncle. There is incidental sphenoidal sinus inflammatory disease.

Cytotoxic oedema is manifest on CT initially as mass effect (Fig. 6.3). The grey matter then decreases in density with loss of definition of the grey–white matter boundary. Both these features may be subtle in early stages and indeed, mass effect may be absent or minimal even in large cerebral infarcts. This can be a useful distinction between infarct and tumour.

In early cerebral infarction MRI is more sensitive than CT.[6,7] The proton density increases and there is lengthening of both T1 and T2 relaxation times. Parenchymal change is well shown on proton density images (Fig. 6.4), mass effect is shown on T1-weighted images (T1WI). As with CT, mass effect precedes signal change that may not be apparent until several hours following the ictus on conventional MRI. Diffusion imaging demonstrates parenchymal change very early in infarction, although this is largely a research tool.

It may be possible to identify an absence of flow void in occluded arteries (Fig. 6.5). The CT corollary of this is the well described but infrequently observed hyperdense middle cerebral artery due to thrombosis which is evident on uncontrasted scans (Fig. 6.6). This is a reliable sign and predicts a large infarct.[8]

Gadolinium enhancement may be helpful in MRI in

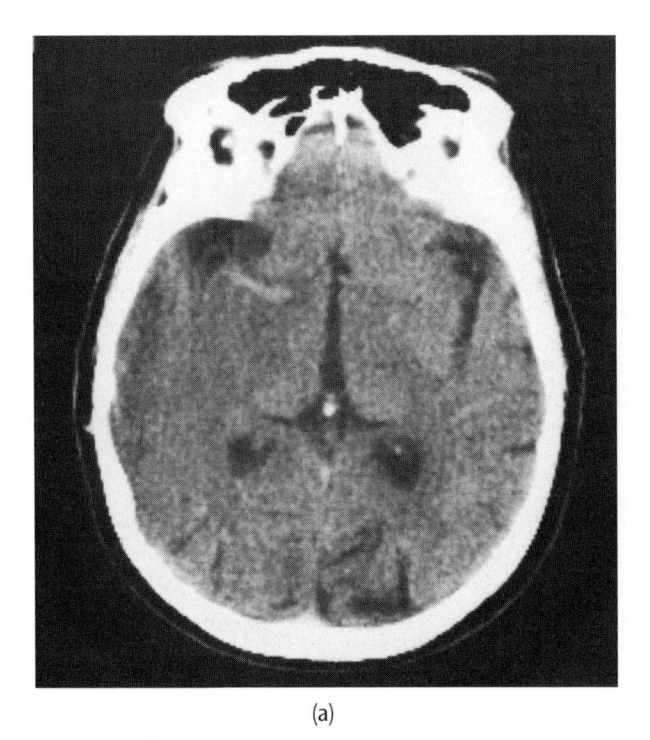

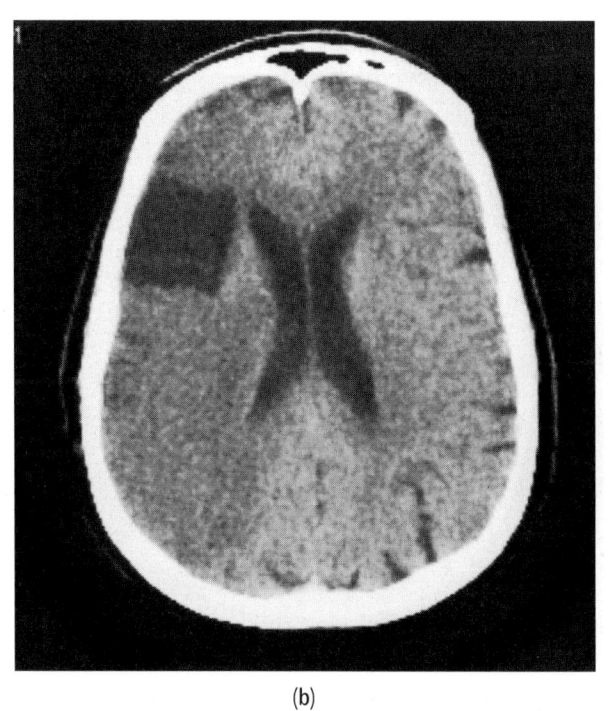

Figure 6.6 Cranial CT without contrast. Hyperdense middle cerebral artery. There has been a recent right hemisphere infarction superimposed on a smaller established infarct.

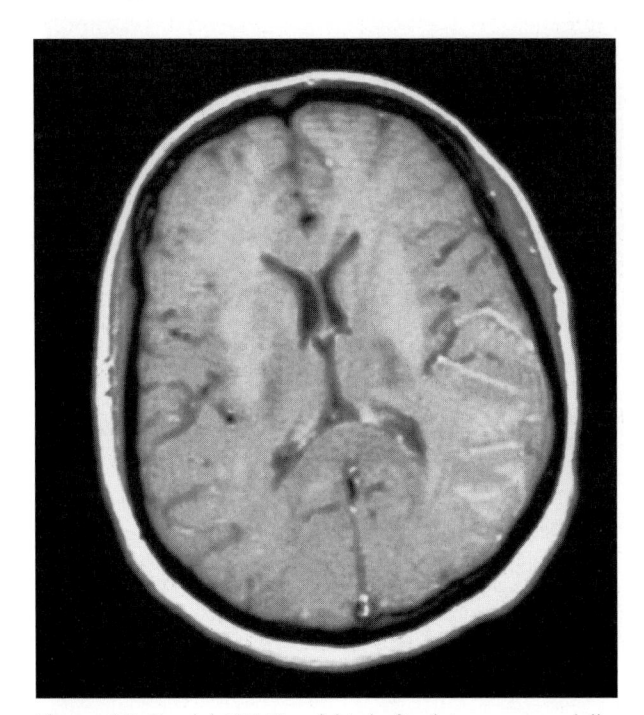

Figure 6.7 Cranial MRI T1-weighted after intravenous gadolinium DTPA. Early enhancement in infarction.

early infarction to show slow flow in affected arteries which may extend to small arteries within cerebral parenchyma (Fig. 6.7). A second type of early MRI contrast-enhancement is meningeal enhancement due to engorgement of meningeal collaterals.[9]

Vascular abnormalities are the earliest changes on MRI in early cerebral infarction, whereas with CT (albeit rather later) it is mass effect.

Within a few hours of arterial occlusion, the endothelial lining of capillaries forming the blood–brain barrier is damaged; however, for this to cause vasogenic oedema there must be perfusion pressure generated either by collateral supply or restoration of flow through the obstructed artery. Vasogenic oedema is therefore seen rather later than cytotoxic oedema but the effects of the two combine to give the typical attenuation or signal change seen in infarction.

Blood–brain barrier breakdown results in parenchymal enhancement seen following intravenous contrast administration in both CT and MRI, though of course more sensitively in the latter (Figs 6.8, 6.9, 6.17). This occurs later than the two types of early enhancement seen with MRI, during the 2nd week following the stroke.[7] It rarely occurs in the first 7 days and it is rare after the 3rd week. Early parenchymal enhancement on MRI is seen in reversible cerebral ischaemia reflecting early reperfusion;[10] conversely the early enhancement seen in watershed infarction does not indicate a benign course.

It is reasonable to state that enhancement seen in relation to a non-haemorrhagic (supposed) infarct of more than 6 week's duration should alert the radiologist to an alternative diagnosis. Ring-enhancement around the site of haemorrhage from whatever cause is known to persist for many months in some cases.[11] It is likely that all infarcts enhance at some stage and variations in the quoted incidence of enhancement most likely reflect its transitory nature.

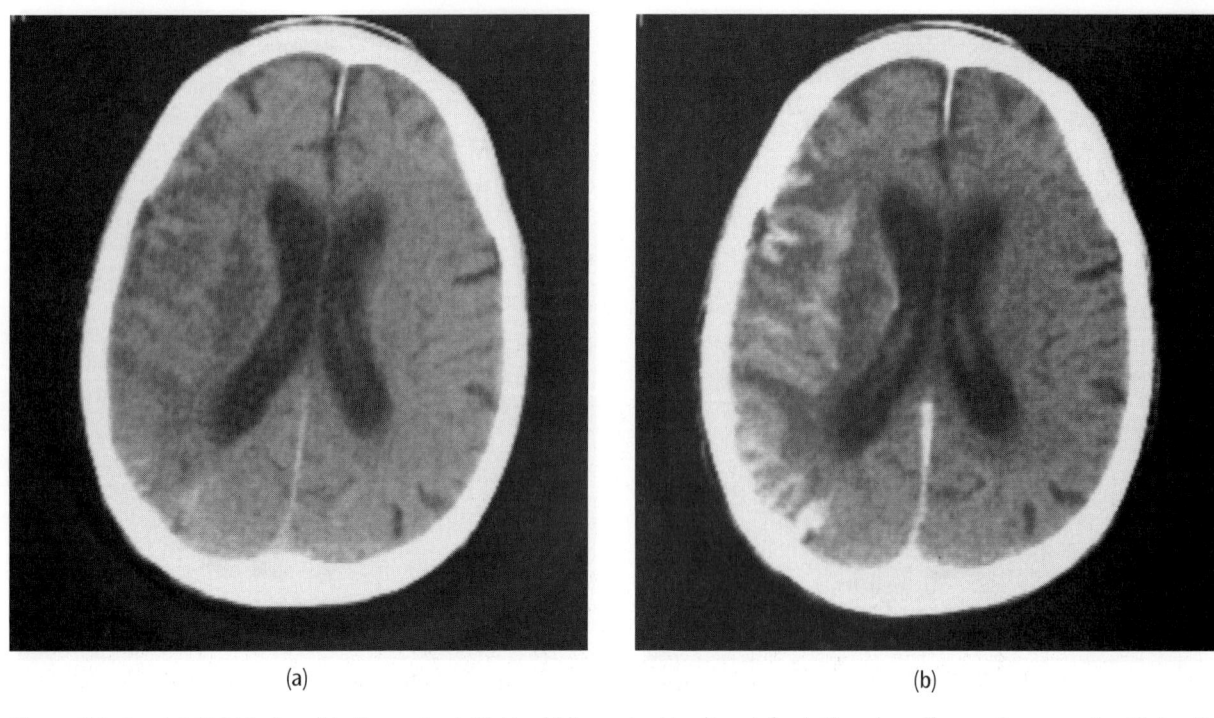

Figure 6.8 Cranial CT (a) before, (b) after contrast. Right middle cerebral territory infarct. There is gyriform enhancement outlining the right insula.

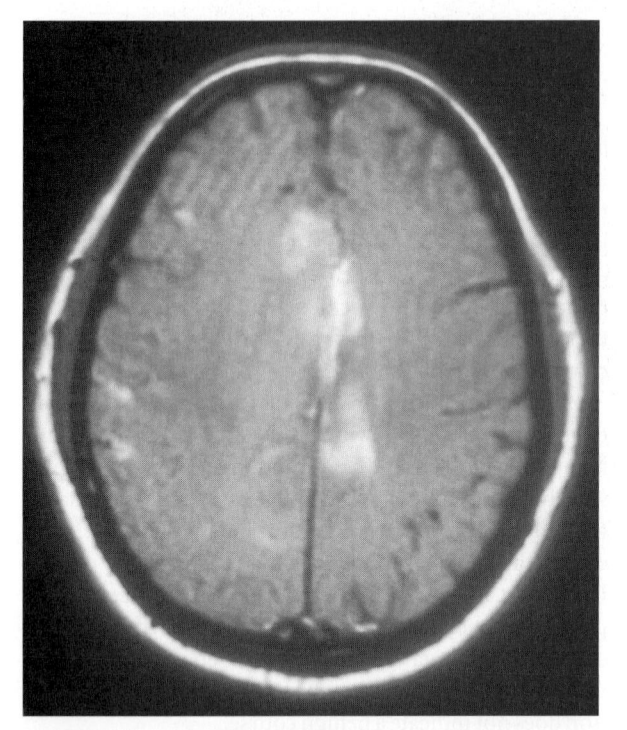

Figure 6.9 Cranial MRI: T1-weighted axial image after intravenous gadolinium DTPA. Enhancing embolic infarction of both anterior cerebral and the right middle cerebral artery territories.

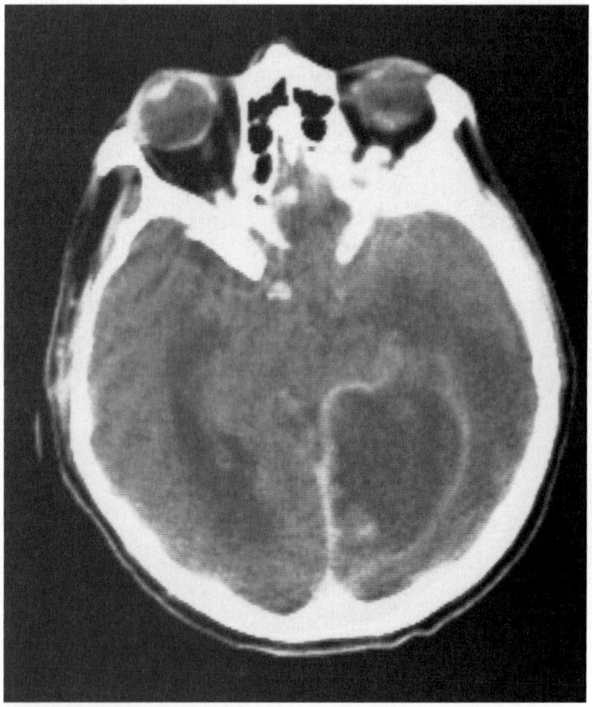

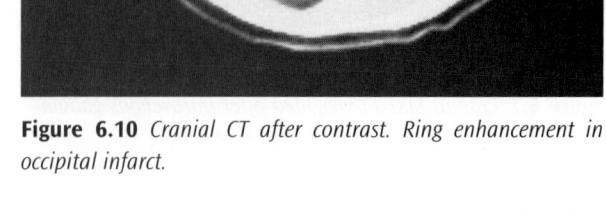

Figure 6.10 Cranial CT after contrast. Ring enhancement in occipital infarct.

The pattern of parenchymal contrast enhancement in cerebral infarction is variable. It may be patchy, gyriform, confluent or conform to a ring pattern (Fig. 6.10). Contrast-enhancement *per se* does not distinguish infarction from other pathologies. Some infarcts can resemble tumour or abscess very closely. Furthermore, administration of intravenous contrast for CT scanning in acute stroke is not usually necessary.

A retrospective study[12] indicated that the administration of iodinated intravenous contrast medium to

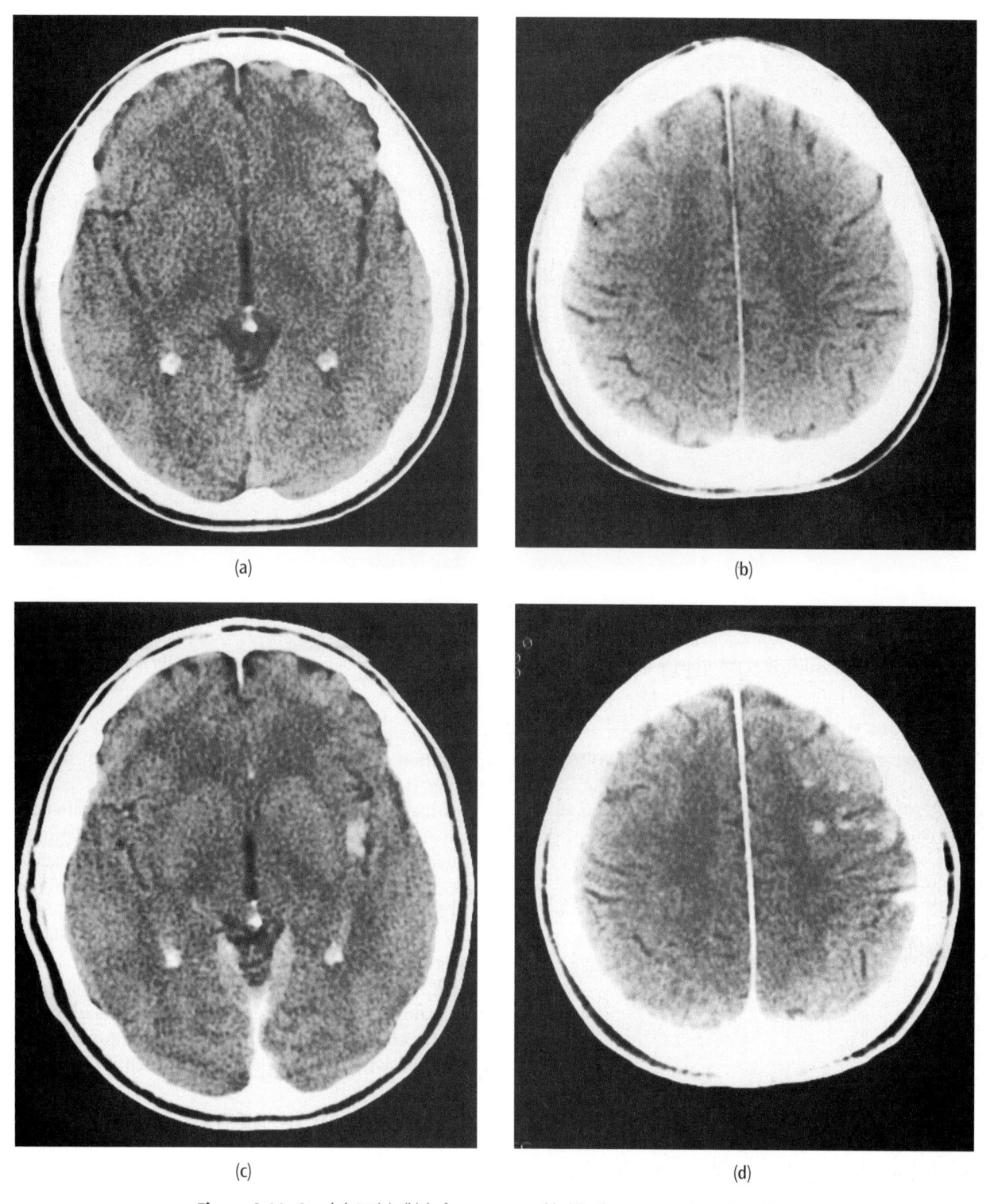

Figure 6.11 *Cranial CT (a), (b) before contrast; (c), (d) after contrast. Fogging effect.*

patients with cerebral infarction may have a detrimental effect on outcome. Although the study has been criticized and involved the use of the older ionic contrast agents, this work provides further reason to avoid contrast agents whenever possible in infarction. The author is unaware of a similar study with gadolinium when enhancement encountered in early infarction may prove helpful.

In perhaps the majority of cerebral infarcts, hypodensity on CT may diminish in the 2nd and 3rd weeks following stroke. This is known as the 'fogging effect' and may result in a normal unenhanced CT scan.[13] Only after intravenous contrast administration is an abnormality apparent (Fig. 6.11). The fogging effect is also found with MRI.[14] It is likely to be due to petechial haemorrhage within the infarct causing an

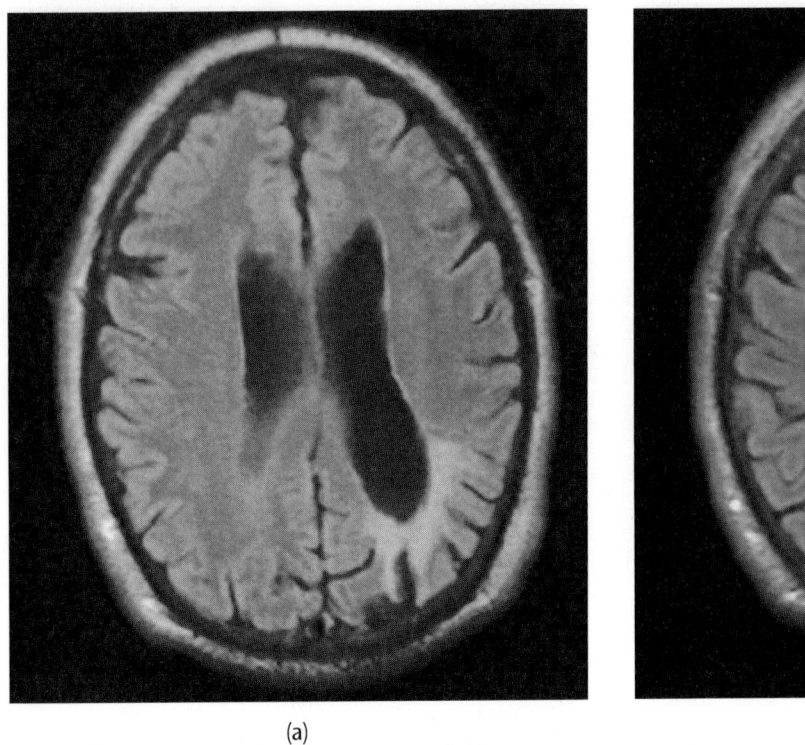

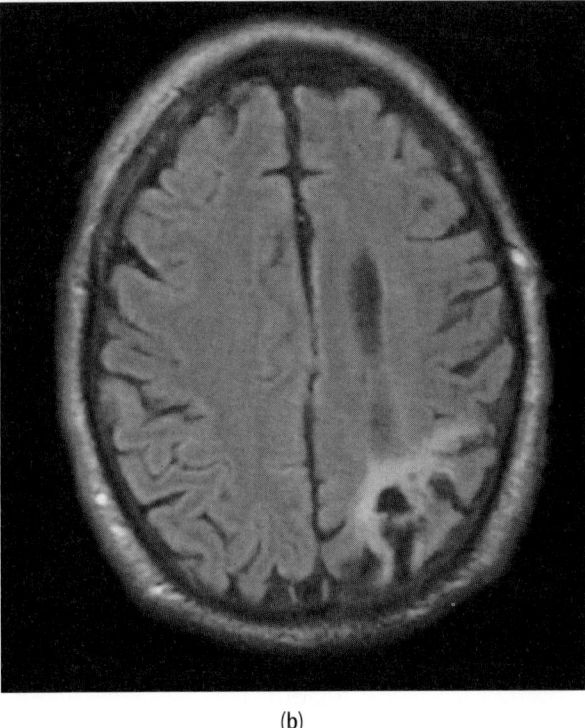

Figure 6.12 *Cranial MRI: FLAIR axial images (a), (b). Established posterior left middle cerebral artery territory infarct. Note the hyperintense gliosis and hypointense cystic change within this established infarct. There is also dilatation of the adjacent lateral ventricle.*

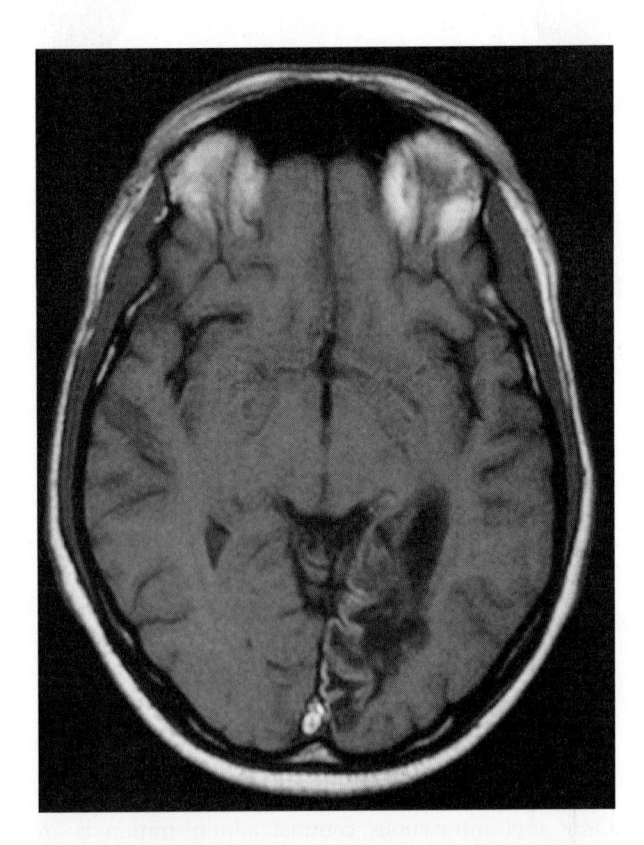

Figure 6.13 *Cranial MRI T1-weighted axial image. Established infarct showing the hyperintensity of laminar necrosis in an established left occipital infarct.*

alteration in attenuation or signal intensity to normal values (see below).

A mature infarct demonstrates parenchymal attenuation or signal change, loss of mass with local sulcal prominence and *ex vacuo* dilatation of the cerebral ventricular system adjacent to the infarct. There will be gliosis and cystic change (Fig. 6.12). On T1WI there may be gyral hyperintensity representing the accumulation of lipid-laden macrophages as part of laminar necrosis, (Fig. 6.13). A cortical infarct causing Wallerian degeneration of motor tracts 'downstream' can lead to atrophy particularly of the ipsilateral cerebral peduncle. Again, although well described, it is observed relatively infrequently (Fig. 6.5).

HAEMORRHAGIC INFARCTS

Haemorrhage has been shown by MRI to be relatively common in infarction (Fig. 6.14). As with the genesis of vasogenic oedema, perfusion is required to allow blood to leave the capillary bed which may come from cortical collateral vessels when there is gyral haemorrhage or alternatively from the restoration of flow in a previously occluded artery.[15]

A proportion of infarcts become frankly haemorrhagic on CT and there is compelling pathological evidence that these are due to initial embolic arterial occlusion which then disperses.[16] Haemorrhagic infarcts enhance following intravenous contrast medium in the usual manner (Fig. 6.15).

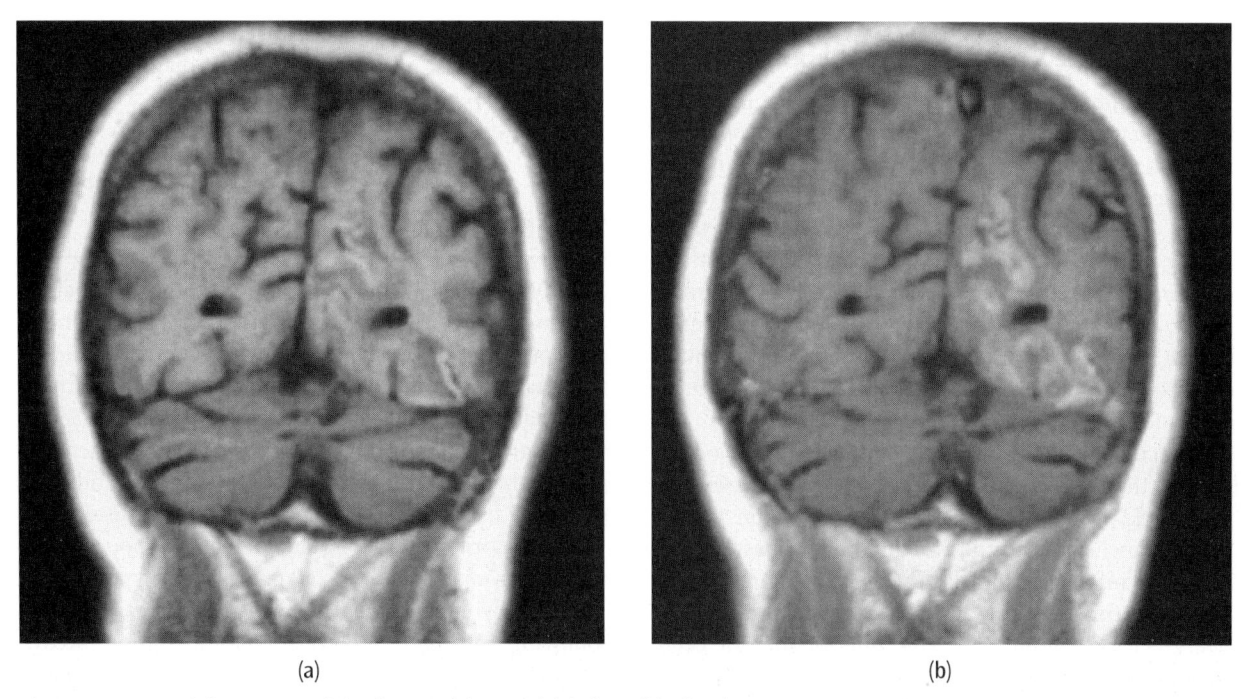

Figure 6.14 Cranial MRI: T1-weighted coronal images (a) before, (b) after intravenous gadolinium DTPA. Enhancing haemorrhagic infarct.

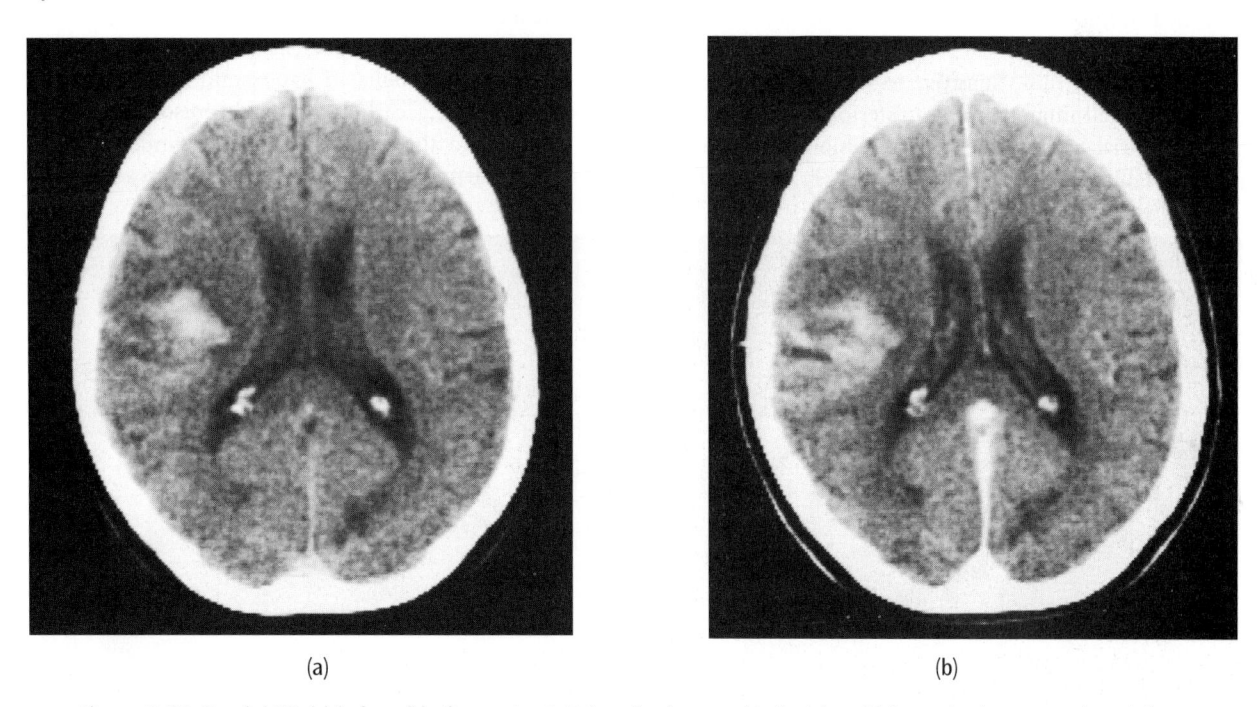

Figure 6.15 Cranial CT: (a) before, (b) after contrast. Enhancing haemorrhagic right middle cerebral artery territory infarct.

It is probable that petechial haemorrhage is part of the normal evolution of a cerebral infarct and should not of itself contraindicate anticoagulation. Larger haematomas are more problematic and the topic is a controversial one.

Infarction with substantial haemorrhage may resemble primary intracerebral haemorrhage or haemorrhagic contusion on CT and head injury may, of course, be a consequence of stroke of whatever cause. Haemorrhage as part of infarction is surrounded by more hypodensity than primary haemorrhage, which dissects through the normal brain.

Primary intracerebral haemorrhage is accompanied by only a thin rim of hypodensity and will be present on the initial scan. Haemorrhagic transformation of an infarct usually results in deterioration in a patient already suffering from stroke.

Haemorrhagic contusion does not respect boundaries of arterial territories and is often multifocal with a number of relatively small haematomas.

POSTERIOR CIRCULATION INFARCTION

It is frequently possible to ascribe infarction of the vertebrobasilar arterial system to the territory of a major arterial branch.[17] It is important to appreciate that this does not necessarily imply disease in that particular artery. There is frequent anatomical variation in the arterial supply to the posterior fossa and collateral circulations may limit the extent of the parenchymal involvement as in the carotid circulation. Even occlusion of the entire basilar artery may result in only a small infarct although catastrophic brainstem and cerebellar infarction usually results (Fig. 6.16).

Infarction of the brainstem may arise from occlusion of the numerous perforating arteries that extend posteriorly from the basilar artery. Occlusion of the larger branches may result in combined brainstem and cerebellar infarction and most cerebellar infarcts occur in the territory of the posterior inferior cerebellar artery (Fig. 6.17). Superior and anterior inferior cerebellar artery territory infarctions are progressively rarer (Fig. 6.18).

Massive cerebellar infarction can result in obstructive hydrocephalus, and ventricular drainage may be required (Fig. 6.19).

MRI is much more sensitive to the identification of the often small infarcts in the posterior fossa. As in the supratentorial compartment, large lesions conforming to a vascular territory can be reliably ascribed to infarction. Accompanying major vessel occlusion may, of course, assist in establishing the diagnosis. Small lesions may need analysing using the criteria for lacunes (see below).

WATERSHED INFARCTION

The hypoxic–ischaemic syndrome results in infarction affecting the so-called 'watershed' regions at the boundaries of the major vascular territories of both the supratentorial and infratentorial compartments. Unless there is unilateral carotid arterial stenosis these ischaemic lesions are bilaterally symmetrical (Fig. 6.20). Watershed infarction in the centrum semiovale may be indistinguishable from intrinsic cerebral small vessel disease.

The majority of cases are due to global hypoperfusion resulting from circulatory arrest or profound hypotension.

The early enhancement seen in watershed infarction following intravenous contrast administration occurs since there is no abrupt cessation of perfusion. Unlike cases of reversible ischaemia due to thromboembolism, the early enhancement of watershed infarcts does not indicate a benign course.

The symmetrical hypodensity seen on CT which affects the basal ganglia in hypoxaemic states without hypoperfusion (e.g. carbon monoxide poisoning) is simply a variant of the hypoxic–ischaemic syndrome. The changes result from the failure to deliver oxygen to the

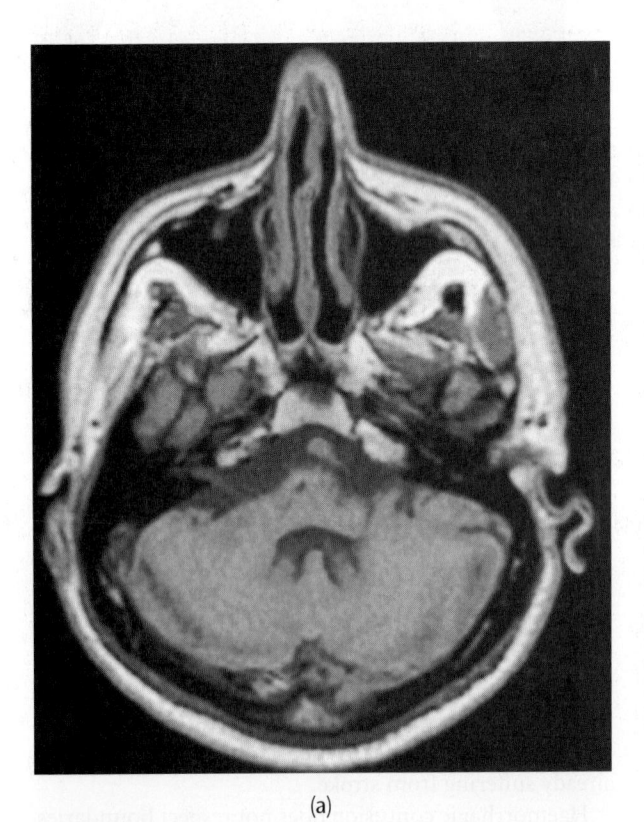

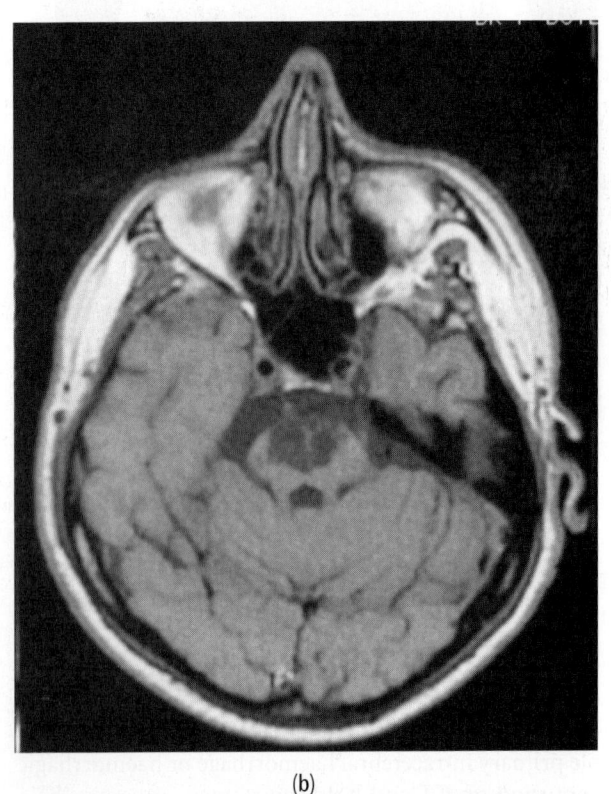

(a) (b)

Figure 6.16 *Cranial MRI: T1-weighted axial images. Basilar artery occlusion – brainstem infarction. Note the absence of signal void within the basilar artery.*

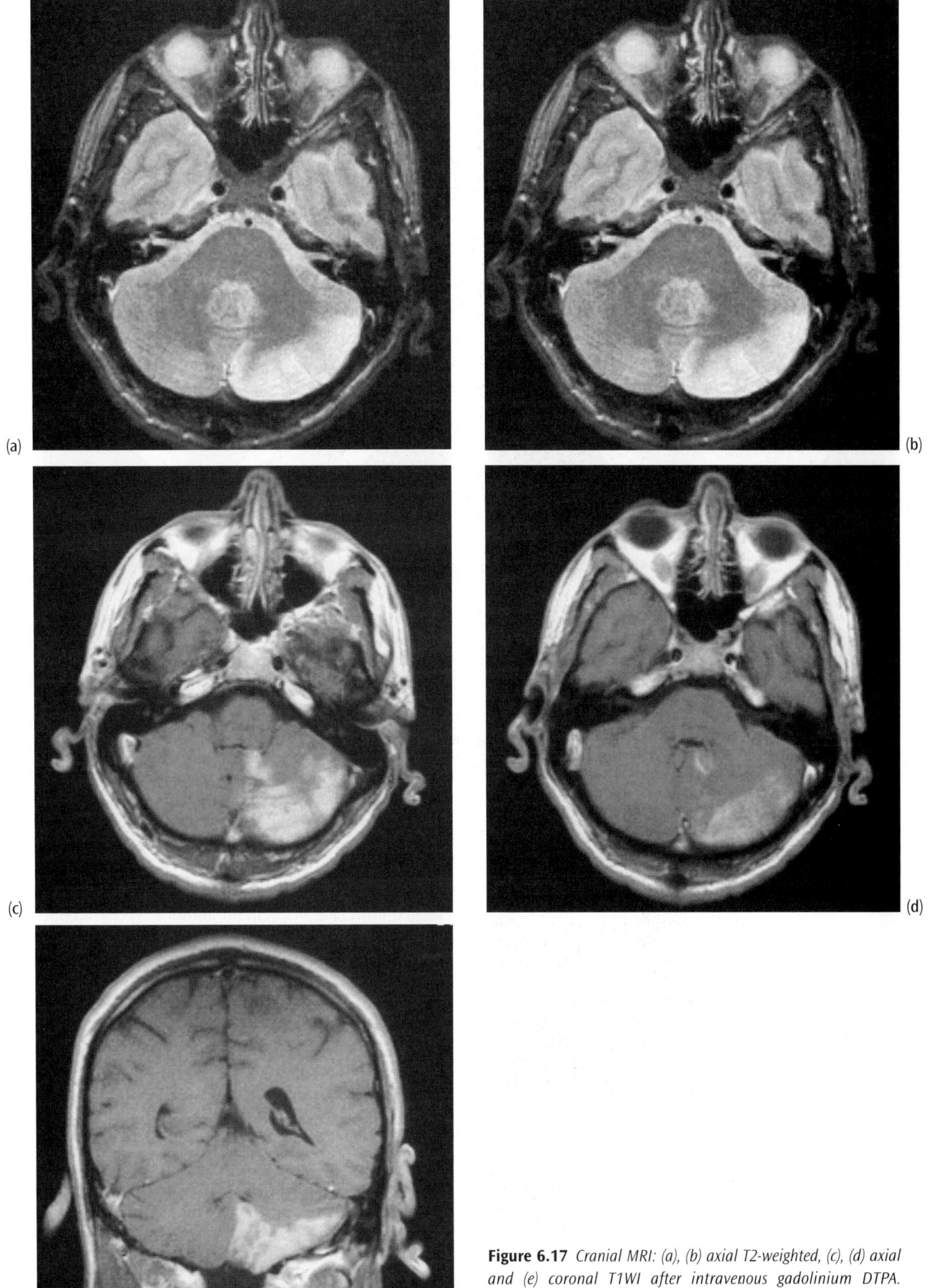

Figure 6.17 Cranial MRI: (a), (b) axial T2-weighted, (c), (d) axial and (e) coronal T1WI after intravenous gadolinium DTPA. Infarction in the territory of the posterior inferior cerebellar artery.

(a)

(b)

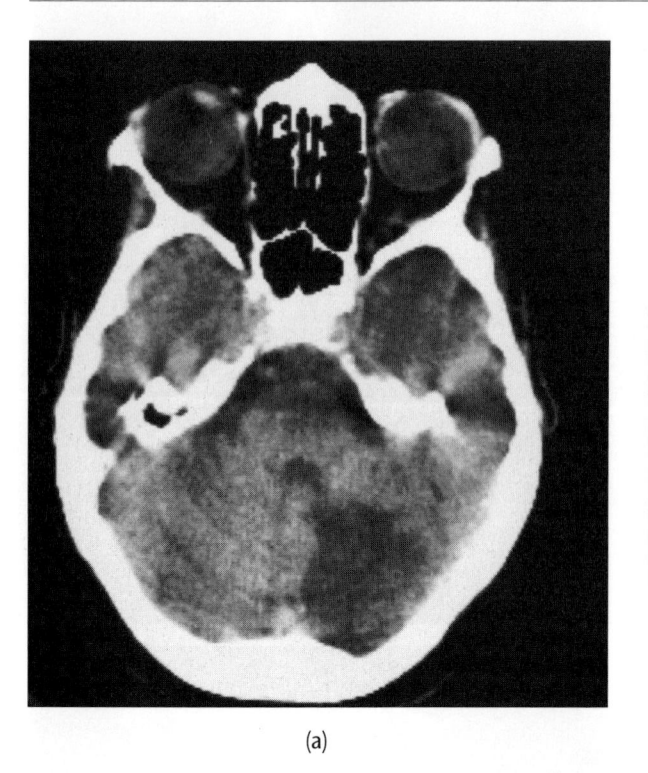

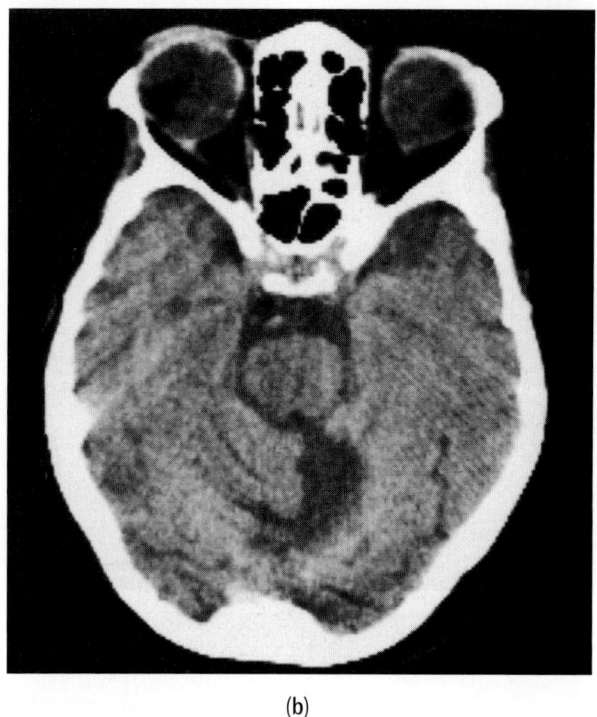

Figure 6.18 *Cranial CT. Left superior cerebellar artery territory infarction.*

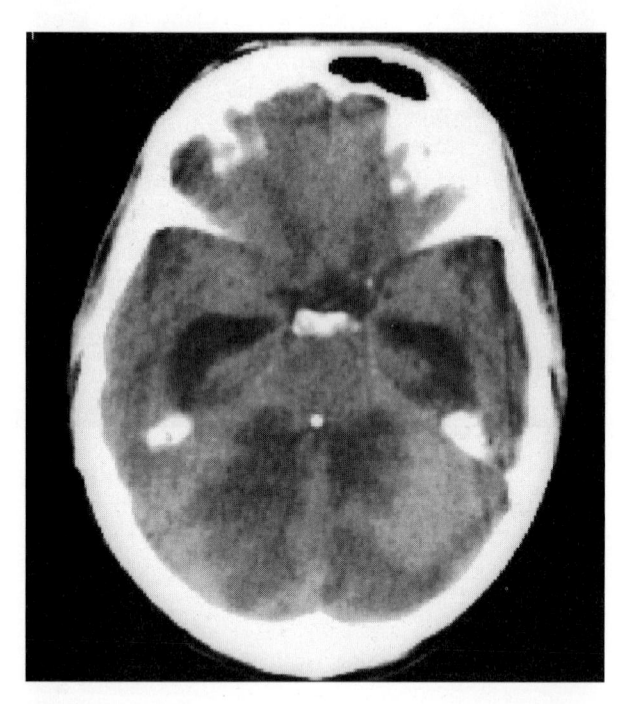

Figure 6.19 *Cranial CT. Large cerebellar infarction with hydrocephalus. The central hyperdensity in the region of the aqueduct is a shunt.*

parenchyma, whether due to a failure of perfusion or oxygenation (Fig. 6.21).

In the hypoxic-ischaemic syndrome MRI has shown evidence of widespread cortical laminar necrosis with gyral haemorrhage and cortical enhancement that may accompany the basal ganglia lesions which will themselves enhance.[18]

LACUNAR INFARCTS

Lacunes are small, deep hemispheric infarcts, defined by Fisher[19] as being between 0.5 and 15mm in diameter, and are said to result from occlusion of small perforating arteries. They are associated with systemic hypertension and diabetes and despite assertions to the contrary, they can be related to extracranial carotid artery disease.[20]

Lacunes may be found within the internal or external capsules, the corona radiata, thalamus and in the basal ganglia (Fig. 6.22). On MRI, which shows many more lacunes than are visible on CT, these appear rather irregular in outline (Fig. 6.23). In the author's experience only very few of the lesions identified as lacunes on CT prove to be sites of previous haemorrhage when studied with MRI. The appearances result therefore from a primary ischaemic process.

Lacunes may evolve in a similar manner to larger infarcts and may show contrast-enhancement. Because of their small size, however, it may not be possible to decide whether a lacune is recent or longstanding.

The normal corticospinal tracts within the internal capsule should not be confused with lacunes (Fig. 6.24). These are seen on MRI in about 50% of normal individuals. They are rounded foci of hyperintensity on T2WI and hypointensity on T1WI, near to the genu.[21]

Lacunar infarcts should also be distinguished from the perivascular (Virchow–Robin) spaces. These become prominent in cerebral atrophy but sometimes also in normal individuals. They are found in relation to the anterior commissure and high in the centrum ovale near

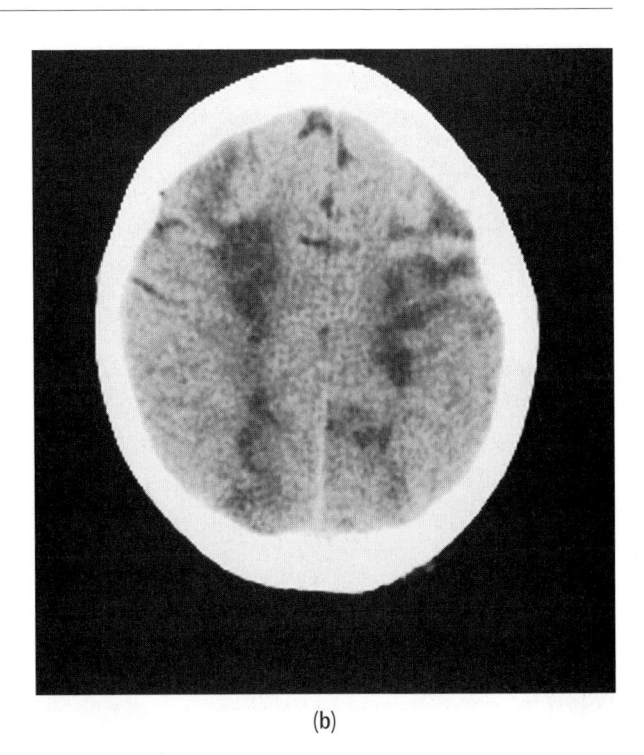

Figure 6.20 *Cranial CT (a), (b). Watershed infarction.*

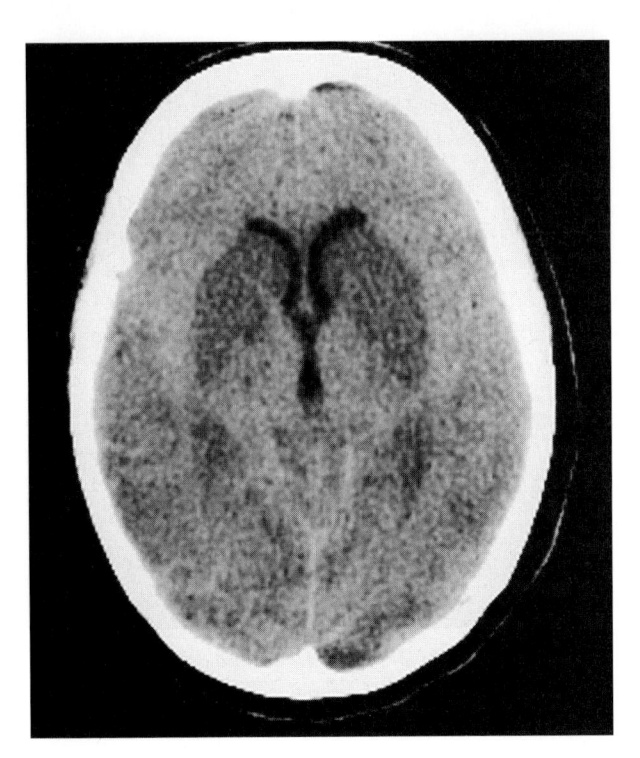

Figure 6.21 *Cranial CT. Global hypoperfusion with bilateral basal ganglial hypodensity.*

to the vertex. Although not in direct continuity with the subarachnoid space, the signal return from the perivascular space is that of cerebrospinal fluid. They are smaller and more rounded than the majority of ischaemic lesions and can also be identified as radial streaks traversing the periventricular white matter on T2-weighted scans (Fig. 6.25).

White matter is less well perfused than grey matter in the adult and generalized intrinsic vascular disease may lead to chronic subcortical ischaemic encephalopathy (or Binswanger disease) (Fig. 6.26). In this condition there is generalized cerebral atrophy and widespread confluent white matter hypodensity. Lacunes may coexist. Sulcal prominence and the absence of temporal horn dilatation in atrophy help to distinguish it from obstructive hydrocephalus. There is also a sharp margin around the periphery of the white matter hypodensity which is not found in that which results from transependymal egress of cerebrospinal fluid in severe hydrocephalus.

Both demyelination and small vessel ischaemic change can lead to similar appearances on MRI. Cerebral atrophy and diffuse, confluent white matter change, is common to the advanced stages of both conditions. Discrete ischaemic lesions tend to be irregular in size and shape and the basal ganglia are involved.

The lesions seen in demyelination are often ovoid with their long axis in a radial distribution due to their perivenous location. This appearance is very well shown on sagittal images in which the lesions of the corpus callosum may also be shown. Indeed, in demyelination atrophy of the corpus callosum may be found disproportionate to atrophy elsewhere. The corpus callosum can also atrophy in isolation. The distinction may not always be straightforward; for instance, infarcts can occur in the corpus callosum and the two conditions may co-exist in the older age-groups.

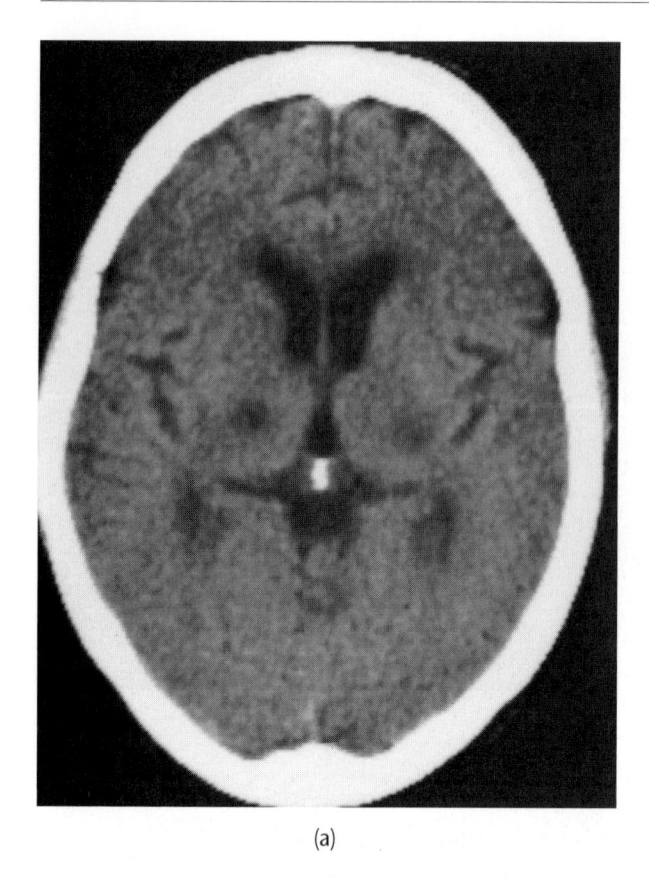

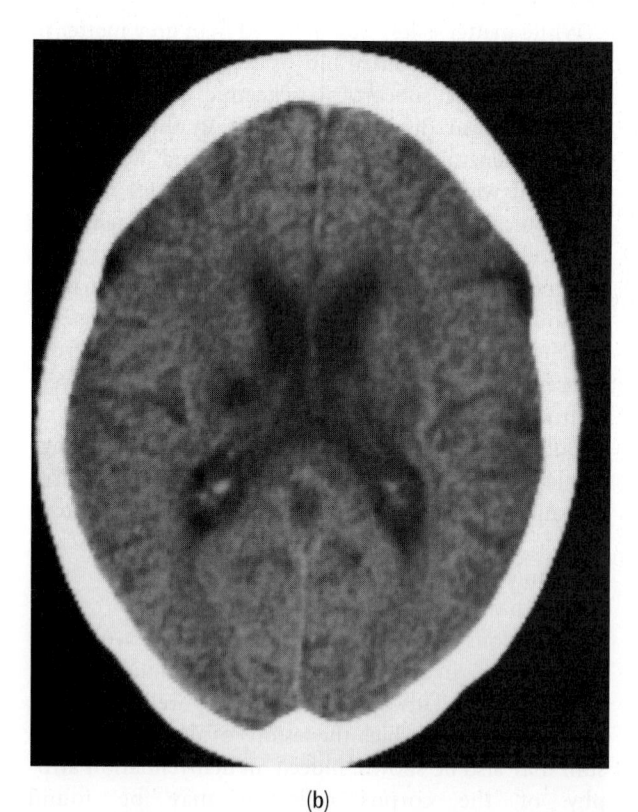

Figure 6.22 Cranial CT. Lacunar infarction. Note the extension into the corona radiata on each side. The normal corticospinal tracts are not identified with clarity on CT in the normal individual, nor can they be traced even with MR into the corona radiata.

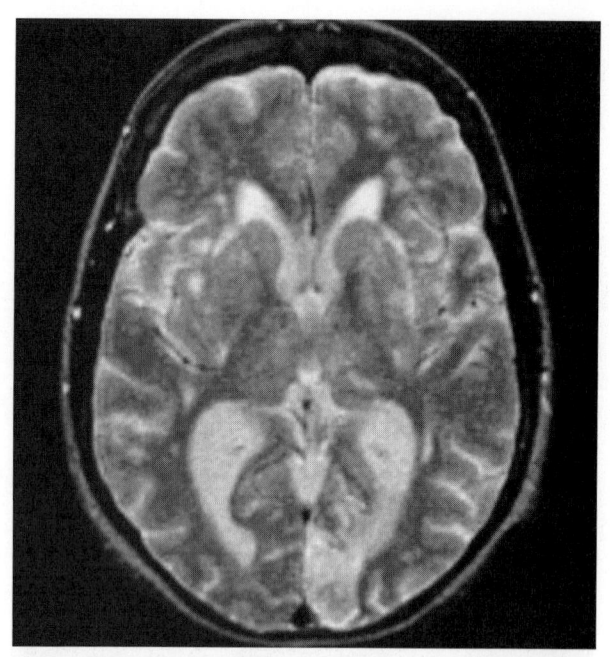

Figure 6.23 Cranial MRI: T2-weighted axial image. Multiple lacunes involving the subinsular and basal ganglial regions. There is also a left occipital infarct.

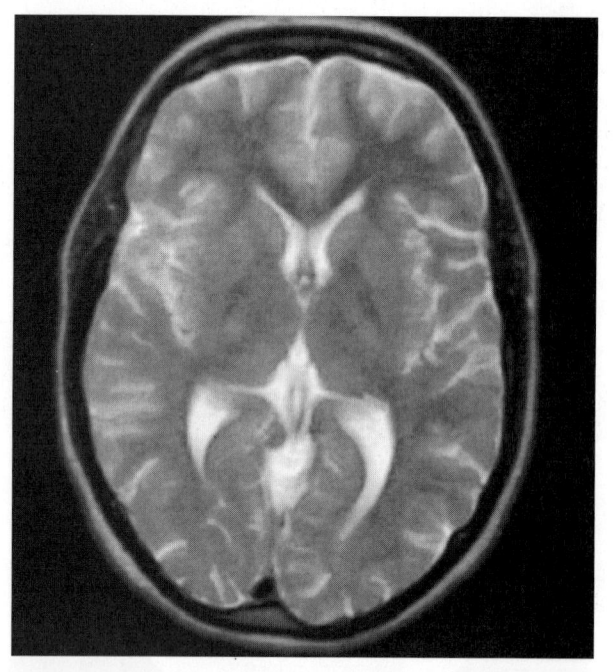

Figure 6.24 Cranial MRI: T2-weighted axial image. Normal corticospinal tracts.

MAGNETIC RESONANCE ANGIOGRAPHY

Two different methods of magnetic resonance angiography (MRA) are commonly employed, namely time-of-flight and phase-contrast.[22]

Flow-related enhancement or the entry slice phenomenon is the basis for time-of-flight MRA.[23] Flowing, unsaturated protons (spins), which are fully magnetized, enter

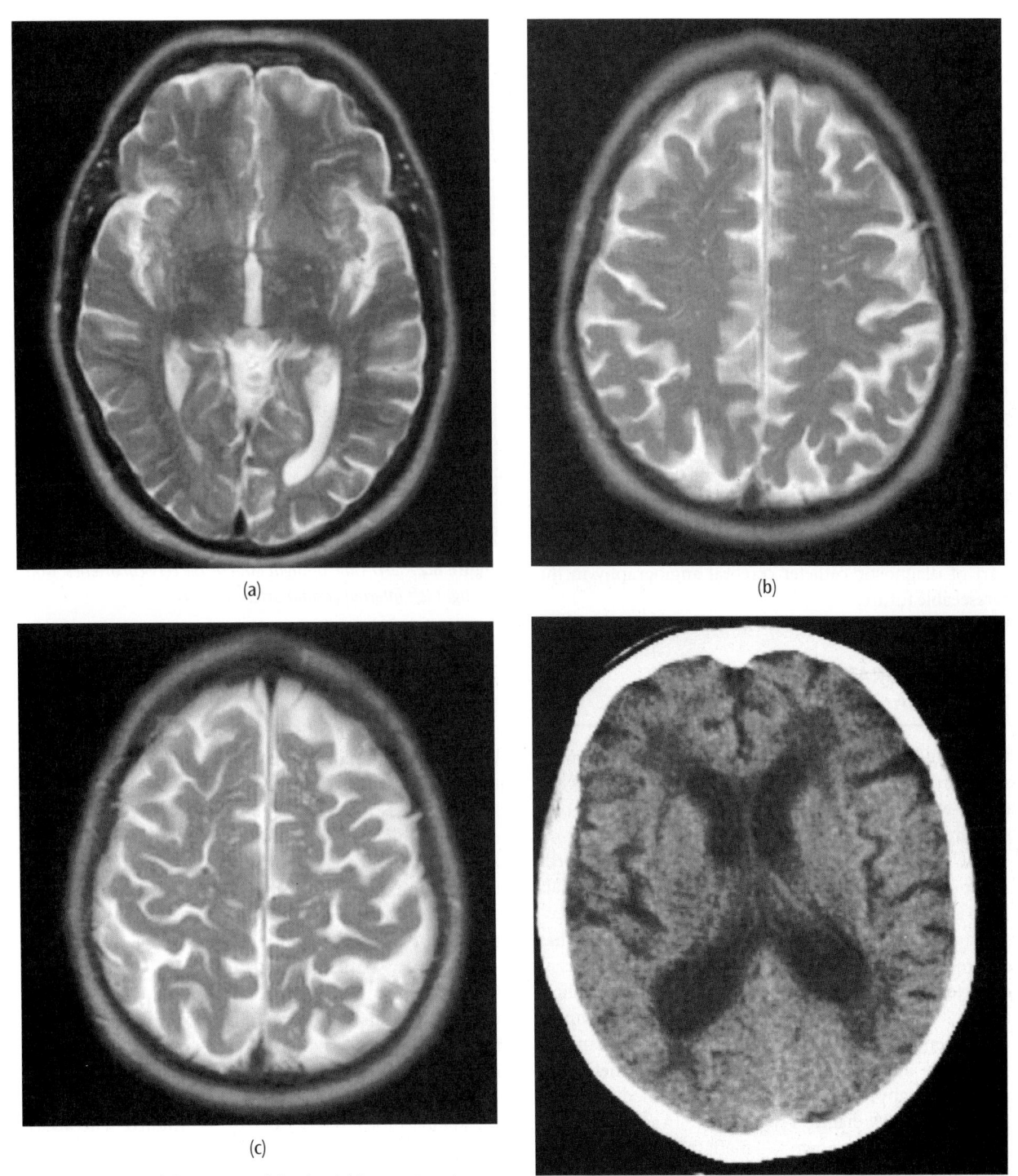

Figure 6.25 *Cranial MRI: T2-weighted axial image. Prominence of the Virchow–Robin spaces.*

Figure 6.26 *Cranial CT. Binswanger disease. There is cerebral atrophy and symmetrical white matter hypodensity.*

an imaging volume and when stimulated return a strong signal and appear bright. Stationary spins in the same volume are stimulated rapidly and repeatedly so that they become saturated and their signal is suppressed.

Spins entering the imaging volume from any direction will appear bright. By placing a saturation band, protons arriving from that direction will become saturated and therefore give no signal. In this way arterial and venous flow can be separated.

Phase-contrast MRA is less often performed but the signal suppression of the background is excellent. In this method appropriate magnetic fields are used so that a phase shift is proportional to velocity and thus flow within certain limited velocity parameters can be studied.

Both time-of-flight and phase-contrast MRA can be undertaken using two- and three-dimensional (2-D, 3-D) techniques. In 2-D MRA, individual slices are excited. In 3-D a volume or slab of tissue is excited simultaneously.

The background suppression of 2-D time-of-flight MRA is superior to that of 3-D time-of-flight. If flow is too slow, protons leaving the imaging volume will become saturated with resultant signal loss. This signal 'drop-out' is more marked with 3-D than 2-D time-of-flight MRA and therefore 3-D time of flight is better for angiography of arteries in which blood flow is high. Magnetic resonance angiography of the cerebral venous system is best accomplished using 2-D time-of-flight MRA. There are nevertheless advantages to 3-D time-of-flight MRA. Its resolution is superior and it is less sensitive to turbulence.

Cervical arterial stenoses investigated using 2-D time-of-flight MRA methods are likely to be overestimated because of sensitivity to turbulence with in-plane saturation leading to signal loss. Nevertheless 2-D time-of-flight is the usual technique used for cervical arteries (Fig. 6.27). The use of intravenous gadolinium administered prior to time-of-flight acquisition largely overcomes the problem of flow-related artefacts encountered in time-of-flight MRA.

At the moment MRA is undergoing continuous refinement and improvement and should replace a substantial part of diagnostic catheter cerebral angiography in the foreseeable future.

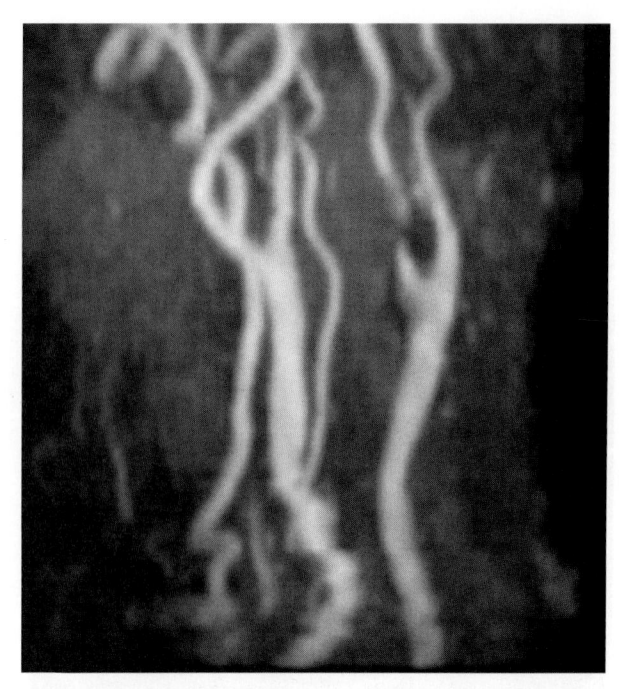

Figure 6.27 *2-D Time-of-flight MRA of the cervical arteries. Note the tight left internal carotid artery stenosis.*

IMAGING STRATEGIES IN CEREBRAL ISCHAEMIA

Following a transient ischaemic attack CT and MRI should be normal. In particular, MRI may show evidence of pre-existing cerebral ischaemic change or, very occasionally, reveal non-vascular pathology.[24]

The interim results of both the European and North American symptomatic carotid endarterectomy trials (ECST and NASCET respectively) have given new direction to imaging in cerebral ischaemia. Using somewhat different methodologies both trials have indicated that endarterectomy results in a better outcome than medical therapy when the carotid artery supplying the symptomatic hemisphere shows a greater than 70% diameter stenosis at angiography. Surgery confers no benefit over medical therapy in the two other groups studied (less than 30% and 30–70% diameter stenoses).[25,26] In asymptomatic groups, surgery was shown to benefit those with a greater than 60% stenosis.[27] Although carotid arterial stenosis is one of several risk factors in stroke, it is potentially treatable and is the factor of most relevance to radiologists.

Catheter angiography has long been regarded as the gold standard for the quantification of arterial stenosis and was employed by both ECET and NASCET. The NASCET triallists pointed out that if the stroke risk from imaging exceeded 1% then this would cancel any benefits of surgery. It is known that patients with arterial degenerative disease are especially prone to morbidity arising from angiography. Surprisingly even arch aortography has not been shown to be safer than selective cerebral arteriography. It is important therefore that the risks of imaging do not outweigh the benefits of treatment and that the radiologist does not become the major risk factor in stroke.

The results obtained and the varying methodologies in both the symptomatic and asymptomatic groups challenge the status of selective angiography as a gold standard. It is known that estimates of stenosis vary between observers even with high quality studies.[28] These are all powerful arguments in favour of non-invasive angiography. From the variations in stenosis assessment, it may also be the case that *all haemodynamically significant* stenoses (i.e. greater than 50% diameter) would benefit from surgery.

Since many patients will require imaging, a screening test is necessary. Duplex carotid ultrasound, ideally with colour, has assumed this role. It is safe and quick to perform. It provides visual information on arterial narrowing and, through Doppler measurements, the identification of any haemodynamic effects of the stenosis. Plaque morphology can also be studied. The accuracy of the examination depends greatly on the skill of the operator and scanning units should validate their results with angiography in the early stages.[29] Haemodynamic disturbance causing increased velocity occurs at greater than 50% diameter stenosis. Below this, one is largely reliant upon measurements from the B-mode images but at the very least high-grade stenoses suitable for surgery should be identified.

Intravenous digital subtraction angiography is not widely used now in the investigation of cerebral ischaemia. It enjoyed popularity in the early to mid 1980s but, although safe and minimally invasive, there are inherent problems of spatial resolution. A poor cardiac output will lead to an inferior study and many patients have combined coronary and cerebral arterial degenerative disease.

Magnetic resonance angiography (MRA) and, perhaps also CT angiography, must be exploited in the imaging of cerebral ischaemia. MRA is safe and either non-invasive or minimally-invasive, depending on whether gadolinium is used. CT angiography unequivocally requires intravenous contrast-medium, which may preclude its use in those at risk of an allergic reaction and in those with renal impairment. Image manipulation with CT is time-consuming but plaque calcification can be identified and the accuracy of CT angiography compares favourably with other techniques.[30] MRA is quicker but more importantly it has been shown that MRA and ultrasound together are more accurate than either alone.[31] The two are therefore complementary. Both MRA and duplex sonography may not distinguish reliably between arterial occlusion and near-occlusion, which may necessitate catheter angiography. In whatever combination, the use of non-invasive methods, at least in the first instance, should be encouraged.[28]

CRANIOCERVICAL ARTERIAL DISSECTION

Arterial dissection is an increasingly recognized cause of cerebral ischaemia particularly in young adults. It can also be responsible for subarachnoid haemorrhage. Although previously described as 'spontaneous', the majority is associated with some form of, often minor, trauma. The association of cervical pain, neurological deficit and trauma should suggest the diagnosis which may involve both intra- and extracranial portions of the carotid and vertebral arteries. A proportion of cases demonstrate underlying fibromuscular hyperplasia in which case more than one artery may undergo dissection.[32]

Angiographically, dissection is shown as a subtle irregularity of the luminal contour, occlusion or pseudo-occlusion and aneurysm formation. With time, unless there is total vessel occlusion, the angiogram can return to normal.

If sought carefully, evidence of cervical arterial dissection can be found on MRI and, less obviously on CT. Axial MRI scans of the brain are usually acquired beginning at a more caudal location than CT. On scans through the skull base the dissected vessel may be seen as a signal void surrounded by thrombus which is hyperintense on dual echo sequences (Fig. 6.28). On intravenous contrast enhanced CT, the enhanced blood within the patent lumen is surrounded by hypodense thrombus. The parenchymal change is that of infarction (Fig. 6.29).

CEREBRAL ARTERIAL ECTASIA

Degenerative disease can lead to arterial dilatation and tortuosity of the cerebral arteries associated with mural calcification. The vertebrobasilar system is more frequently involved than the carotid arteries and can be sufficient to cause brainstem compression and even hydrocephalus.

Figure 6.28 *Cranial MRI: axial proton density image. Dissection of the right internal carotid artery. Note the hyperintense thrombus surrounding the signal void of the patent lumen (arrow).*

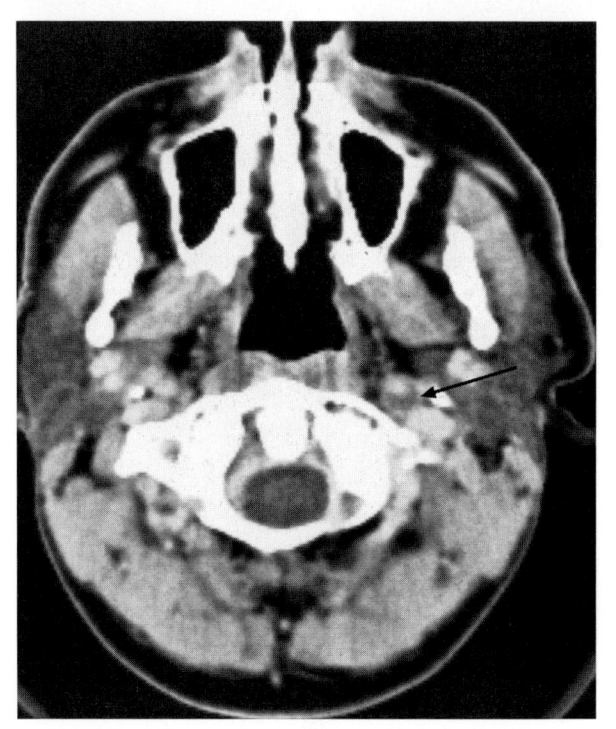

Figure 6.29 *Cranial CT after contrast. Dissection of the left internal carotid artery. Note the hypodense crescentic thrombus posterior to the enhancing lumen (arrow).*

Ectasia is also associated with rare conditions such as pseudoxanthoma elasticum and Ehlers–Danlos syndrome.

On CT, degenerative vertebrobasilar ectasia is shown as enlarged calcified arteries anterior and sometimes lateral to the brainstem (Fig. 6.30). Although there may be mural thrombus, flow-related effects may lead to regions of luminal hyperintensity on MRI in the absence of occlusion.

CEREBAL VASCULITIS AND OTHER ANGIOPATHIES

Many conditions are associated with cerebral vasculitis. Unfortunately the changes seen on CT and MRI may be identical to those of 'small vessel' ischaemia already described and even those appearances may not be distinguishable from inflammatory causes such as demyelination.

Moyamoya disease

Moyamoya disease is an obliterative angiopathy first described amongst the Japanese but it is not exclusive to that race. It is an angiographic diagnosis and consists of progressive narrowing and ultimately occlusion of the basal cerebral arteries. Interestingly the vertebrobasilar circulation is spared. Numerous collateral pathways open up and these may form an array of signal voids within the basal ganglia on MRI.[33] In the 'idiopathic' form, cerebral haemorrhage due to vessel fragility occurs in affected adults. Cerebral infarction is commoner in children.

Similar angiographic appearances are seen in association with sickle cell disease, basal meningiomas and arteriovenous malformations.

Systemic lupus erythematosus

Cerebral atrophy, small vessel ischaemic change, major territory infarction and venous sinus occlusion may be found in this condition.

Sickle cell disease

Neurological complications of sickle cell disease are usually encountered in the young. Cerebral atrophy may develop and there may be widespread white matter ischaemia. Affected individuals may develop an obliterative angiopathy conforming to a moyamoya pattern (Fig. 6.31). The administration of contrast agents, especially when hyperosmolar, to those with sickle cell disease should be undertaken with caution because of the risk of precipitating a crisis.

Drug abuse

Substance abuse can lead to neurological complications resulting from cerebral infarction or haemorrhage.

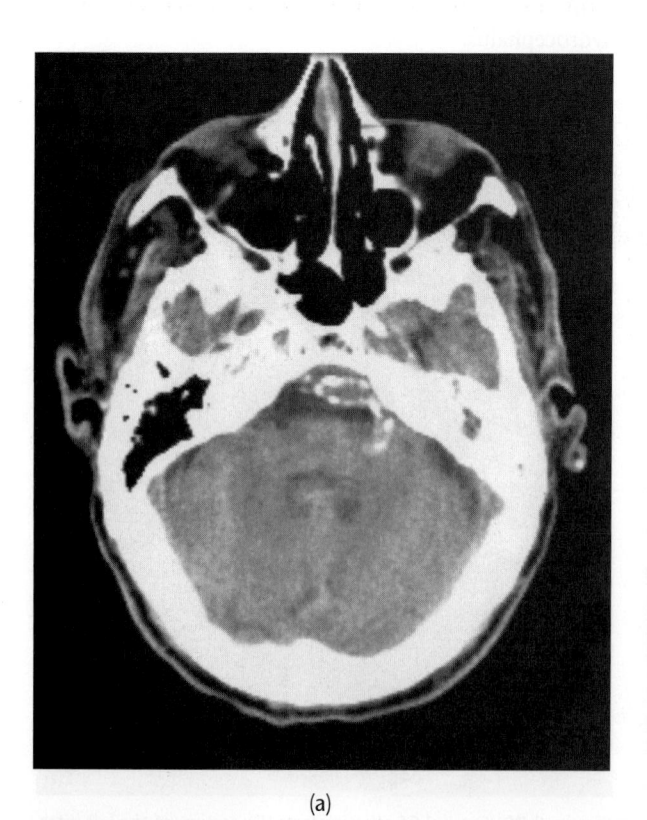

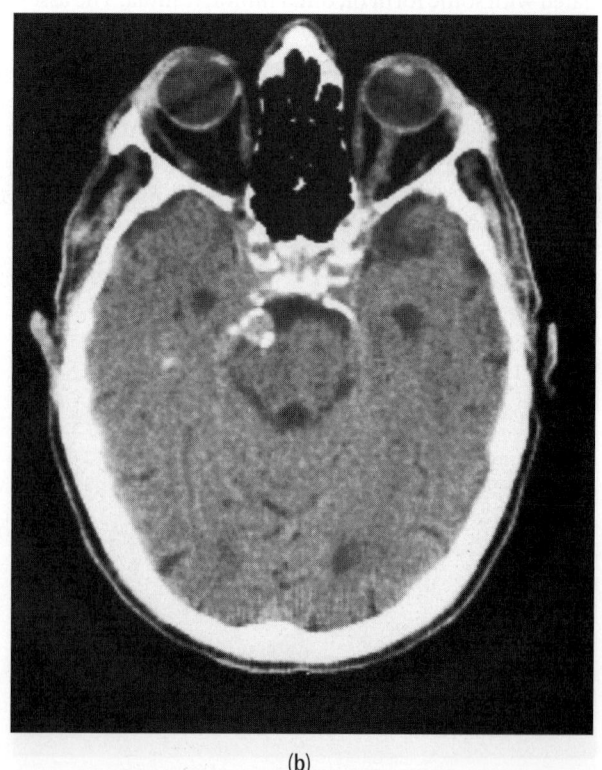

(a)   (b)

Figure 6.30 *Cranial CT (a), (b). Basilar artery ectasia. The basilar artery is enlarged and has a calcified wall. Calcification is also seen in the carotid siphons.*

Although cocaine and methamphetamine can cause a vasculitis with multiple focal aneurysmal dilatations, haemorrhage may be related to hypertensive crises.[34]

CEREBRAL VENOUS INFARCTION

Cerebral venous infarction is much less common than arterial infarction and may arise from either cortical venous or dural venous sinus occlusion or a combination of the two. Usually thrombosis of the venous sinus occurs first with extension into cortical veins and it is the cortical venous involvement that determines the clinical severity. Often no predisposing cause is found but venous occlusion may occur in pregnancy and the puerperium and be related to oral contraception. The common denominator in many cases is a hypercoagulability state. In the neonate,

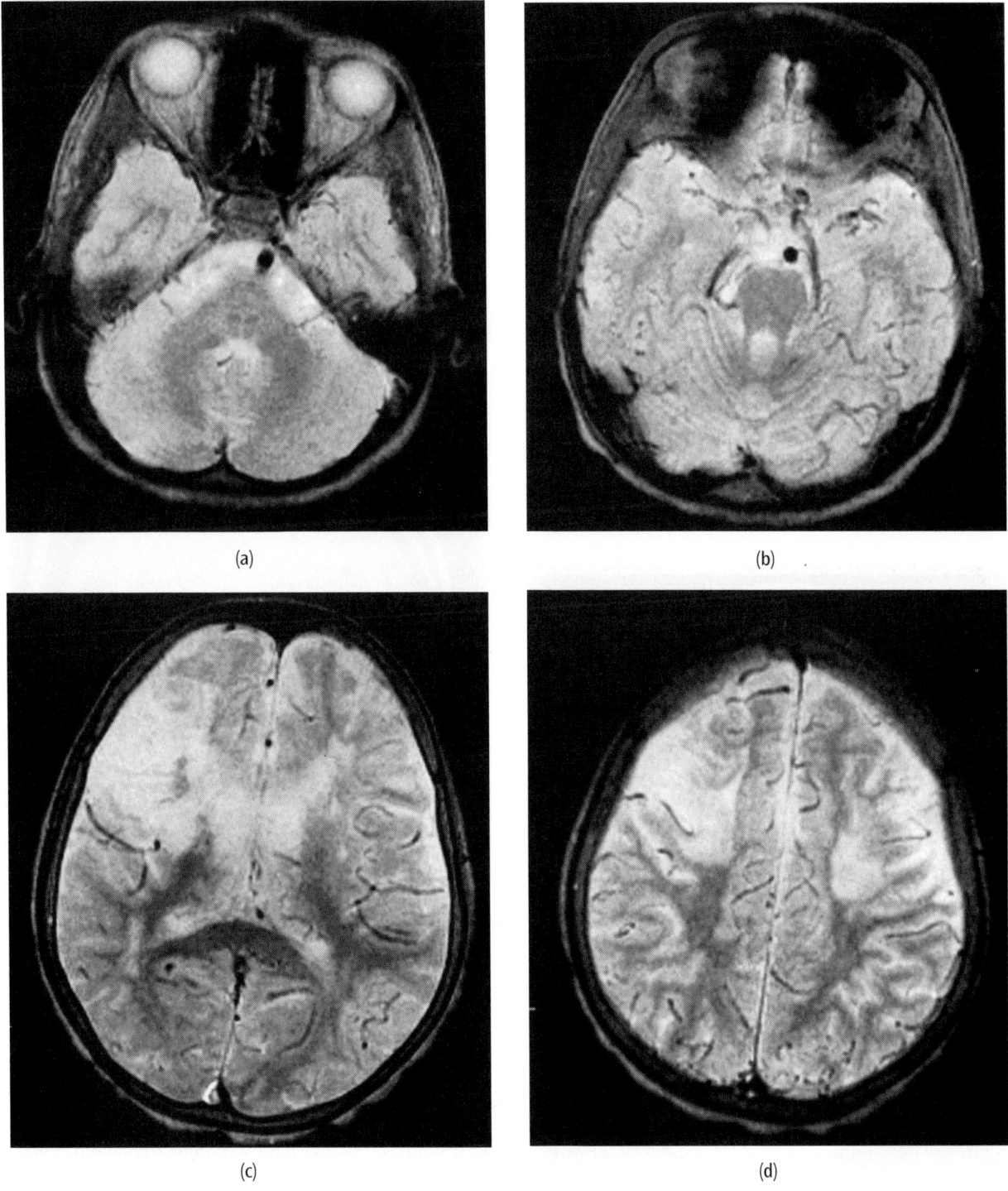

Figure 6.31 *Cranial MRI: axial proton density images (a)–(d). Sickle cell disease. Note: the parenchymal ischaemic change and the profusion of flow-voids due to collateral pathways. This patient has a moyamoya angiographic pattern. The carotid arteries are vestigial. The basilar artery is prominent.*

dehydration is a well recognized cause. Several causes are listed in Table 6.2. Up to 25% may be idiopathic but such patients should be kept under review since they may develop a systemic illness later.[35]

Venous infarcts may resemble their arterial counterparts in exerting mass effect and exhibiting contrast-enhancement. They can also be haemorrhagic but ultimately may resolve to leave a normal CT scan. Their typical location is described as within the subcortical white matter and if the superior sagittal sinus is involved, then infarction may be bilateral. Haemorrhage within the thalamus or basal ganglia, especially when bilateral, should alert the physician to deep cerebral venous thrombosis.

MRI findings in venous sinus occlusive disease show three patterns:[36]

- mass effect but no parenchymal signal change thought to be due to dilatation of the venous bed;
- both mass effect and signal alteration explained by rising venous pressure causing fluid movement out into the interstitium;
- the third, most severely affected group of patients show haematoma formation consequent upon very high venous pressure.

The normal appearance of the patent superior sagittal sinus on intravenous contrast-enhanced axial CT is of a uniformly enhancing triangle seen posteriorly in cross-section. When there is thrombosis the lumen remains hypodense and only the meningeal rim enhances. This is

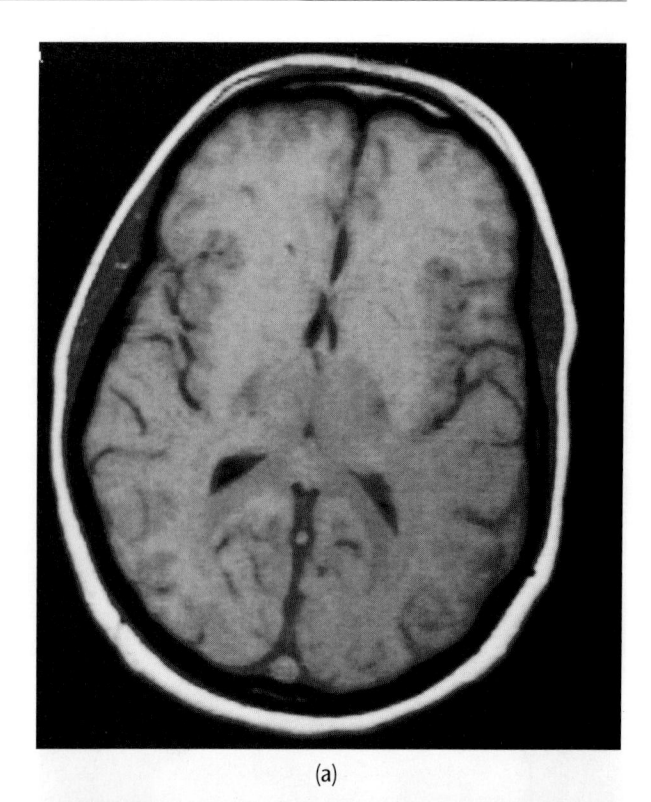

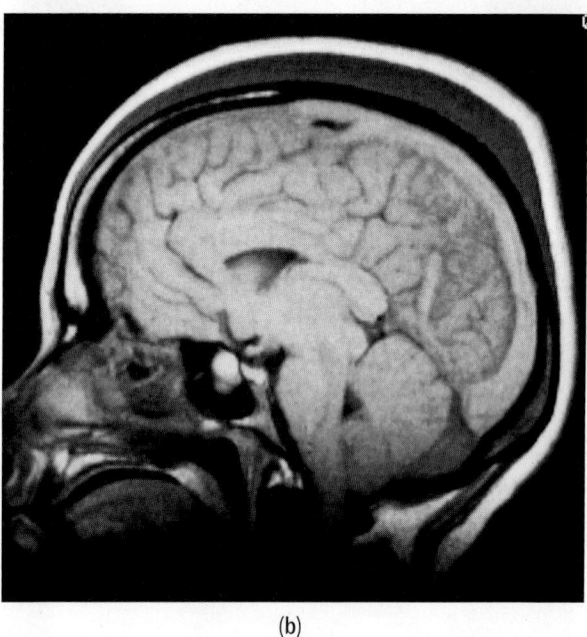

Figure 6.33 *Cranial MRI: T1-weighted (a) axial, (b) sagittal images Dural venous sinus thrombosis. Note hyperintensity within the superior sagittal sinus.*

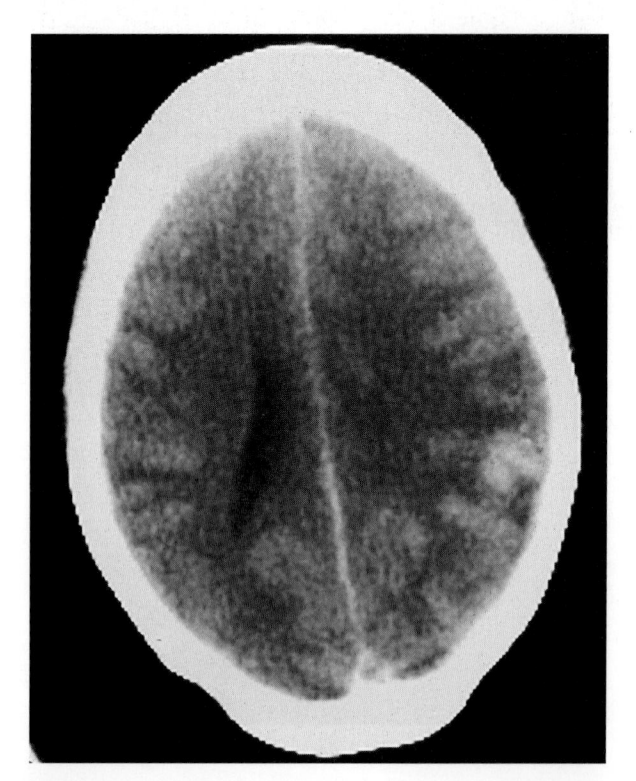

Figure 6.32 *Cranial CT after contrast. Empty triangle sign. Note the haemorrhagic foci due to venous infarction in the left hemisphere.*

the 'empty triangle' or 'empty delta' sign described by Buonanno[37] (Fig. 6.32). A superior sagittal sinus which bifurcates more superiorly than normal may give rise to what is a false positive empty triangle sign and this sign should therefore be interpreted with some caution. Using these criteria there may also be difficulty in appreciating thrombosis situated more anteriorly in the superior sagittal sinus. In this case the sinus seen along its

Table 6.2 *Causes of cerebral sinovenous occlusion*

Pregnancy and the puerperium
Craniofacial infections and tumours
Blood dyscrasia leading to hypercoagulable states
    polycythaemia (including cyanotic congenital heart disease)
    leukaemias and lymphomas
    sickle cell disease.
Systemic lupus erythematosus
Behçet's disease
Homocystinuria
Dehydration (in infants)

length may be hyperdense on unenhanced CT and enlarged with a 'shaggy' margin.[38] A thrombosed vein is sometimes seen on CT or T1-weighted MRI as a hyperdense or hyperintense (respectively) 'cord'.

Thrombus within the dural venous sinuses on MRI may be easy to detect (Fig. 6.33) but the normal patent lumen can be rendered hyperintense by various flow-related phenomena, most notably flow-related enhancement and the 'entry slice phenomenon'. Multislice acquisition of spin-echo sequences in particular may be responsible. Reviewing all the sequences obtained during an examination and performing scans in different planes generally avoids errors. T2-weighted sequences tend to be flow-sensitive but conversely, hypointensity within a sinus need not necessarily imply patency since deoxyhaemoglobin in fresh thrombus may be hypointense. In the acute stage of dural venous sinus thrombosis thrombus is isointense with brain on T1WI and relatively hypointense on T2WI. Later T2 relaxation lengthens to give hyperintensity on T2WI whilst the thrombus remains isointense on T1WI.

In chronic dural venous sinus thrombosis (months or years old) the organized thrombus enhances with gadolinium so that contrast-enhanced 2-D time-of-flight-MRA, which is T1 sensitive, can be falsely negative.[39]

The administration of intravenous gadolinium DTPA causes luminal enhancement of the patent sinus where blood is relatively slow-flowing. Magnetic resonance angiography of the dural venous sinuses is undertaken using 2-D time-of-flight techniques at least in the first instance for the reasons given previously[40,41] (Fig. 6.34). It can be difficult when in the presence of an adjacent meningioma to decide whether the dural venous sinus is effaced due to extrinsic compression or occluded. In the author's experience, angiography by whatever means may be equivocal. However, when studied alongside a conventional T1-weighted study, with gadolinium DTPA, the answer is usually becomes clear.

CEREBROVASCULAR DISEASE IN CHILDREN

Cerebral infarcts may occur in children and are usually due to thrombosis in the middle cerebral artery territory (Fig. 6.35). The evolution of childhood infarction resembles that in adults. Affected children have usually been healthy but amongst possible underlying conditions one must consider sickle cell disease, cyanotic congenital heart disease and moyamoya disease.

Neonatal hypoxic damage is influenced by the degree of maturity of the brain. In the immature neonate (less than 34 weeks gestation), the vessels are prominent in the region of the basal ganglia and in particular the germinal matrix. This is the site of origin of neuronal tissue and is located in subependymal region over the head and body of the caudate nucleus. The germinal matrix involutes between 32 weeks and term.

The cortex is thin and supplied by peripheral vessels with numerous anastomotic channels to the leptomeningeal vessels. The watershed zone between these central and peripheral vessels is within the periventricular white matter.

Cerebral development in the last trimester is rapid and the vascular anatomy comes to resemble that in the adult. At birth the white matter is more active metabolically than grey matter since myelination is proceeding apace.

(a)

(b)

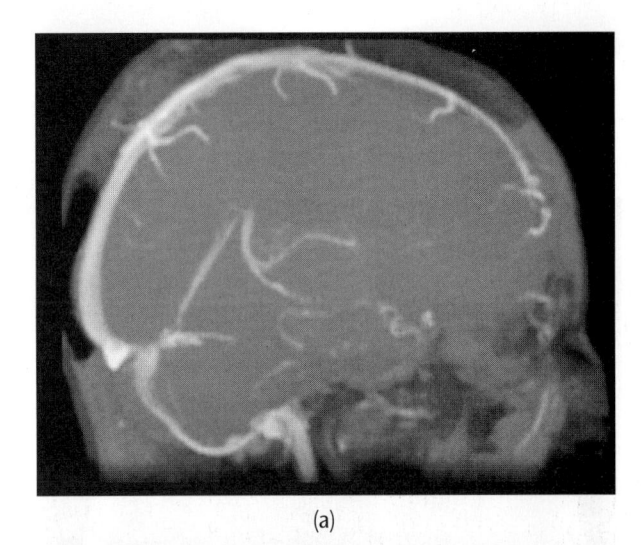

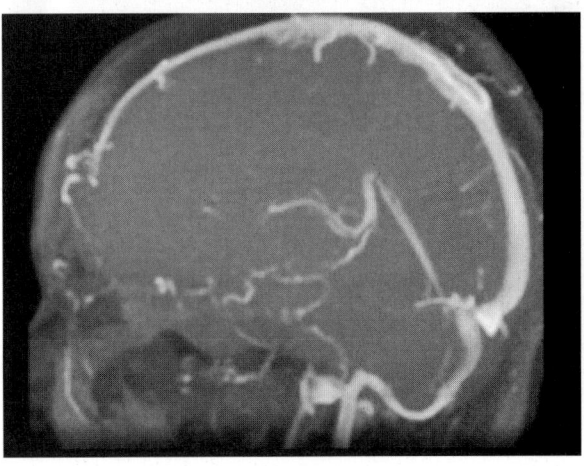

Figure 6.34 *2-D Time-of-flight MRA of the dural venous sinuses. Note the occluded right transverse sinus.*

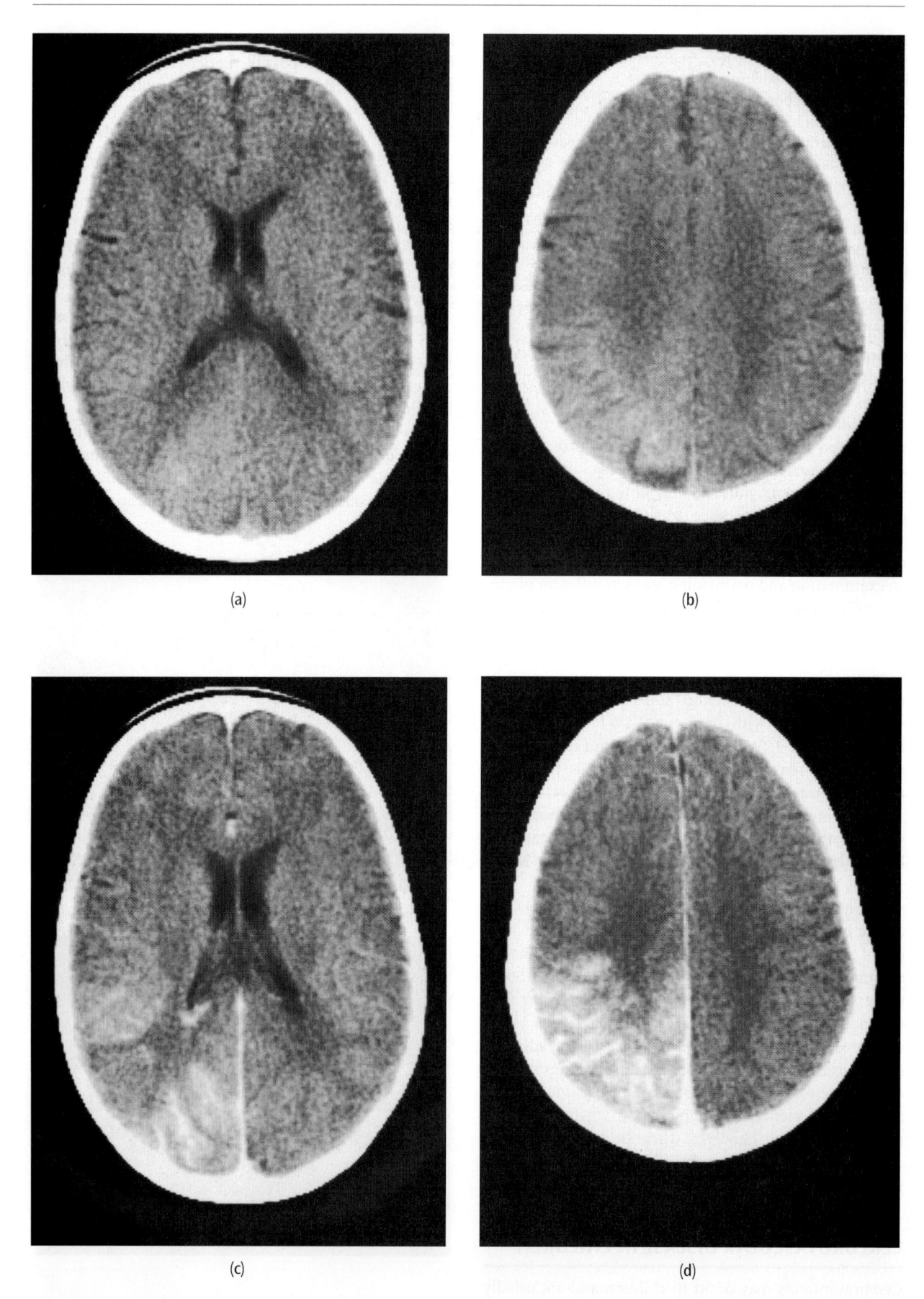

Figure 6.35 *Cranial CT (a), (b) before contrast; (c), (d) after contrast. Enhancing haemorrhagic right posterior cerebral artery territory infarct in a 3-year-old child.*

Cerebrovascular disease in children 209

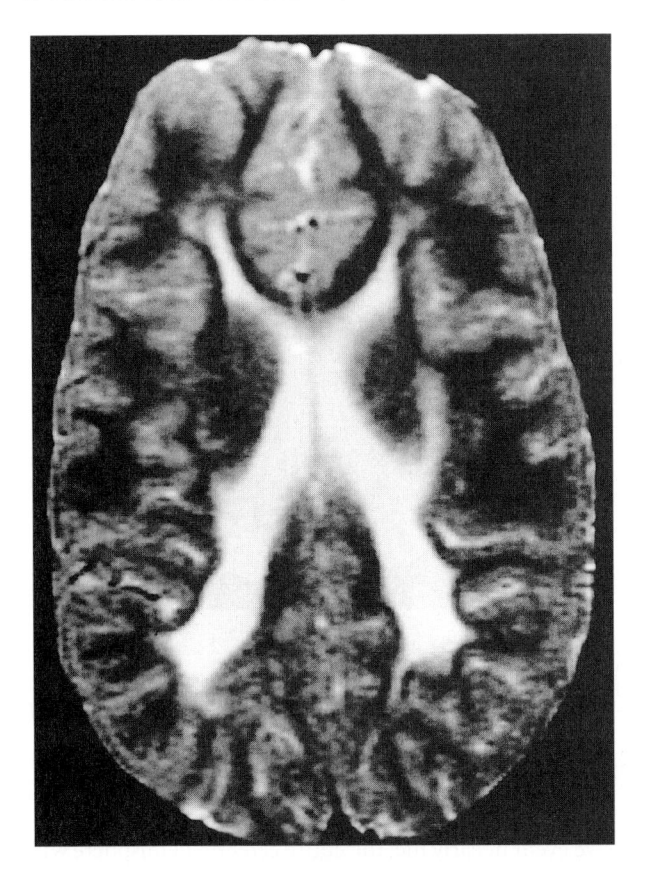

Figure 6.36 *Periventricular leukomalacia (end-stage). Axial T2-weighted demonstrating lateral ventricular enlargement with irregularity of outlining and diminishing volume of cerebral white matter. (Courtesy of Dr WK Chong, Consultant Neuroradiologist, Great Ormond Street Hospital for Children, London, UK.)*

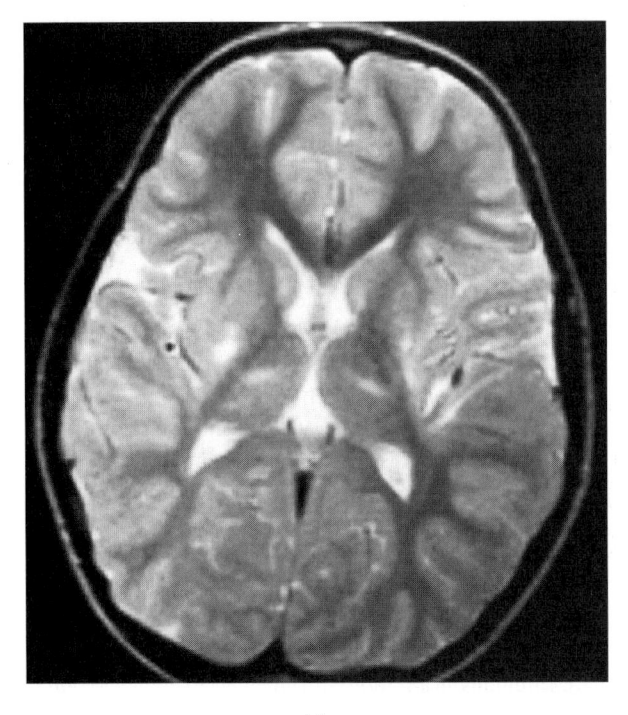

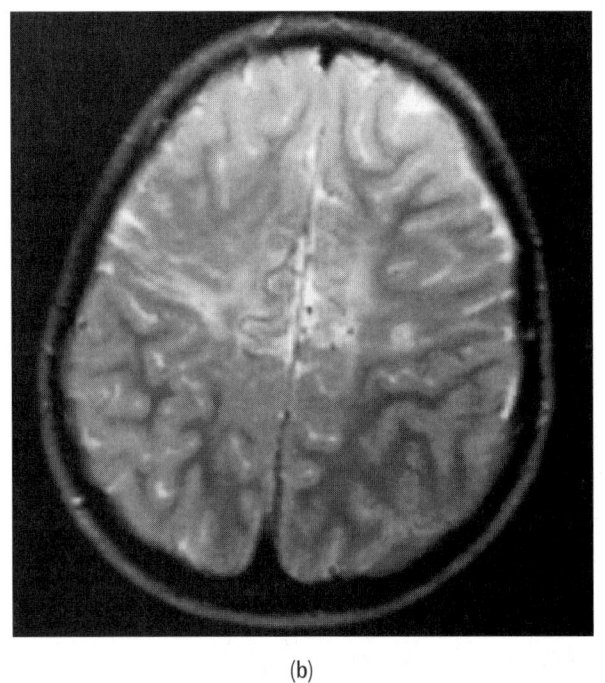

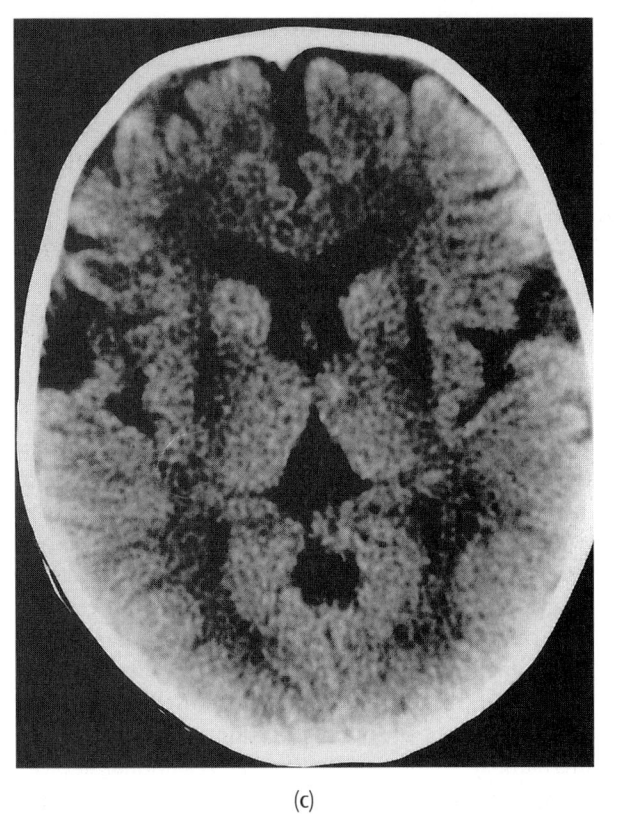

Figure 6.37 (a–c) (above and left) *Cranial MRI T2-weighted axial images showing typical changes of profound perinatal asphyxia (a) in the basal ganglia, thalami and (b) perirolandic regions. (c) Axial CT (different patient) showing bilateral striated necrosis.*

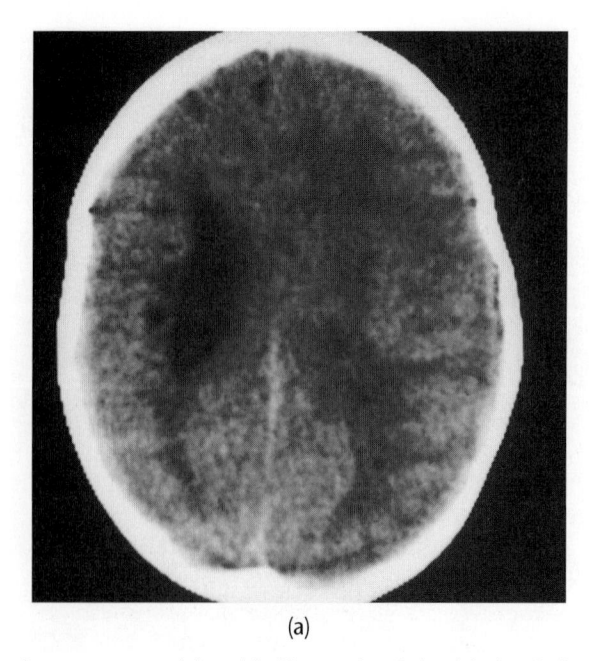

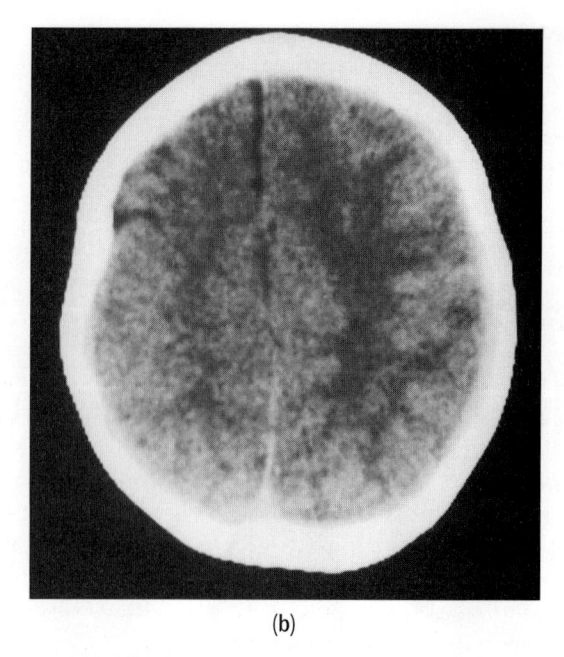

Figure 6.38 *Cranial CT (a), (b). Atrophy of the right hemisphere in a 7-year-old child due to a cerebrovascular accident early in life. There are ischaemic lesions adjacent to an enlarged lateral ventricle. This should not be confused with a contralateral isodense subdural collection.*

In the premature neonate, fluctuation in the vascular regulation may give rise to cerebral haemorrhage but hypotension leading to hypoperfusion results in damage mainly to the watershed areas (i.e. the periventricular white matter). The regions usually affected are close to the trigones but also adjacent to the frontal horns of the lateral ventricles. Cyst-like areas develop within the damaged white matter, which regress between 1 and 3 months after injury to leave a reduced amount of white matter as the legacy of periventricular leukomalacia (Fig. 6.36). The cerebral ventricles are enlarged and irregular. If cerebral injury occurs in the first two trimesters damaged cells are simply resorbed with no gliosis. There will thus be no signal abnormality on MR.

In the term neonate, mild-to-moderate hypoxic ischaemic damage affects the adult watershed regions, as 'parasagittal infarctions'. Profound hypoxia in the term neonate can lead to very specific MR changes, which persist into adult life and which can be used retrospectively as evidence of perinatal asphyxia. Often quite subtle abnormal signal on T2WI is shown within the thalami, basal ganglia, hippocampi and cortex around the central sulcus (Fig. 6.37). These are the most metabolically active regions of the brain at this time. It is emphasized that similar change at a particular gestational age can occur either *in utero* or postnatally.

In the older child profound asphyxia results in diffuse oedema with hypodensity on CT, beginning in the basal ganglia and insula, ultimately becoming diffuse. In a subgroup of severely affected patients, the white matter shows increased density compared with the grey matter, the so-called 'reversal sign'.[42] Ultimately atrophy and perhaps cystic degeneration supervene.

If there has been some sort of cerebrovascular occlusive event in early life, the entire cerebral hemisphere will ultimately be smaller, the lateral ventricle enlarged and a variable degree of ischaemic parenchymal change will be present (Fig. 6.38). This should not be confused, in the context of trauma, with a contralateral isodense subdural collection (i.e. occurring on the normal side).

REFERENCES

1 Hise JH, Nipper NL, Schnitker JC. Stroke associated with coronary artery bypass surgery. *Am J Neuroradiol* 1991; **12**: 811–14.
2 Bousser MG, Baron JC, Chiras J. Ischemic strokes and migraine. *Neuroradiology* 1985; **27**: 583–7.
3 Peatfield R. *Headache and Other Head Pain* pp. 67–8. Berlin: Springer Verlag, 1986.
4 Godon-Hardy S, Meder JF, Dilouya A *et al*. Ischemic strokes and oral contraception. *Neuroradiology* 1985; **27**: 588–92.
5 Masdeu JC. Infarct versus neoplasm on CT: four helpful signs. *Am J Neuroradiol* 1983; **4**: 525–8.
6 Bryan RN, Levy LM, Whitlow WD, Killian JM, Preziosi TJ, Rosario JA. Diagnosis of acute cerebral infarction: comparison of CT and MR imaging. *Am J Neuroradiol* 1991; **12**: 611–20.
7 Yuh WTC, Crain MR, Loes DG, Greene GM, Ryals TJ, Sato Y. MR Imaging of cerebral ischaemia: findings in the first 24 hours. *Am J Neuroradiol* 1991; **12**: 621–9.
8 Thomsick T, Brott T, Barsan W, Roderick J, Haley EC, Spilker J. Thrombus localization with emergency cerebral CT. *Am J Neuroradiol* 1992; **13**: 257–63.

9. Elster AD, Moody DM. Early cerebral infarction: gadopentate dimeglumine enhancement. *Radiology* 1990; **177**: 627–32.
10. Crain MR, Yuh WTC, Greene GM, Loes DJ, Ryals TJ et al. Cerebral ischaemia: evaluation of contrast-enhanced MR imaging. *Am J Neuroradiol* 1991; **12**: 631–9.
11. Zimmerman RD, Leeds NE, Naidich TP. Ring blush associated with intracranial hematoma. *Radiology* 1977; **122**: 707–11.
12. Kendall BE, Pullicino P. Intravascular contrast injection in ischaemic lesions. *Neuroradiology* 1980; **19**: 241–3.
13. Skriver EB, Olsen TS. Transient disappearance of infarcts on CT scan: the so-called fogging effect. *Neuroradiology* 1981; **22**: 61–5.
14. Asato R, Okumura R, Konishi J. Fogging effect in MR of cerebral infarct. *J Comput Assist Tomogr* 1991; **15**: 160–2.
15. Bozzao L, Angeloni U, Bastianello S, Fantozi M, Pierallini A, Fieschi C. Early angiographic and CT findings in patients with haemorrhagic infarction in the distribution of the middle cerebral artery. *Am J Neuroradiol* 1992; **12**: 1115–21.
16. Fisher CM, Adams RD. Observations on brain embolism – with special reference to haemorrhagic infarction. In: *The Heart and Stroke*. Furlan AJ (Ed), Berlin: Springer Verlag, 1987.
17. Savoiardo M, Bracchi M, Passerini A et al. The vascular territories in the cerebellum and brainstem. *Am J Neuroradiol* 1987; **8**: 199–209.
18. Osborn AG. *Diagnostic Neuroradiology* p. 355. Chicago: Mosby, 1994
19. Fisher CM. Lacunes:small, deep cerebral infarcts. *Neurology* 1965; **15**: 774–84.
20. Waterston JA, Brown MM, Butler P, Swash M. Small deep cerebral infarcts associated with occlusive internal carotid artery disease: a hemodynamic phenomenon? *Arch Neurol* 1990; **47**: 935–57.
21. Yagashita A, Nakano I, Oda M et al. Location of corticospinal tract in the internal capsule at MR imaging. *Radiology* 1994; **191**: 455–60.
22. Rosovsky MA, Litt AW. MR angiography of the extracranial carotid arteries. *MRI Clin N Amer* 1995; **3**: 439–54.
23. Bradley WG. Basic flow phenomena. *MRI Clin N Amer* 1995; **3**: 375–90.
24. Dennis MS, Bamford JM, Sandercock PAG, Molyneux A, Warlow CP. Computerized tomography in patients with transient ischaemic attacks: when is a transient ischaemic attack not a transient ischaemic attack but a stroke? *J Neurol* 1990; **237**: 257–61.
25. North American Symptomatic Carotid Endartorectomy Trial Collaborators: Beneficial effect of carotid endarterectomy in symptomatic patients with high-grade carotid stenosis. *New Engl J Med* 1991; **325**: 453–5.
26. European Carotid Surgery Triallist Collaboration Group. MRC European Carotid Surgery Trial: Interim results of symptomatic patients all severe (70–99%) or with mild (0–29%) carotid stenosis. *Lancet* 1991; **337**: 1235–43.
27. Hobson RW, Weiss DG, Fields WS. Efficacy of carotid endartorectomy for asymptomatic carotid stenosis. *New Engl J Med* 1993; **328**: 221–7.
28. Stevens JM. Imaging carotid stenosis (Editorial). *Clin Radiol* 1995; **50**: 821–2.
29. Mattle HP, Kent KC, Edelman RR et al. Evaluation of the intracranial carotid arteries: Correlation of magnetic resonance angiography, duplex ultrasonography and conventional angiography *J Vasc Surg* 1991; **13**: 838–45.
30. Vieco PT. CT angiography of the carotid artery. *Neuroimaging Clin N Amer* 1998; **6**: 593–605.
31. Turnipseed WD, Kennel TW, Turski PA et al. Combined use of duplex imaging and magnetic resonance angiography for evaluation of patients with symptomatic ipsilateral high-grade stenosis. *J Vasc Surg* 1993; **17**: 832–40.
32. Houser UW, Mokri B, Sundt T, Baker HL, Reese DF. Spontaneous cervical cephalic arterial dissection: angiographic spectrum. *Am J Neuroradiol* 1984; **5**: 27–34.
33. Fujisawa I, Asato R, Nishimara K et al. Moya-moya disease: MR imaging *Radiology* 1987; **164**: 103–5.
34. Jacobs IG, Roszler MH, Kelly JK et al. Cocaine abuse: neurovascular complications. *Radiology* 1989; **170**: 223–7.
35. Bousser MG, Chiras J, Bories J et al. Cerebral venous thrombosis – a review of 38 cases *Stroke* 1985; **16**: 199–213.
36. Yuh WTC, Simonson TM, Wang Am, Kochi TM, Tali ET et al. Venous sinus occlusive disease: MR findings. *Am J Neuroradiol* 1992; **15**: 309–16.
37. Buonanno FS, Moody DM, Ball MR et al. Computed cranial tomographic findings in cerebral sinovenous occlusion. *J Comput Assist Tomogr* 1978; **2**: 281–90.
38. Zimmerman RD, Ernst RJ. Neuroimaging of cerebral venous thrombosis. *Neuroimag Clin North Amer* 1992; **2**: 463–85.
39. Dormont D, Sag K, Biondi A et al. Gadolinium enhanced MR of chronic dural sinus thrombosis. *Am J Neuroradiol* 1995; **16**: 1347–52.
40. Cure JK, Van Tassel P. Congenital and acquired abnormalities of the dural venous sinuses *Semin US, CT, MRI* 1994; **15**: 520–39.
41. Cure JK, Van Tassel P, Smith MT. Normal and variant anatomy of the dural venous sinuses. *Semin US, CT, MRI* **15**: 499–519.
42. Han BK, Towbin RB, de Courten-Myers G, McLaurin RL, Ball WS. Reversal sign on CT: effect of anoxic ischemic cerebral injury in children. *Am J Neuroradiol* 1989; **10**: 1191–8.

FURTHER READING

Barkovich AJ. Destructive brain disorders of childhood. In: *Pediatric Neuroimaging* 2nd edn. New York: Lippincott–Raven, 1996: Ch. 4.

7

Infections and inflammatory diseases

CHARLES A J ROMANOWSKI

Introduction	212	Encephalitis	232
Congenital infection	212	Post-infective encephalitis	235
Cerebral AIDS and HIV infection	215	Tuberculosis, fungal and parasitic infections	236
Meningitis	222	Sarcoidosis	239
Cerebral abscess	230	References	239

INTRODUCTION

Infections involving the central nervous system (CNS) have significantly increased in recent years largely due to the increased number of immunocompromised patients. Neuroimaging plays an important role in these conditions. Some diseases have specific features on imaging; however, there may be a significant overlap in the appearances on computed tomography (CT) and magnetic resonance imaging (MRI). The aim of this chapter is to highlight the important neuroimaging features of infections of the CNS in children and adults and in both immunocompetent and immunocompromised patients. Initially, however, the effects of infection on the developing CNS are discussed.

CONGENITAL INFECTION

Infections that involve the developing fetus *in utero* have a markedly different effect upon the brain when compared with infections occurring in the older child or the adult.[1] Infections occurring during the first and second trimesters result in congenital malformations of the brain whereas those infections occurring in the third trimester typically result in destructive lesions of the brain. The timing of the particular insult to the brain is more important than the nature of the insult itself. In many cases the infection is not apparent in the mother.

Congenital infections of the brain may be acquired via transplacental spread. This is the case with most of the viral infections and toxoplasmosis. Alternatively the infection may be acquired at the time of birth during passage through the birth canal. This is the usual pattern with herpes simplex infection. Finally neonatal bacterial meningitis is usually secondary to ascending infection, particularly in the context of early rupture of membranes. A useful mnemonic for congenital infections is TORCH – Toxoplasmosis, Other (e.g. syphilis), Rubella, Cytomegalovirus and Herpes simplex virus. As HIV (human immunodeficiency virus) is now becoming the commonest maternally transmitted infection perhaps this mnemonic should become 'A TORCH' to signify the importance of AIDS (acquired immunodeficiency syndrome).[2]

CYTOMEGALOVIRUS

Cytomegalovirus (CMV) is a DNA virus in the herpes group. It results in the most common serious viral infection of the CNS in the newborn. The infection is acquired via the transplacental route when there is maternal infection or reactivation. Maternal infection is more commonly identified in lower socioeconomic groups and CMV infection can be identified in approximately 1% of all births. Of those neonates infected, approximately 10% will have significant abnormalities. Generalized infection results in hepatosplenomegaly, microcephaly and cardiac anomalies. If the infection is acquired later in pregnancy then sensorineural hearing loss is an important feature. Of those children showing signs and symptoms of significant infection, between 55 and 70% have involvement of the CNS. CMV infection has a predelection for the germinal matrix, although primary vascular involvement with secondary brain damage has been suggested.

Pathologically there is evidence of microcephaly together with polymicrogyria. There is a decrease in the amount of white matter which may be gliotic and myelination is often delayed. There is periventricular calcification although basal ganglia calcification can also occur. With early (i.e. first trimester and early second trimester) and severe infection there is often marked thick periventricular calcification together with ventriculomegaly. The brain may show signs of a thin cortex with lissencephaly and a hypoplastic cerebellum. If infection occurs in the latter portion of the second trimester there is polymicrogyria with a lesser degree of ventricular dilatation. When infection occurs even later in pregnancy there is normal gyral pattern with only mild atrophy. The periventricular calcification, however, remains prominent and CT is superior at showing this (Fig. 7.1). However, MRI is better at showing the associated areas of cortical dysplasia and may also demonstrate small subependymal cysts in the occipital horns which may be specific for CMV.[2] The presence of cortical dysplasia is particularly important in differentiating CMV from toxoplasmosis, the second most common congenitally acquired CNS infection.

Toxoplasmosis

Toxoplasma gondii results in the second most common CNS congenital infection. The organism is an obligate intracellular parasite and the oocytes are ingested in either undercooked meat or cat faeces. Congenital infection only occurs when the mother herself is infected during pregnancy. Toxoplasmosis can be identified in between 1000 and 3000 live births. If still births are included, then toxoplasmosis may be identified in up to 1% of all pregnancies. In some countries the rate of infection is very high; for example in France 90% of adult women are seropositive and toxoplasmosis is said to affect 3% of all pregnancies.[2] More than 50% of infected fetuses develop CNS disease. This manifests as bilateral chorioretinitis, hydrocephalus and microcephaly with a spectrum of atrophic changes. There is a relatively wide range of clinical manifestations from only very mild disease presenting later in life to more severe disease with a significant mortality. Of those children surviving the infection there may be mental retardation, seizures or spasticity.

Pathologically there is diffuse inflammation of the

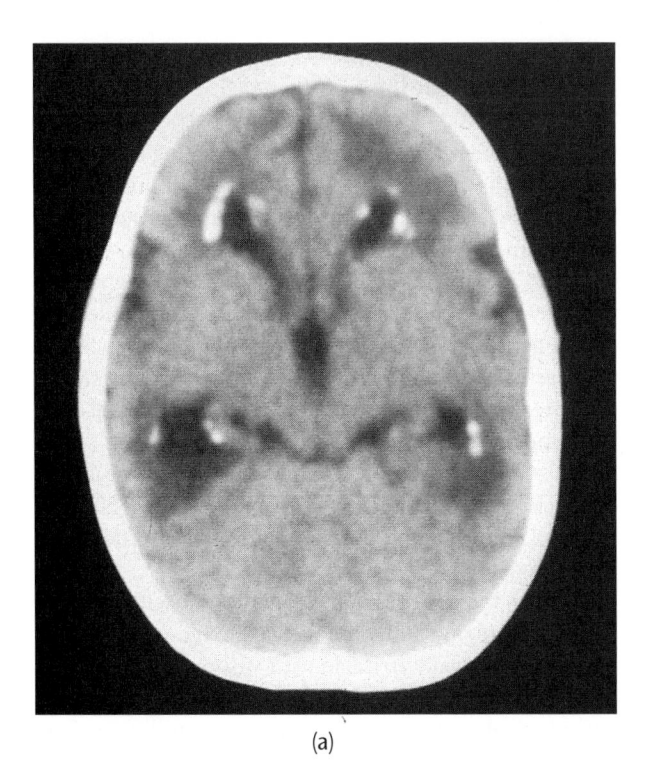

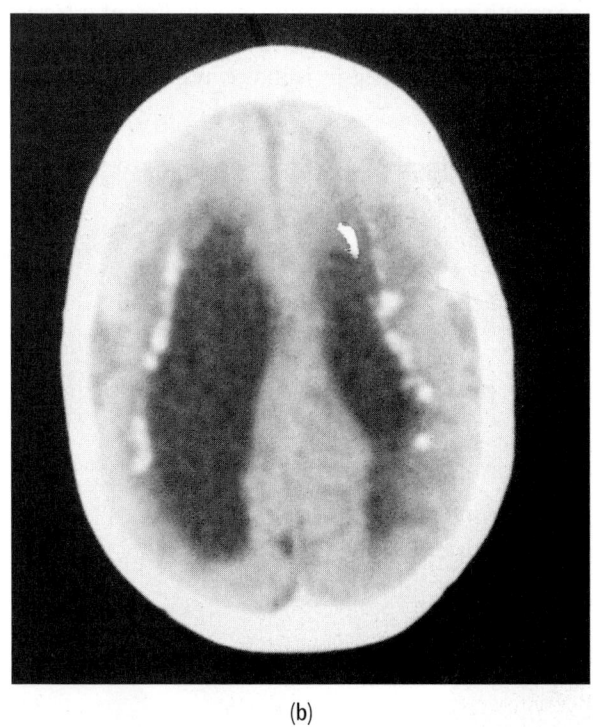

Figure 7.1 *(a), (b) Congenital cytomegalovirus (CMV) infection. There is prominent periventricular calcification with loss of brain substance, particularly involving the white matter, more marked on the right than the left. The cortex over the left frontal lobe appears abnormal and may be dysplastic although MRI would demonstrate this more clearly. (Reproduced courtesy of Dr A Sprigg, Consultant Paediatric Radiologist, Sheffield Children's Hospital.)*

meninges and the brain with granulomatous lesions and associated giant cells. Hydrocephalus occurs secondary to ependymitis resulting in aqueductal stenosis. With early infection there may be severe brain destruction resulting in hydrancephaly.

On CT there is evidence of scattered calcification. This is usually more diffusely distributed than that seen with CMV. Calcification is therefore seen not only in a periventricular distribution but also peripherally within the cortex and the basal ganglia (Fig. 7.2). There may well be significant hydrocephalus and microcephaly with atrophy ranging from mild to severe. This tends to reflect the timing of the insult with earlier infection resulting in more severe brain destruction. The cortical dysplasia which is often seen in association with CMV is not seen with toxoplasmosis. This is an important consideration in a differential diagnosis.

Herpes simplex virus (HSV)

This infection is due to the herpes simplex type 2 virus, the agent responsible for genital herpes. The infection is seen in one child in every 2000–5000 deliveries and is usually acquired at the time of passage through the birth canal. Rarely, it occurs as an ascending infection following earlier rupture of the membranes and, very rarely, may be acquired postnatally from oral lesions (HSV type 1) on visitors to the new baby. The most common manifestation is mild cutaneous infection possibly involving the mouth and also eyes. Approximately 30% of infected infants develop CNS infection. There may well be generalized disease resulting in jaundice, respiratory distress and fever. Symptoms usually develop within the 2nd to 4th weeks of life and result from meningoencephalitis producing lethargy, fever and focal or generalized seizures. If left untreated there is a poor prognosis with up to 80% mortality.

Imaging studies show widespread patchy abnormal areas mainly within the white matter. On CT there is decreased attenuation of the white matter which may be rapidly progressive. Also there is increased attenuation identified in the grey matter which may persist for weeks or months. There may be evidence of meningeal enhancement. Perhaps MRI is less useful in this age-group. The white matter is largely unmyelinated and is of low signal on T1-weighted images (T1WI) and high signal on T2-weighted images (T2WI). It is therefore difficult to confidently identify diffuse white matter oedema.

With untreated disease there is rapidly progressive brain destruction resulting in severe atrophy, profound cortical thinning, multicystic encephalomalacia involving the white matter and gyriform or punctate calcification. The suspicion of herpes simplex encephalitis should be raised in the presence of relatively increased attenuation of the grey matter together with meningeal enhancement. The pattern of congenital encephalitis is more diffuse and widespread than the pattern of encephalitis occuring due to herpes in adults and older children. There is also a predilection for vascular endothelium which results in thrombosis or haemorrhagic infarction.

Congenital rubella

The development of maternal rubella during early pregnancy results in devastating congenitial abnormalities. This has led to widespread screening and immunization programmes which have now resulted in congenital rubella CNS infection being very rare. When rubella does involve the developing brain there is predilection for the germinal matrix where it has an antimitotic effect with resultant inhibition of cell development and subsequent reduction in the number of neurons and glial cells. The most severe abnormalities result from early intrauterine infection. Congenital rubella also results in cataracts, glaucoma and cardiac abnormalities. Hearing loss is the most common manifestation of infection later on in pregnancy.

At birth the patient is usually hypotonic with lethargy and large bulging fontanelles. By the age of 4 months children are usually irritable with vasomotor instability, psychomotor retardation and seizures in up to 25%. Pathologically there is microcephaly and ventriculomegaly secondary to atrophy. There is evidence of involvement of the eyes with cataracts, glaucoma and chorioretinitis as well as microphthalmia.

On imaging there are congenital anomalies and microcephaly. The brain is atrophic with calcification

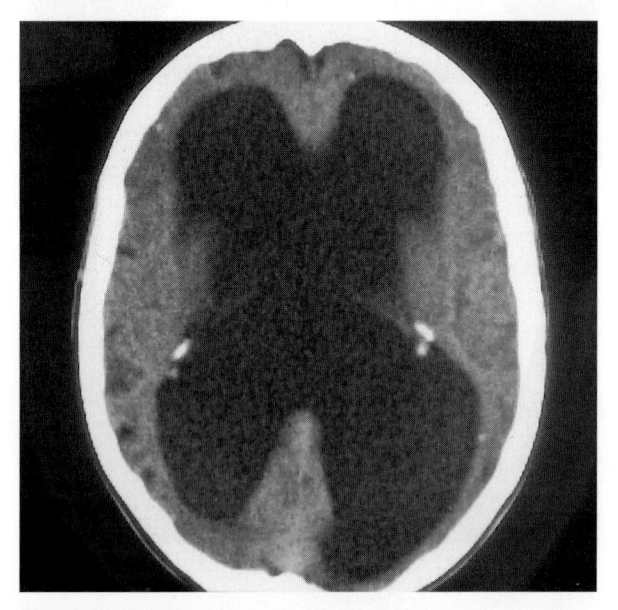

Figure 7.2 *Congenital toxoplasmosis. There is marked ventricular dilatation together with periventricular calcification. There are also smaller more peripherally placed foci of calcification present.*

particularly in the basal ganglia and cortex. There is delayed myelination which is a manifestation of the reduced number of oligodendrocytes. In severe cases there is near total brain destruction.

Congenital HIV

Congenital HIV infection is usually caused by perinatal transmission most commonly from the mother. Indeed 80% of childhood cases of HIV infection are maternally transmitted. However, only one-third of HIV-positive mothers actually pass on the infection to their children. A seemingly high proportion of seropositive cases in children appear to be related to drug abuse in either the mother or her partner. Congenital HIV results in atrophy of the neonatal brain and calcification particularly within the basal ganglia.

Clinically there is failure to thrive with diarrhoea, chronic fever and decrease in weight. There is lymphadenopathy and repeated infections, in particular with oral thrush. About 30–50% of such patients develop encephalopathy with progressive spasticity and ataxia. There is developmental delay with cognitive and psychomotor impairment. In addition to the encephalopathy there may also be an arteriopathy which results in dilatation of the vessels around the circle of Willis which predisposes to thrombosis and embolic disease. Haemorrhage can occur secondary to thrombocytopenia. Most children die in the first year.

On imaging the most common finding is diffuse atrophy. Basal ganglia (Fig. 7.3) and subcortical calcification can be identified which is especially prominent in the white matter of the frontal lobes. Calcification can also be seen within vessel walls. The intracranial calcification is only identified in those children who are infected whilst still *in utero*. Opportunistic infections such as toxoplasmosis are much less common in children. The commonest infection that does occur is progressive multifocal leucoencephalopathy. Tumours of the CNS are also uncommon in childhood cases of AIDS. When a mass does occur this is usually non-Hodgkin lymphoma and is often sited on the basal ganglia and thalamus. HIV also causes myelopathy and corticospinal tract degeneration with relative sparing of the dorsal columns.

CEREBRAL AIDS AND HIV INFECTION

It is known that AIDS is caused by HIV, a retrovirus which as well as having profound effects upon the immune system is also neurotropic and therefore directly involves the CNS. Up to 40% of patients with AIDS develop significant neurological symptoms at some point; 75% of patients have abnormalities of the CNS at autopsy. As well as direct involvement of the CNS by the HIV virus, opportunistic infections of the CNS

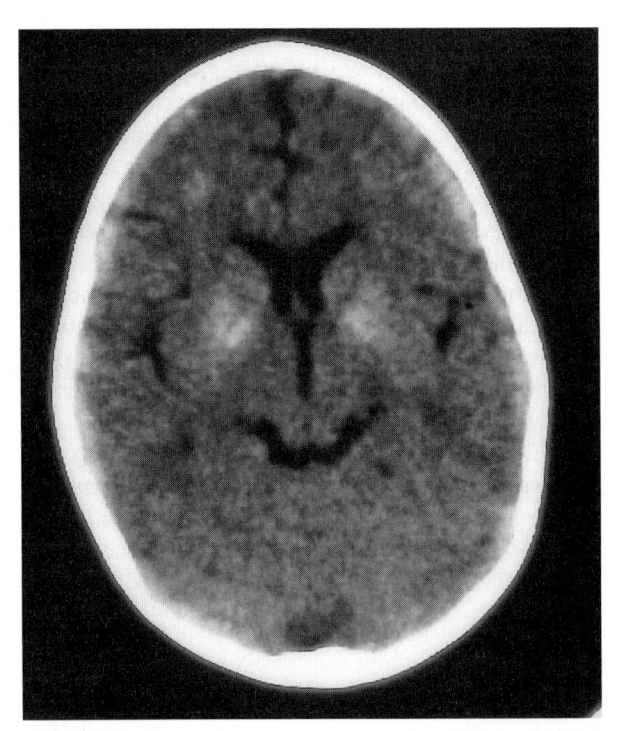

Figure 7.3 *Basal ganglia calcification in congenital HIV infection. A small amount of calcification is also identified within the white matter of the right frontal lobe. (Reproduced courtesy of Dr A Sprigg, Consultant Paediatric Radiologist, Sheffield Children's Hospital.)*

are important manifestations of AIDS. Imaging of the CNS is therefore taking on an increasingly important role in AIDS especially as new treatments are developed and patients survive longer.[3]

Toxoplasmosis is the commonest cause of focal lesions of the brain in AIDS patients, accounting for 50–70% of such focal abnormalities. The second most common cause, lymphoma, accounts for 20–30% of focal brain lesions. The third most commonly encountered focal abnormality is progressive multifocal leucoencephalopathy (PML) which accounts for 10–20% of focal lesions.

HIV Encephalopathy

The HIV virus itself is the most common agent to involve the CNS in patients who are HIV-positive resulting in HIV-encephalopathy which is present in up to 60% of AIDS patients. Indeed neurological signs are the first indicator of disease in up to 10% of AIDS cases. Direct involvement of the CNS results in subacute encephalitis which results in a subcortical dementia. This is termed AIDS dementia complex (ADC) or HIV-associated cognitive/motor complex.

Pathologically there is evidence of atrophy with decrease in the number of axons and demyelination. Microglial nodules and multinucleated giant cells occur.

On imaging with CT there is evidence of generalized

atrophy (Fig. 7.4) and multifocal areas of reduced attenuation within the central white matter. MRI is more sensitive in demonstrating the white matter changes. These comprise ill defined diffuse and confluent areas of increased T2 signal within the white matter (Fig. 7.5) which represent secondary demyelination and gliosis.[4,5] The changes are commonest in the frontal lobes and are usually bilateral yet asymmetrical. High signal identified in the fornix/subcallosal area in particular is associated with early cognitive impairment.[6] The grey matter is spared and there is no mass effect and no evidence of enhancement. Other opportunistic infections may co-exist with HIV encephalopathy (Fig. 7.6).

Proton MR spectroscopy shows a decrease in the relative levels of N-acetyl aspartate (NAA). This is present only in neurons and axons and is therefore an indicator of neuronal loss. These spectroscopic changes of reduced NAA are probably more sensitive than conventional imaging.[7,8]

Toxoplasmosis

Toxoplasmosis is the most common opportunistic infection of the CNS in AIDS. This may be seen in up to 25% of all AIDS patients. The organism *Toxoplasma gondii* is an obligate intracellular parasite. Infection of the CNS with this results in either focal lesions or a diffuse encephalitis The commonest site of infection is within the basal ganglia or at the grey white matter interface. Lesions also occur in the brainstem.[9]

On CT there are solitary or multiple ring-enhancing masses which have substantial peripheral oedema. There may sometimes be a central area of high attenuation giving a target lesion appearance. On MRI these lesions are slightly reduced or isointense on T1 and show focal nodular and/or rim enhancement following intravenous gadolinium (Fig. 7.7). However, T2WI are more sensitive than enhanced T1WI at showing multiple lesions. Treatment consists of two drugs, sulphadiazine and pyrimethamine. Improvement is usually seen in 1–2 weeks both clinically and on CT or MRI (Fig. 7.8). At follow-up there may be complete resolution; however, there may also be evidence of calcification or haemorrhage. Persistence of enhancement in treated lesions correlates with subsequent recurrence of the disease.[10]

One of the major diagnostic challenges in imaging patients with AIDS is differentiating between toxoplasmosis and primary CNS lymphoma. In some circumstances it is not possible on imaging alone to make this distinction. It is also of note that toxoplasmosis and lymphoma may co-exist in the same patient.[11] Other factors are important in the diagnosis such as rising titres of *Toxoplasma* antibodies. Haemorrhage is uncommon in primary lymphoma in immunocompetent patients. Haemorrhage does occur in lesions of toxoplasmosis (Fig. 7.9). This, however, can be an unreliable finding because in AIDS patients lymphoma behaves somewhat differently from that seen in the immunocompetent population. Hence haemorrhage can occur in lymphoma in patients with AIDS.

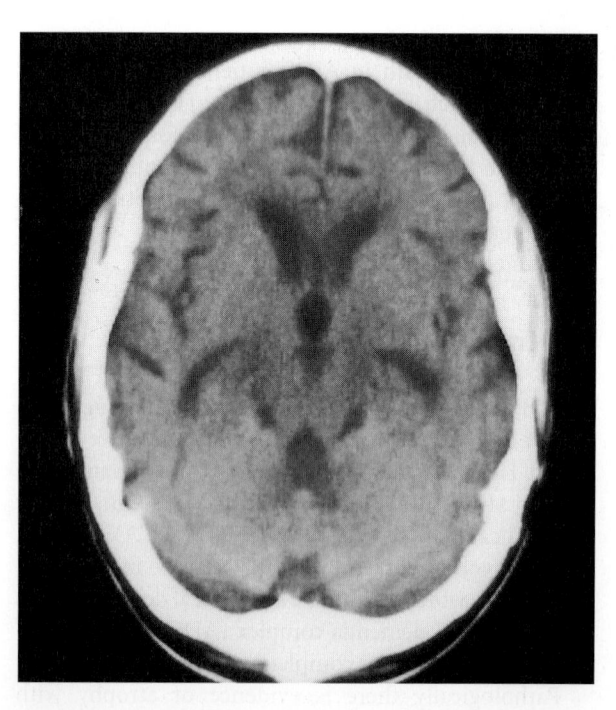

Figure 7.4 *HIV infection. CT scan of a young patient with moderate generalized atrophic change out of proportion to the patient's young age. No focal abnormality.*

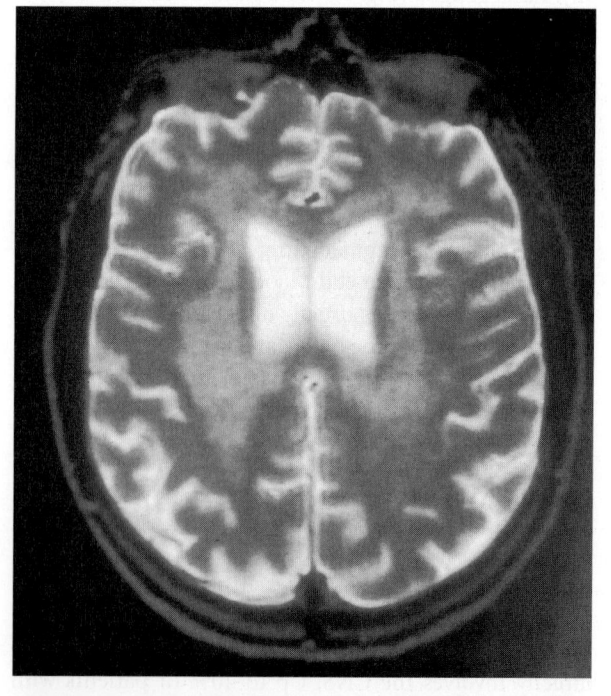

Figure 7.5 *HIV encephalopathy. T2-weighted MRI scan shows diffuse increased signal within the central white matter. (Reproduced courtesy of Dr W K Chong, Consultant Neuroradiologist, Great Ormond Street Hospital for Children.)*

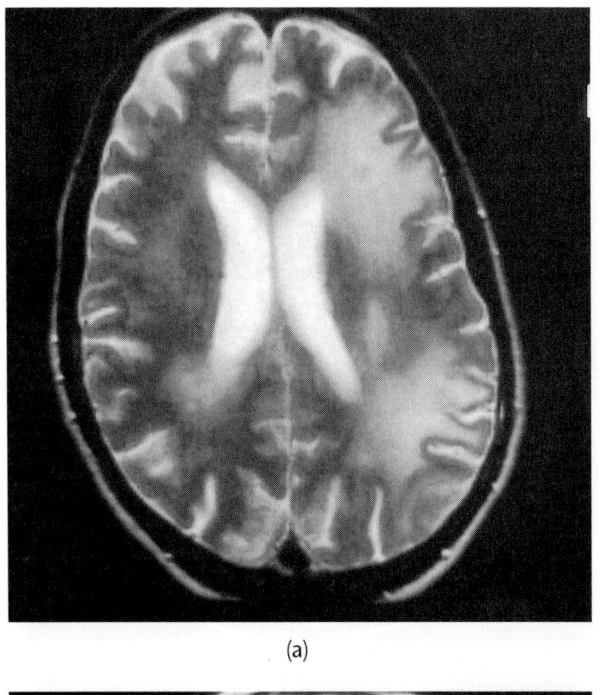

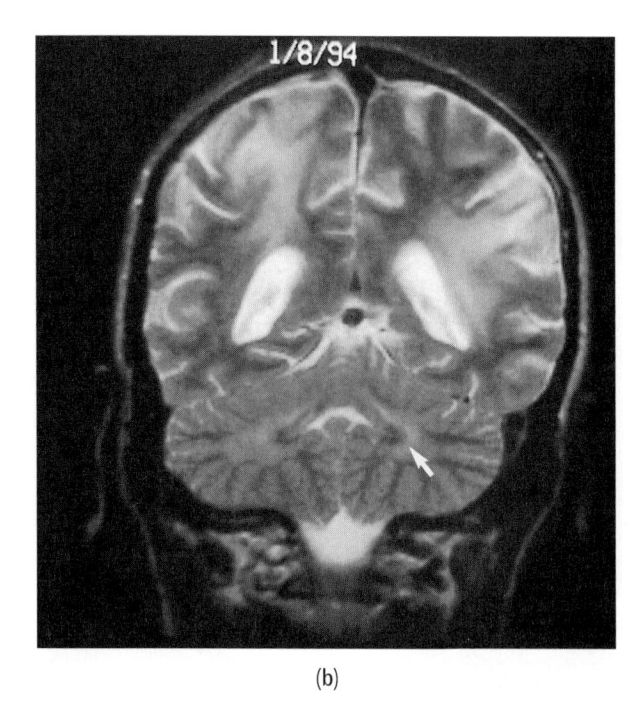

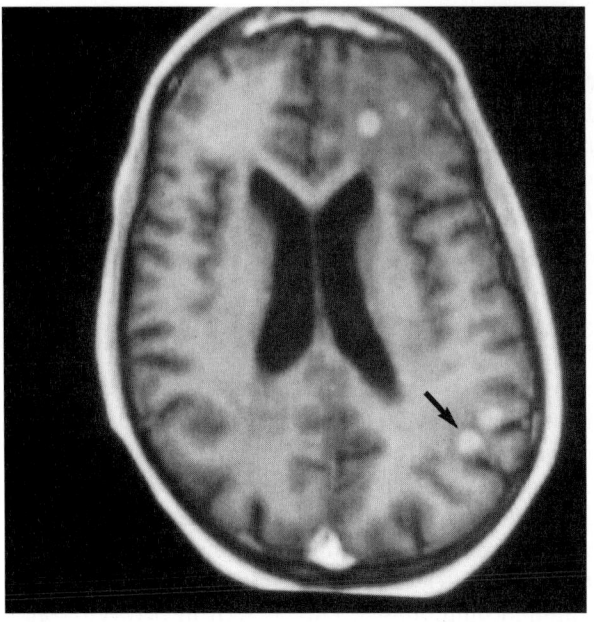

Figure 7.6 HIV encephalopathy with co-existent toxoplasmosis. On the T2WI (a), (b) there are large diffuse areas of white matter involvement. Involvement of the cerebellar white matter with sparing of the dentate nuclei (b) can also be seen (white arrow). In addition to the changes of the encephalopathy, however, there are some small foci of lower signal on the T2WI at the grey–white matter interface (black arrow) which show signs of enhancement following intravenous gadolinium (c). These multiple lesions are in keeping with Toxoplasma infection.

Some features, however, can be useful in distinguishing toxoplasmosis from lymphoma. Multiple lesions favour the diagnosis of toxoplasmosis although lymphoma may also be multifocal in up to 50% of cases (Fig. 7.10). In general, however, *Toxoplasma* lesions are more numerous and smaller than lymphoma. On the other hand 70% of solitary lesions are lymphomas.[12] Biopsy of solitary lesions (rather than the empirical use of anti-*Toxoplasma* chemotherapy) is therefore advocated by some with early use of radiotherapy. This may prolong the mean survival in patients with lymphoma by a factor of three. Delaying radiotherapy results in a poorer response. In addition to this, delaying biopsy until after an empirical trial of anti-*Toxoplasma* chemotherapy may allow some fulminant lymphomas to progress rapidly with doubling times of less than 2 weeks.[13] *Toxoplasma* lesions typically occur at the grey–white matter interface or in the basal ganglia whilst periventricular lesions are more typical of lymphoma (compare the small multiple lesions of *Toxoplasma* with the grey–white matter interface in Fig. 7.6(c) with the two large periventricular lesions of lymphoma in Fig. 7.10). Indeed periventricular lesions with subependymal spread and ventricular encasement occur only with lymphoma[14] (Fig. 7.11).

The eccentric target sign[15] is said to be highly suggestive of a toxoplasmosis abscess. This consists of ring

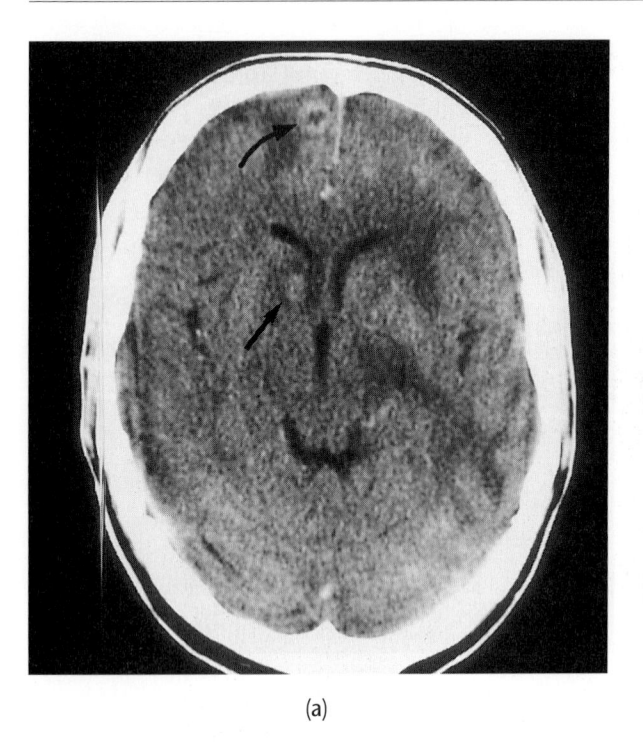

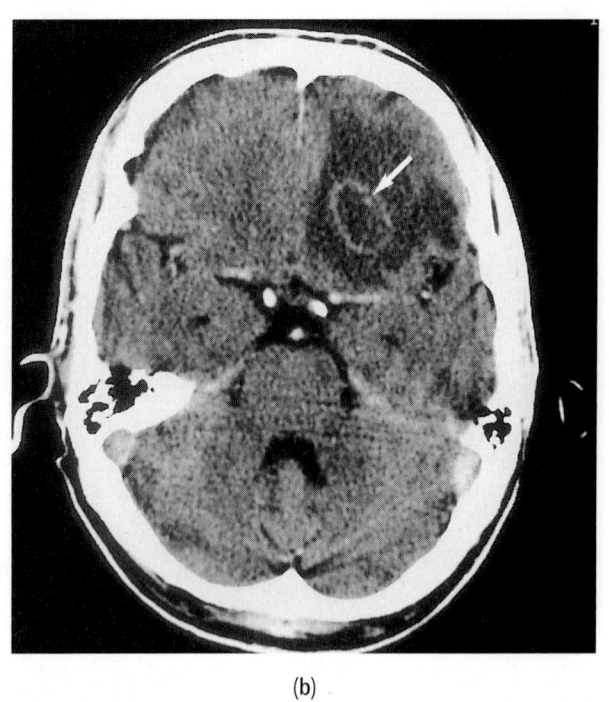

Figure 7.7 *Toxoplasmosis in HIV infection. Contrast-enhanced CT scans (a), (b), unenhanced* **facing page** *(c) and enhanced (d) T1-weighted MRI scans (in a different patient). Multiple nodular or ring enhanced lesions are seen within the brain involving caudate nucleus, (straight black arrow) grey–white matter interface at the frontal lobe on the right (curved black arrow) and the inferior regions of the basal ganglia on the left. Further lesions at the grey–white matter interface are identified on other sections. Note the eccentric nodule sign in (b) (straight white arrow). The MRI scans show a large mass with ring enhancement in the right basal ganglia with a further lesion identified within the cerebellum. (Parts (c), (d) reproduced courtesy of Dr W K Chong, Consultant Neuroradiologist, Great Ormond Street Hospital for Children.)*

enhancement with a small eccentric nodule along its wall. Even though virtually pathognomonic of toxoplasmosis it is only seen in approximately 30% of cases (see Fig. 7.7b).

Thallium single photon emission computed tomography (SPECT) scanning may be a useful tool.[16] There is increased uptake in lymphomas with no uptake in toxoplasmosis lesions or other abscesses such as tuberculosis. Proton spectroscopy, however, shows an overlap between the spectra from toxoplasmosis and lymphoma. Hence this technique is of little value in the differentiation of these lesions.[17]

Recently it has been suggested that perfusion MRI may help to differentiate cerebral toxoplasmosis from lymphoma. The regional cerebral blood volume (rCBV) is decreased in lesions of toxoplasmosis probably due to reduced vascularity of such abscesses. On the other hand rCBV is increased in the actively growing tumour regions of lymphoma.[18]

Progressive multifocal leukoencephalopathy

Progressive multifocal leukoencephalopathy (PML) is caused by the group B human papova virus and as the name suggests it consists of a triad of features: 1) white matter involvement; 2) multiple lesions; and 3) a progressive course. The virus has a predilection for oligodendrocytes which results in their destruction and hence leads on to extensive demyelination. There are multifocal areas of axonal and myelin loss with sparing of the cortical grey matter. Only ever identified in patients who are immunocompromised, PML is seen in between 1 and 4% of AIDS patients. Initially there are multifocal areas of subcortical involvement; however, these become large and confluent (Fig. 7.12) resulting in bilateral somewhat asymmetrical lesions which are most commonly centred on the centrum semiovale in the parietal and occipital lobes.

On MRI there are areas of increased signal on T2WI which are round and oval shaped. These become confluent and at the late stage there may even be cavity formation. Occasionally, with extensive disease, lesions may be seen in the thalamus and basal ganglia. PML demonstrates changes on T1WI and T2WI. This can be used to differentiate PML from HIV encephalopathy which shows changes only on T2WI. On MRI subacute infarcts may have a similar appearance to PML.

(c)

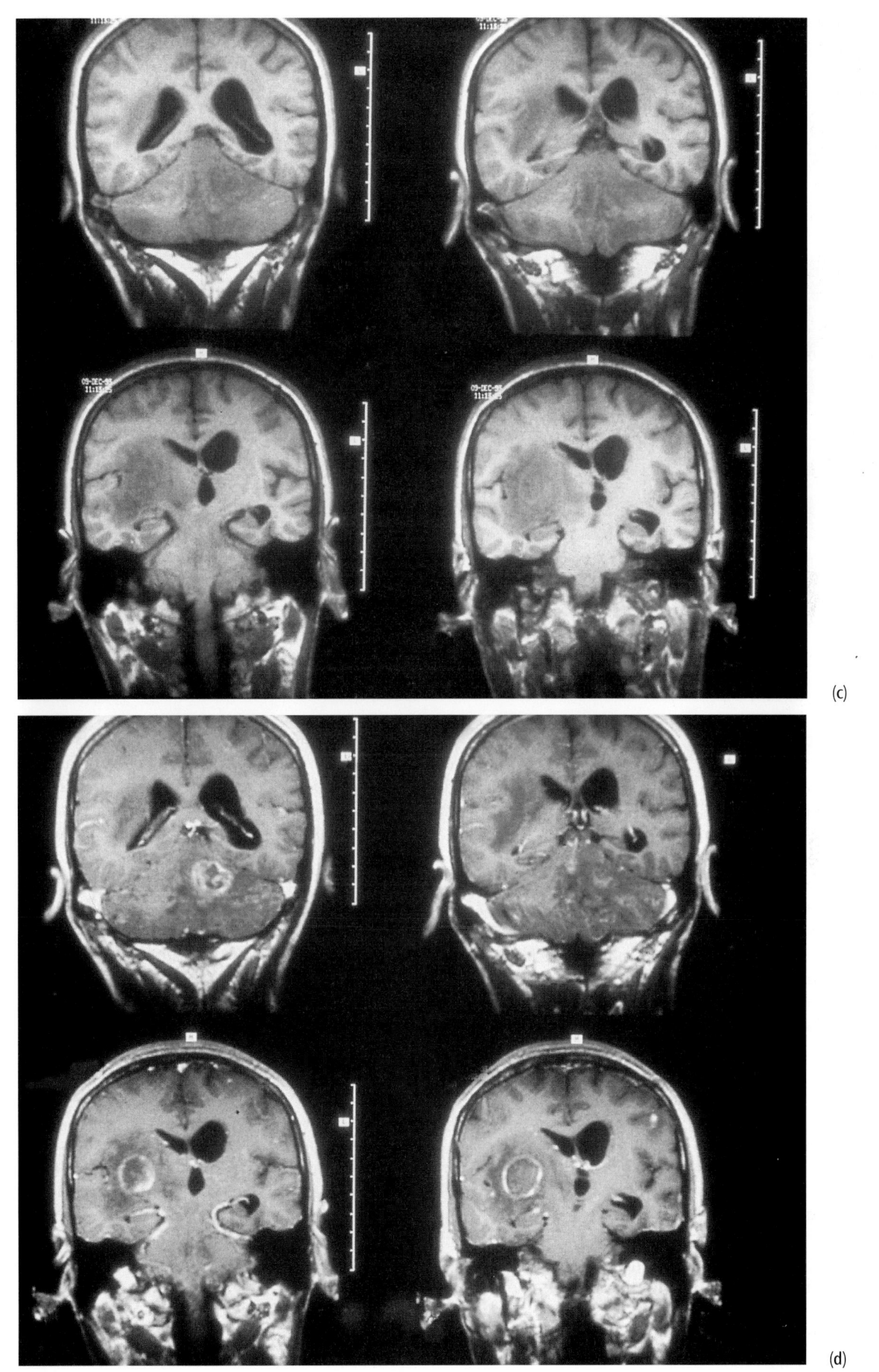

(d)

Figure 7.7 (*Continued*)

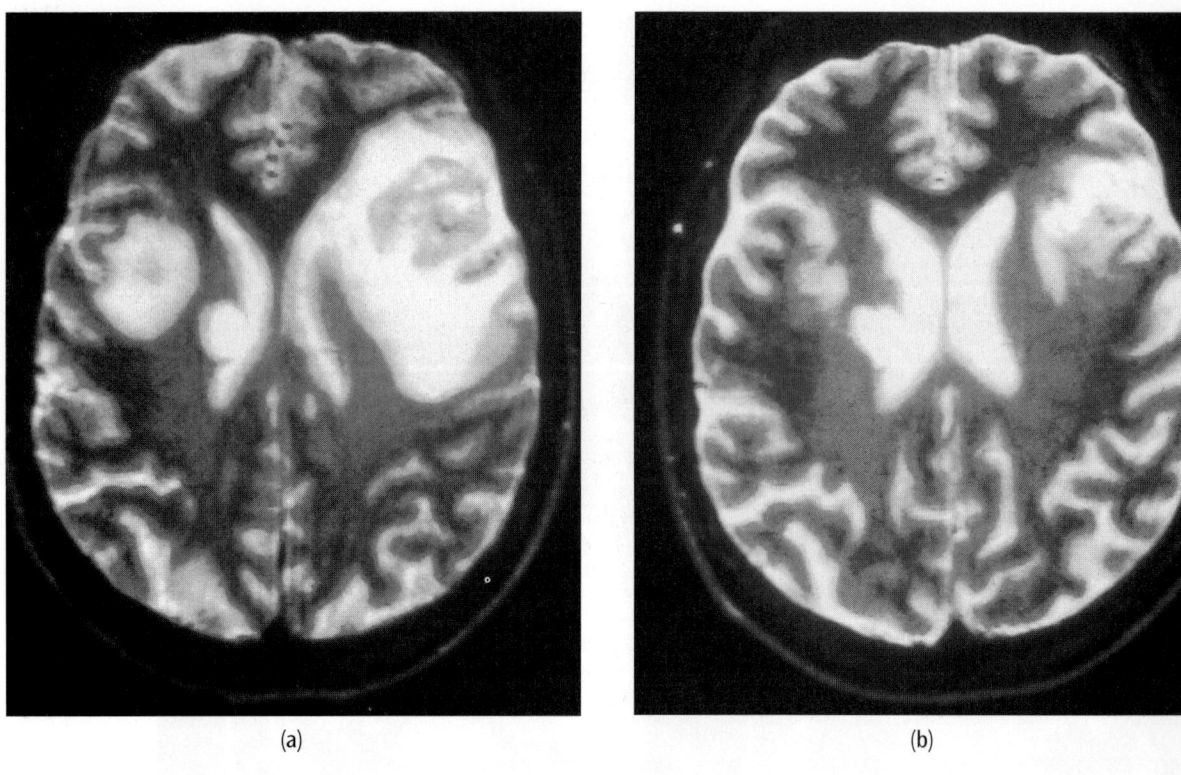

Figure 7.8 *T2-weighted MRI scan shows lesions of toxoplasmosis in HIV infection. Following treatment there has been significant reduction in the size of these lesions (b). (Reproduced courtesy of Dr W K Chong, Consultant Neuroradiologist, Great Ormond Street Hospital for Children.)*

Cryptococcus

Cryptococcus neoformans is a fungus that is usually acquired through the respiratory tract. Haematogenous spread then occurs leading ultimately to CNS infection. In immunocompetent patients the commonest manifestation of cryptococcosis is as a meningitis. In AIDS patients, however, disseminated disease is the commonest manifestion. This usually results in dilated perivascular spaces containing organisms, inflammatory cells and mucoid material.

On MRI there is evidence of multifocal increased T2 signal in the basal ganglia and midbrain together with gelatinous pseudocysts and dilated Virchow–Robin spaces (Fig. 7.13). There is a variable degree of meningeal enhancement. In patients who present purely with crytococcal meningitis there is often no specific imaging feature.

Other organisms

Pyogenic infection of the CNS is uncommon in AIDS patients except in intravenous drug abusers using non-sterile needles.

Neurosyphilis is caused by the spirochete *Treponaema pallidum*. Neurosyphilis may manifest from weeks to decades following the initial infection. There has been a dramatic increase in the incidence of neurosyphilis in the AIDS population.[19] The picture is confused by a high incidence of false negative Venereal Disease Research Laboratories results on testing CSF.

Neurosyphilis results in a small vessel endarteritis. This pattern of meningovascular syphilis results in infarctions within the basal ganglia and other vascular territories particularly the middle cerebral artery. Indeed it is necessary to consider neurosyphilis in any young patient presenting with a stroke. Such infarctions may also present atypically with a subacute syndrome. White matter lesions are also seen, presumably being related to ischaemia. Cerebral gummas may also occur but are very rare. These are manifest as peripheral enhancing masses. Cranial nerve involvement may occur, particularly the optic and vestibulocochlear nerves.

Tuberculosis is a disease which is seen with increasing frequency, particularly within the AIDS population.[20] The incidence of tuberculosis depends on the local prevalence. There is a strong correlation, however, with intravenous drug abuse. In tuberculous meningitis MR- and CT show signs of hydrocephalus with marked meningeal enhancment (Fig. 7.14). Areas of ischaemia may be seen especially in the basal ganglia due to involvement of the lenticulostriate arteries by the thick exudate in the basal cisterns. Parenchymal lesions occur

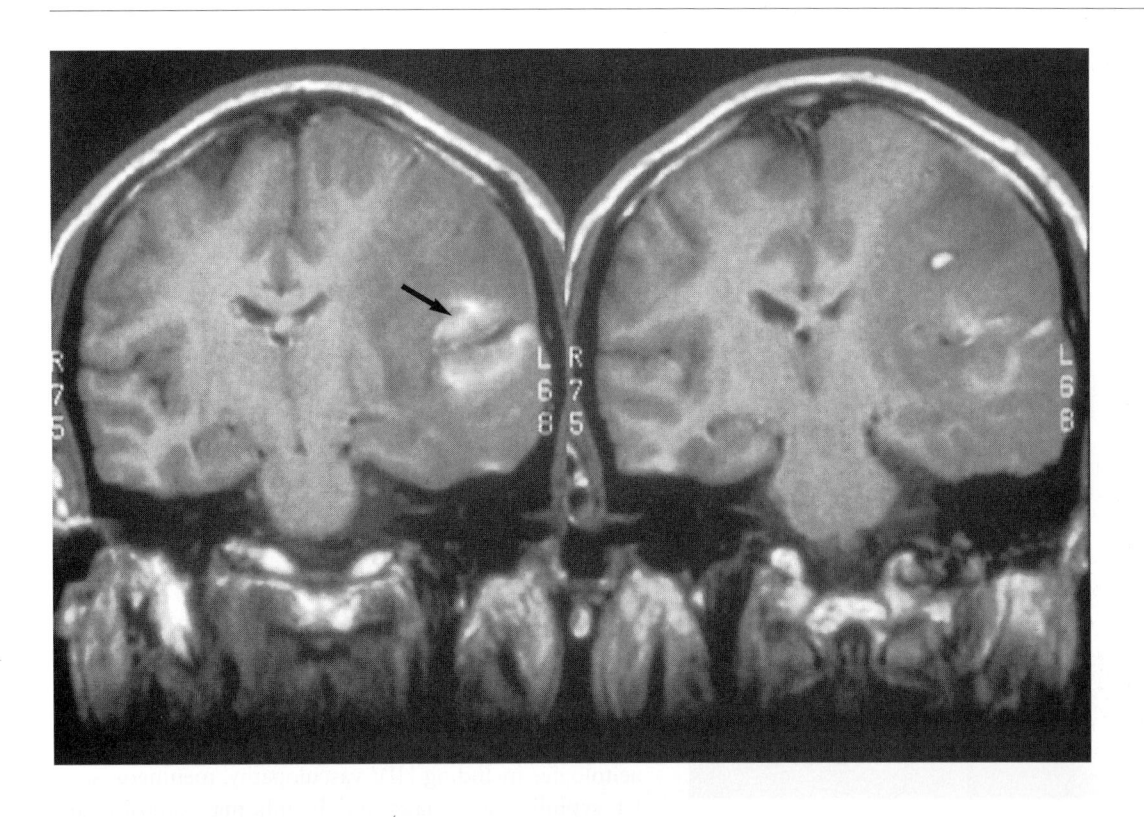

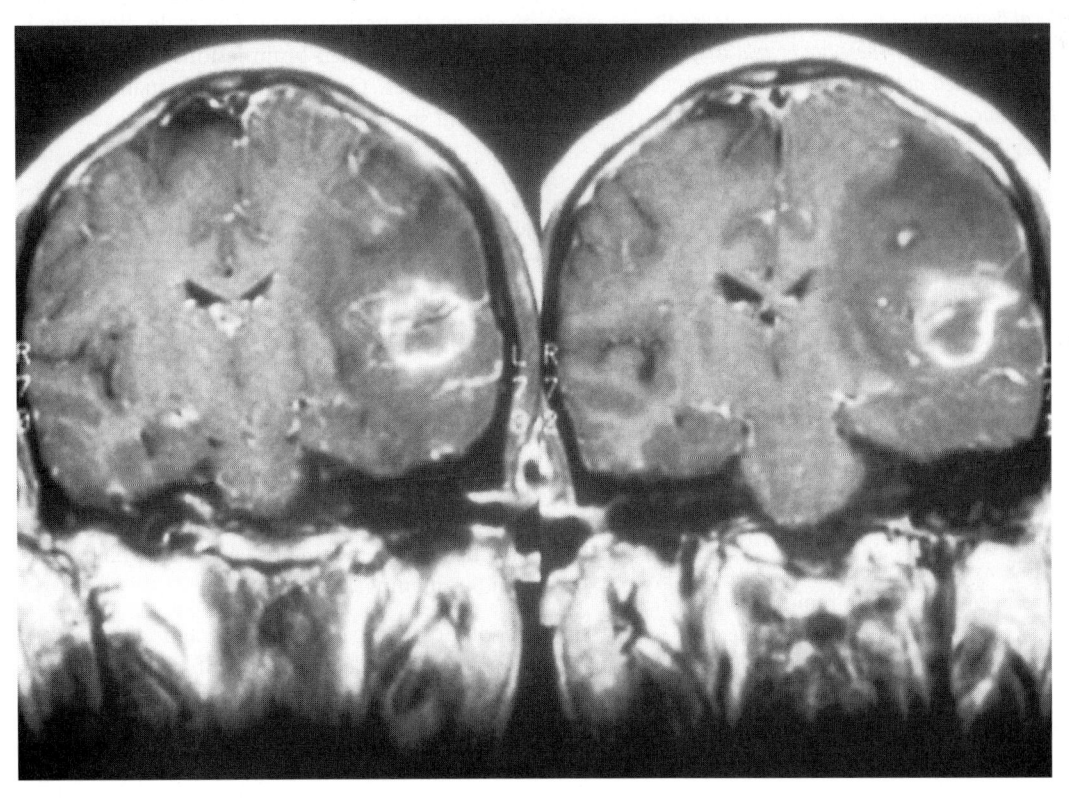

Figure 7.9 *T1WI before (a) and after (b) intravenous gadolinium in a patient with a large single focus of toxoplasmosis. This is situated at the grey–white matter interface in the region of the left sylvian fissure. Before gadolinium (a) there is evidence of high signal which is indicative of haemorrhage into the lesion (black arrow). (Reproduced courtesy of Dr T J Hodgson, Consultant Neuroradiologist, Royal Hallamshire Hospital, Sheffield.)*

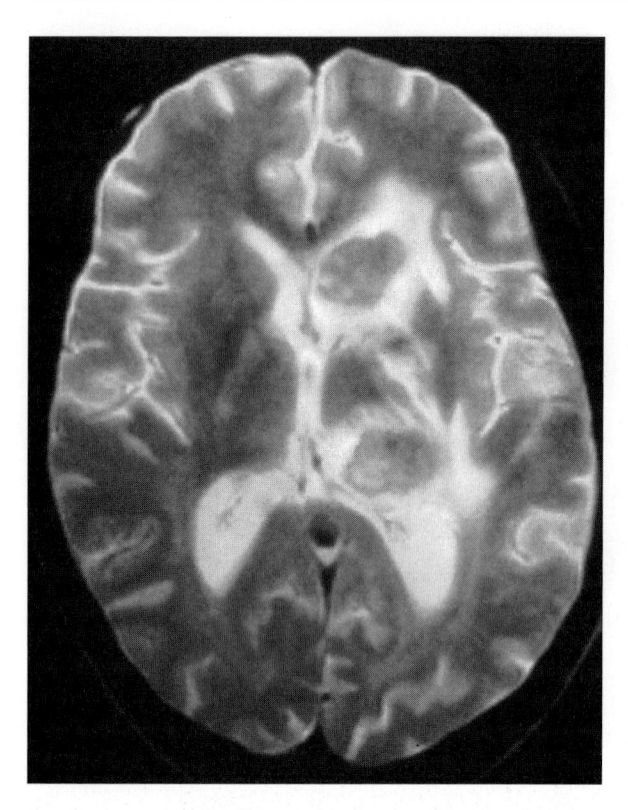

Figure 7.10 *Multifocal lymphoma. Two large lesions are identified in a periventricular distribution. These are of relatively low signal on the T2WI and are well defined by the adjacent white matter oedema. (Reproduced courtesy of Dr T J Hodgson, Consultant Neuroradiologist, Royal Hallamshire Hospital, Sheffield.)*

Varicela zoster is an organism that remains dormant for many years but may be reactivated particularly when there is decreased cell mediate immunity. Reactivation is therefore commonly seen in patients with lymphopreliferative malignancies, immunosuppresive treatments, radiotherapy, AIDS and with increasing age. The disease often results in plaque-like myelin loss at the grey–white matter interface. These progress and coalesce with evidence also of necrosis and haemorrhage. On MRI multiple lesions may be identified which have subtle ring enhancement characteristics.

Cytomegalovirus may cause an encephalitis in patients with reduced immunity. It is unclear whether this represents a true reactivation of dormant virus particles. The imaging features are similar to CNS lymphoma with nodular periventricular and subependymal enhancement. This may result in a diffuse ependymitis.

Other CNS features of AIDS

Infarction of the brain is relatively common, occuring in up to 20% of AIDS patients. There is a wide range of aeitologies including HIV vasculopathy, meningovascular syphilis, candidiasis and lymphoma. Kaposi's sarcoma involving the brain is rare. The scalp, however, is commonly involved. When brain lesions are seen these represent metastases. On CT they are usually of high attenuation and show contrast enhancement.

MENINGITIS

Meningitis is the most common infection to involve the central nervous system. There are three main categories of infection:

1. acute pyogenic meningitis caused mainly by bacterial infections;
2. lymphocytic meningitis which is a more benign entity and is usually caused by viral infections;
3. the chronic form of meningitis which is typified by tuberculous meningitis.

The type of organism that causes meningitis is very much dependant on the age-group of the patient. For example infections within the neonatal period are most commonly caused by group B streptococcus, *E. coli* or *Listeria monocytogenes*. These are usually acquired at the time of delivery either as a consequence of early rupture

in approximately 40% of patients. Tuberculomas (granulomas) may occur with solid central casseous necrosis. These have a hypointense centre on T2WI due to the solid centre. Tuberculous abscesses are rare in the general population but are seen with increasing frequency in the AIDS population. These have a semiliquid centre teaming with bacilli. They are often larger than tuberculomas and are multiloculated.

Diagnosis of tuberculosis is aided by the CSF findings of a low glucose and high protein. Culture of the bacilli takes a long time (6–8 weeks); however, the technique of polymerase chain reaction may give a rapid answer.

Herpes simplex (type 1 and type 2) viral infection is relatively uncommon in patients with reduced immunity. In these patients with reduced immunity the temporal lobe predilection seen in an immunocompetent patient is not present and hence there is a diffuse encephalitis.

Figure 7.11 (facing page) *Lymphoma in HIV infection. Contrast-enhanced CT scan (a), (b), T2-weighted MRI (c), contrast-enhanced T1-weighted MRI scans (d), (e), (f). There is a large mass with irregular contrast enhancement in the right frontal lobe causing significant mass effect. On the CT scan there is evidence of minor subependymal enhancement in the right frontal horn (black arrow (b)). The MRI scan shows a mass of relatively low intensity surrounded by oedema on T2WI. Following gadolinium there is irregular enhancement of the mass within the frontal lobe together with marked subependymal enhancement resulting in encasement of the right frontal horn (black arrow heads (d,e)). This feature is very typical of lymphoma.*

Meningitis 223

(a)

(b)

(c)

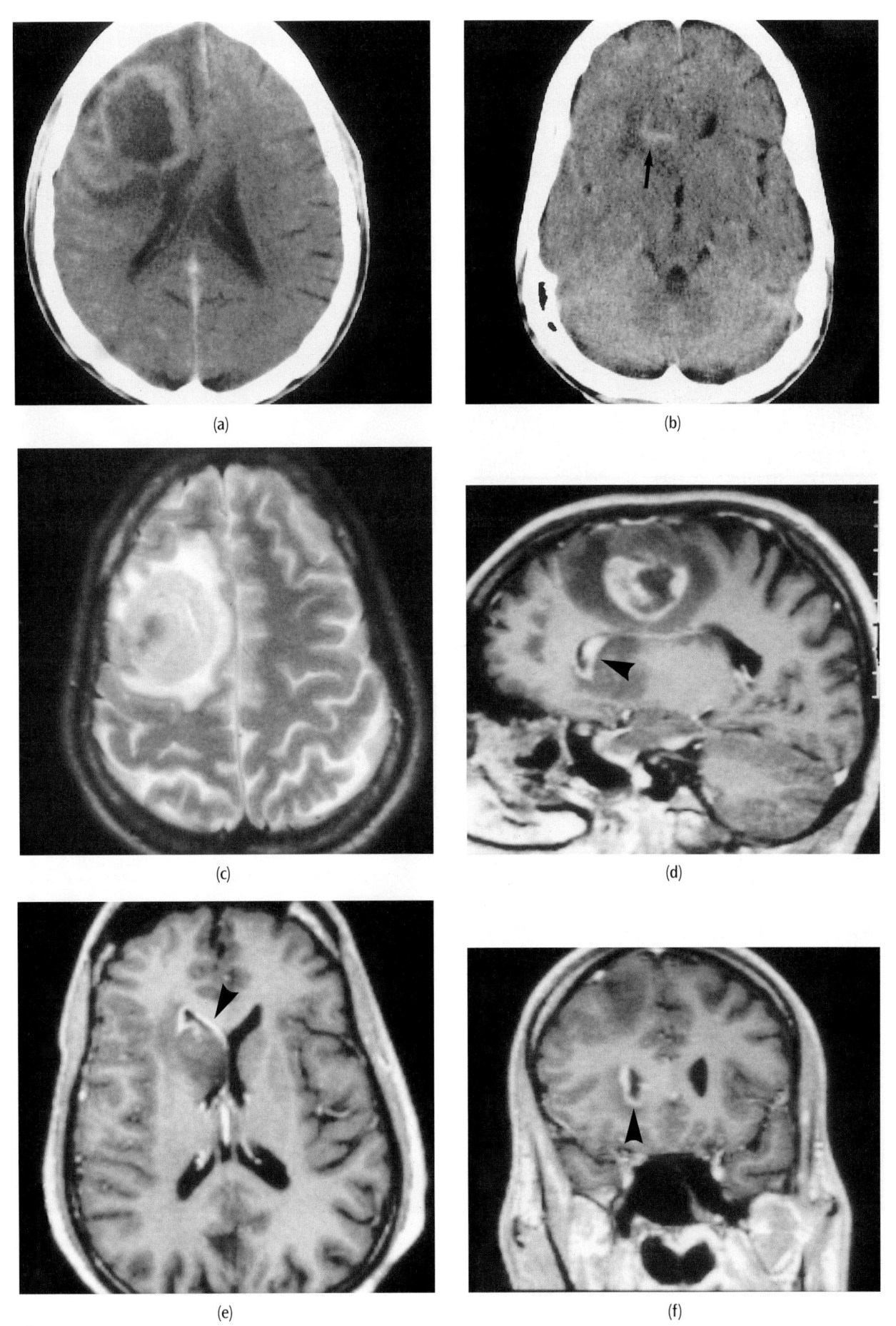

(d)

(e)

(f)

Figure 7.11

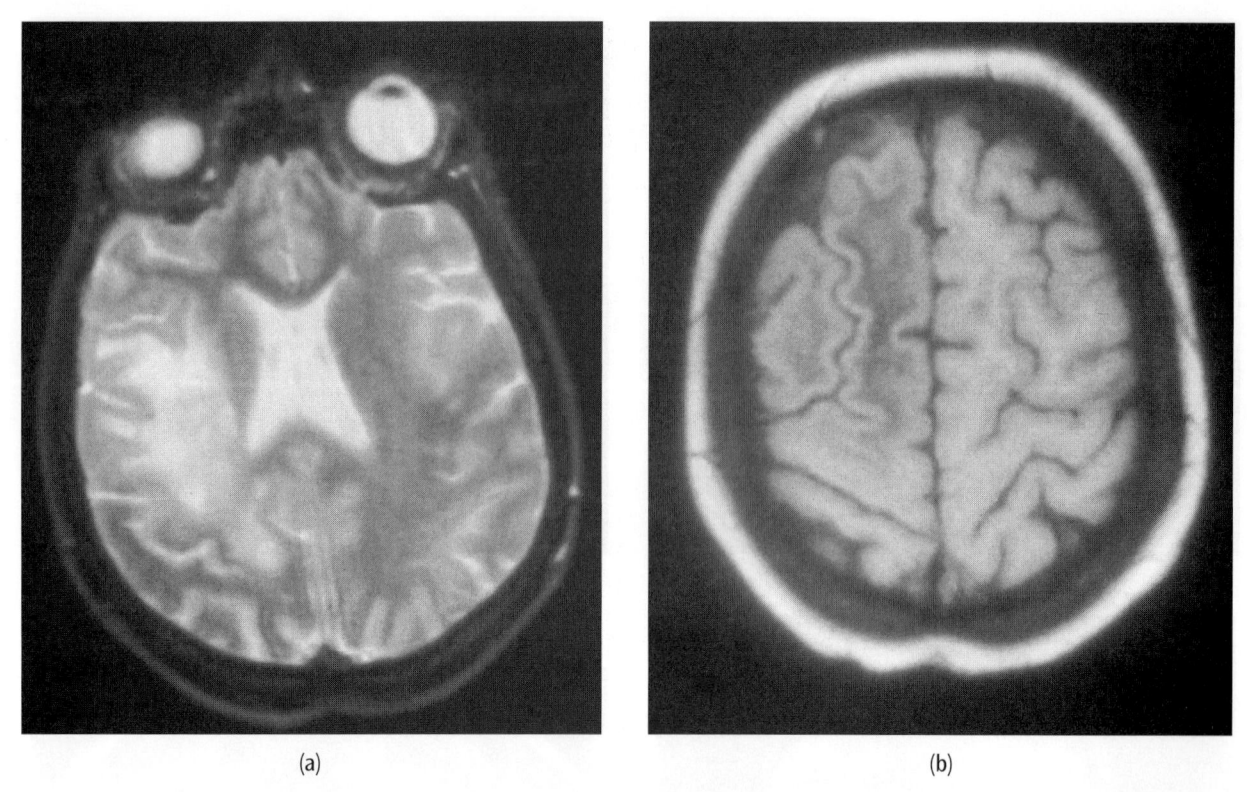

Figure 7.12 *Progressive multifocal leucoencephalopathy (PML) showing involvement of the white matter in the right hemisphere. (Reproduced courtesy of Dr W K Chong, Consultant Neuroradiologist, Great Ormond Street Hospital for Children.)*

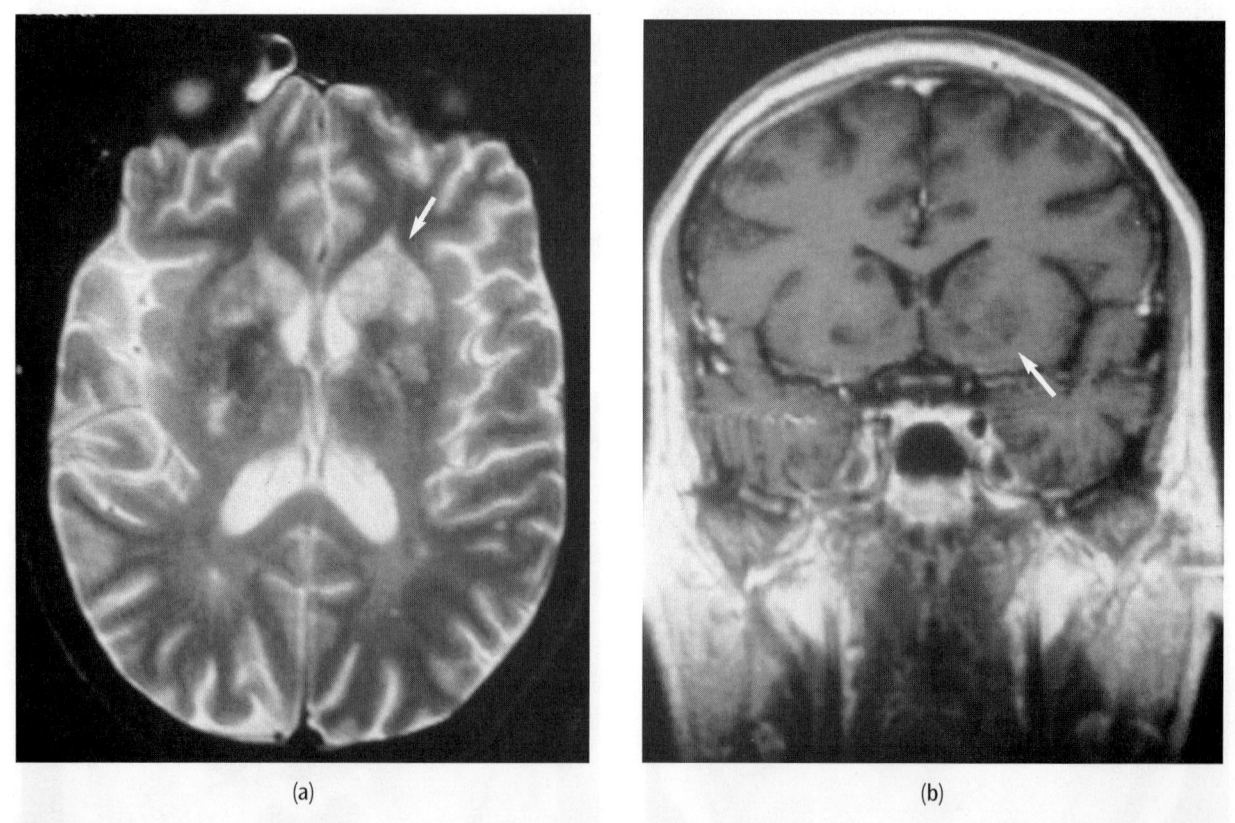

Figure 7.13 *Cryptococcosis in AIDS. T2WI (a) and T1WI (b) show gelatinous pseudocysts extending up into the basal ganglia due to involvement of the Virchow–Robin spaces (white arrows). (Reproduced courtesy of Dr W K Chong, Consultant Neuroradiologist, Great Ormond Street Hospital for Children.)*

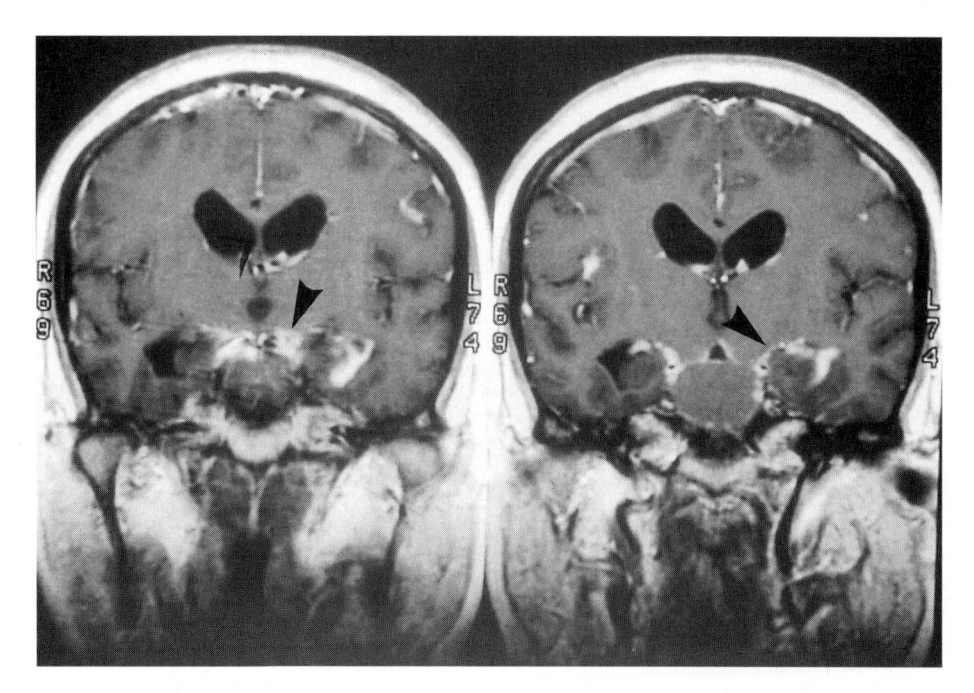

Figure 7.14 *Marked meningeal enhancement in a patient with tuberculous meningitis complicating HIV infection (black arrow heads). (Reproduced courtesy of Dr T J Hodgson, Consultant Neuroradiologist, Royal Hallamshire Hospital, Sheffield.)*

of the membranes or maternal genitourinary tract infection. Alternatively they may be related to reduced immunity in the immature neonate or they may be related to indwelling catheters etc in patients being intensively cared for in special care baby units. In children under the age of 7 years *Haemophilus influenzae* is the most important organism. In adults and older children *Neisseria meningitidis* is the main cause of infection whereas in older adults *Streptococcus pneumoniae* is the most common organism.

Most infections resulting in meningitis reach the meninges via haematogenous spread. Alternatively infection may be acquired by spread from local extension of an otitis media, mastoiditis or sinusitis. Head injury in which there is a compound skull fracture may result in infection of the meninges. In children the subarachnoid space does tend to resist infection and even when there are significant predisposing factors an infection tends to be uncommon.

The clinical presentation is that of fever, headache, nausea, vomiting, neck stiffness, occasionally convulsions and papilloedema may also be seen. Particularly in children this is often preceded by an upper respiratory tract or a gastrointestinal tract infection. In the neonate there is a very different presentation. There are non-specific signs of sepsis and it is unusual to detect neck stiffness. Fever and bulging of the anterior fontanelle may also be absent. Seizures may well be the presenting complaint in up to 40% neonates and younger children.

Pathologically there is a thick purulent exudate identified around the brain particularly within the basal cisterns but extending down into the spinal subarachnoid space and also up over the higher convexities. This results in perivascular inflammation and there may be associated vasospasm. These together result in secondary venous or arterial infarction. Venous infarction tends to be more common and occurs especially in cases of meningitis complicated with empyema. Subdural effusions or empyema may also be identified as may cerebritis and abscess formation. Ventriculitis and hydrocephalus are also features that are seen. The hydrocephalus may either be a communicating hydrocephalus due to thick exudate within the basal cisterns and subarachnoid space. Alternatively there may be a true obstructive hydrocephalus secondary to ependymitis involving the aqueduct. The inflammatory response microscopically is seen to spread into the brain along Virchow–Robin spaces.

Early diagnosis is important and treatment with antibiotics has resulted in a significant decrease in the mortality and morbidity associated with the disease.

Imaging of meningitis in the uncomplicated case is usually normal. Imaging is often therefore performed in cases where there are complications. Imaging is also used if the diagnosis is uncertain, if there is a neurological deterioration secondary to raised intracranial pressure or if there is an associated focal neurological deficit. In the majority of cases CT scanning is unremarkable although there may be mild ventricular dilatation (Fig. 7.15). The basal cisterns may be effaced due to the presence of a thick exudate which may occasionally be of high attenuation. In demonstrating the presence of exudate obliterating the cisterns, MRI is superior to CT. Contrast-enhancement of the meninges may occur (Fig. 7.16) but this is uncommon even with MRI.

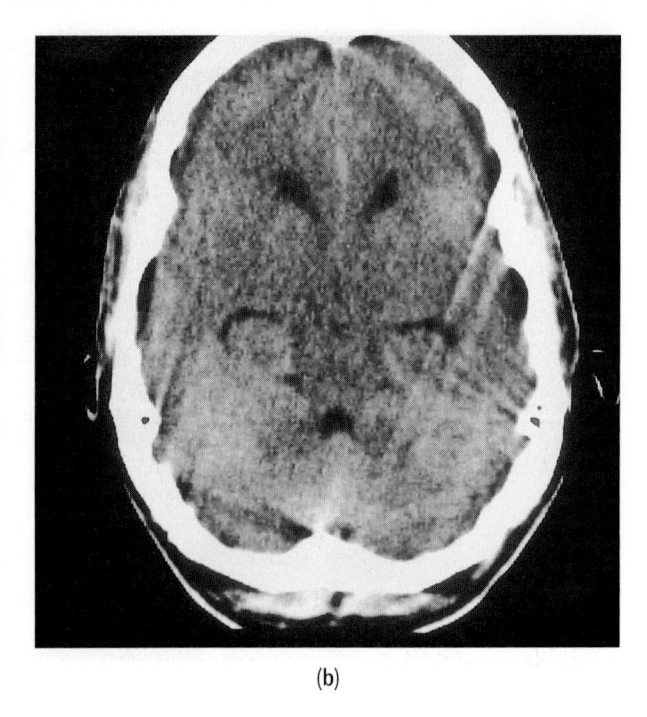

Figure 7.15 *Unenhanced CT scan in a patient with severe meningitis. There is obliteration of the third ventricle indicating generalized brain swelling with raised intracranial pressure. There is prominence of the temporal horns of the lateral ventricles indicating early ventricular dilatation. There is material of high attenuation within the anterior interhemispheric fissure and other subarachnoid spaces which is probably due to haemorrhagic exudate.*

There are some important clinical features that do need to be stressed. The intracranial pressure is virtually always raised in patients with meningitis, particularly children. This may have a number of causes including occlusion of the arachnoid granulations, generalized cerebral oedema and hydrocephalus. The intracranial pressure is also raised following major seizures. The result of the raised intracranial pressure is coning which is a common cause of death due to meningitis. The risk of coning significantly increases following lumbar puncture. This may be delayed due to the slow leakage of CSF through the dural tear at the site of lumbar puncture. Often CT scans are requested prior to lumbar puncture in these patients. Most of these scans will be normal. A normal CT scan **DOES NOT** indicate that it is safe to do a lumbar puncture. The clinical condition of the patient is the most important factor to consider. Even though most children with meningitis are drowsy, a deteriorating level of consciousness suggests raised intracranial pressure.[21,22] Bacteriological confirmation of the organism responsible can often be obtained from throat swabs or blood cultures.

A CT scan may show that it is positively unsafe to do a lumbar puncture. Occasionally other pathologies that mimic meningitis with raised intracranial pressure will be identified, such as posterior fossa tumours, acute hydrocephalus or a cerebral abscess. With generalized brain swelling the third ventricle is obliterated early followed by the perimesencephalic cisterns (ambient and quadrigeminal cisterns) and then the suprasellar cistern (see Figs 7.15, 7.16). Even in children and young adults where the brain is, relatively speaking at its largest volume, the third ventricle is always normally visible. Obliteration of the third ventricle on a CT scan therefore indicates raised intracranial pressure, whatever the age of the patient.

Complications

Complications may be identified in up to 50% of adults with meningitis. The most common complications encountered include hydrocephalus (see Fig. 7.15), ventriculitis, subdural effusion or subdural empyema. Lesions involving the brain *per se* such as cerebritis, abscess formation and infarction may also be identified.

Hydrocephalus may either be a communicating hydrocephalus due to the thick exudate within the basal cisterns and subarachnoid spaces, or alternatively it may be secondary to ependymitis and consequent obstruction of the aqueduct. The hydrocephalus usually clears spontaneously following resolution of infection. Ventriculitis is particularly common in young children, especially so in neonates where it is identified in more than 90% of cases. The ventricles are usually dilated and there is associated ependymal enhancement. Loculations may be identified within the ventricles and occasionally fluid collections are seen outside of the ventricular sys-

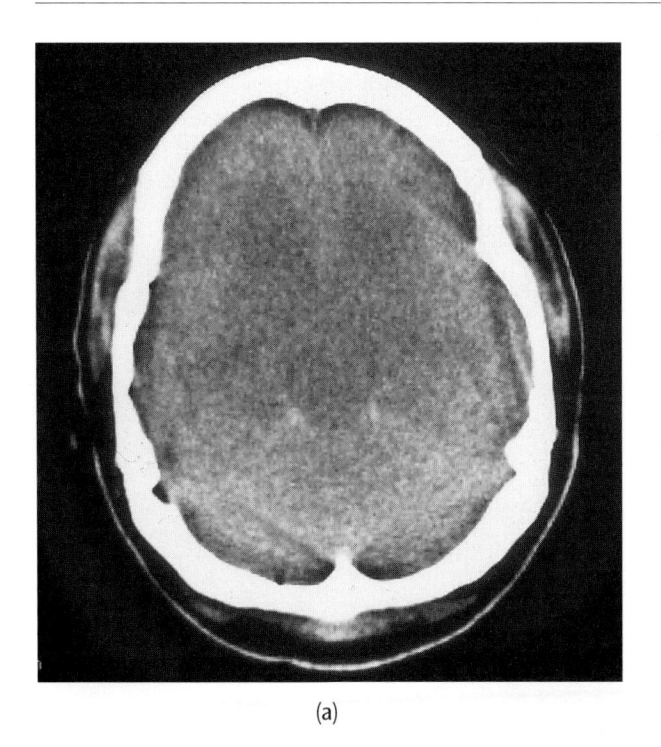

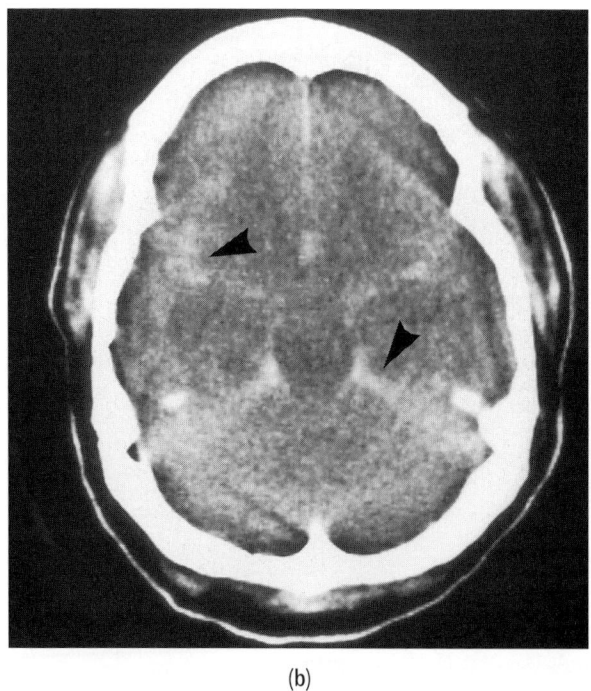

Figure 7.16 *Unenhanced and (a) enhanced (b) CT scans in a patient with severe meningitis. On the unenhanced scan there is evidence of generalized brain swelling with obliteration of the third ventricle and the basal cisterns. Following contrast enhancement there is a moderate degree of meningeal enhancement (black arrow heads).*

tem. This is presumed to be due to necrosis within the periventricular tissues. Enhancement of the choroid plexus resulting in a plexitis can occasionally be seen in these patients.

Subdural effusions are particularly common in children, especially when *Haemophilus influenzae* is the infecting organism. Between 20% and 50% of children under 1 year of age develop these sterile subdural effusions. Some of these may become secondarily infected. Usually the subdural effusions resolve spontaneously. The differential diagnosis for this appearance includes the normal prominent subarachnoid spaces identified in children under 1 year of age.

Empyema may be a complication of meningitis (Fig. 7.17). Alternatively the empyema may be acquired from adjacent sinusitis particularly the frontal sinus. Empyemas also occur as a postoperative complication. The imaging features of an empyema are a cresentic or lentiform collection which is of low density on CT and hyperintense with respect to CSF on T2-weighted MRI. These are usually situated over the high convexities or within the interhemispheric fissure (Fig. 7.18). There is marked enhancement on both CT and MR of the membrane around the collection. Cortical vein thrombosis and infarction are an important complication of an empyema.

Focal cerebritis may occur as a complication of meningitis. Organisms enter the brain via thrombosed venules leading into the parenchyma. A focal area of cerebritis may then develop into an abscess (see subsequent discussion). Cerebrovascular disease is one of the most common complications identified in adults and may be either due to small or large arterial occlusion or venous thrombosis and infarction. In children there may also be evidence of cerebrovascular disease complicating meningitis (Fig. 7.19). Indeed meningitis is one of the more common causes of cerebrovascular disease within the childhood population. Venous infarctions have a typical distribution. With thrombosis of the superior sagittal sinus there are usually parasagittal areas of infarction. The thalami are typically involved with infarction of the straight sinus, vein of Galen or internal cerebral veins. The temporal lobe is typically involved with venous infarctions of the vein of Labbé or with involvement of the transverse or sigmoid sinuses. Venous infarctions are usually manifest as somewhat poorly defined areas of focal oedema with areas of associated haemorrhage. The haemorrhage typically occurs at the grey–white matter interface and may have somewhat irregular margins. These features can be clearly identified both on MR and CT. There may be gyral enhancment following contrast.

228 Infections and inflammatory diseases

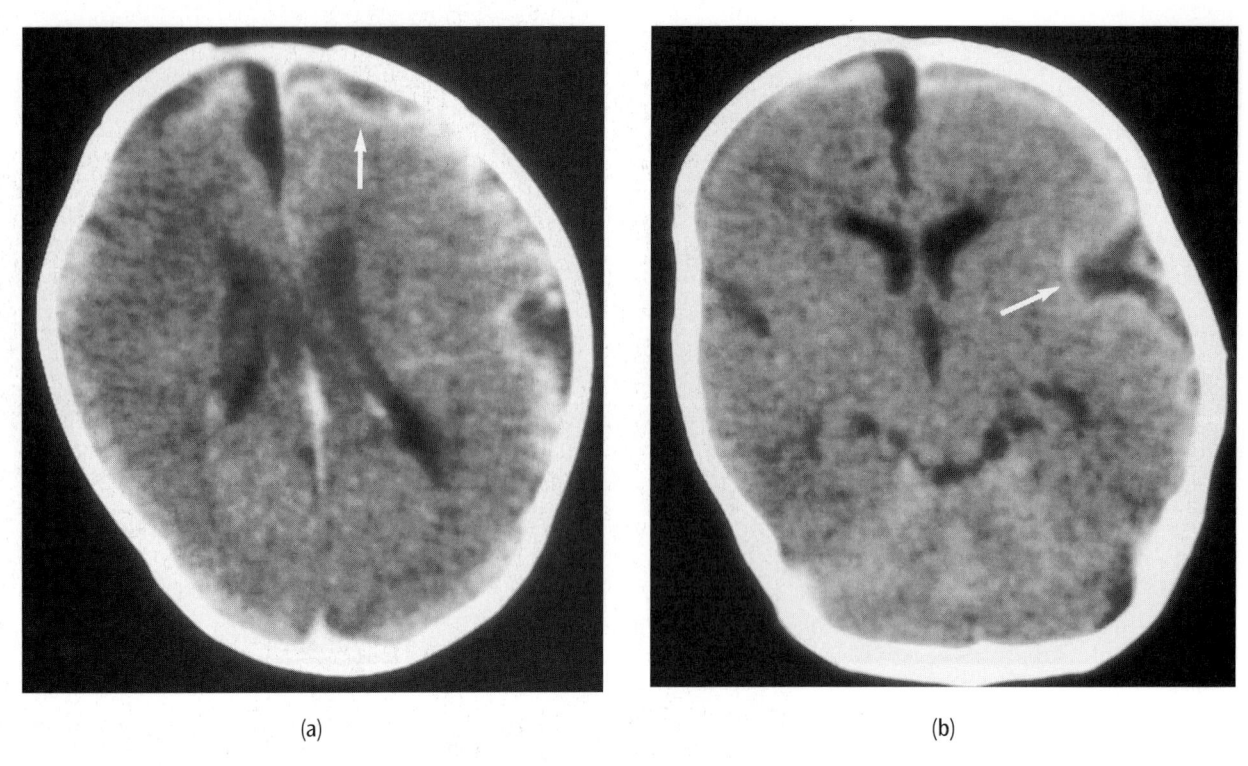

(a) (b)

Figure 7.17 *Subdural empyema complicating meningitis in a young child. Enhanced CT scans (a), (b). Note the enlarged CSF spaces over the frontal and temporal lobe with marked meningeal enhancement (white arrows).*

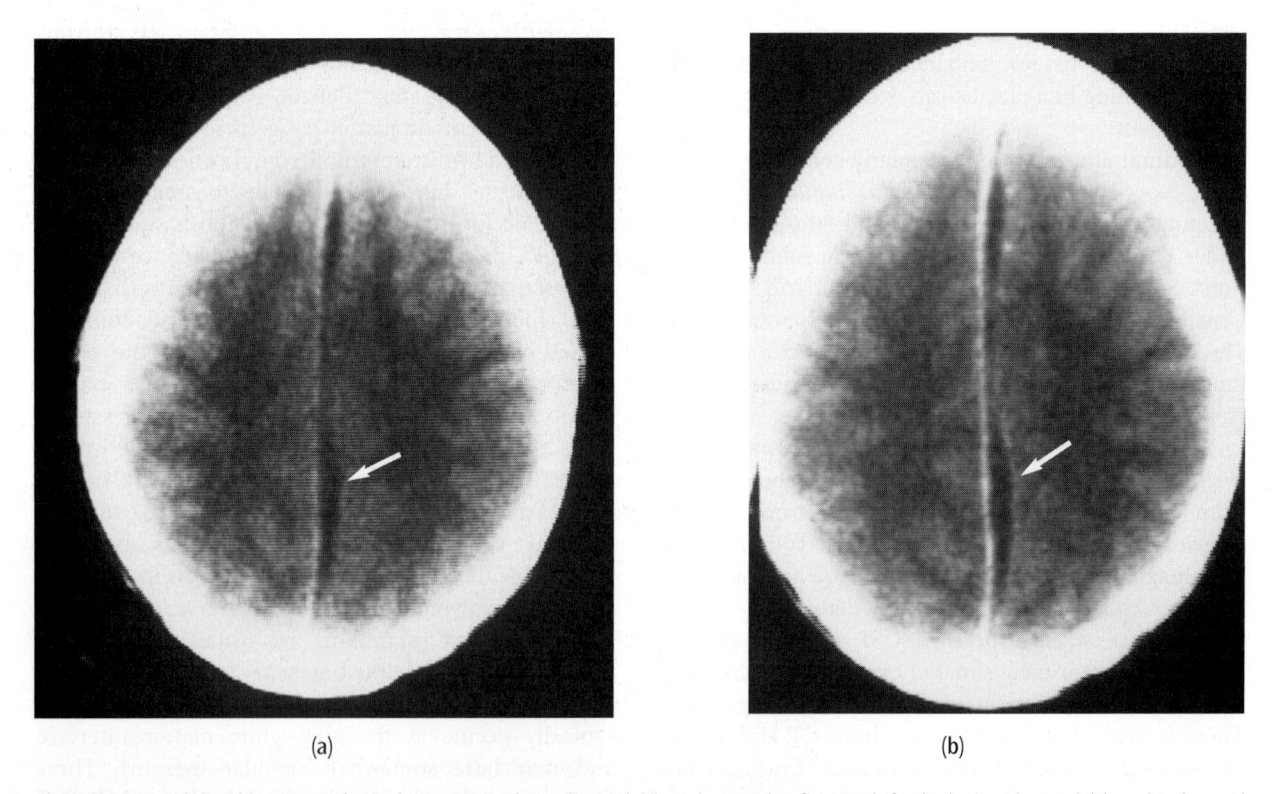

(a) (b)

Figure 7.18 *Subdural empyema in an intravenous drug abuser (although negative for HIV infection). Unenhanced (a) and enhanced (b) CT scans. There is low density collection in the interhemispheric fissure (white arrows) which shows signs of meningeal enhancement following intravenous contrast.*

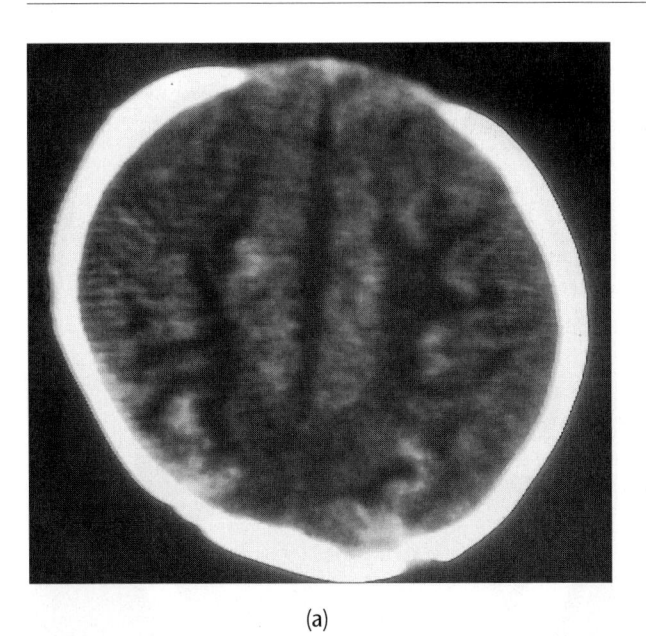

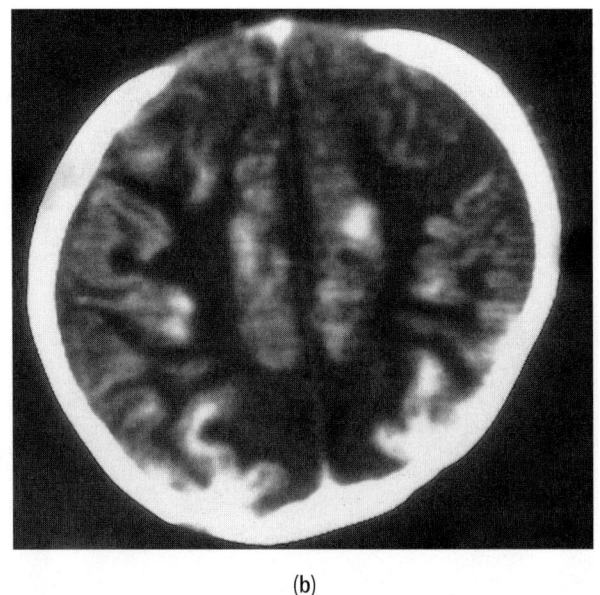

Figure 7.19 CT before (a) and after (b) contrast in an infant with severe meningococcal septicaemia and meningitis showing cortical laminar necrosis. On the unenhanced scan the high attenuation within the cortex may represent either haemorrhage or calcification. Following intravenous contrast there is a typical gyriform pattern of enhancement.

Acute lymphocytic meningitis

Clinically this is a benign and self-limiting disease caused by viruses of which the enteroviruses form the most common group. These include the echo virus and the coxsackie virus. Other agents such as mumps, the Epstein–Barr or arboviruses may also cause meningitis. Imaging in these patients is usually normal.

Chronic meningitis

This condition is typified by tuberculous meningitis although other organisms such as *Cryptococcus neoformans* or fungal diseases such as coccidiodomycosis may also result in a chronic menigitis. Tuberculous meningitis is a major disease on a worldwide scale but is also now seen with an increasing incidence within Western countries due to an increase in the population of immigrants, the homeless, intravenous drug abusers and patients with HIV infection. There is also an increasing incidence of tuberculosis within nursing homes and prisons. Clinically, tuberculous meningitis does not have the typical pattern associated with acute pyogenic meningitic disease. Fever for example may be absent in more than 50%. A high index of suspicion is needed clinically. Pathologically there is a thick gelatinous exudate which is mainly centred on the basal cisterns. There is deposition of fibrin and chronic granulomas with associated caseous necrosis. Haemorrhage, endarteritis and perivascular inflammation are also typical. In children tuberculous meningitis is almost always a consequence of miliary tuberculous. There are often therefore multiple parenchymal abnormalities present in these patients. Children also may have a fairly rapid progression of the disease with death occurring rapidly if untreated. There is a significant morbidity in those patients surviving.

Sequele of the infection are common. These include pachymeningitis, ischaemia secondary to lenticulostriate infarction (which is secondary to perivasculitis), hydrocephalus and atrophy. Calcification is identified particularly around the basal cisterns which may have a 'popcorn' appearance; CT and MRI reveal exudate in the basal cisterns together with meningeal thickening (Fig. 7.20). There is intense basal meningeal enhancement following intravenous contrast. Enhancement may also be seen within the spinal subarachnoid space. Atrophic changes and areas of infarction may be identified. The areas of infarction typically occur within the basal ganglia or the thalamus in the distribution of the lenticulostriate or thalamic perforating branches. Hydrocephalus is very common particularly in children where it may be seen in up to 70%. Since miliary tuberculosis is the most common cause of tuberculous meningitis in children, multiple small foci may be identified within the brain parenchyma itself. These are typically high signal on T2WI and show marked enhancement following intravenous contrast. They occur at the grey–white matter interface and within the distribution of the perforating arteries.

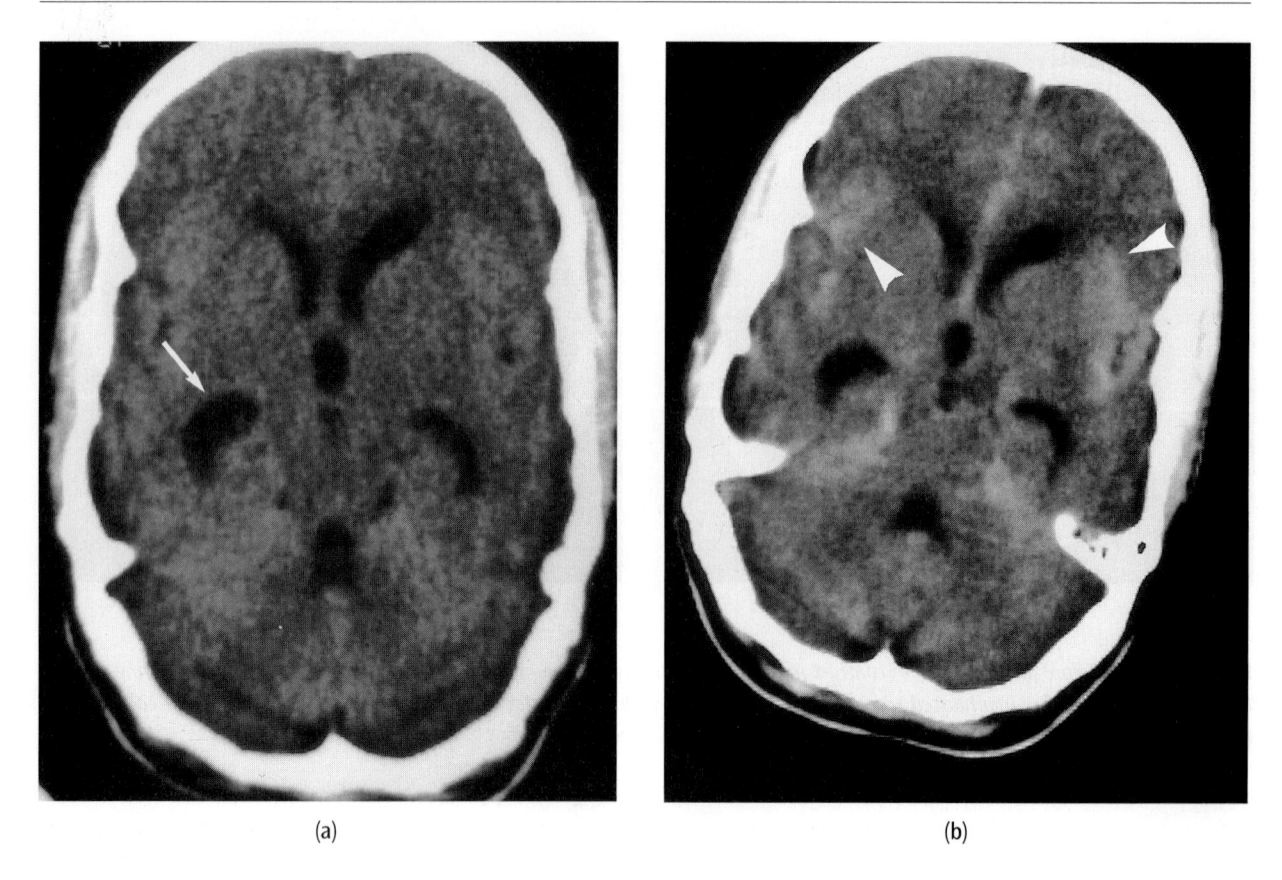

Figure 7.20 *Tuberculous meningitis in a young female immigrant from India with a known previous history of pulmonary tuberculosis. CT scans unenhanced (a) and enhanced (b). There is hydrocephalus with dilatation of the ventricular system, in particular the temporal horns of the lateral ventricles (white arrow in (a)). Following intravenous contrast there is marked meningeal enhancement (arrow heads in (b)).*

CEREBRAL ABSCESS

Cerebral abscesses occur either by haematogenous spread which is the most common route or by local extension from adjacent sinus infection. The commonest organisms are usually mixed aerobic and anaerobic streptococci or staphyloccocus. *Staphyloccocus aureus* is particularly common after trauma or surgery. In up to one-third of patients multiple organisms can be identified. With the increase in the immunocompromised population there has also been an increase in the number of Gram-negative organisms identified. In children and neonates other organisms such as pneumococci, *Proteus* and *Pseudomonas* can also be identified. Indeed in neonates there is often a slightly different pattern with large abscesses with relatively poorly formed capsules. Tuberculosis, parasites and fungi such as *Actinomyces* may occasionally be responsible for intracerebral abscesses.

Cerebritis is the earliest form of infection. This results in a focal yet poorly demarcated area of oedema and vascular congestion with small areas of necrosis and petechial haemorrhage. There is no capsule at this stage. This focus of cerebritis then progresses to become more focally demarcated with coalescence of the areas of necrosis. Eventually a capsule develops with a collagenous rim surrounding a liquified and necrotic centre. There is marked adjacent oedema throughout these stages although the oedema does begin to decrease as the capsule matures and thickens. Most patients present either at the stage of late cerebritis or with a mature abscess.

The most common site of involvement is at the corticomedullary junction particularly in the frontal and parietal lobes. Only a small proportion (2–14%) occur within the posterior fossa. Multiple lesions are uncommon except when septic emboli are the underlying cause (see later).

On imaging studies there may be little to see in the very earlier stages of cerebritis. The first changes are those of mild oedema with possible enhancement. As the lesion progresses the mass effect becomes marked with increasing oedema and development of a central necrotic area. Eventually after a variable time period of between weeks and months there is a well defined rim of surrounding oedema and liquified contents. The content of the abscess is a highly proteinaceous liquid which is therefore hyperintense on T1 relative to CSF. The rim of the capsule can usually be identified as an area of iso- or hyperintensity relative to white matter on T1-weighted sections and is of hypointensity on T2-weighted sections. These signal changes are due to collagen, haemorrhage or possibly free radicles within macrophages. Since the hypointensity of the rim reflects the phagocytic activity of macrophages it has been suggested that resolution of this hypointense rim on T2-weighted sections is a better indicator of successful response to treatment than the degree of contrast-enhancement.

The enhancing capsule is usually smooth and thin-walled (Fig. 7.21) and tends to be thinner towards the ventricular surface than towards the cortical surface. The enhancment may persist for months despite clinical improvement. It is also of note that the volume of vasogenic oedema associated with an abscess may be greater than the actual volume of the abscess itself. Following treatment with steroids there is often reduction in the oedema and thinning of the capsule with decreasing enhancement. In patients with AIDS despite the decreased immunity pyogenic abscesses remain relatively rare.

There is a wide differential diagnosis for ring-enhancing lesions within the brain including primary brain tumours, metastases, resolving haematomas, infarctions, demyelination, thrombosed aneurysms and thrombosed vascular malformations.

Small daughter lesions may be occasionally seen as complications. These tend to develop medially where the wall is thinnest or they may develop from adjacent cerebritis. If there is rupture of the abscess into the ventricle then a ventriculitis and ependymitis ensues. There is intense enhancement of the ependyma in this circumstance which is associated with a very poor prognosis.

Intracerebral abscesses require surgical drainage in most instances. On serial scans following drainage there is reduction in the oedema, mass effect and enhancement. Residual enhancement may persist but is usually resolved after 3–4 months. There is a residual gliotic scar which may occasionally be associated with some calcification.

Septic emboli may occur in intravenous drug abusers (Fig. 7.22), patients with bacterial endocarditis (Fig. 7.23) and in the context of congenitial cyanotic heart disease. With the variable size of these emboli there are either small multiple small abscesses or else large vessel occlusion. Mycotic aneurysms also may occur. These tend to occur on intermediate to small sized arteries and are therefore more peripherally placed within the intracranial circulation as opposed to the more typical

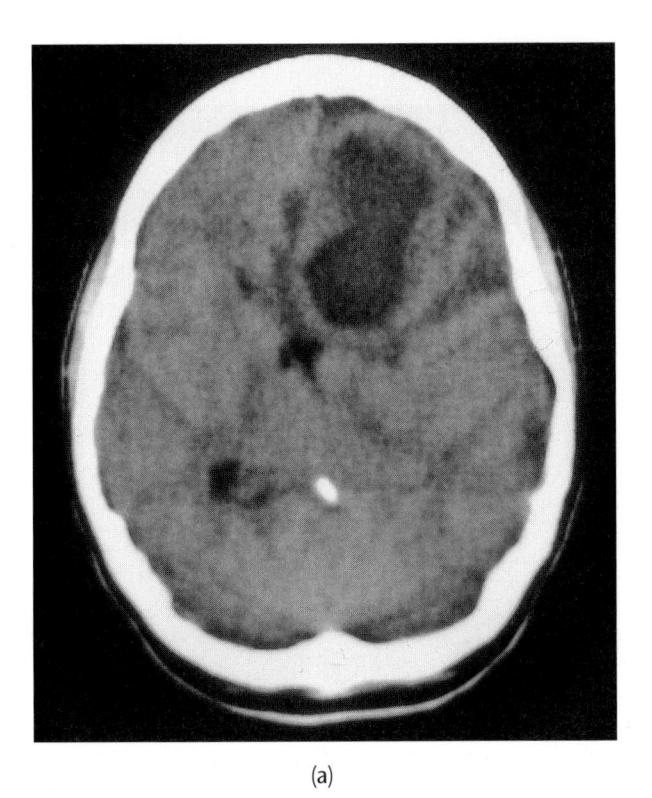

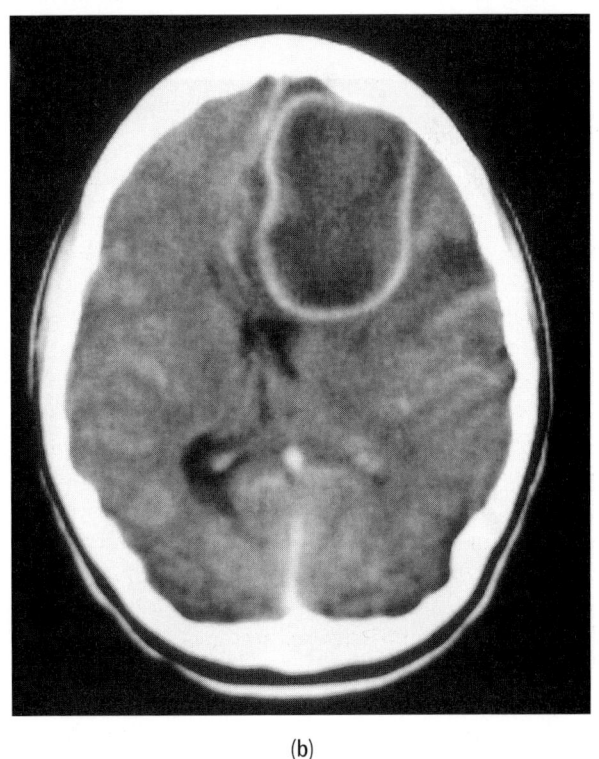

Figure 7.21 *Unenhanced (a) and enhanced (b) CT scans of a patient with a large left frontal abscess There is a well defined smooth and thin walled enhancing capsule with a low density centre and surrounding oedema.*

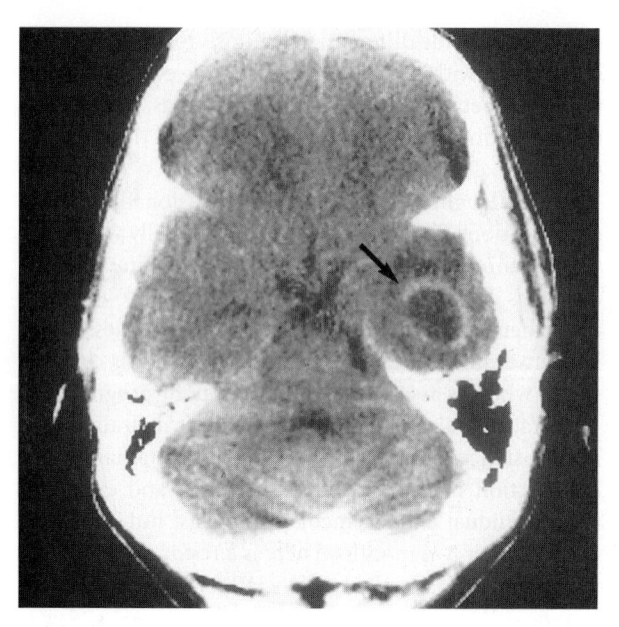

Figure 7.22 *Small left temporal lobe abscess in an intravenous drug abuser (black arrow).*

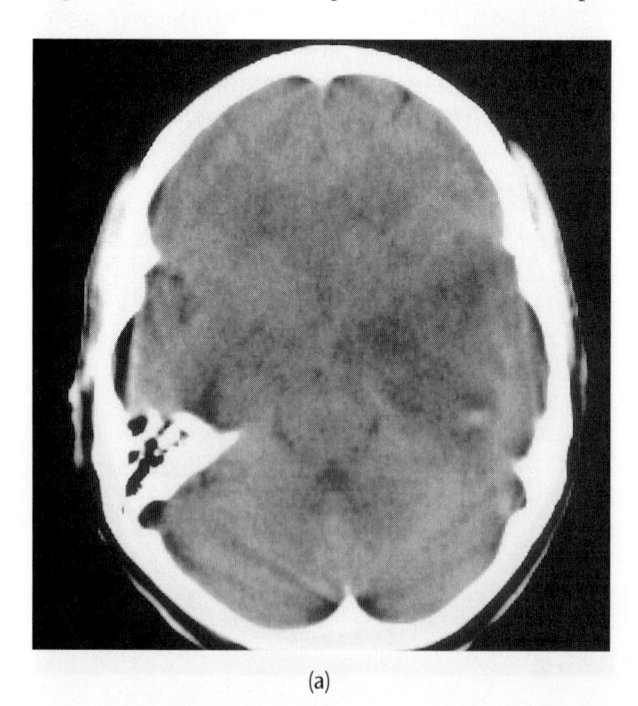

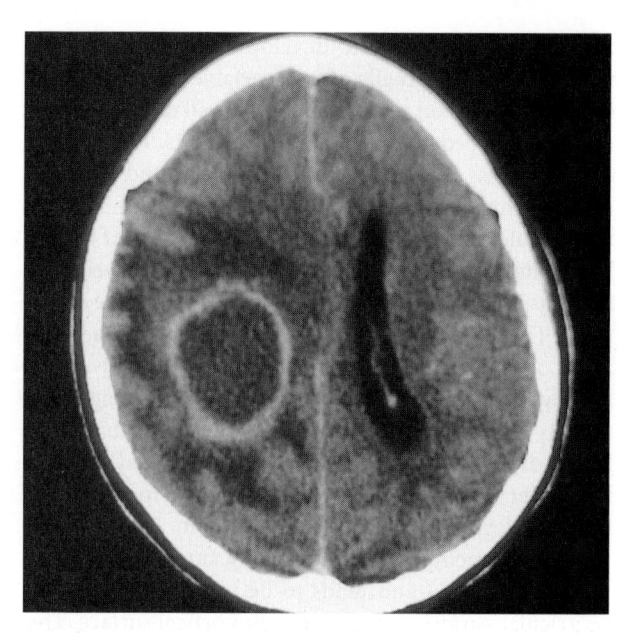

Figure 7.23 *Right frontoparietal abscess in a patient with bacterial endocarditis.*

berry aneurysms. There is usually high mortality should these mycotic aneurysm rupture.

ENCEPHALITIS

Encephalitis is a diffuse infection of the brain parenchyma resulting in a marked inflammatory response. The commonest agent involved is the herpes simplex type 1 virus although other viruses such as the Epstien–Barr virus and mumps virus may also be causative agents.

Herpes simplex encephalitis

The herpes simplex type 1 virus is the commonest agent to cause encephalitis in adults and children. The type 2 virus is the commonest agent in the neonatal period. The

(a)

(b)

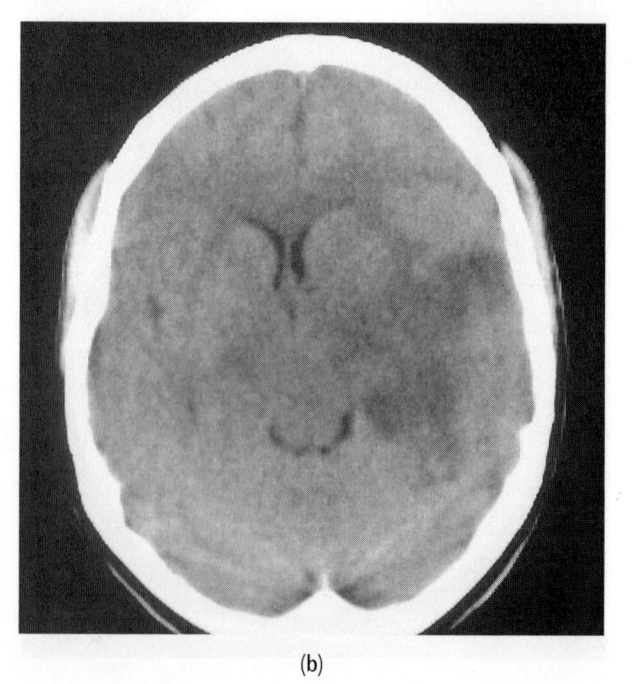

Figure 7.24 *Herpes simplex encephalitis. Unenhanced CT scans show low density within the medial portion of the temporal lobe on the left with some associated mass effect. T2-weighted MRI* **facing page** *(c)–(e) in a different patient with marked involvement of right medial temporal lobe and cingulate gyrus. Note the sparing of the putamen on the axial T2WI.*

(c)

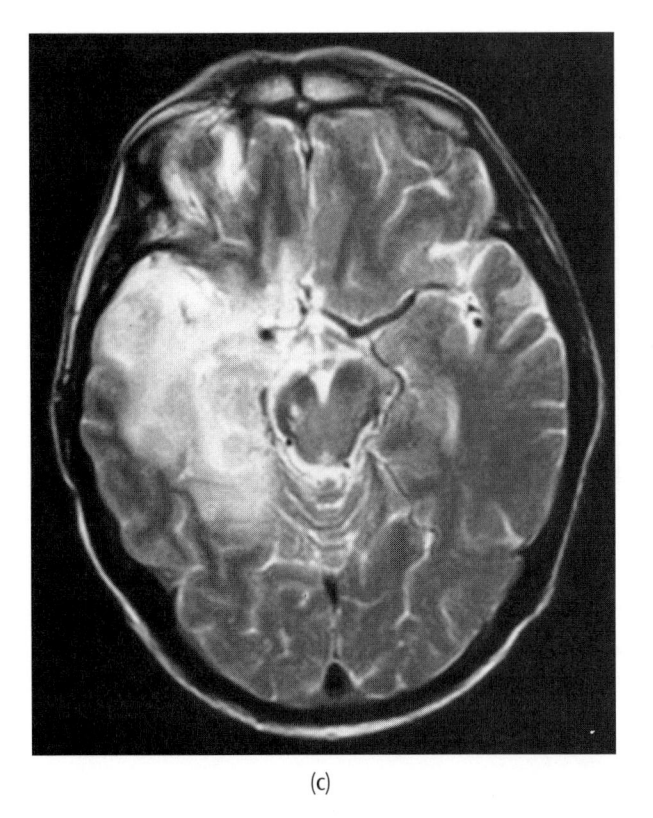

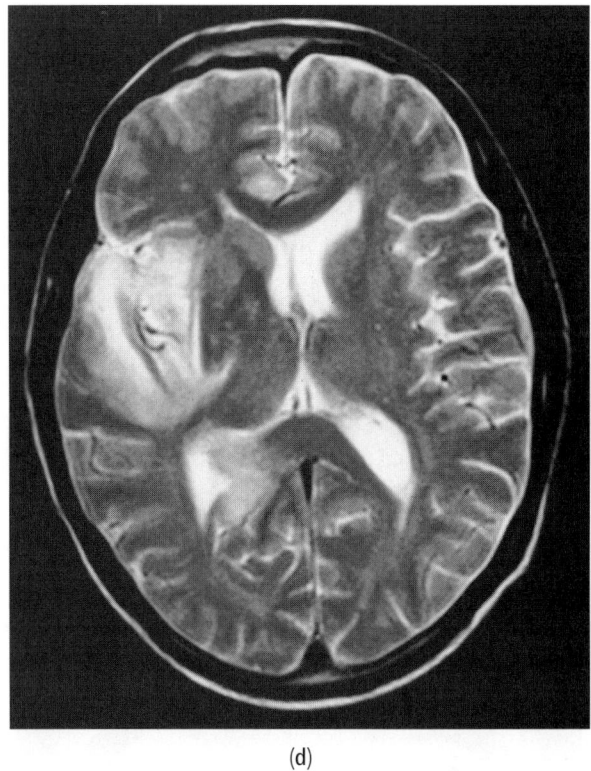

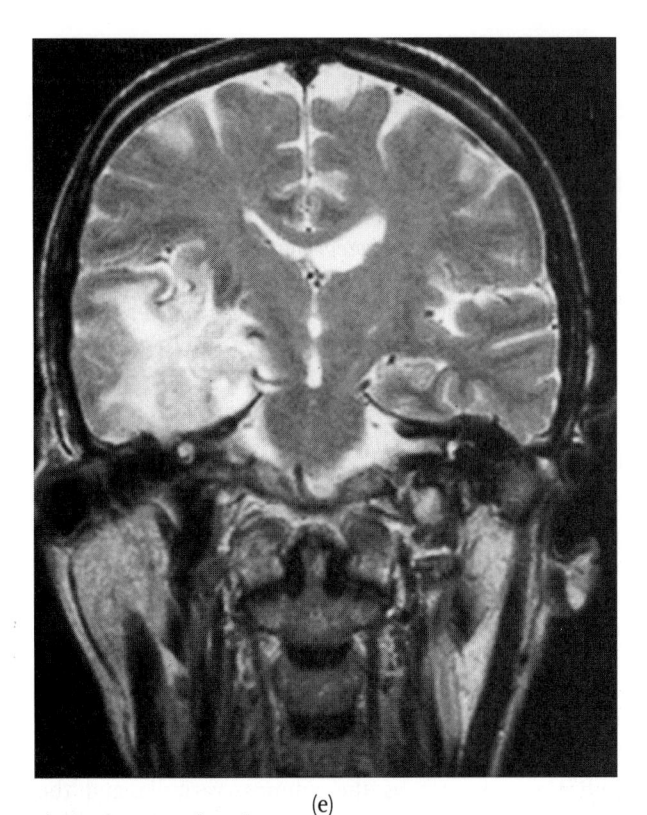

(d)

(e)

Figure 7.24 *Continued*

encephalitis produced by the herpes simplex virus may be acquired at the time of primary infection. Most commonly, however, it is caused by reactivation of latent infection. The virus lies dormant within the Gasserian ganglion and causes encephalitis by retrograde spread initially involving the meninges but then extending into the adjacent brain parenchyma. This meningoencephalitis is a fulminant process with haemorrhage, necrosis and marked local oedema. Histologically there are eosinophilic intranuclear inclusions within infected glial cells or neurons.

Herpes simplex infection usually involves the temporal lobes, insular cortex, subfrontal region and cingulate gyri (i.e. limbic structures). Initially the infection is unilateral but bilateral and asymmetric changes develop. In some instances there may be direct involvement of the mesencephalon and pons.

Encephalitis can occur at any age but one-third of patients are under the age of 20. Clinically the patients present with altered mental state, headache, fever and possibly seizures. It is necessary to maintain a high degree of clinical suspicion as early diagnosis is vital. Untreated the disease is rapidly progressive with up to 70% mortality. Those patients surviving may have marked changes within the temporal lobes with resultant severe memory disorders. Even with immediate and optimal therapy severe structural changes may persist at long-term follow-up.[23]

Serology and CSF analysis are important investigations; however, negative results cannot exclude the diagnosis. Modern techniques such as polymerase chain reaction (PCR) are rapid and sensitive means of detecting viral DNA particles; EEG changes occur but these can be non-specific in the early phase. In the past, brain biopsy was regarded as the means of obtaining a definitive diagnosis; however, there is now often reluctance on

234 Infections and inflammatory diseases

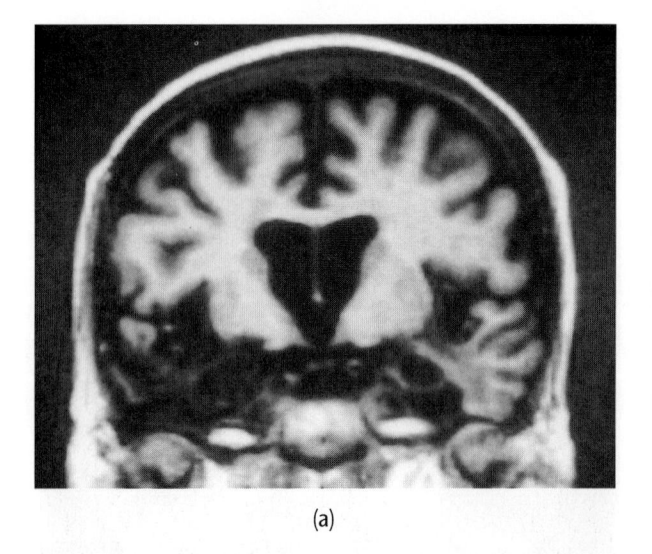

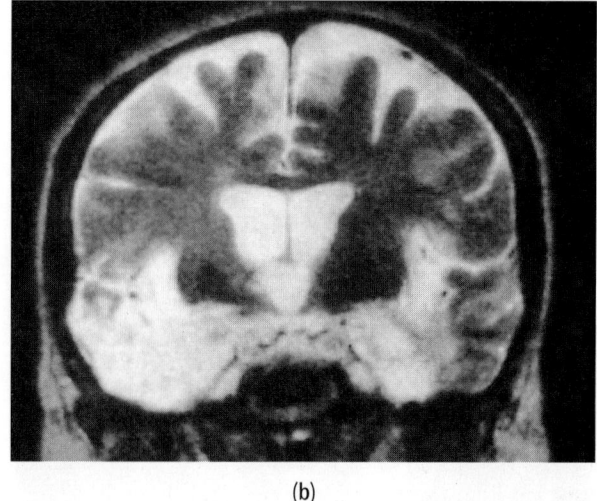

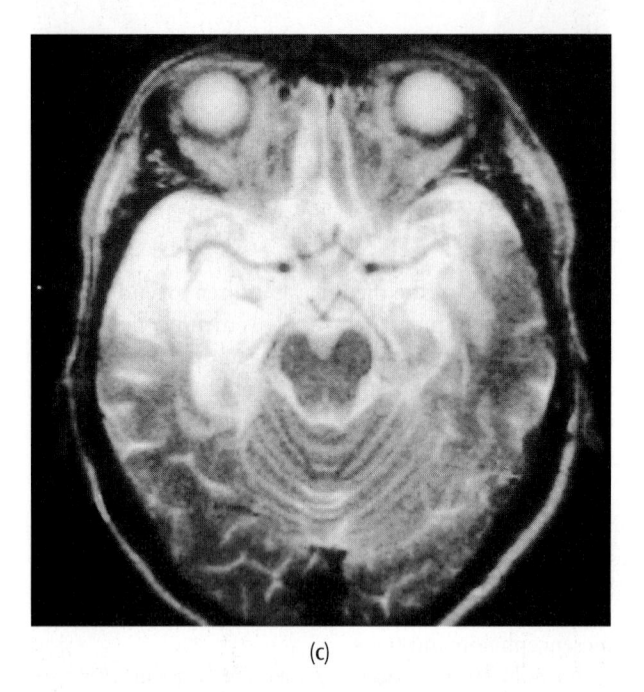

Figure 7.25 *T1-weighted (a) and T2-weighted (b), (c) MRI scans in a patient with severe atrophic changes as a consequence of previous of herpes simplex encephalitis. There is marked atrophic change within the medial portions of both temporal lobes. There is more extensive involvement of the right side compared with the left. This patient had a moderately severe memory disorder due to the temporal lobe damage.*

the part of the neurosurgeons to obtain biopsies particularly in eloquent areas.

In the first few days CT scans are usually normal. Changes, however, do occur after 5 or 6 days with low density and mass effect within the temporal lobes (Fig. 7.24). Haemorrhage may be seen but this is a late feature. Patchy gyriform enhancement may also be identified. MRI, however, is more sensitive than CT especially in the early phase. The grey matter is usually involved initially with thickening of the cortical mantle and sulcal effacement due to oedema. The thickened cortex is therefore of high signal on T2WI. Involvement of the underlying white matter is also seen. The oedema commonly involves the insular region with sparing of the putamen. Gyriform enhancement can be seen after a few days. Haemorrhage occurs later and is best detected on gradient echo sequences. Severe atrophic change (possibly with calcification) is seen at the long-term follow-up of these patients (Fig. 7.25). It is important to note, however, that the imaging features particularly in the acute phase may be modified with the early use of aciclovir in cases where there is a high clinical suspicion.

Other types of viral encephalitis

Other agents such as the mumps, varicella and the measles virus may cause acute viral encephalitis. Different patterns of infection occur on a worldwide scale including the tick-borne viral encephalitides such as Eastern or Western equine encephalities.

The Epstein–Barr virus causes infectious mononucleosis can result in an acute illness or chronic or recurrent encephalitis. The virus causes a direct meningoencephalitis or alternatively can result in acute disseminated encephalomyelitis (see later).

Slow viruses result in spongiform encephalopathy – a transmissible neurodegenerative disease. Creutzfeldt–Jakob (CJD) disease is a devastating condition which clinically resembles Alzheimer's disease and is due to a primitive infective particle termed a prion. Pathologically the disease appears similar to Scrapie in sheep and bovine spongiform encephalopathy (BSE or 'mad cow disease'). The responsible organism is very resistant to more conventional forms of sterilization of equipment and has in the past been transmitted between patients following neurosurgical procedures. The disease results in a progressive dementia. A similar disease Kuru has been identified in tribes within New Guinea and is said to be related to ritualistic cannibalism.

Imaging by MR of CJD disease shows cortical atrophy and white matter degeneration which develop relatively quickly. Scans at presentation may be within normal limits and follow up imaging is advised.[24] High signal changes in the cortex on T2WI have recently been described,[25] possibly within a different subgroup of the disease.

New variant CJD was first described in the UK in 1996.[26] The link between BSE and new variant CJD has been proven beyond reasonable doubt.[27] It affects young patients and has a more rapidly progressive course. Signal changes in the pulvinar of the thalamus have been described in some cases of new variant CJD.[28]

POST-INFECTIVE ENCEPHALITIS

Subacute sclerosing panencephalitis

There are a number of conditions that involve the brain as an immune consequence of previous viral infection. The most devastating of these is subacute sclerosing panencephalitis. This occurs many years following measles infection. Antibodies to the measles virus are identified within the serum and the CSF in infected patients. The disease usually involves children or young adults and presents wth progressive mental and behavioural abnormality. This is followed by myclonic jerks, tremors and seizures. The condition is uniformly fatal within 2–6 years. Pathologically there is gross atrophy with neuronal loss, patchy demyelination, gliosis and perivascular inflammatory change; MRI shows widespread atrophic change with multifocal areas of increased T2 signal.[29]

Acute disseminated encephalomyelitis (ADEM)

This is an immune-mediated reaction involving the CNS which follows specific viral infections (such as chilhood exanthemata) or non-specific infections. It may also occur after vaccination and is due to an antibody–antigen complex reaction. Some cases occur spontaneously. Demyelination, gliosis and perivenular inflammation are the typical pathological changes. The disease is most commonly seen in children and young adults and presents acutely. ADEM has a monophasic course, unlike the relapsing clinical pattern of multiple sclerosis. The

(a)

(b)

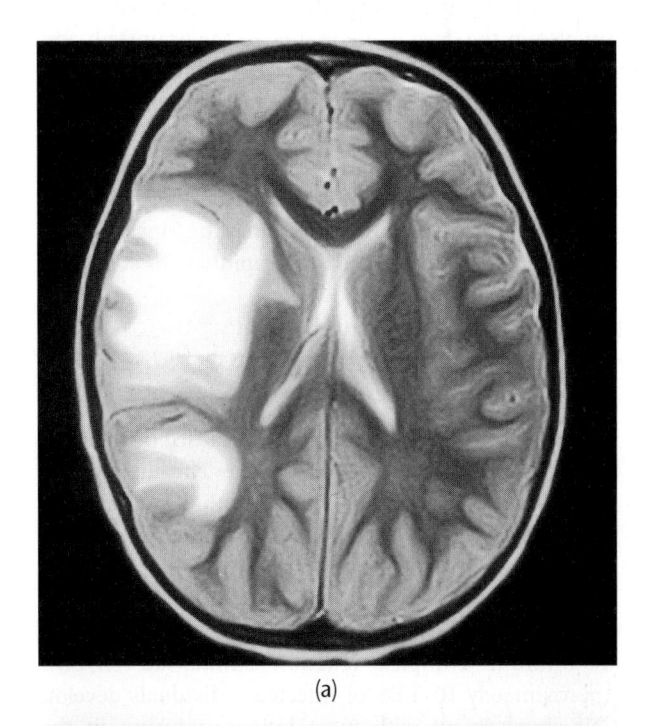

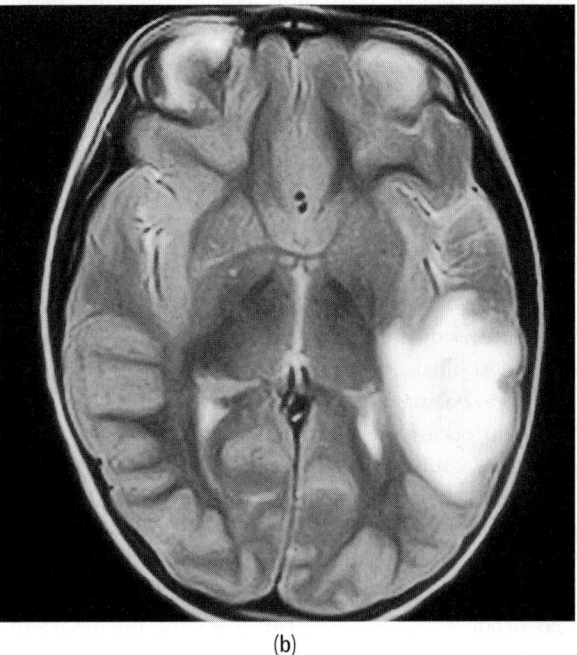

Figure 7.26 *Acute disseminated encephalomyelitis (ADEM). T2-weighted MRI scans in a teenage boy presenting with neurological symptoms, 2 weeks after an upper respiratory tract infection. Large areas of high signal within the white matter are identified in both hemispheres.*

onset of symptoms occurs between 10 and 21 days following the initial infection. Some prodromal features of headache, fever and drowsiness may occur with rapid progression to multifocal neurological deficits and occasional seizures. In severe cases coma and ultimately death may occur. Most patients recover fully; however, some may be left with permanent neurological deficits.

The imaging modality of choice is MRI. Increased T2 signal is seen particularly in the subcortical white matter but also in the deep white matter of the brainstem and cerebellum. These changes are bilateral but asymmetrical. Large confluent areas of white matter hyperintensity may be seen (Fig. 7.26). Basal ganglia involvement may also occur, occasionally resulting in necrosis. Haemorrhagic change is often seen pathologically but is rarely identified on MRI. There may be ring or solid enhancement which can subside rapidly with steroids.[30] Most lesions ultimately resolve.

Lyme disease

This is a multisystem disease which is caused by the tick-borne spirochete *Borrelia burgdorferi*. The disease was first described in 1977 following an outbreak of arthritis in children in the town of Old Lyme, Connecticut, USA. It is endemic in several European countries (especially around the Black Forest) and clusters of the disease occur within the USA. The cerebral involvement may be an immune complex reaction similar to ADEM. Approximately 10–15% of infected individuals develop CNS involvement with most lesions occuring in the white matter. Cranial nerve and peripheral nerve neuropathies also occur.[31]

TUBERCULOSIS, FUNGAL AND PARASITIC INFECTIONS

Tuberculosis

The features of tuberculous meningitis have been previously described. Parenchymal lesions i.e. tuberculomas are due to haematogenous spread. These are granulomas with central casseous necrosis. Lesions are uncommon in developed countries but there is an increasing incidence in patients with decreased immunity and also in immigrants (see section on HIV infection, p. 215). Tuberculomas are commonly seen at the grey–white matter interface in the hemispheres (Fig. 7.27) but also may occur within the posterior fossa and the basal ganglia. Ventricular or brainstem lesions occur less commonly. In children with miliary tuberculosis there may be multiple small parenchymal lesions which are often associated with tuberculous meningitis. On imaging there is evidence of a round or oval ring-enhancing lesion. The capsule is usually thicker and more irregular than that associated with a pyogenic abscess. There also tends to be less oedema than is associated with a pyogenic abscess. Calcification is unusual in the acute lesion although is commonly seen in healed tuberculomas.

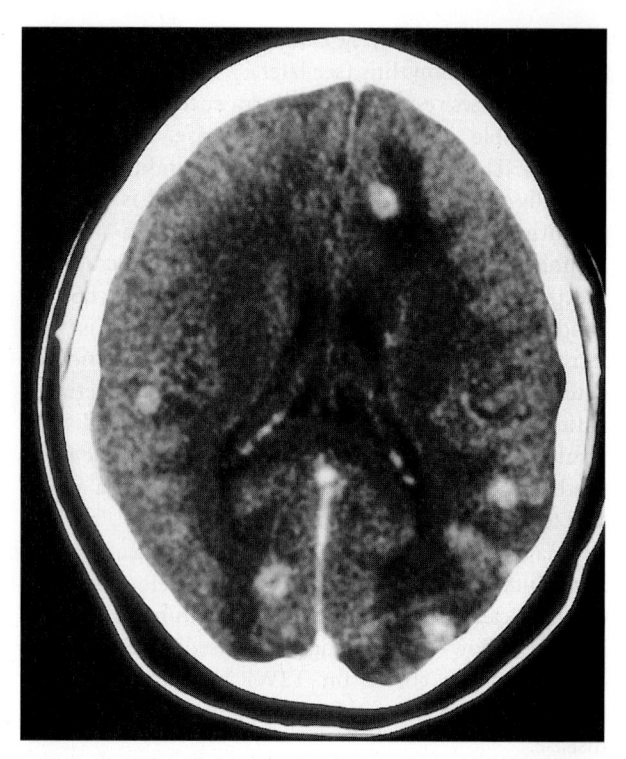

Figure 7.27 *Multiple tuberculomas. There are multiple-enhancing lesions identified at the grey–white matter interface. (Reproduced courtesy of Dr A Sprigg, Consultant Paediatric Radiologist, Sheffield Children's Hospital.)*

FUNGAL INFECTIONS

Fungal infections may involve the brain parenchyma, leptomeninges or blood vessels. In some ways the findings are similar to infection with tuberculosis. Fungal infections can be divided into those which involve patients with normal immunity. These include histoplasma, blastomyces and coccidiodes. In patients with decreased immunity other fungi such as *Aspergillus fumigatus*, *Candida albicans* and *Cryptococcus neoformans* are responsible. In general, fungal infections are rare; however, there is an increasing incidence due to the increase in the immunocompromised population.

Different features are typically seen with different organisms. For example cryptococcus causes a meningitis with a thick gelatinous exudate. This exudate extends into the dilated Virchow–Robin spaces resulting in large pseudo cysts along the perforating lenticulostriate vessels in the basal ganglia. Mucormycosis and aspergillosis can spread into the frontal lobes through the cribriform plate from the nasal cavity and paranasal sinuses.

Extension through the orbital apex into the cavernous sinus can occur. Involvement of large or small vessels at the base of the brain is seen with mucormycosis and aspergillosis. This can lead to infarction or haemorrhagic mycetomas. Coccidiodomycosis usually results in a thick, purulent basal meningitis. Because of this meningeal thickening communicating hydrocephalus is commonly encountered.

Neurocysticercosis

The human is a definitive host for the adult pork tapeworm (*Taenia solium*). The adult tapeworm lives in the small intestine and sheds eggs. These are then shed in the faeces where they may be ingested by pigs or man. The eggs may then hatch within the human gut giving rise to primary larvae (oncospheres) which in turn bore through the intestinal mucosa and are distributed via the circulation to the brain, muscle and the eye. These oncospheres then develop into secondary larvae – the cysticerci within the brain resulting in neurocysticercosis.

Neurocysticercosis is the most common CNS infection on a worldwide scale. It is endemic in Africa, Central and South America and parts of Eastern Europe as well as Asia. Involvement of the CNS occurs in 90% of infected individuals. Parenchymal disease is the most common type with lesions occurring at the corticomedullary junction. Intraventricular cysts are also relatively common especially with involvement of the fourth ventricle. Subarachnoid involvement also occurs.

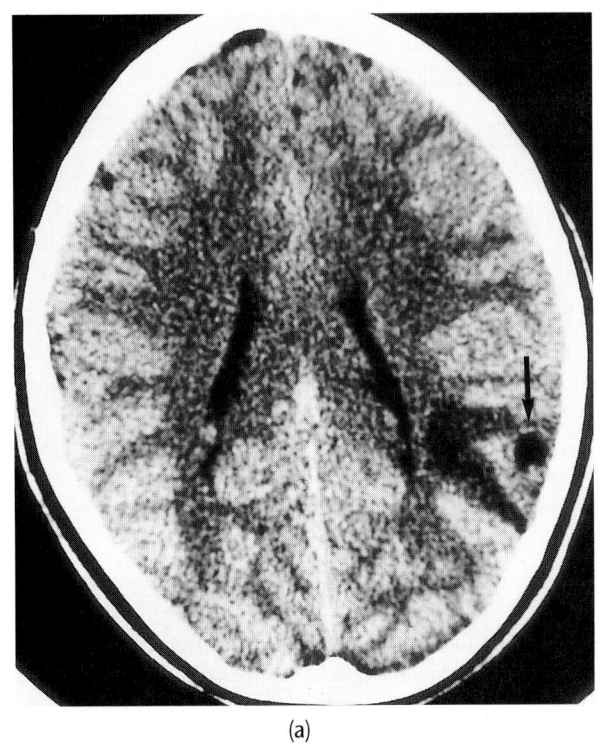

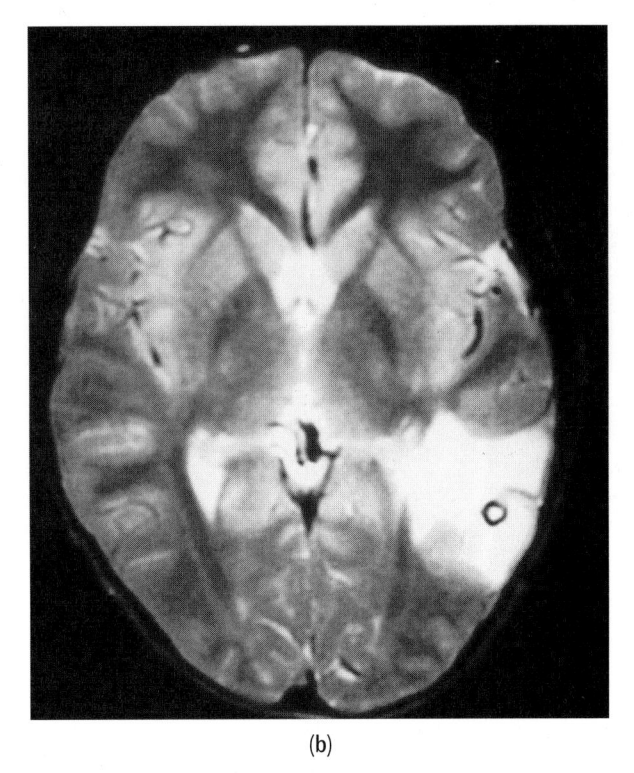

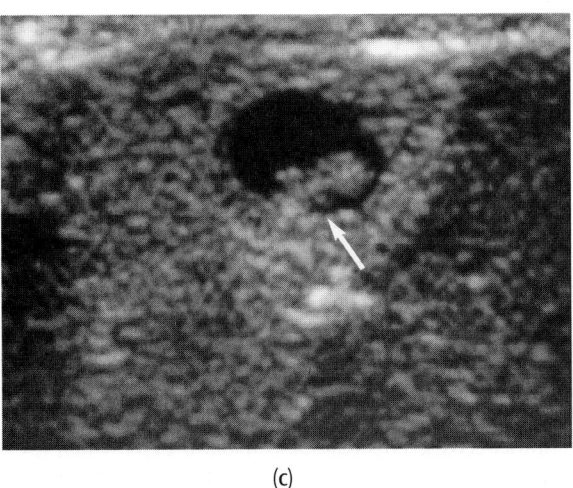

Figure 7.28 *Neurocysticercosis. Unenhanced CT scan (a) shows a peripherally placed cyst (black arrow) with local surrounding oedema. Posteriorly a tiny mural nodule can be identified representing the scolex. T2-weighted MRI scan (b) shows very low signal intensity capsule surrounded by a marked degree of oedema. Intraoperative ultrasound (c) shows a cystic lesion which contains a small mural nodule (white arrow). (Reproduced courtesy of Dr A Sprigg, Consultant Paediatric Radiologist, Sheffield Children's Hospital.)*

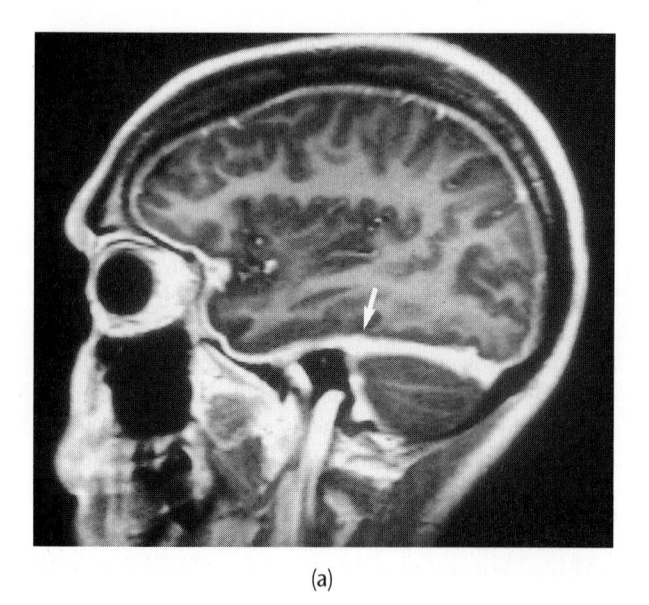

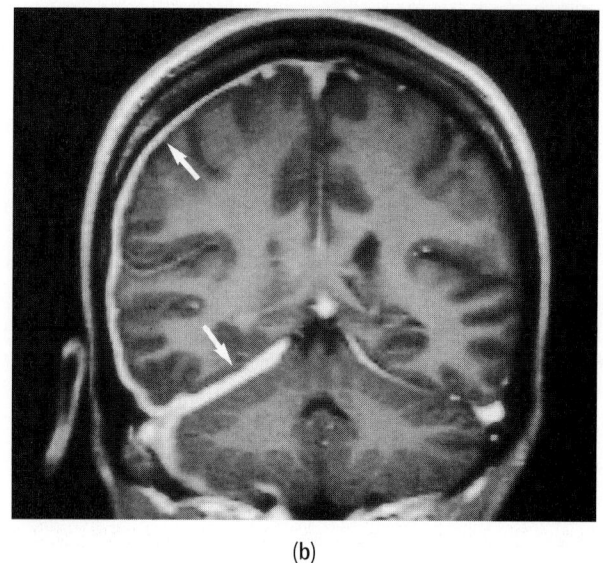

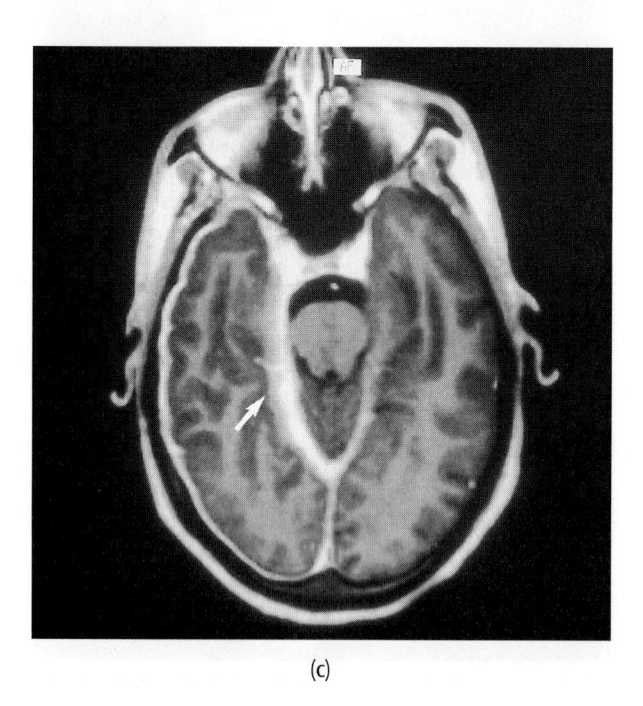

Figure 7.29 *Gadolinium-enhanced T1WI (a)–(c) showing marked leptomeningeal enhancement in neurosarcoidosis (white arrows).*

The larvae progress through various stages and it is fairly common to find multiple stages within the same patient. The initial stage is the vesicular phase where there is a thin capsule surrounding a viable larva. This incites little or no inflammatory reaction and the fluid contained within the bladder of the larva is clear. A small mural nodule may be identified on imaging which represents the scolex (head) of the larva. At this stage there is little evidence of oedema and usually no enhancement.

When the larva dies, however, the fluid within the cyst becomes turbid and gelatinous. As the body of the larva degenerates metabolic products are released causing disruption of the blood–brain barrier and an intense host inflammatory reaction. This results in local oedema (Fig. 7.28). Enhancement of the cyst wall can be identified at this stage. As the lesion progresses the capsule thickens, the cyst retracts and the scolex calcifies. This is termed the granular nodular stage. Oedema and enhancement remain. The final nodular calcified stage occurs when the lesion has contracted to a fraction of its original size and is completely calcified. At this stage there is no mass effect with no oedema and no enhancement. In the detection of the associated calcifications CT is superior to MRI. However, MRI is more sensitive in the detection of parenchymal cysts and the pericystic oedema.

Other parasites that involve the CNS include echinococcosis. This results in hydatid cysts which most commonly occur in the liver and the lung but may also

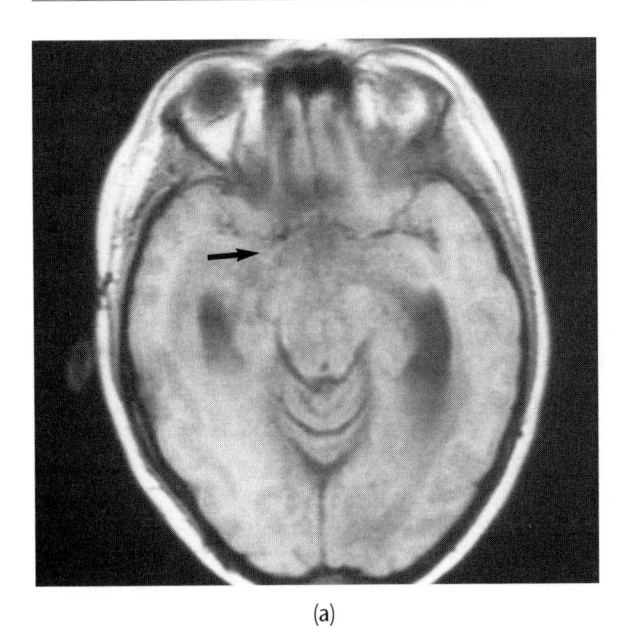

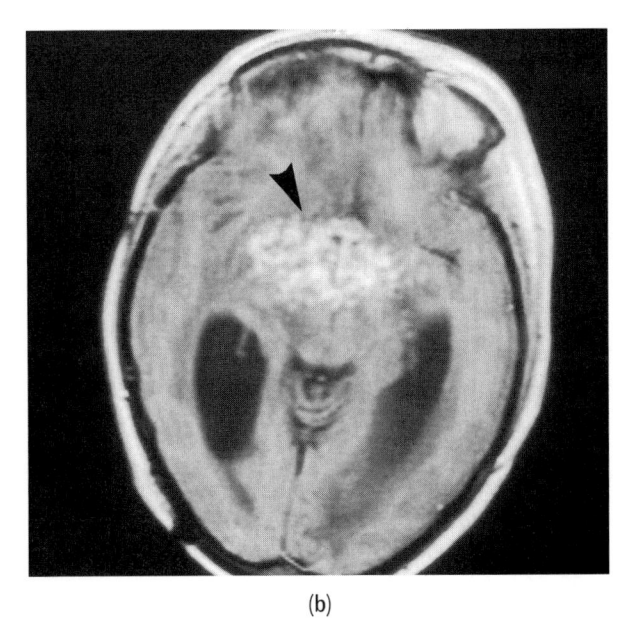

Figure 7.30 *T1-weighted MRI scans before (a) and after (b) intravenous gadolinium. This is a young patient with severe infiltrating neurosarcoidosis. On the unenhanced scans the suprasellar cistern is obliterated (black arrow) and there is evidence of hydrocephalus. Following gadolinium there is marked basal meningeal enhancement which extends into the brain substance along the line of Virchow–Robin spaces (black arrow head).*

involve the brain. This results usually in the single thin-walled CSF density cyst most often within the parietal lobe. Within endemic areas (regions associated with sheep farming), however, intracranial hydatid cysts do contribute a significant percentage to the overall number of intracranial masses.

SARCOIDOSIS

Sarcoidosis is granulomatous disease with involvement of multiple systems throughout the body. Neurosarcoidosis occurs when the CNS is involved and can be seen in between 5 and 16% of patients with systemic sarcoid. Involvement of the CNS typically occurs with systemic disease; however, it may also occur in the absence of systemic involvement. Neurosarcoidosis commonly involves young to middle-aged adults although children may be affected.

Neurosarcoidosis is one of the great mimics of alternative pathology. There may be marked leptomeningeal involvement mimicking tuberculous meningitis or meningeal carcinomatosis. Neurosarcoidosis may result in mass lesions that can mimic gliomas, lymphoma or metastases. Finally diffuse white matter disease may be difficult to distinguish from multiple sclerosis.

Clinically, neurosarcoidosis classically presents with cranial nerve palsies although more acute meningitic symptoms may be present. The intracranial lesions may result in raised intracranial pressure, focal neurologial deficits or seizure disorders. There may also be a vasculitic process resulting in cerebral infarction.

Pathologically there is thickening of the leptomeninges, in particular the arachnoid around the basal cisterns. The meningeal thickening may extend over the remainder of the brain or down the spinal cord. Occasional involvement of the ependyma and the choroid plexus may also be identified. On CT and MRI there is intense meningeal enhancement following intravenous contrast (Fig. 7.29).

Parenchymal lesions are typically seen as extensions of basal meningeal infiltration through the Virchow–Robin spaces at the base of the brain (Fig. 7.30). Parenchymal abnormalities may, however, occur anywhere in the brain resulting in solitary enhancing mass lesions. These can therefore be confused with other causes of mass lesions such as lymphoma, metastases or gliomas. Extensive white matter changes may occur within the centrum semi ovale but also in a periventricular distribution. This may therefore lead to confusion with multiple sclerosis. The vasculitis may be identified as areas of non-specific stenosis on cerebral angiography. This may then give rise to areas of infarction.

REFERENCES

1 Becker LE. Infections in the developing brain. *Am J Neuroradiol* 1992; **13**: 537–49.
2 Fitz CR. Inflammatory diseases of the brain in childhood. *Am J Neuroradiol* 1992; **13**: 551–67.

3 Ketonen L, Tuite MJ. Brain imaging in human immunodeficiency virus infection. *Semin Neurol* 1992; **12**: 57–69.
4 Olsen WL, Longo FM, Mills CM, Norman D. White matter diseases in AIDS: findings at MR imaging. *Radiology* 1988; **169**: 445–8.
5 Olson EM, Healy JF, Wong WHM, Youmans DC, Hessenlink JR. MR detection of white matter disease of the brain in patients with HIV infection: fast spin-echo vs conventional spin-echo pulse sequences. *Am J Prentgenol* 1994; **162**: 1199–204.
6 Kierburtz KD, Ketonen I, Zettelmaier AE *et al*. MRI findings in HIV cognitive impairment. *Arch Neurol* 1990; **47**: 643–5.
7 Chong WK, Paley M, Wilkinson ID, Hall-Craggs MA, Sweeney B *et al*. Localized cerebral proton spectroscopy in HIV infection and AIDS. *Am J Neuroradiol* 1994; **15**: 21–25.
8 Barker PB, Lee RR, McArthur JC. AIDS. *Radiology* 1995; **195**: 58–64.
9 Daras M, Koppel BS, Samkoff L, Marc J. Brainstem toxoplasmosis in patients with acquired immunodeficiency syndrome. *J Neuroimag* 1994; **4**: 85–90.
10 Laissy JP, Soyer P, Partier C, Lariven S, Benmelha Z *et al*. Persistent enhancement after treatment for cerebral toxoplasmosis in patient with AIDS: predictive value for subsequent recurrence. *Am J Neuroradiol* 1994; **15**: 1773–8.
11 Chang L, Cornford ME, Chiang FL, Ernst TM, Sun NCJ, Miller BL. Cerebral toxoplasmosis and lymphoma in AIDS: radiologic-pathologic correlation. *Am J Neuroradiol* 1995; **16**: 1653–63.
12 Ciricillo SF, Rosenblum ML. Use of CT and MR imaging to distinguish intracranial lesions and to define the need for biopsy in AIDS patients. *J Neurosurg* 1990; **73**: 720–4.
13 Chiang F L, Miller B L, Chang L, McBride D, Cornford M, Mehringer CM. Fulminant cerebral lymphoma in AIDS. *Am J Neuroradiol* 1996; **17**: 157–60.
14 Dina TS. Primary central nervous system lymphoma versus toxoplasmosis in AIDS. *Radiology* 1991; **179**: 823–8.
15 Ramsey RG, Gean AD. Central nervous system toxoplasmosis. *Neuroimag Clin N Amer* 1997; **7**: 171–86.
16 Ruiz A, Ganz WI, Donovan Post J, Camp A, Landy H. Use of thallium-201 brain SPECT to differentiate cerebral lymphoma from toxoplasma encephalitis in AIDS patients. *Am J Neuroradiol* 1994; **15**: 1885–94.
17 Chinn RJS, Wilkinson ID, Hall-Craggs MA, Paley MNJ, Miller RF *et al*. Toxoplasmosis and primary central nervous system lymphoma in HIV infection: diagnosis with MR spectroscopy. *Radiology* 1995; **197**: 649–54.
18 Ernst TM, Chang L, Witt MD, Aronow HA, Cornford ME *et al*. Cerebral toxoplasmosis and lymphoma in AIDS: perfusion MR imaging experience in 13 patients. *Radiology* 1998; **208**: 663–9.
19 Brightbill TC, Ihmeidan H, Post JD, Berger JR, Katz DA. Neurosyphlilis in HIV-positive and HIV-negative patients: neuroimaging findings. *Am J Neuroradiol* 1995; **16**: 703–11.
20 Whiteman M, Luis Espinoza M, Donovan Post J, Bell MD, Falcone S. Central nervous system tuberculosis in HIV-infected patients: clinical and radiographic findings. *Am J Neuroradiol* 1995; **16**: 1319–27.
21 Mellor DH. The place of computed tomography and lumbar puncture in suspected bacterial meningitis. *Arch Dis Child* 1992; **67**: 1417–9.
22 Rennick G, Shann F, de Campo J. Cerebral herniation during bacterial meningitis in children. *Br Med J* 1993; **306**: 953–5.
23 Koelfen W, Freund M, Guckel F, Rohr H, Schultze C. MRI of encephalitis in children: comparison of CT and MRI in the acute stage with long-term follow-up. *Neuroradiology* 1996; **38**: 73–9.
24 Uchino A, Yoshinaga M, Shiokawa O, Hata H. Ohno M. Serial MR imaging in Creutzfeldt-Jakob disease. *Neuroradiology* 1991; **33**: 364–7.
25 Ishida S, Sugino M, Koizumi N, Shinoda K, Ohsawa N *et al*. Serial MRI in early Creutzfeldt-Jakob disease with a point mutation of prion protein at codon 180. *Neuroradiology* 1995; **37**: 531–4.
26 Will RG, Ironside JW, Zeidler M, Cousens SN, Estibeiro K *et al*. A new variant of Creuzfeld-Jakob disease in the UK. *Lancet* 1996; **347**: 921–5.
27 Ironside JW, Knight RSG, Will RG, Smith PG, Cousens SN. New variant Creutzfeldt-Jakob disease ia more common in Britain than elsewhere. *Br Med J* 1998; **317**: 352.
28 Sellar RJ, Will W, Zeidler M. MR imaging in new variant Creuzfeldt disease: the pulvinar sign. European Society of Neuroradiology Annual Congress, Oxford 1997.
29 Bohlega S, Al-Kawi MZ. Subacute sclerosing panencephalitis: imaging and clinical correlation. *J Neuroimag* 1994; **4**: 71–6.
30 Mader I, Stock K W, Ettlin T, Probst A. Acute disseminated encephalomyelitis: MR and CT features. *Am J Neuroradiol* 1996; **17**: 104–9.
31 Demaerel P, Wilms G, Van Lierde S, Delanote J, Baert AL. Lyme disease in childhood presenting as a primary leptomeningeal enhancement with parenchymal findings on MR. *Am J Neuroradiol* 1994; **15**: 302–4.

8

Neurodegenerative and white matter diseases

ALAN JACKSON

Introduction	241	White matter diseases	254
The ageing brain	241	References	264
Neurodegenerative diseases	245		

INTRODUCTION

The neurodegenerative diseases present an increasingly important clinical problem as improvements in longevity lead to an increase in the average age of the population. Normal ageing of the brain is characterized by programmed death of neurons and neuroglial cells known as apoptosis. This cell loss leads to increasing cerebral atrophy which is often accompanied by the development of areas of abnormal cortical high signal on T2-weighted images (T2WI). Neurodegenerative diseases result from premature death of brain cells of one or more specific subtypes. This loss leads to focal or diffuse atrophy that is more pronounced, and progresses at a greater rate, than that seen with the normal ageing process. High signal abnormalities on T2WI are also a common feature in a wide range of these diseases.

Diseases of white matter are also typified by areas of high signal abnormality on T2WI. Although multiple sclerosis is the archetypal white matter disease, white matter damage can result from a wide range of acquired metabolic and physical insults and can be the result of abnormalities in myelin development and distribution known as dysmyelination.

When faced with a brain scan, in which the abnormalities are characterized by cerebral atrophy and/or white matter abnormality, it is essential that the radiologists have insight into the changes that occur with the normal ageing process.

THE AGEING BRAIN

The normal magnetic resonance (MR) appearances of the brain in the elderly differ in a number of ways from those in young adults. Some of these changes can easily be mistaken as part of a pathological process.

Cerebral atrophy starts in the fifth decade with slowly progressive and generalized loss of brain substance. The rate of loss is approximately 1% of brain volume per annum and by the age of 60, dilatation of the third ventricle and mild widening of peripheral sulci is often apparent. It should be noted that there is commonly asymmetry in sulcal width, which becomes more prominent as normal atrophy progresses so that, for instance, the left sylvian fissure often appears to be somewhat larger than that of the right. By the late part of the sixth decade, sulcal prominence and third ventricular dilatation is more evident and lateral ventricular dilatation with blunting of the anterior and a posterior horn is common.[1]

Areas of high signal abnormality on T2-weighted lesions are common with increasing age and are more apparent on fluid attenuated inversion recovery (FLAIR) sequences than on conventional. Even the normal white matter of the young adult is not uniform on T2WI. Areas of terminal myelination in the posterior parts of the occipital radiation may be seen up to the fourth decade. Hyperintense foci anterior to the frontal horns of the lateral ventricles relate to areas of decreased myelin content and breakdown of the ependymal linings of the lateral ventricles which causes increased interstitial fluid (Fig. 8.1). This region is believed to act as a drainage channel for excess extracellular fluid produced in the brain, which has no lymphatic drainage system. Up to 50% of normal subjects have well-circumscribed high signal areas in the posterior part of the internal capsule. These are symmetrical and it has been suggested that they correspond to the parietopontine tracts, which contain decreased amounts of myelin or possibly to the retrolenticular portion of the optic tract (Fig. 8.2).

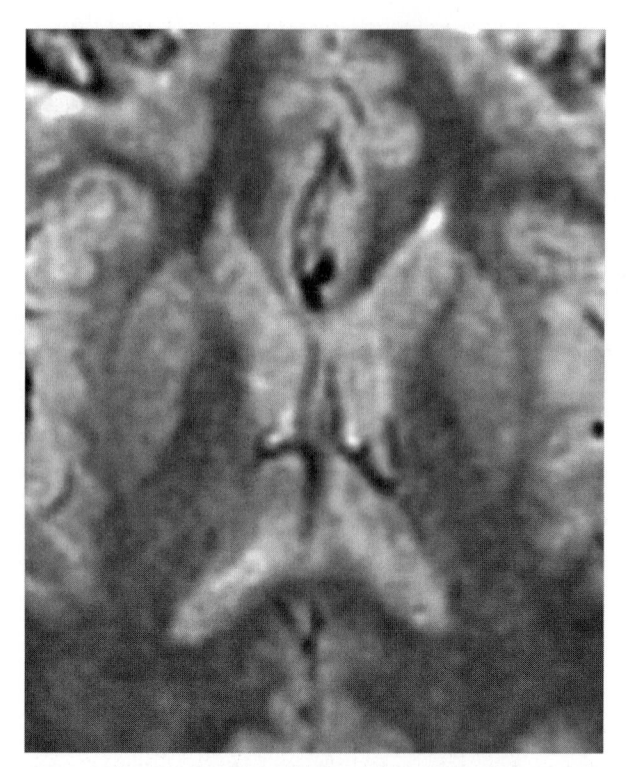

242 Neurodegenerative and white matter diseases

Figure 8.1 *T2-Weighted axial images through the lateral ventricles in a young normal adult. Note the focal areas of high signal at the anterior border of the lateral ventricles due to ependymitis granularis. These are normal findings.*

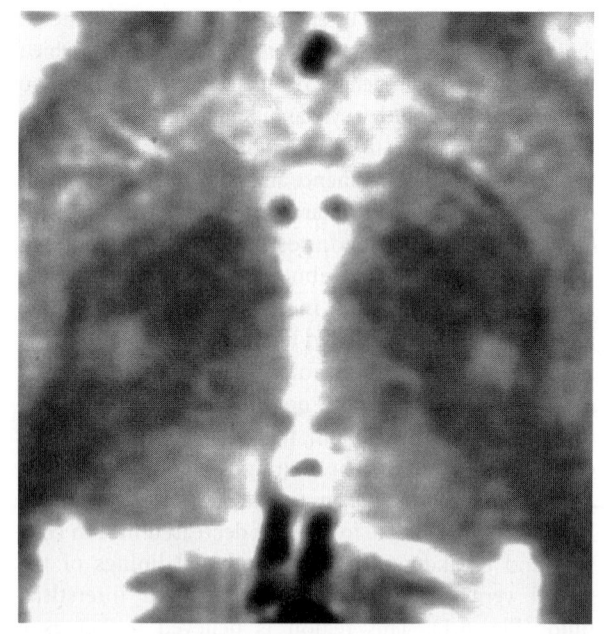

Figure 8.2 *Axial T2WI through the thalamus and third ventricle in a normal subject showing well-defined bilateral areas of high signal in the posterior interior capsule.*

Virchow–Robin spaces

Involution of the pia mater around penetrating cerebral arteries produces a potential intracerebral extension of the subarachnoid space known as a Virchow–Robin space. This potential space may dilate to contain cerebral spinal fluid (CSF) and so appear as a small area of high signal on T2WI.[2,3] Typically, Virchow–Robin spaces are isointense to CSF on all sequences and therefore appear low signal on T1WI in distinction to areas of gliosis or infarction. The high sensitivity of magnetic resonance imaging (MRI) allows the demonstration of normal Virchow–Robin space, even in the young adult. These are seen, on T2WI, as

(a)

(b)

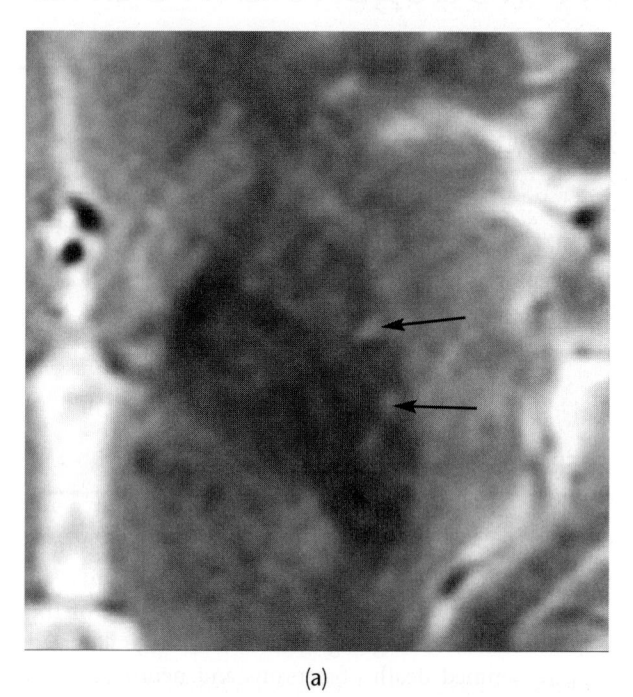

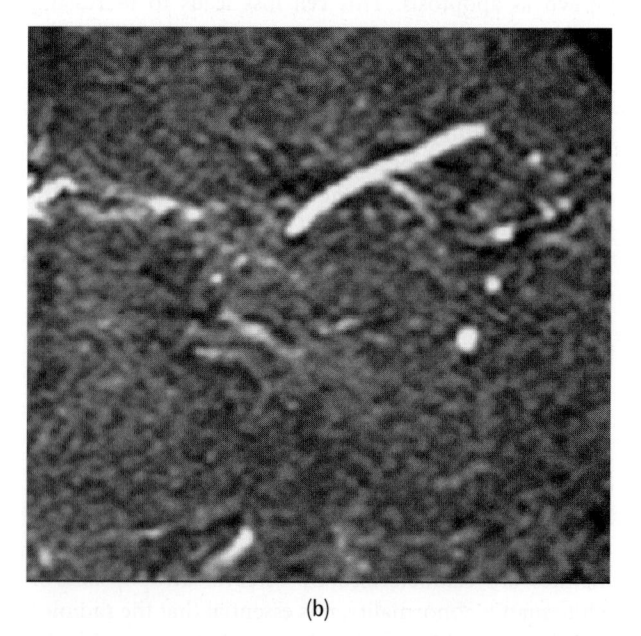

Figure 8.3 *Virchow–Robin spaces in the basal ganglia. (a) T2-Weighted axial image showing the lentiform nucleus with a darker medial globus pallidus. Tiny areas of high signal are seen within the putamen (arrows) indicating the position of Virchow–Robin spaces. (b) Matched slice from a time-of-flight magnetic resonance angiogram shows the penetrating vessels in these positions.*

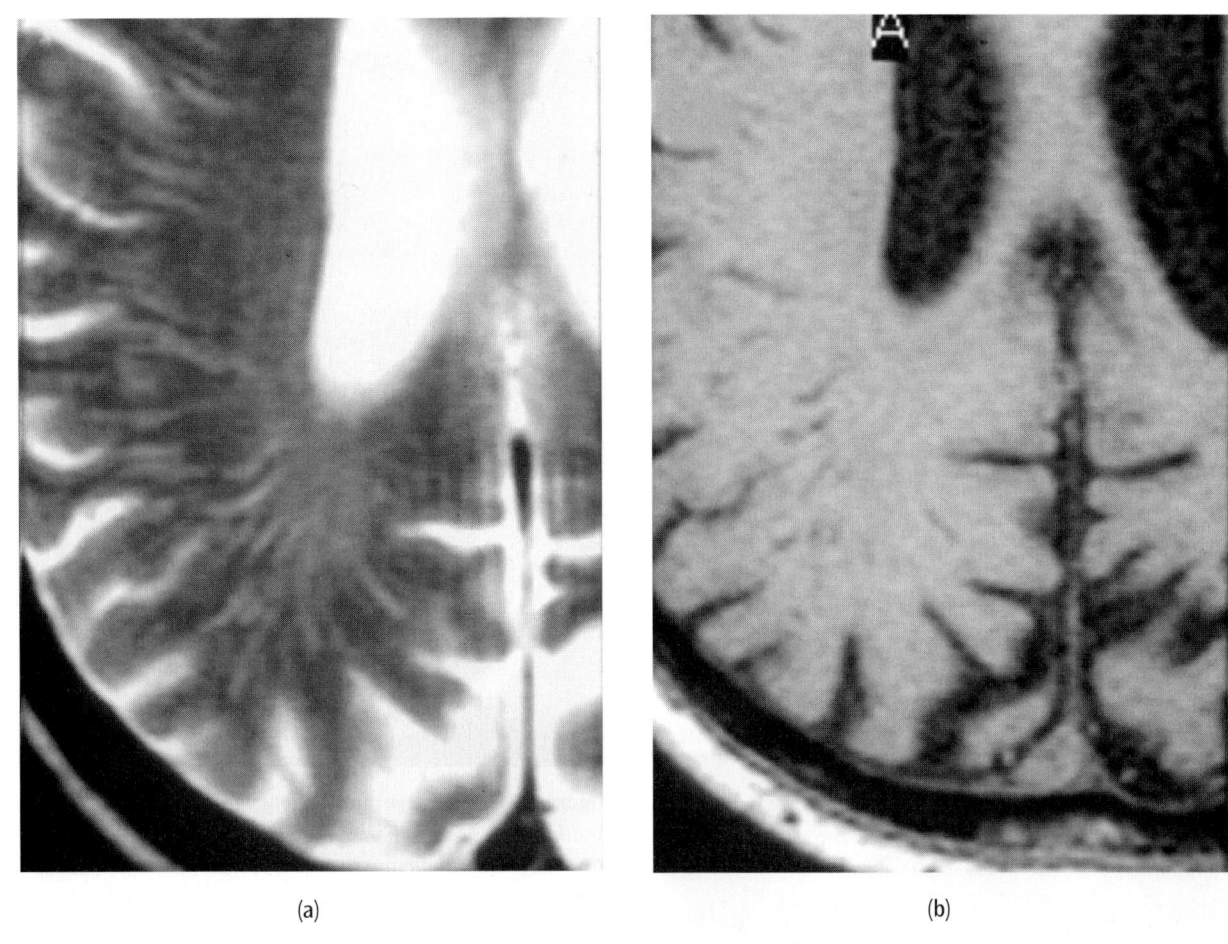

Figure 8.4 Matched axial T2WI (a) and T1WI (b) through the corona radiata and occipital radiation in an elderly patient with established small vessel brain disease. Note the multiple dilated perivascular spaces seen as a medusa-like radiation of high signal on the T2WI with matched low signal areas on T1WI.

small (less than 2 mm) areas of high signal at the base of the brain, lateral to the anterior commisure (Fig. 8.3). With increasing age, these lesions are more frequently observed and large in size. Virchow–Robin spaces may also be seen with increasing age in the cerebral hemispheres where draining veins penetrate the centrum semiovale (Fig. 8.4) and in the upper mesencephalic tegmentum (Fig. 8.5). Although they become more prominent with age, they may also be exaggerated in some disease states, particularly in patients with hypertension or diffuse vascular disease. In severe cases, dilated Virchow–Robin spaces may extend through the substance of the brain and into the basal ganglia following the root of the penetrating lenticulostriate vessels. This vacuolated appearance has been described as status cribrosus or état criblé and is a pathological finding.

Periventricular white matter hyperintensities

Areas of high signal on T2-weighted lesions, which are contiguous with the margins of the lateral ventricles, are commonly observed over the age of 50 and increase in incidence with increasing age (Fig. 8.6).[4] They are present in up to 30% of normal elderly patients, but are also commonly associated with a wide range of pathological cerebral processes. Areas of increased signal may result from increased local extracellular water content. In normal ageing, this is felt to represent a change in the dynamics of extracellular fluid transudation and reabsorbtion, which is secondary to changes in autoregulatory control of cerebral blood flow. Periventricular white matter hyperintensities (PVH) are also a common feature of demyelinating diseases due to loss of myelin content in the periventricular white matter. In these patients, the areas of high signal represent loss of myelin and secondary gliosis.

Deep white matter hyperintensities

Areas of increased signal on T2WI are commonly seen in the deep white matter of the corona radiata and centrum semiovale (Fig. 8.7).[5] These lesions are hyperintense on both proton density and T2WI distinguishing them

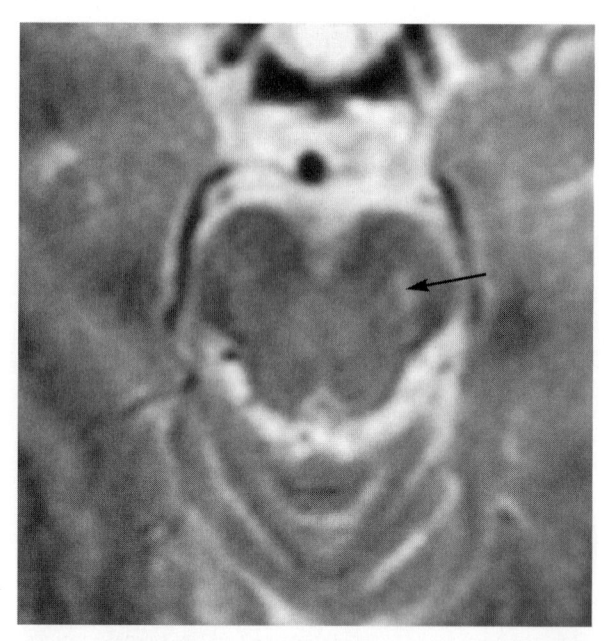

Figure 8.5 *The typical position of dilated Virchow–Robin spaces in the mesencephalon (arrow).*

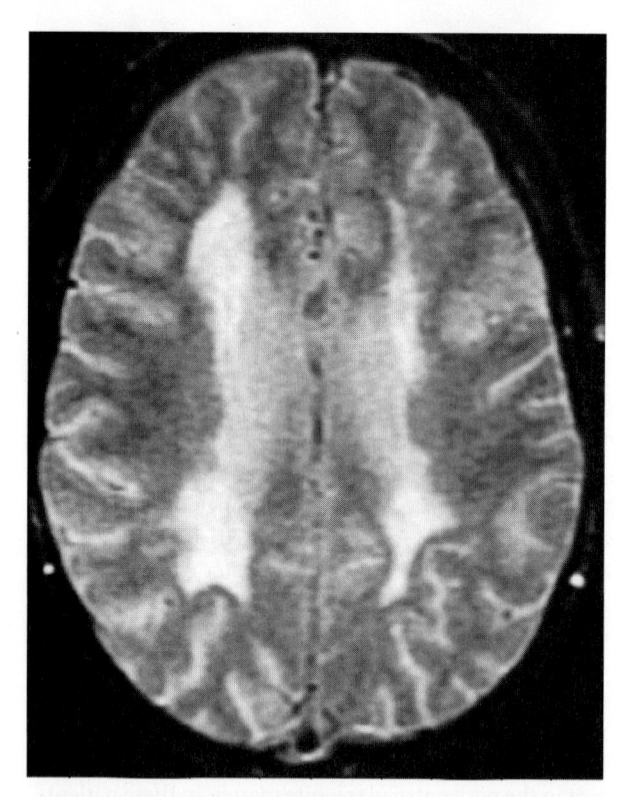

Figure 8.6 *Axial T2WI demonstrating extensive confluent areas of periventricular hyperintensity. These abnormalities were associated with established cerebrovascular disease in an elderly patient with Binswanger's syndrome.*

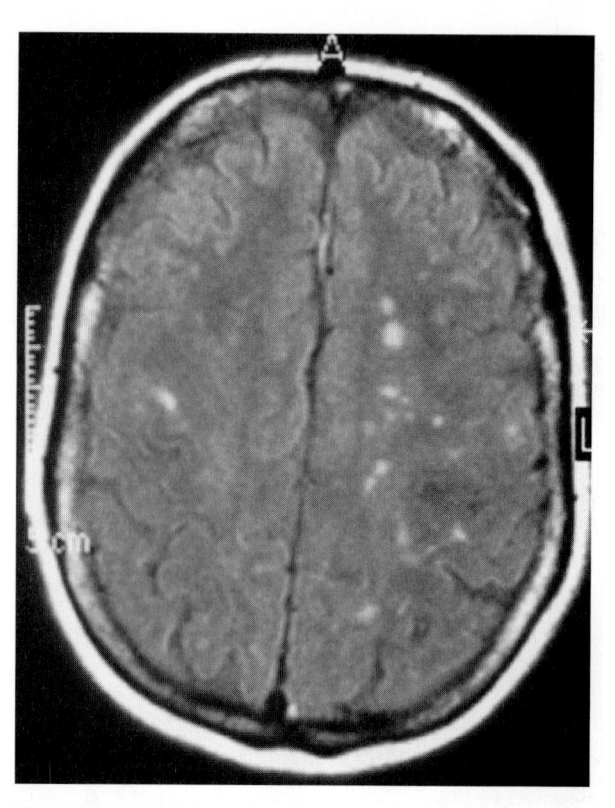

Figure 8.7 *FLAIR image through the centrum semiovale showing multiple high signal abnormalities within the deep white matter. This image is taken from a scan of a 70-year-old normal asymptomatic individual.*

lesions remains vague. Histologically, areas of high signal may demonstrate appearances similar to infarction or incomplete demyelination, which may be associated with increased glial cell content often described as isomorphic gliosis. These lesions are strongly correlated with cerebrovascular risk factors and decreased regional perfusion has been demonstrated on positron emission tomography (PET) studies. This has led to the hypothesis that these lesions are primarily ischaemic in nature.[6]

The suggestion that leukoaraiosis has an ischaemic aetiology is further supported by the distribution of lesions. The deep white matter intensities are rarely seen in areas with significant collateral supply such as the cortex subcortical U fibres or Rolandic fissure. They are similarly rare in areas supplied by short arterial vessels such as the medial corpus callosum, medulla and midbrain. The lesions are, however, common in areas supplied by long arteries and with little or no collateralization such as the corona radiata, centrum semiovale, lateral corpus callosum and central pons.

Iron deposition

In many individuals the globus pallidus, red nucleus and pars compacta of the substantia nigra (Fig. 8.8) become progressively hypointense on T2WI. This change begins

from the dilated Virchow–Robin spaces described above. This pattern of high signal white matter abnormalities increasing with age is often referred to as leukoaraiosis although the aetiology and clinical correlation of the

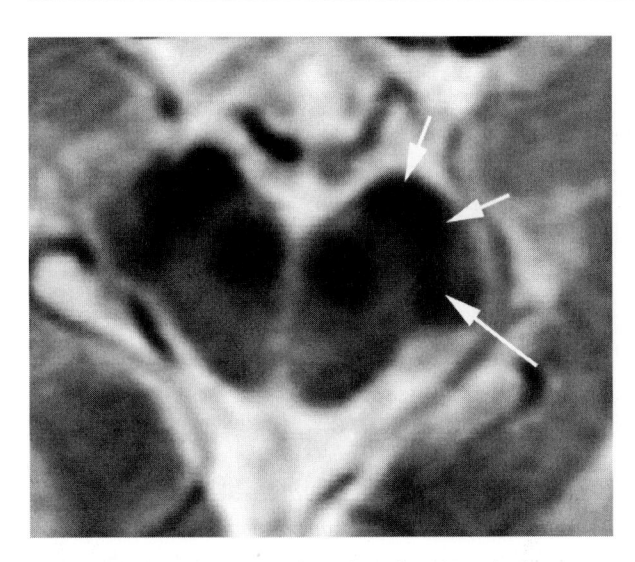

Figure 8.8 *Transverse T2-weighted section through the mesencephalon showing loss of signal in the red nucleus (long arrow) and pars compacta of the substantia nigra (short arrows) due to iron deposition.*

in early adulthood and is usually visible by the third decade. Within increasing age, the change becomes more marked and the signal within the putamen also falls. By the eighth decade, the signal in the putamen and globus pallidus is similar. These changes mirror the increase in iron deposition, which occurs in these areas with advancing age. The change is more evident at higher field strength and on long TE (echo time), long TR (repetition time) and gradient echo sequences due to increased sensitivity to paramagnetic (T2*) effects. The mechanism of iron deposition is complex, but similar changes may also occur, with an accelerated time course in a number of disease, including demyelination, trauma and cerebral infarction.

NEURODEGENERATIVE DISEASES

Neurodegenerative diseases form a wide spectrum of abnormality characterized by progressive cerebral degeneration. The classification of neurodegenerative diseases is complex, but it is common to identify diseases that affect primarily the grey matter or white matter respectively. Although in many cases the aetiology of the disease is unknown, in others, there is a clear genetic vascular or metabolic mechanism. In this chapter, we will describe the grey matter and white matter disorders separately, concentrating on those most commonly experienced in clinical practice. Descriptions of the rarer and in particular, the inherited disorders will concentrate on typical or distinctive radiological features only and references to more specialist texts will be provided in these cases.

Grey matter neurodegenerative diseases

Degenerative diseases affecting primarily grey matter are typified by loss of one or more specific neuronal subtype resulting in distinctive patterns of cerebral atrophy or signal change. The diseases are generally classified according to their pathological anatomy and the clinical syndromes that consequently result.

Dementing disease

Dementia occurs in 15–20% of the population over the age of 65, rising to in excess of 35% over the age 85. The role of neuroimaging in the investigation of dementing illnesses remains unclear since diagnosis is commonly based on typical clinical and neuropsychological features. Nonetheless, imaging is commonly undertaken, particularly when the diagnosis is uncertain or where there is a suspicion of a treatable disorder such as chronic subdural haematoma, normal pressure hydrocephalus or neoplasm.[7]

ALZHEIMER'S DISEASE

Alzheimer's disease is the most common neurodegenerative disease of the brain and the most common cause of dementia. Although rare cases may be familial, the majority are sporadic and onset of symptoms may occur as early as 40 years of age.

Patients become gradually cognitively impaired exhibiting problems with memory, language and visuospatial co-ordination. The illness normally lasts for 5 years or more with progressive deterioration in all higher cognitive functions. Differentiation from vascular dementia can be difficult and currently relies on the use of clinical scoring systems, which have a specificity of approximately 80%. Single photon emission computed tomography (SPECT) imaging also has a role in diagnosis demonstrating typical perfusion defects in the temporal and posterior parietal cortices in most cases.

Neuroimaging in Alzheimer's disease

Alzheimer's disease is characterized by rapid and progressive cerebral atrophy affecting specifically the temporal and frontal lobes. Symmetrical bilateral hippocampal cell loss is a particularly striking feature (Fig. 8.9), which results in hippocampal shrinkage and enlargement of temporal horns of the lateral ventricles.[8] Atrophy is far more rapidly progressive than that seen in normal ageing, but despite this, there is significant overlap in most objective indicators of atrophy between Alzheimer's and normal ageing individuals.[9] Measurements of intra-uncal distance,[10] medial temporal lobe and temporal horn volume reflect hippocampal atrophy and have been shown to reliably distinguish patients with Alzheimer's disease from normal age-matched controls.[11] Similarly, measurements of the

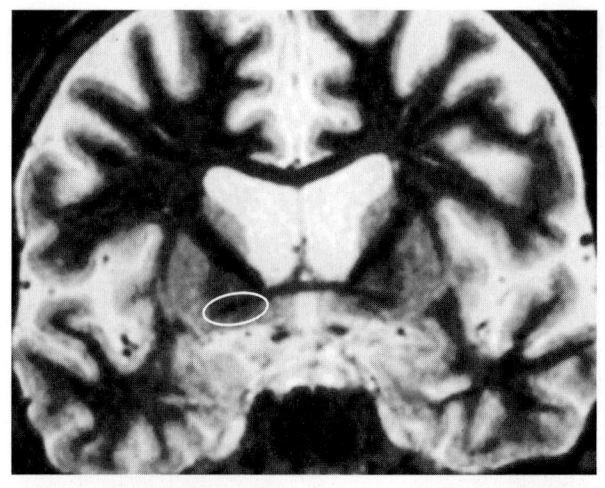

Figure 8.10 *Coronal T2WI in a patient with advanced Alzheimer's disease showing generalized cerebral atrophy affecting the parietal and temporal lobes. This section is at the level of the amygdala anterior to the hippocampus. The anterior commissure can be seen extending across the midline and lying below the lentiform nucleus. On the left side a white outline indicates the position of the substantia innominata.*

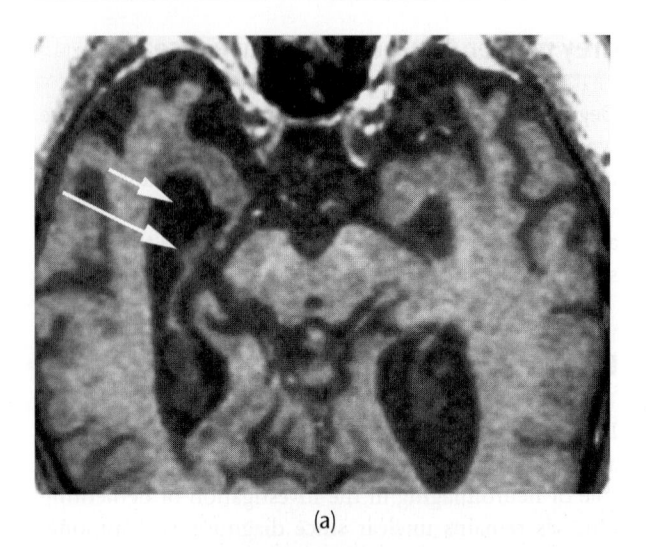

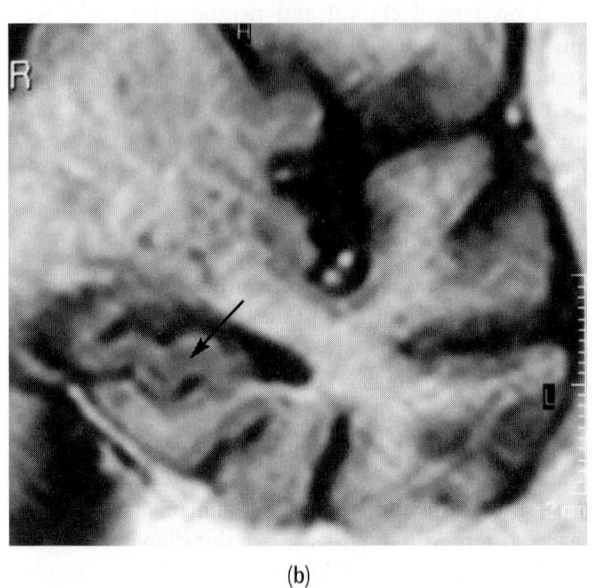

Figure 8.9 *Axial (a) and coronal (b) T1-weighted sections through the hippocampus in a patient with Alzheimer's disease. On the axial image marked dilatation of the temporal horn of the lateral ventricle (short arrow (a)) is clearly seen and the hippocampus is seen as a thin ribbon-like structure forming the medial border of the temporal horn (long arrow (a)). Coronal images show a small atrophic hippocampus (arrow (b)). The associated lateral recess of the temporal horn is markedly dilated and there is loss of internal structure of the hippocampus.*

substantia innominata which contains the cholinergic basal nucleus of Meynert, which is specifically affected early in Alzheimer's disease, appear to differentiate between Alzheimer's disease and controls (Fig. 8.10). Unfortunately, little information is available concerning the ability of these measures to distinguish between patients with Alzheimer's disease and other dementing illnesses, particularly frontotemporal and vascular dementias which form the principle differential diagnoses. Consequently, at the present time, no volumetric measurement is in routine clinical use.

Up to 60% of patients with Alzheimer's disease show periventricular and deep white matter hyperintensities on T2WI. The incidence of these appears to be slightly greater than in aged-matched controls but less than in patients with cerebral vascular disease or multi-infarct dementia. The aetiology of high signal T2-lesions in Alzheimer's disease is unknown. Pathological studies do indicate that concomitant vascular abnormality is not uncommon giving a combination of multi-infarct dementia and Alzheimer's disease.[12]

FRONTOTEMPORAL DEMENTIA

Frontotemporal dementias form a relatively broad spectrum of neurodegenerative disease primarily affecting the temporal and frontal lobes. Histologically, they are characterized by neuronal loss, spongiform changes and astrocytosis in the outer cortical layers and white matter.[13] It is thought that frontotemporal dementias represents approximately 10% of patients presenting with pre-senile dementia. The histological classification of frontotemporal dementias includes the classical description of Pick's disease, which is typified by the presence of Pick bodies in affected areas. Clinical presentation depends on the actual distribution of degenerative changes and the clinical diagnosis is based on the Lund/Manchester clinical criteria. Neuroimaging appearances may differ from those of Alzheimer's disease. Cerebral atrophy affecting the frontal and temporal lobes can be severe and commonly affect the lateral and inferior portions of the temporal lobe to an equal or

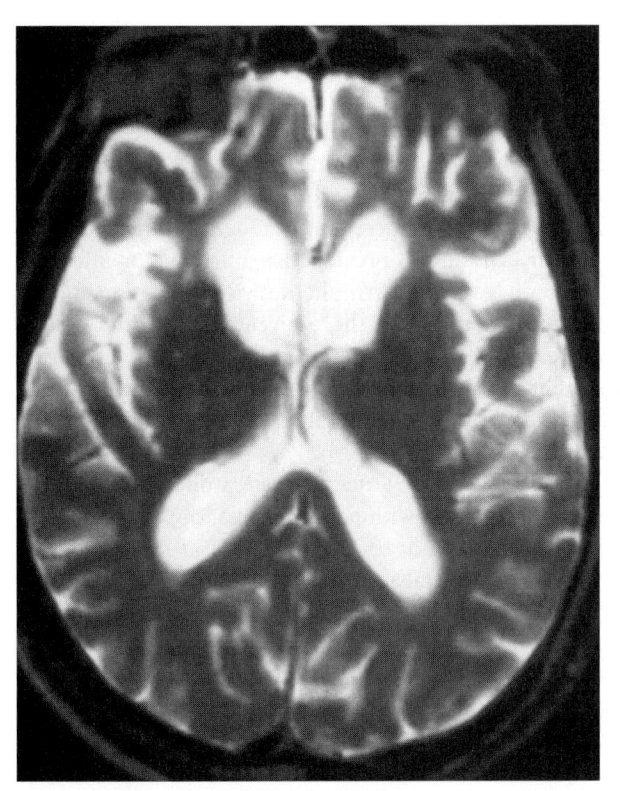

Figure 8.11 *Axial T2WI from a patient with frontotemporal dementia. Note the severe frontal and temporal atrophy and relative preservation in the posterior parietal and occipital areas.*

even greater degree than the medial temporal gyrus and hippocampus (Fig. 8.11).[14] Asymmetrical atrophy is common and increased MR signal intensity may be seen in the frontotemporal white matter on T2- and proton density-weighted images. These white matter signal changes have been suggested as a method for differentiating between frontotemporal and Alzheimer dementia. Regional atrophy in frontotemporal dementias may be severe and marked sulcal widening can give rise to the knife-blade gyri typically associated with pathological descriptions of Pick's disease (Fig. 8.12).

CEREBRAL AMYLOID ANGIOPATHY

Vascular deposition of amyloid is more common in the elderly and particularly in patients with Alzheimer's disease. The incidence of cerebral amyloid angiopathy is in excess of 20% over the age 60 and over 50% over the age of 80. The disease shows no correlation with classical cerebral vascular risk factors. The typical presentation of cerebral amyloid angiopathy is with intracerebral haemorrhage, although some patients present with slowly progressive dementia or multiple infarcts. It is believed to account for as many as 10% of sporadic cerebral haemorrhages in the elderly. In the absence of haemorrhage, no specific imaging findings have been described. Typical imaging descriptions are of single or multiple superficial lobar haematomas, although haemorrhage may occur anywhere within the brain.[15]

VASCULAR DEMENTIA

Vascular insults can result in dementing illness through a number of disease mechanisms. Patients with multiple, small or large infarcts present primarily with symptoms of cognitive disturbance and it is estimated that up to a quarter of elderly patients with a history of stroke fulfil the criteria of vascular dementia. A dementia syndrome may also result from diffuse small vessel disease typified by subcortical arteriosclerotic encephalopathy often called Binswanger's syndrome.[16] Characterized by arteriosclerotic changes in small vessels, this syndrome is seen in 3–5% of individuals over the age of 60 years, although most will not present with dementia. A third form of vascular dementia is typified by perivascular atrophy with marked dilatation of perivascular spaces in the basal ganglia and throughout the corona radiata. These appearances are commonly described as état lacunaire or état criblé.[17]

All forms of vascular dementia are strongly associated with increased vascular risk scores. The most commonly used clinical scoring system for vascular risk was described by Hachinski (Table 8.1). Clinically, the picture of vascular dementia is usually more stepwise than is seen in Alzheimer's disease or frontotemporal dementia. A history of a focal defect and stroke is common and pseudobulbar palsy and motor signs tend to be more prominent. The syndrome of état lacunaire is classically associated with pseudobulbar palsy, a short mincing gait (marche à petits pas), incontinence, imbalance and emotional lability.

Imaging features which favour a diagnosis of vascular dementia rather than a pure neurodegenerative syndrome include established cortical or basal ganglia

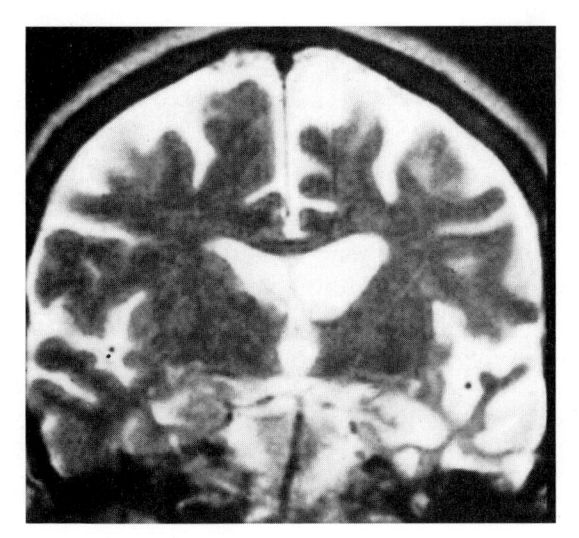

Figure 8.12 *Coronal T2WI through a patient with severe frontotemporal degeneration. Note the knife-blade gyri in the left temporal lobe typically associated with pathological descriptions of Pick's disease.*

Table 8.1 *Features suggesting high risk of cerebrovascular disease*

Clinical features	Score
Abrupt onset	2
Stepwise deterioration	1
Fluctuating cause	2
Nocturnal confusion	1
Relative preservation of personality	1
Depression	1
Somatic complaints	1
Emotional incontinence	1
History of hypertension	1
History of strokes	2
Evidence of associated atherosclerosis	1
Focal neurological symptoms	2
Focal neurological signs	2

infarcts, dilated Virchow-Robin spaces and high T2 signal in the basal ganglia and extensive periventricular hyperintensity (Fig. 8.13).

NORMAL PRESSURE HYDROCEPHALUS

Normal pressure hydrocephalus first described in 1965 is an important and potentially treatable cause of presenile and senile dementia. Clinically, the classic triad of symptoms is dementia, gait disturbance and urinary incontinence. The disease is characterized by increased pulsativity of CSF with a significant increase in the stroke volume of CSF passing through the cerebral aqueduct and fourth ventricle during the cardiac cycle. The aetiology remains uncertain, although, failure of absorption of CSF due to previous haemorrhage or infection has been suggested. An alternative explanation is that ischaemic damage to the periventricular white matter decreases the strength of the ventricular walls leading to systolic ventricular dilatation. All of the symptoms may be reversed or progress halted by ventriculoperitoneal shunting.

Both MR and CT demonstrate a dilated ventricular system associated with periventricular hyperintensity on T2WI (Fig. 8.14 a, b).[7] The increase in stroke volume within the cerebral aqueduct and lower third and fourth ventricles may be seen as an increased signal void on proton density and T2WI (Fig. 8.14c). Measurements of cerebral aqueduct CSF stroke volume, using quantified phase contrast flow imaging, can confirm the diagnosis and have been suggested to be of value in predicting response to treatment. Deep white matter hyperintensities are common in this disease and response to shunting is less common when these changes are extensive.

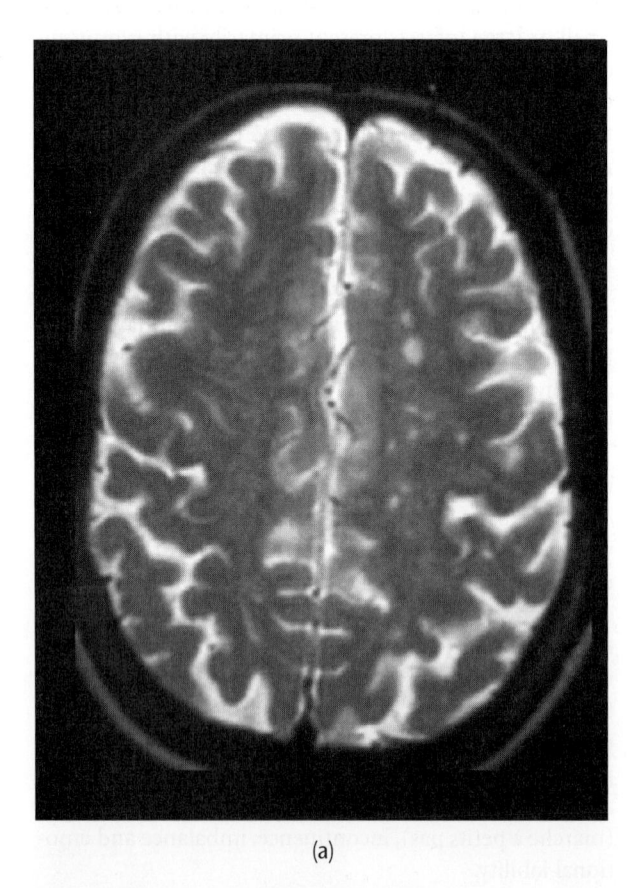

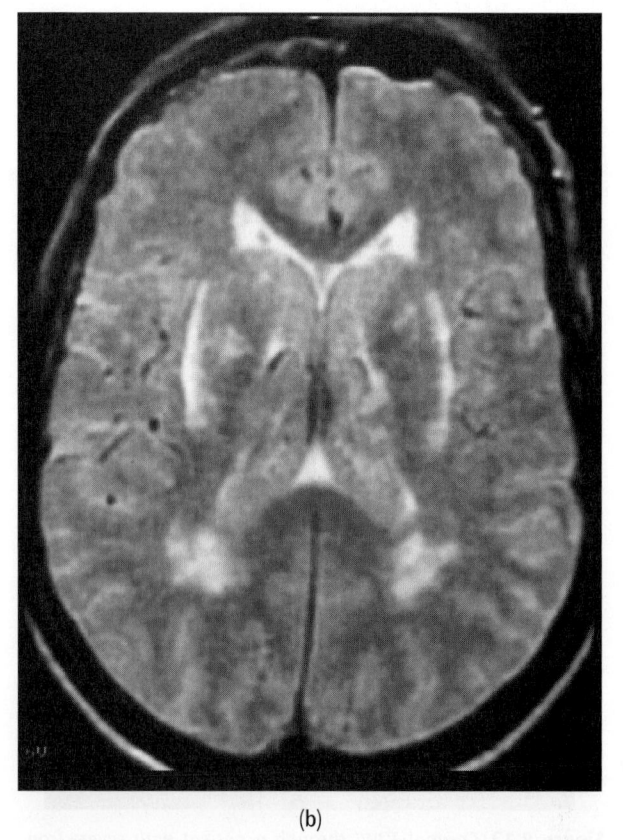

Figure 8.13 *Axial T2-weighted (a) sequence through the corona radiata and FLAIR sequence (b) through the basal ganglia demonstrating extensive white matter abnormality in a patient with Binswanger's disease. Note the involvement of the external capsules and areas of high signal within the basal ganglia themselves, which are typical features of small vessel cerebrovascular disease.*

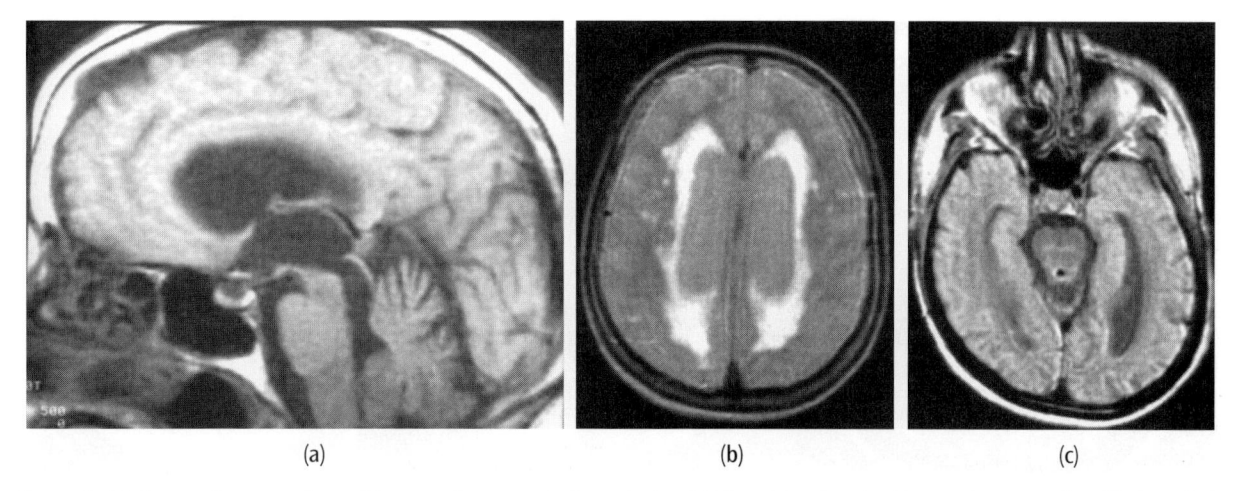

Figure 8.14 *Images from a patient with normal pressure hydrocephalus. (a) T1-weighted sagittal image demonstrating dilation of the third ventricle cerebral aqueduct and thinning of the tectal plate which is a typical feature resulting from the increase flux of CSF through the cerebral aqueduct during systole. (b) FLAIR image demonstrating dilated ventricles, extensive periventricular hyperintensity and areas of high signal within the corona radiata bilaterally. (c) Proton density weighted image showing an area of flow related signal void in the lower border of the cerebral aqueduct.*

Neurodegenerative diseases of the basal ganglia

HUNTINGTON'S DISEASE

Named after the description by George Huntington in 1872, Huntington's disease has an incidence of approximately 5 per 100 000. The age of onset is in the fourth to fifth decades and the disease is inherited in autosomal dominant fashion with complete penetrance. Carriers of the defective gene can be detected by means of a marker linked to the Huntington's gene on the short arm of chromosome 4. Patients present with gradually worsening choreoathetosis, emotional disturbance and dementia. Death occurs 10–15 years after onset and progress is relentless.

The disease is characterized by loss of volume of the caudate nucleus and putamen. Generalized cerebral atrophy also occurs at a greater rate than in normal ageing. Gliotic changes and loss of myelinated fibres in the striatum give rise to increase signal on T2WI, which may be reversed in some patients by iron accumulation.[18,19]

HALLERVORDEN–SPATZ DISEASE

Hallervorden-Spatz disease is a metabolic disorder occurring in adolescence and young adults. In 50% of cases autosomal recessive inheritance is seen and the remainder are sporadic. Clinical features include rigidity, dystonia, chorea, athetosis, gait impairment, mental deterioration, dysarthria and dysphasia.

Two types of Hallervorden-Spatz disease exist – the first affects the globus pallidus and pars reticulata of the substantia nigra, the second only the globus pallidus. A mixture of hypo- and hyperintense changes are seen on T2WI in the affected nuclei due to a mixture of demyelination, gliosis and iron deposition. Initial changes are characterized by high signal on T2WI with gradual loss of signal, particularly at the periphery of the lentiform nucleus.

WILSON'S DISEASE

Wilson's disease is an autosomal recessive disorder carried by chromosome 13. It is characterized by deficiency of ceruloplasmin, which is responsible for plasma transport of copper, leading to copper deposition in normal tissues. Patients present between 5 and 50 years of age with liver disease and neurological signs. Neurological defects include tremor, gait ataxia, rigidity, incoordination and dysarthria. The CT and MRI abnormalities, which are due to copper deposition and gliosis, are symmetrical and involve the basal ganglia thalamus dentate nuclei, pons, substantia nigra, peri-aqueductal grey matter, tectum and red nucleus. The lesions are of decreased attenuation on CT and of variable high and low intensity on T2WI (Fig. 8.15). Most patients show significant generalized cerebral atrophy and the extent of imaging changes shows a close correlation with severity of symptomatology.[18,19]

PARKINSON'S DISEASE

Parkinson described a syndrome of involuntary tremor, rigidity and akinesia. These symptoms result from damage to the dopaminergic nigrostriatal tract. This may be idiopathic or may result from vascular injury or, rarely, from specific drug or toxic insults. Idiopathic

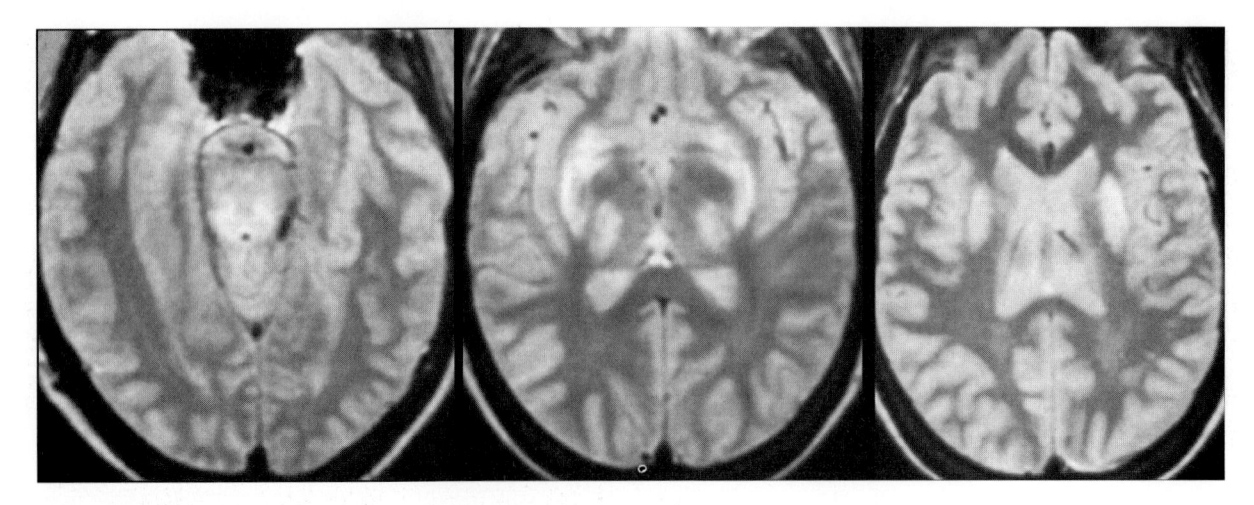

Figure 8.15 *Axial T2WI from a patient with Wilson's disease showing extensive areas of high signal in the lentiform nuclei, thalamus and pontine tegmentum.*

neurodegenerative Parkinsonian syndromes include classical Parkinson's disease, striatonigral degeneration and progressive supranuclear palsy.

Parkinson's disease has a clinical onset between 40 and 60 years of age with an incidence of approximately 0.5–1% over the age of 50 years. Patients develop problems with the generation of spontaneous movements associated with rigidity and spontaneous tremor at rest. Symptoms progress slowly and may respond well to cholinergic and dopaminergic medication, particularly in the early phases.

Imaging changes are non-specific. Loss of width to the melanin containing dopaminergic pars compacta of the substantia nigra, together with areas of increased signal on T2WI within the nigra may be apparent. Depletion of iron from the substantia nigra leads to loss of the low signal, which is commonly present in patients of this age. Cerebral atrophy is also a feature and is more rapid than in age-matched controls.[1]

PARKINSON PLUS SYNDROMES

Approximately 20% of patients with Parkinson's disease have distinctive syndromes typified by more severe Parkinsonian symptoms and a poor response to dopaminergic medications. These disorders are commonly referred to as Parkinsonian plus syndromes or multisystem atrophy. They include striatonigral degeneration, Shy–Drager syndrome, progressive supranuclear palsy and olivopontocerebellar degeneration .

Striatonigral degeneration

Striatonigral degeneration is characterized by Parkinsonian symptoms dominated by severe rigidity and poor response to dopaminergic therapy. Imaging features differ from classical Parkinson's disease in showing very severe atrophy of the striatum (caudate nucleus and putamen). In addition, the putamen and substantia nigra show hypointense signal changes on T2WI which are dependent on magnetic field strength. At 1.5 TESLA progressive hypointensity develops which will render the putamen lower in signal than the adjacent globus pallidus. On lower field systems, the putamen may appear to be high intensity because of increased local water due to gliosis and degeneration.[20]

Shy–Drager syndrome

Shy–Drager syndrome is a further Parkinsonian variant associated with failure of autonomic nervous system functions. Patients suffer from urinary incontinence, postural hypotension, and show inability to sweat. Imaging features do not distinguish this syndrome from striatonigral degeneration.[20]

Progressive supranuclear palsy

Beginning between the ages of 40 and 70 this Parkinsonian variant is characterized by predominant involvement of the brainstem with impairment of vertical eye movements, supranuclear ophthalmaplegia, pseudobulbar palsy and associated extrapyramidal symptoms.

Neuroimaging may show atrophy of the superior colliculus with areas of high signal on T2WI which may extend into the periaqueductal grey matter of the mesencephalon and pons. These changes occur in addition to the loss of substantia nigra volume seen in classical Parkinson's disease and may be associated with signal abnormalities in the putamen similar to striatonigral degeneration.[20]

Olivopontocerebellar degeneration

This disorder has both familial and sporadic forms clinically presenting anywhere between infancy and old age. Commonest age of onset is mid-adulthood. Patients develop slowly progressive cerebellar ataxia associated with typical speech disorder. Neuroimaging shows loss of cerebellar folia, particularly affecting the vermis (Fig. 8.16).[20–22] The differential diagnosis of focal cerebellar and brainstem degeneration is shown in Table 8.2.

Neurodegenerative diseases 251

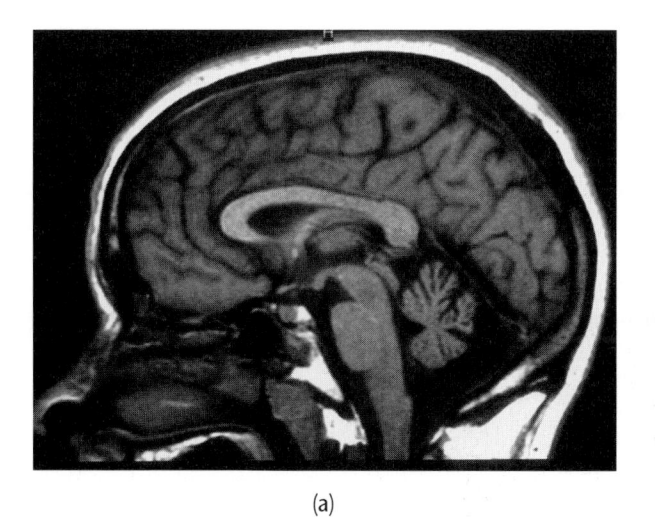

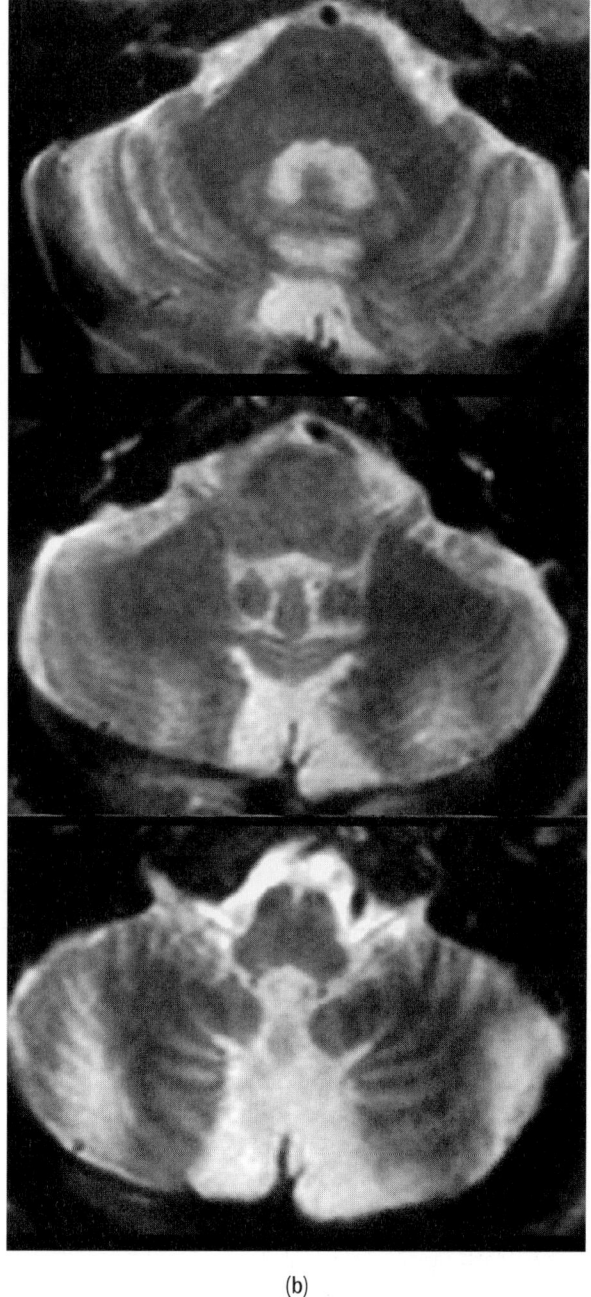

Figure 8.16 *Images from a patient with olivopontocerebellar degeneration. (a) Sagittal image showing gross atrophy of the midline cerebellar structures. (b) Axial images throughout the cerebellum showing gross central vermian atrophy and less severe but pronounced atrophy of the cerebellar hemispheres.*

Leigh's syndrome

Subacute necrotizing encephalomyelopathy known as Leigh's syndrome presents in childhood or more rarely in early adulthood and is inherited in an autosomal recessive manner. Symptoms include widespread neurological dysfunction with abnormalities of psychological and motor function weakness, dystonia and focal brainstem and cerebellar symptoms. Diagnosis is based on clinical symptoms, together with metabolic abnormalities and findings on neuroimaging.

Magnetic resonance shows areas of abnormal high signal intensity in the basal ganglia, corpus callosum, brainstem and periventricular white matter on T2WI. Lesions are commonly seen in the brainstem spinal cord and optic pathways. These areas of signal change correspond to focal spongiform degeneration and demyelination. Although individual lesions may show partial resolution, the disease shows overall progression until death.[18,19]

Other grey matter degenerations

TEMPORAL MESIAL SCLEROSIS

Temporal mesial sclerosis, also known as hippocampal sclerosis is the most common cause of temporal lobe epilepsy found in surgical resection specimens. There is

Table 8.2 Differential diagnosis of brainstem and cerebellar atrophy

Disorder	Cause	Pathological and MRI features
Acquired cerebellar degenerations		
Toxic	Alcohol	Primary cerebellar cortical atrophy results from direct toxic effects. Vermian atrophy is greater than hemispheric involvement.
	Toluene	
Drugs	Phenytoin	
	Diphenylhydantion	
	High dose cytosine arabinoside	
	Thallium	
Paraneoplastic		
Autoimmune	Influenza vaccine	
Inherited disorders		
Olivopontocerebellar atrophy	Autosomal dominant and sporadic forms	Atrophy results from loss of pontine nuclei and projections to cortex. Cerebellar atrophy greatest in the hemispheres. Associated pontine and middle cerebellar peduncle atrophy.
Cerebello-olivary degeneration	Familial and sporadic forms	Cerebellar atrophy worst in vermis. Relatively slow progression and good prognosis.
Fragile X syndrome	X-linked	Marked atrophy of posterior cerebellar vermis.
Autism		Reports of cerebellar atrophy in autism remain contentious.
Friedreich's ataxia		Primarily marked by spinal cord atrophy. Cerebellar atrophy principally affects the superior vermis but is commonly mild or absent.

loss of hippocampal neurons most marked in the pyramidal cell layer of the cornu ammonis and the granular cell layer of the dentate gyrus.[23] The aetiology and pathogenesis of these changes is not understood. It is believed that a developmental insult such as a complicated febrile seizure or encephalitis damages the dentate interneuron system. Surgical resection of the affected hippocampus is the only reliable therapy and MR is the investigation of choice for its diagnosis. The affected hippocampus appears high signal on T2WI and is atrophic (Fig. 8.17). Formal measurements of hippocampal volume may be helpful but are time consuming. The diagnosis may be supported by associated loss of the collateral white matter tracts in the temporal radiation and the fornix (Fig. 8.17).[24] The presence of bilateral hippocampal sclerosis can be a relative contraindication to surgery and the MRI diagnosis must lead to extensive presurgical functional investigations including WADA testing to predict potential functional loss which may result from surgery.

WERNICKE'S ENCEPHALOPATHY

Wernicke's encephalopathy is a neurodegenerative disorder resulting from thiamine deficiency usually resulting from chronic alcoholism. The clinical syndrome reflects neuronal death in the mamillary bodies, periaqueductal grey matter and hypothalamus. Clinically, the patients present with Korsakoff's dysmenesis characterized by retrograde amnesia and confabulation, opthalmoplegia, ataxia and nystagmus. Typically, MRI demonstrates areas of high signal on T2WI in the mamillary bodies and similar changes may be seen in the periaqueductal grey. The mamillary bodies undergo quite severe atrophy, particularly in the late stages of the disease.[19]

MITOCHONDRIAL ENCEPHALOMYELOPATHIES

These diseases are linked by the presence of mitochondrial abnormalities. Clinically, patients have multisystem disorders involving gut, heart, muscle, kidney and central nervous system. All the mitochondrial encephalomyelopathies are rare. Two of these are described in more detail due to distinctive neuroimaging features.

MELAS syndrome

The MELAS syndrome describes a combination of Mitochondrial myopathy, Encephalopathy, Lactic Acidosis and Stroke. Patients present in adulthood with stroke-like lesions that do not conform strictly to vascu-

Neurodegenerative diseases

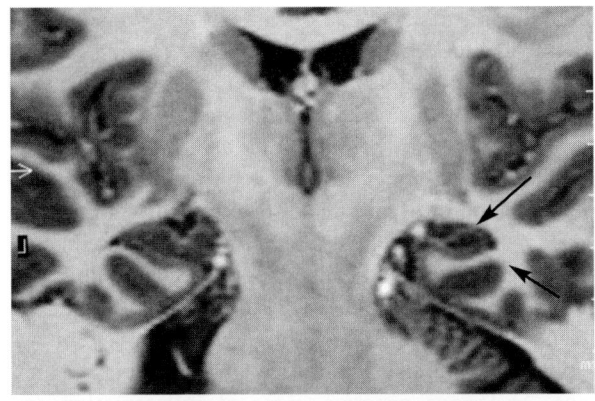

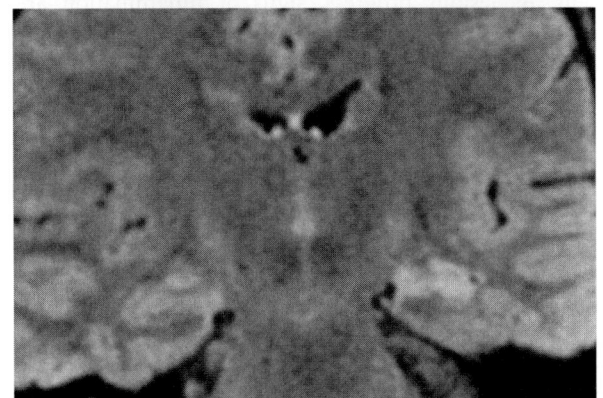

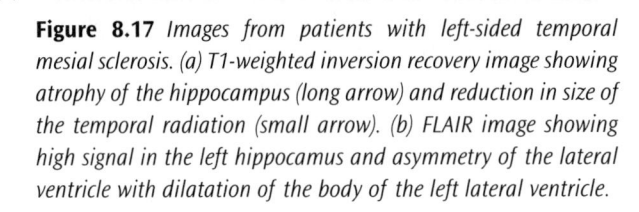

Figure 8.17 Images from patients with left-sided temporal mesial sclerosis. (a) T1-weighted inversion recovery image showing atrophy of the hippocampus (long arrow) and reduction in size of the temporal radiation (small arrow). (b) FLAIR image showing high signal in the left hippocamus and asymmetry of the lateral ventricle with dilatation of the body of the left lateral ventricle.

lar territories. Cortical blindness is common and any area of the brain may be involved, although the brainstem and frontal lobes are typically spared (Fig. 8.18). Lesions occur acutely and result in progressive focal regional atrophy.[18,19]

MERRF syndrome

The MERRF (Myoclonic Epilepsy with Ragged Red Fibres) syndrome is a mitochondrial encephalomyopathy that presents with myoclonic epilepsy, weakness and ophthalmoplegia. Patients commonly are of short stature and the syndrome is associated with cardiac conduction abnormalities and endocrine disorders. Imaging appearances are similar to MELAS.

Figure 8.18 Images from a patient with proven MELAS syndrome. (a) CT scan and (b) T2-weighted MR demonstrate posterior cerebral infarction involving white matter and grey matter and extending to the visual cortex. This distribution is typically associated with MELAS. Other imaging findings such as low signal in the basal ganglia were not present in this patient.

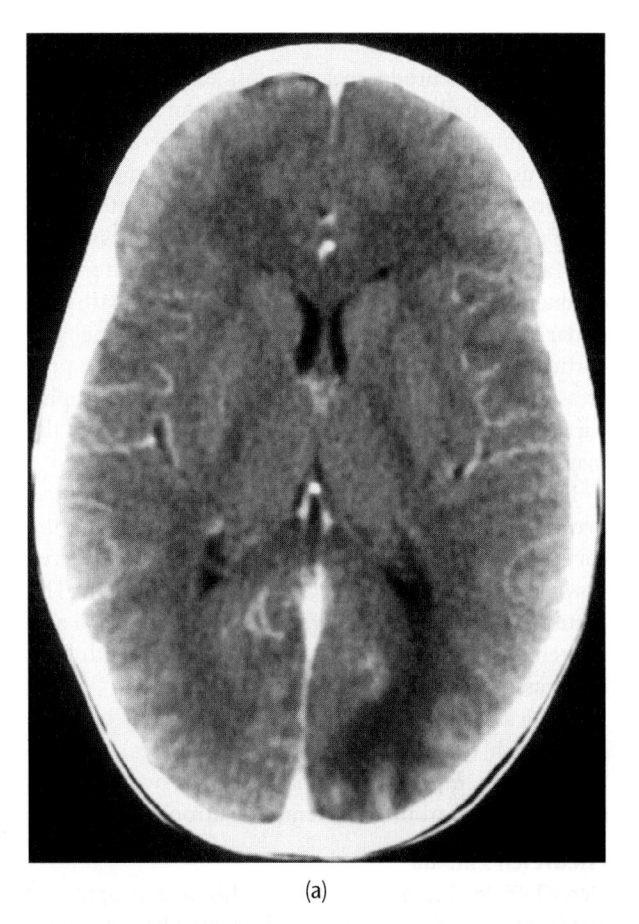

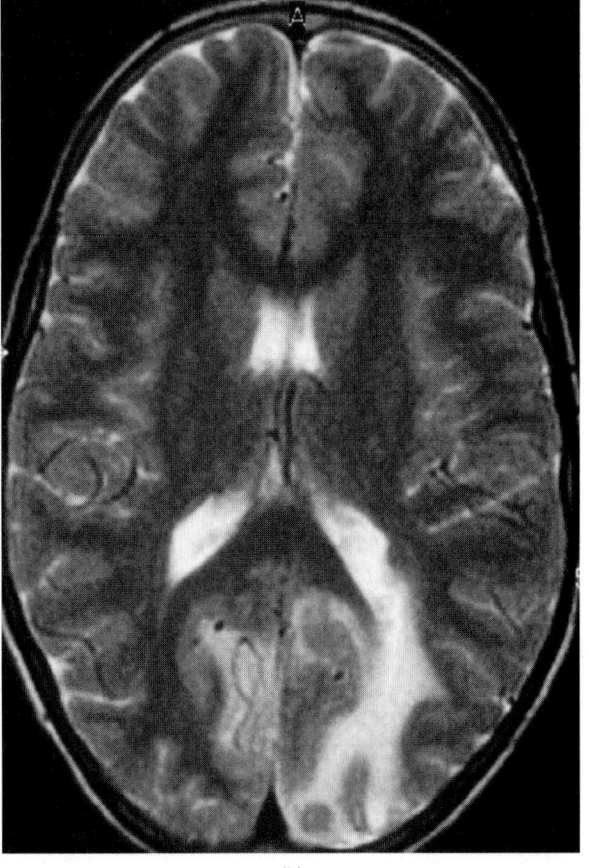

Motor neuron disease
Spontaneous neurodegenerative loss of primary motor cortex is the hallmark of the motor neuron diseases. The most common of these is amyotrophic lateral sclerosis which usually presents in the fifth decade and has an incidence of 1.5/100 000. Autosomal dominant inheritance is seen in 5% but most are sporadic and its aetiology and pathogenesis are unknown. Spontaneous degeneration of the motor cortex cell bodies with secondary Wallerian degeneration of the corticospinal and corticobulbar pathways lead to relentless disease progression. Patients present with weakness and atrophy, particularly affecting the arms in the early stages and the majority die within 5 years of onset.

Neuroimaging shows focal atrophy of the pre-central gyrus with areas of high signal on T2WI following the cortical spinal tract course from the pre-central gyrus down through the internal capsule and brainstem. The cortex itself may be of relatively low signal on T2WI and the remainder of the brain is relatively spared with little or no associated generalized atrophy.[25]

Clinically, amyotrophic lateral sclerosis may be associated with other neurodegenerative diseases, particularly, frontotemporal dementia where an overlap form with associated frontal and temporal atrophy is seen.

Friedreich's ataxia
Described by Friedreich in 1861 this is a progressive ataxia, often of familial origin which may be autosomal recessive or dominant. Patients become symptomatic between the ages of 10 and 20 years with early ataxia of gait and dysarthria. They become unable to walk within 4 years and develop kyphoscoliosis. Meanwhile, life expectancy is decreased with death typically occurring between the ages of 20 and 40. Imaging shows marked spinal cord atrophy with variable degrees of brainstem and cerebellar atrophy.

WHITE MATTER DISEASES

Diseases affecting white matter typically reflect disordered formation or abnormal breakdown of myelin. Although CT shows abnormalities in many of these diseases, there is no doubt that MR has a far higher sensitivity to white matter lesions. This sensitivity together with the specific patterns of lesions in white matter diseases has given MR a significant clinical role in their diagnosis and management.

Multiple sclerosis

Multiple sclerosis is the archetypal demyelinating disease. It is the most common of all the demyelinating diseases occurring most commonly in young adults, usually presenting between the ages of 20 and 40 years. It is more common in females (1.5–2:1) and may also occur in children where the female to male ratio is even higher.

The origin of multiple sclerosis is unknown. The disease appears to be an autoimmune mediated demyelination, which occurs, primarily in genetically susceptible individuals. Pathologically, the multiple sclerosis brain shows 'plaques' of disease distributed throughout the white matter. Plaques are typified by loss of myelin and the myelin-producing oligodendrocytes. In the early phases when the plaques are active, there is localized loss of the endothelial blood–brain barrier and macrophage infiltration and other inflammatory changes may be present. As lesions progress, signs of inflammation are reduced and astrocytic gliosis occurs. Plaques commonly develop in sites related to subependymal veins giving rise to a distribution of lesions that can be distinctive and aid in diagnosis.

Clinical features and diagnosis
The clinical presentation of multiple sclerosis is variable. The first symptom is often painful visual loss due to optic neuritis. Up to 45% of these patients will have evidence of multiple sclerosis plaques elsewhere in the brain at presentation and progression to multiple sclerosis is the rule in this group. As the disease progresses, neurological symptoms and signs typical of multiple white matter lesions occur. Visual disturbance, loss of sphincter control, sensory abnormalities, muscle spasm, regional paralyses, and cognitive dysfunction may develop. Other than that associated with optic neuritis, pain is extremely rare. Most patients experience a relapsing, remitting disease with periods of exacerbation and remission of their neurological deficits. Recovery between episodes may be complete, particularly in the early phase, but as the disease progresses, the patient is left with increasing sequellae of the recurrent attacks. Some patients exhibit a chronic, progressive pattern, often typified by spinal cord and motor involvement. Both forms can progress to a severe endstage with extensive neurological disability and cognitive impairment.

Diagnosis is based on typical clinical features combined with laboratory and imaging confirmation. A number of clinical criteria exist of which the commonest are the Poser and Bartel criteria. Originally these criteria were entirely clinical but have been modified to include elements based on CSF analysis and imaging studies.

Neuroimaging findings
The classical MRI features of the multiple sclerosis plaque are an increased signal on T2WI and a decrease in signal on T1WI (Fig. 8.19). It must be appreciated that up to 15% of patients with clear established clinical multiple sclerosis will have normal MR scans and that this does not invalidate the clinical diagnosis. The disease is also characterized by cerebral atrophy that may be very severe particularly in progressive or longstanding cases. Secondary degeneration of pathways gives rise to increased signal distal to plaques on T2WI that may be

seen as abnormalities in entire fibre tracts in established cases.

The T2 imaging features of multiple sclerosis are the most commonly used diagnostic indicators in clinical practice. Despite this, it should be recognized that the extent and distribution of lesions correlates poorly with the clinical picture or severity of disease. The exceptions to this are lesions in the optic nerve, spinal cord and brainstem, which tend to be associated with predictable neurological deficit. Some workers have found that the identification of lesions on T1WI has a closer relationship with the degree of disability than the lesions identified on T2-weighted sequences. This is believed to reflect the fact that T1WI represent areas of established necrosis and therefore highlight those lesions of clinical importance.[26]

The demonstration of plaques on MRI is extremely technique dependent. The use of thin contiguous sections (3 mm or less) significantly increases the number of plaques identified due to reduction in partial volume averaging effects. The fluid suppressed T2WI (FLAIR) increases the conspicuity of lesions in the forebrain and considerably increases the sensitivity of scanning to lesions within the grey matter of the cerebral cortex (Fig. 8.20). Nonetheless, several groups have shown that FLAIR is less sensitive to lesions in the brainstem than conventional spin echo techniques.[27,28] The use of a conventional spin echo technique should include both proton density and T2WI usually obtained as a dual echo sequence. The sensitivity of proton density weighted images to MR plaques is higher than that of the associated T2WI although the conspicuity of the lesions tends to be lower.

The diagnosis of multiple sclerosis on MRI can be difficult particularly in those patients with few lesions and, in older patients where leukoaraiosis or vascular lesions within the brain may be difficult or impossible to distinguish from multiple sclerosis plaques. This distinction is possible in many cases due to the different distribution of vascular and demyelinating lesions. The vascular white matter lesions seen in the elderly tend to occur in areas where deep penetrating arteries with little or no collateral supply are prejudiced by systemic physiological changes affecting flow. Lesions are therefore typically seen in the depth of the corona radiata and central portions of the pontine reticular formation. Multiple sclerosis plaque represents an inflammatory lesion of white matter that is commonly perivenular. This pathological process leads to a distinctive distribution of lesions in multiple sclerosis affecting areas that are typically spared by diffuse vascular disease. Demyelinating plaques are commonly found around the penetrating veins on the ventral surface of the central corpus callosum where it is joined to the septum pellucidum. These callosal–septal interface lesions have a high specificity (> 90%) for a diagnosis of multiple sclerosis (Fig. 8.21).[29] Lesions in the cerebellar white matter, cerebellar peduncles, spinal cord, and adjacent to the CSF surfaces of the brain stem are also unusual in vascular brain disease (Fig. 8.22).[30] Perivenular lesions, following the penetrating veins in the corona radiata, give rise to the classic Dawson's finger described by pathologists.[31] These lesions may be seen on MR scans as an area of high signal on T2WI passing through the corona radiata perpendicular to the lateral margin of the lateral ventricles. Periventricular lesions are also common and may be confluent around the entire lateral ventricle. The presence of focal gliosis gives rise to a distinctive 'lumpy bumpy' appearance of the periventricular hyperintensity which may help distinguish it from the periventricular hyperintensity seen in vascular disease (Fig. 8.23).[32] Multiple sclerosis lesions may be seen in both white and grey matter and grey matter lesions are increasingly recognized with the introduction of long TR/long TE FLAIR sequences.[27]

Enhancement of multiple sclerosis lesions with contrast is an indication of blood–brain barrier breakdown. Enhancement is believed to indicate inflammatory activity within the plaque and provide some indication of activity although this is of little clinical benefit in most cases. Large lesions may show a ring-like pattern and areas of decreased signal at the margins of these on

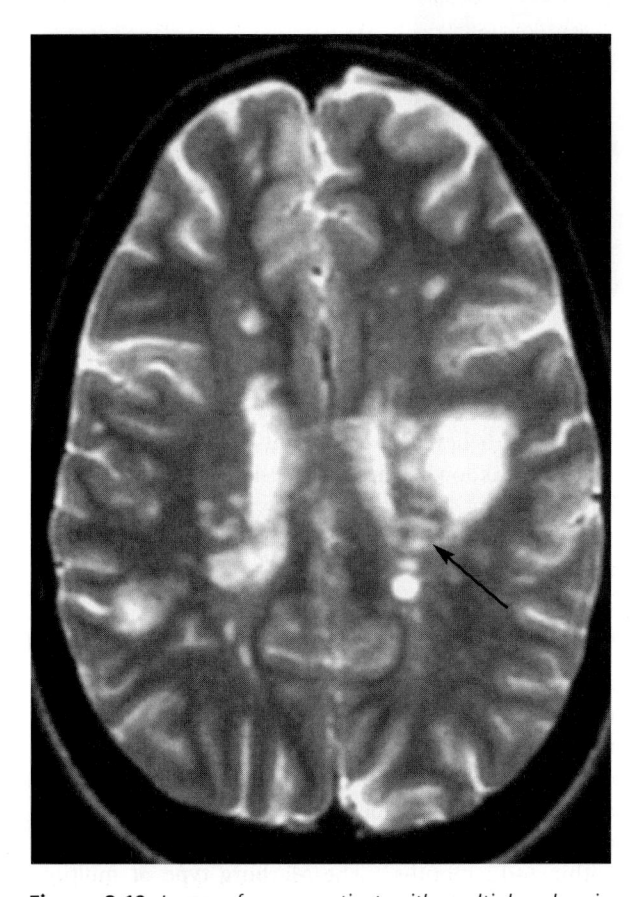

Figure 8.19 *Images from a patient with multiple sclerosis. Extensive areas of confluent white matter demyelination are seen around the top of the lateral ventricles throughout the centrum semiovale. Some of the white matter abnormalities in the left side are typical ovoid lesions lying perpendicular to the anteroposterior axis of the brain (arrow).*

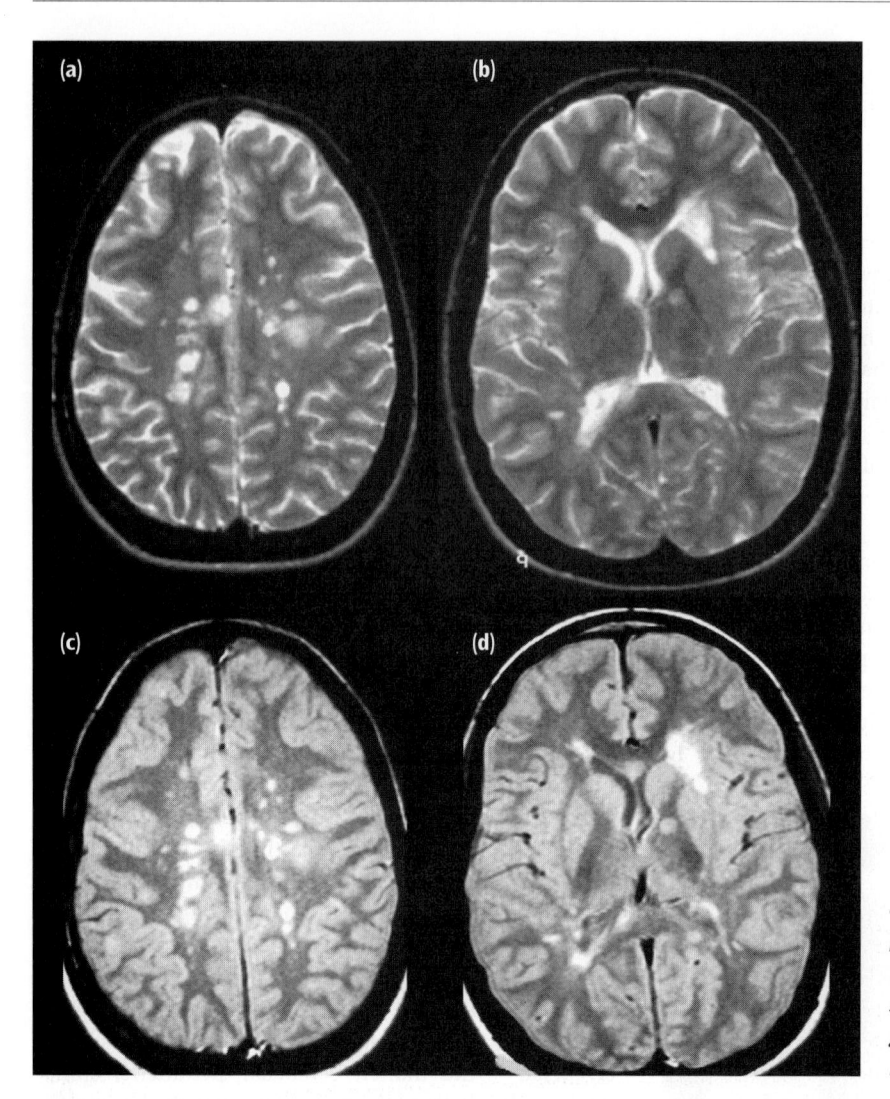

Figure 8.20 *T2-weighted (top row) and FLAIR (bottom row) images from a patient with multiple sclerosis. Slice thickness is 3 mm for both image acquisitions. FLAIR images show lesions with greater conspicuity particularly where lesions lie adjacent to CSF spaces.*

T1WI are believed to represent areas of incomplete myelin breakdown. These ring lesions may cavitate and chronic cystic lesions secondary to demyelination are not uncommon, particularly in the periventricular regions (Fig. 8.24).[33]

ATYPICAL FORMS OF MULTIPLE SCLEROSIS

A number of rare but distinctive clinical presentations of multiple sclerosis are recognized. Devic's disease (neuromyelitis optica) presents as a combination of severe optic neuritis and spinal cord demyelination. These appear around the same time and are the predominant clinical features. Approximately 50% of the patients die within 6–12 months.[34] The Marburg type of multiple sclerosis sometimes known as acute MS is rare, occurring in young patients and is often associated with a preceding febrile illness. The disease is rapidly and inexorably progressive and death usually occurs within months. Diffuse sclerosis or Schilder type multiple sclerosis is very rare and is characterized by asymmetric

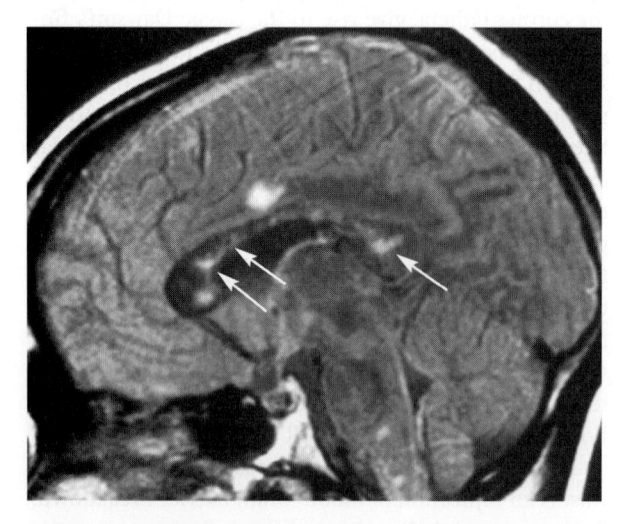

Figure 8.21 *Sagittal FLAIR image from a patient with multiple sclerosis showing typical calloso–septal interface lesions. These lesions extend from the ventral surface of the corpus callosum into its depth and lying within 5 mm of the midline (arrows). Lesions are also seen in the pons and medulla.*

White matter diseases 257

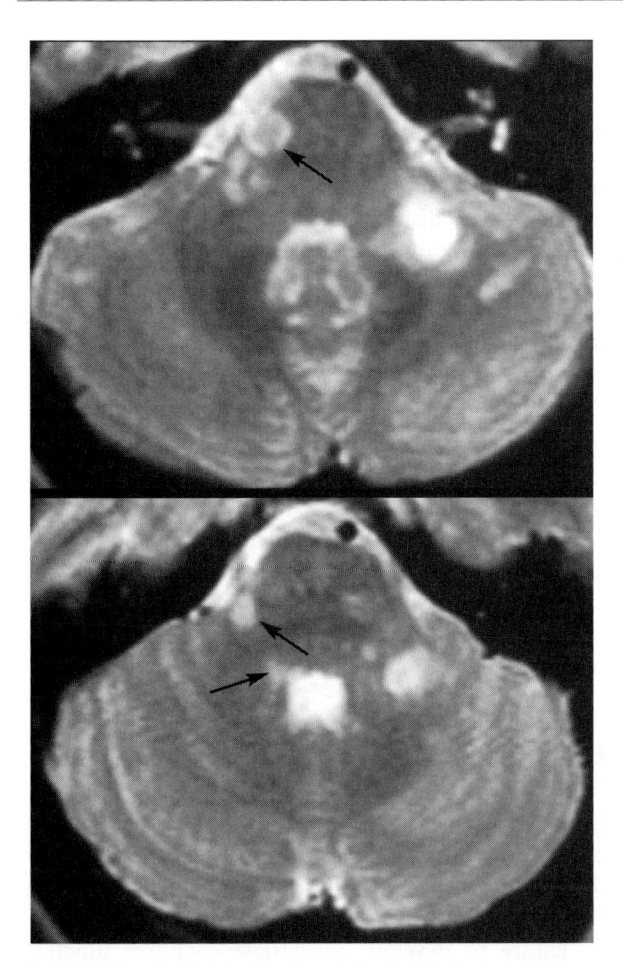

Figure 8.22 Images showing lesions in the brainstem and cerebellum in a patient with multiple sclerosis. The appearance of high signal lesions adjacent to the white matter CSF surface of the brainstem (arrows) are typical of multiple sclerosis although they are also seen in other demyelinating diseases.

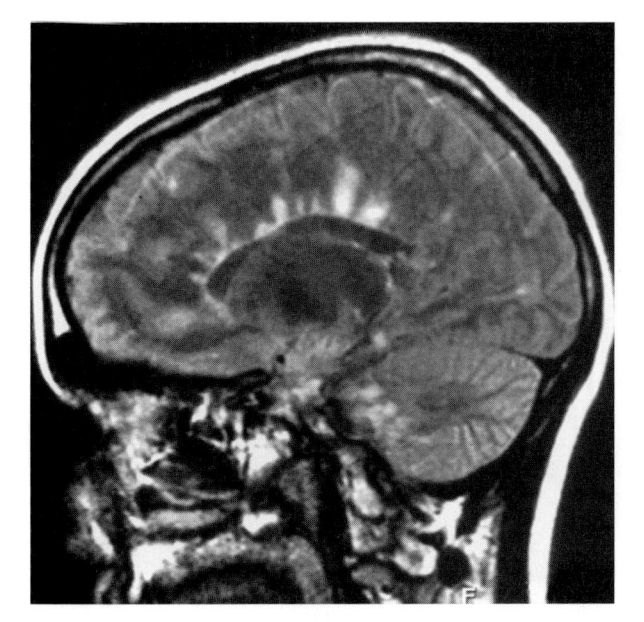

Figure 8.23 Parasagittal FLAIR image of a patient with multiple sclerosis showing the 'lumpy bumpy' appearance of periventricular lesions.

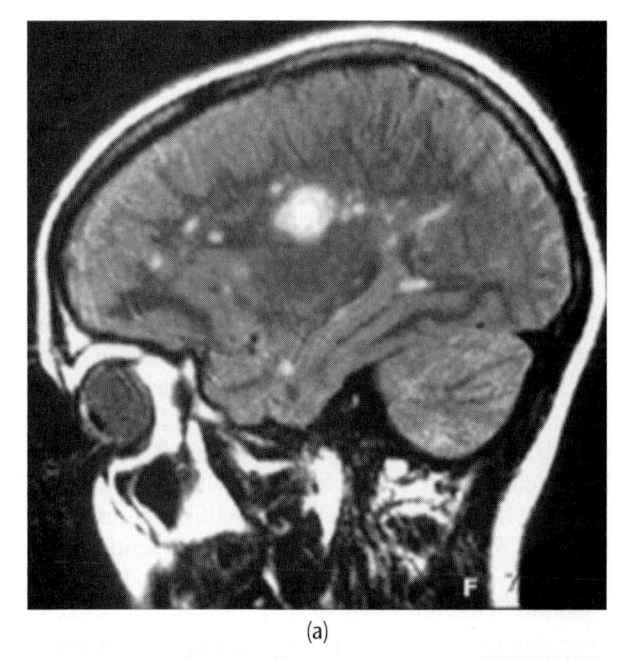

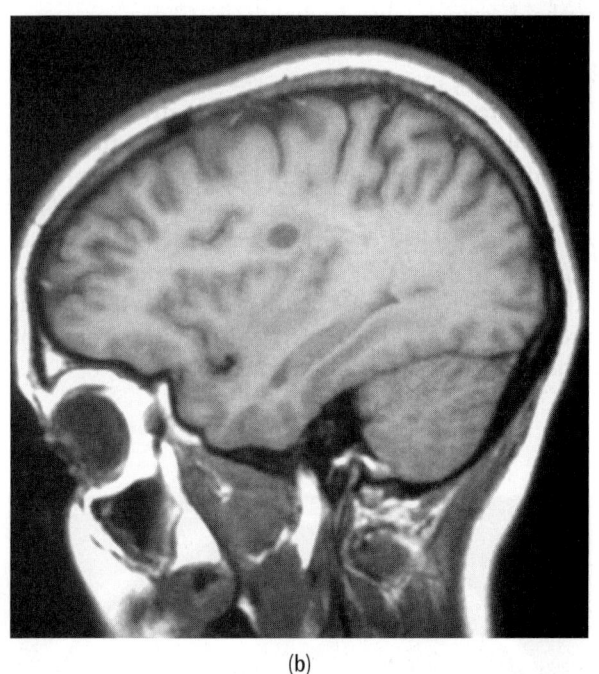

Figure 8.24 Cystic lesion in a patient with multiple sclerosis shown on FLAIR (a) and T1 (b) images. Note the area of decreased signal surrounding the cyst on the T1WI and the central area of low signal corresponding to the cyst itself.

bilateral demyelination of the hemispheres, cerebellum and brainstem which is extensive and may be associated with cavitating lesions.

Infective demyelination

A number of viral infections can cause demyelinating syndromes, the most common of which is progressive multifocal leukoencephalopathy which is due to reactivation of a latent virus infection (the JC papovirus). Progressive multifocal leukoencephalopathy presents in immunocompressed patients particularly those with AIDS, leukaemia or lymphoma[35] and is also associated with other causes of immunocompromise such as immunosuppressive therapy, sarcoidosis, neoplastic disease and tuberculosis. Clinically, patients present with a slowly progressive dementia associated with other neurological defects including visual loss and ataxia. On MRI, confluent areas of high signal due to demyelination are demonstrated. These are seen as asymmetric large patchy areas of demyelination usually in the subcortical white matter and corona radiata (Fig. 8.25). Some of these lesions may be associated with mass effect and may be difficult to differentiate from neoplastic lesions.

Acute disseminated encephalomyelitis is an immune mediated form of demyelination usually presenting clinically 1–2 weeks after a flu-like illness. It may also follow childhood viral infections such as measles and chickenpox and can occur after vaccination for influenza, typhoid, tetanus, rabies or diphtheria. Clinical presentation is usually with onset of seizures or focal defects, which resolve in over 80% of cases within 1–2 months. The syndrome most commonly follows measles, rubella, chickenpox or mumps. On MRI, lesions of acute disseminated encephalomyelitis are indistinguishable from those of multiple sclerosis. Lesions are usually bilateral, asymmetrical and are widely distributed, usually affecting deep white matter, cerebellum and brainstem (Fig. 8.26). These lesions may rarely enhance and the natural progression is for all lesions to regress over a period of months.[36–38]

Central pontine myelinosis

Central pontine myelinosis is a demyelinating disease caused by electrolyte imbalances leading to osmotic injury. It is commonly associated with drug overdose, diabetes, liver disease, kidney disease and neoplasia. Pontine myelinosis is common particularly following profound hyponatraemia and presents with typical features of an extensive pontine lesion. Patients develop quadriparesis, pseudobulbar palsies and depression of conscious level and may go on to coma and death. Central pontine lesions may lead to a locked-in syndrome where patient's conscious level is maintained but in association with complete paralysis which may spare some ocular movements. On MRI, high signal T2-weighted confluent lesions are demonstrated in the mid portion of the pons (Fig. 8.27). These may be associated with lesions elsewhere particularly in the posterior part of the thalamus and internal capsule although they may be anywhere within the brain.[18,19]

Leukodystrophies

Leukodystrophies form a group of inherited diseases characterized by failure of formation or premature destruction of myelin. The clinical picture varies only slightly from case to case and is characterized by a loss of or failure to develop appropriate cognitive function associated with motor visual and auditory defects. Most of these are diseases of childhood presenting under the age of 10 years. Detailed description of these diseases is beyond the scope of this chapter and summary informa-

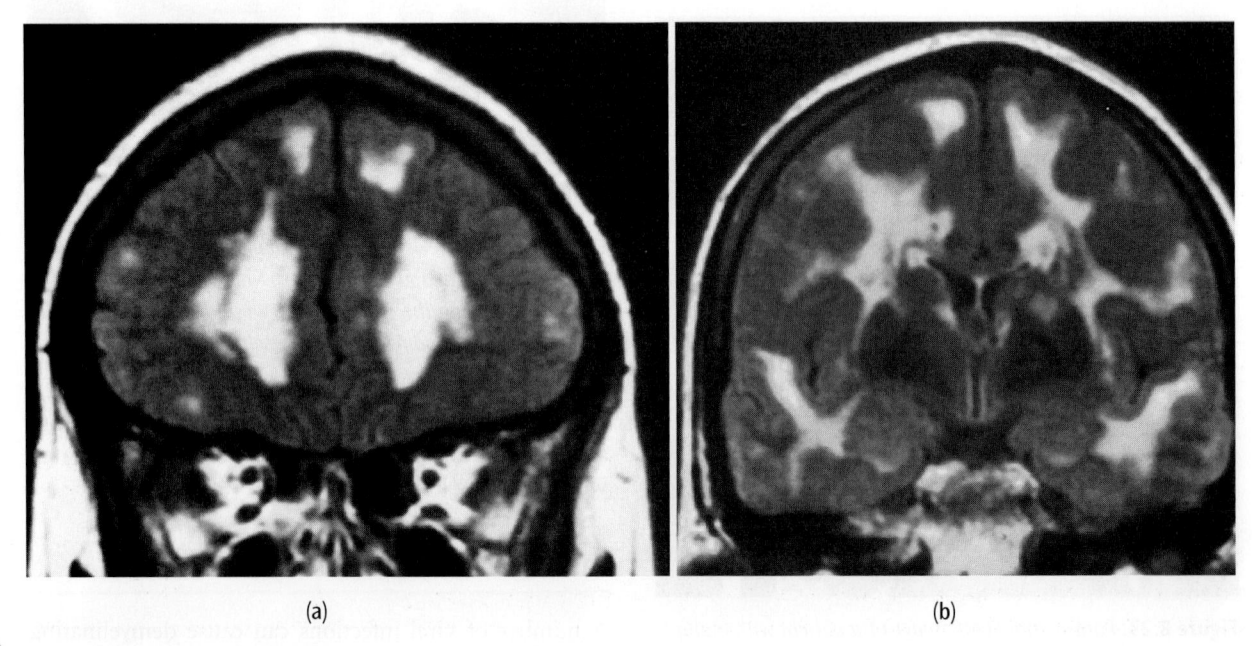

(a)   (b)

Figure 8.25 *Coronal FLAIR images showing extensive white matter demyelination in a patient with progressive multifocal leukoencephalopathy occurring as a complication of lymphoma.*

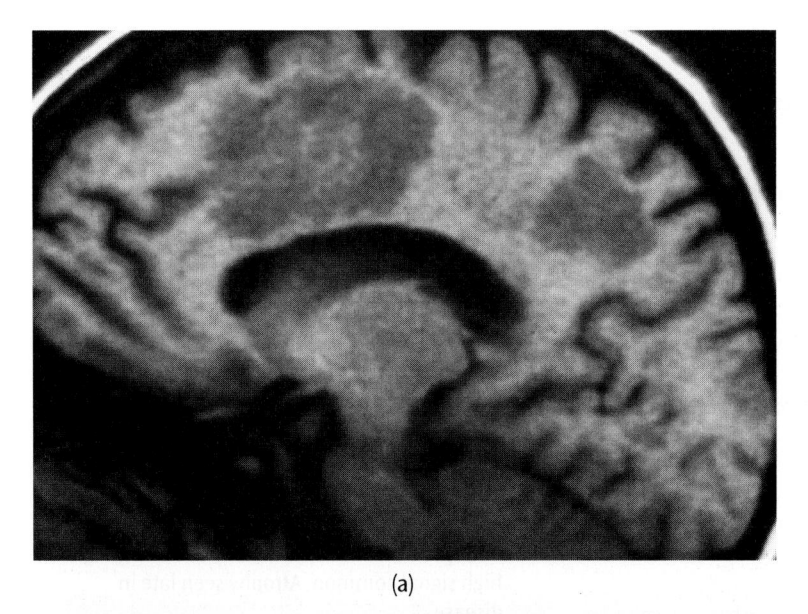

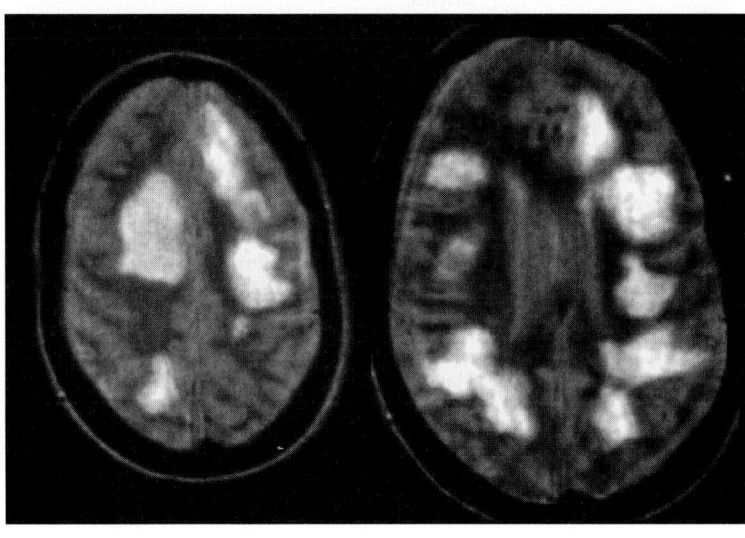

Figure 8.26 *Images from a patient with acute disseminated encephalomyelitis. (a) Sagittal T1WI showing large confluent areas of low signal due to demyelination. (b) Axial T2WI showing widespread multiple areas of confluent demyelination. This patient contracted acute disseminated encephalomyelitis following a non-specific flu-like illness. Viral titres were positive for chickenpox and the patient made an uneventful recovery over a period of several months.*

tion has been provided in Table 8.3. Brief descriptions will be given below simply to highlight the typical or distinctive imaging features in the more common diseases.[18,19]

Sudanophilic leukodystrophies

These disorders are characterized by accumulation of cholesterol and triglyceride containing sudanophylic droplets in the white matter. The group includes Pelizaeus–Merzbacher syndrome and Cockayne's syndrome. The former presents in the neonatal period and death occurs in the first decade. Imaging shows severe brain atrophy particularly affecting the hindbrain. Widespread demyelination with small islands of normal myelin gives rise to a tigroid appearance on histology that may also occasionally be seen on MRI. Cockayne's syndrome presents in early to late infancy with ataxia, delayed development and abnormal eye movement.

Children may survive into adolescence. On MR and CT basal ganglia may be demonstrated and cerebellar calcification associated with replacement of the entire white matter throughout the brain by high signal on T2-weighted lesions.

Canavan's disease

Canavan's disease is an autosomal recessive inherited disease most common in children of Ashkanazi Jewish descent. The brain undergoes widespread cystic spongiform degeneration. MRI shows diffuse high signal throughout the brain white matter but with a relatively typical sparing of the internal capsule.

Krabbe's disease

Krabbe's disease is an autosomal recessive inherited disease presenting at 2–6 months of age with increasing

Table 8.3 *Imaging features of the leukodystrophies*

Disorder	Cause	Pathological and MRI features
Sudanophilic leukodystrophies		
Pelizaeus–Merzbacher disease	Sporadic	Cerebral atrophy, severe in posterior fossa. Symmetric extensive demyelination, may have 'tigroid' appearance. Variable calcification in basal ganglia, commonest in Cockayne's syndrome
Cockayne's syndrome	Sporadic	
Other leukodystrophies		
Canavan's disease	Autosomal dominant	Macrocephaly progressing to atrophy in late stages. Extensive symmetric demyelination with distinctive sparing of internal capsule.
Krabbe's disease	Sporadic	Increased signal in periventricular white matter and splenium of corpus callosum. Basal ganglia high signal common. Atrophy seen late in disease.
Metachromatic leukodystrophy	Autosomal recessive	Symmetric extensive white matter high signal progressing from front to back of brain. Cerebellum commonly involved, arcuate U fibres spared.
Adrenoleukodystrophy	X-linked recessive	Specific appearances. Symmetric white matter high signal around atria of lateral ventricles and splenium of corpus callosum. Marginal areas of high signal area enhance due to active demyelination.
Alexander's disease	Sporadic	Macrocephaly progressing to atrophy in late stages. Extensive symmetric demyelination involving internal capsule (see Canavan's disease).

(a)

(b)

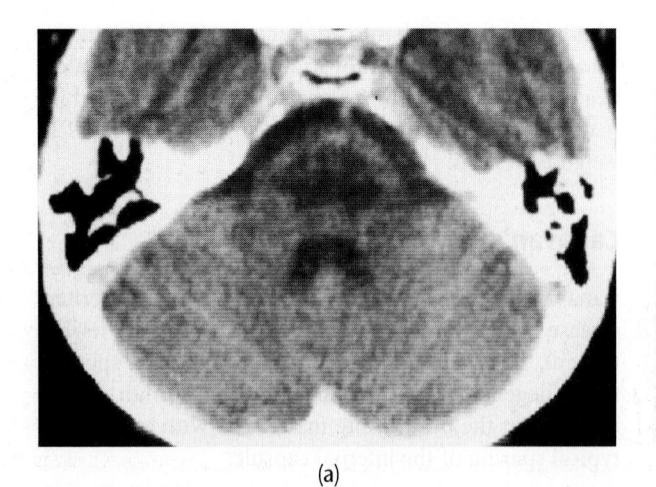

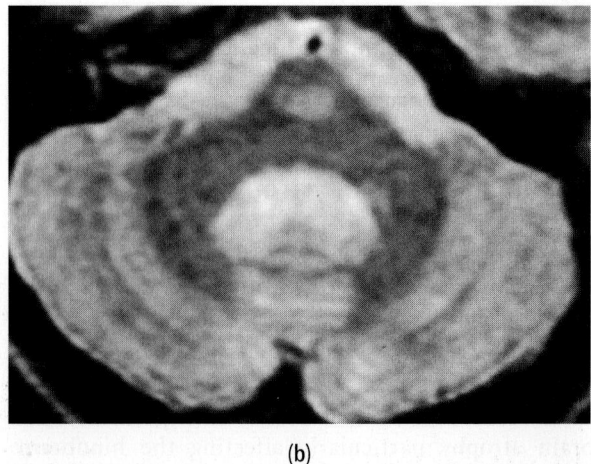

Figure 8.27 *Images from patients with central pontine myelinosis. (a) CT scan from an alcoholic patient presenting with central pontine signs. This image was taken during the recovery phase of the illness and the patient at the time of this image was asymptomatic. Lesions may persist for long periods of time despite apparent symptomatic improvement. (b) T2-weighted MR scan from a diabetic patient showing a central area of high signal within the pons.*

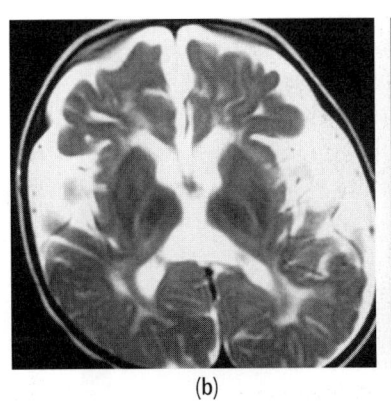

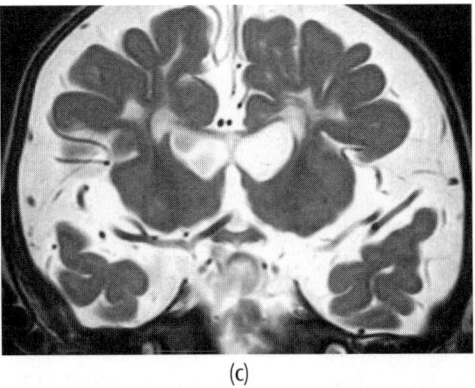

Figure 8.28 Images from a patient with Krabbe's disease. Parasagittal T1 (a) shows abnormal cerebral development, marked cerebral atrophy particularly affecting the occipital poles and resultant microcephaly. T2-weighted axial (b) and coronal (c) images show white matter signal changes particularly in the periventricular and occipital regions together with severe cerebral atrophy. (Image courtesy of Dr S Sheppard.)

spasticity which may be associated with episodes of fever. As this disease progresses spasticity leads to opisthotonus and myoclonic jerks occur combined with hyperpyrexia. In the late stage the child becomes decerebrate and death occurs due to aspiration or infection in many cases. Increased density in the thalamus, caudate nucleus and corona radiata is shown on CT; MRI shows white matter signal change initially affecting the occipital lobes and and anterior corpus callosum which is associated with quite severe atrophy particularly in later phases (Fig. 8.28).

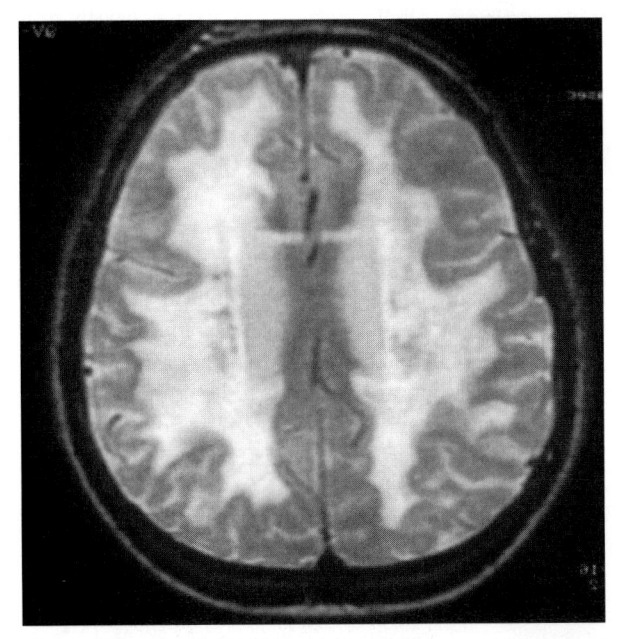

Figure 8.29 T2-weighted MR axial image from an adult patient with late onset metachromatic leukodystrophy. Note extensive high signal abnormality affecting the entire visualized white matter.

Metachromatic leukodystrophy

Metachromatic leukodystrophy is actually a group of autosomally recessive inherited diseases. The disorder results from deficiency of a single enzyme, arylsulphatase A. Four forms of the disease occur distinguished by age of onset. Patients may present at birth, during infancy, in early childhood (4–6 years of age) or in adulthood (up to age 70).[39,40] On MRI, symmetrical extensive white matter abnormalities are seen, commonly commencing anteriorly (Fig. 8.29). High signal changes typically spare the subcortical U fibres and, unlike other leukodystrophies, cerebellar involvement is common.[19]

Adrenoleukodystrophy

Adrenoleukodystrophy is an X-linked recessive disorder presenting in boys in late childhood. Presentation is with mental deterioration and is often associated with visual or hearing disorders. Later stages of the disease are typified by ataxia and it is often associated with Addison's syndrome due to adrenal involvement. Progression of the disease often occurs over 3–4 years and at the end-stage patients are usually quadriplegic, spastic and decorticate; MRI and CT have a distinctive appearance with symmetrical white matter abnormality favouring the posterior part of the cortical white matter around the lateral ventricles and involving the corpus callosum (Fig. 8.30). The demyelinating lesions may appear to be stratified with inner areas of cellular destruction, intermediate areas of demyelination and peripheral areas of myelin repair.[41–43]

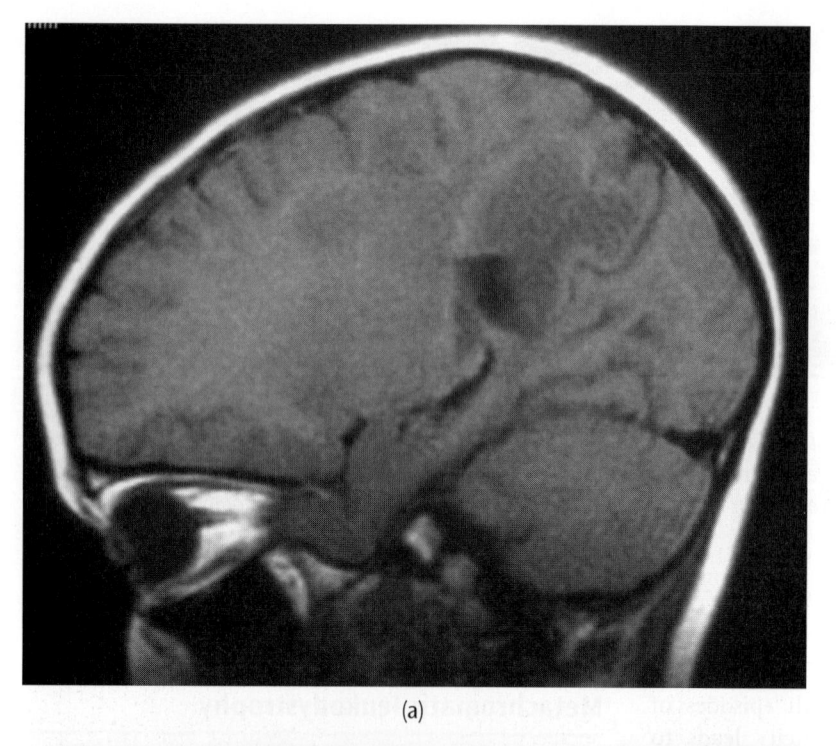

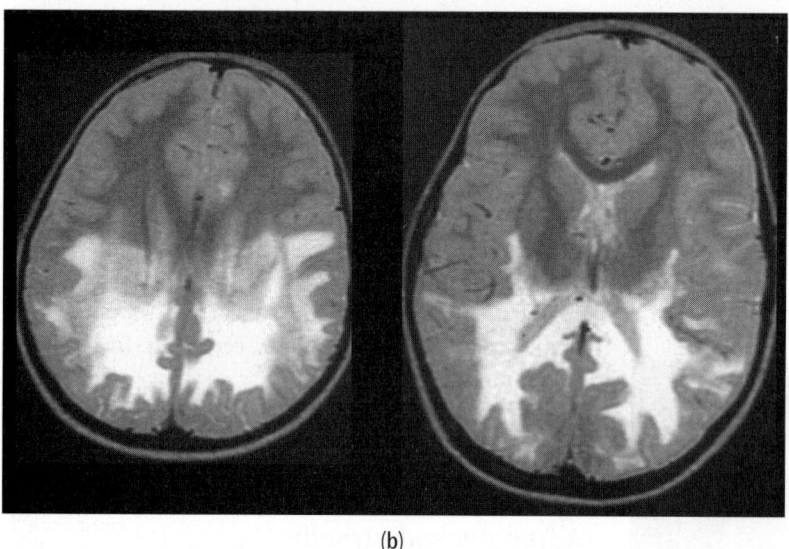

Figure 8.30 *Images from a patient with adrenoleukodystrophy. Sagittal T1 (a) and axial T2 (b) images demonstrate symmetrical white matter abnormality affecting principally the cortical white matter around the posterior part of the lateral ventricles and the corpus callosum.*

Other inherited brain diseases

A wide range of inherited diseases of lipid metabolism and lysosomal function give rise to imaging abnormalities within the brain. These diseases are rare and the cerebral appearances are relatively non-specific and are rarely seen outside specialist centres. A brief overview of some of these is presented in Table 8.4.

Chemotherapy and radiotherapy

Radiation and chemotherapy may induce a secondary arteritis in the brain, which can give rise to cerebral lesions. Clinically these may present with seizures, headaches, cognitive impairment and focal neurological deficits. The arteritis may be associated with mass effect and signal change which can make distinction from residual tumour impossible. Radiation-induced arteritis may give rise to severe chronic damage resulting in regional necrosis, leukomalacia or microangiopathy. This can result in focal atrophy or infarction of any area of the nervous system depending on the area of radiation field.

Radiation necrosis may be seen in white matter and in the acute phase may be associated with oedema and mass effect (Fig. 8.31). In the later phase, secondary atrophic changes occur with dilatation of CSF spaces.

Use of intrathecal methotraxate may give rise to subacute leukoencephalopathy with extensive diffuse white matter abnormality characterized by signal increase on

Table 8.4 *Other rare inherited brain disorders*

Disorder	Cause	Pathological and MRI features
Disorders of lipid metabolism		
Fabry's disease	X-linked recessive	Multiple small infarctions commonest in basal ganglia. Progressive atrophy, occasional haemorrhage.
Gaucher's disease	Autosomal recessive	
Mucopolysaccharidoses (with cerebral involvement)		
Hurler's disease (I)	Autosomal recessive	Variable cerebral MRI features include: • hydrocephalus
Hunter's disease (II)	X-linked recessive	• periventricular white matter lesions due to mucopolysaccharide deposition
Sanfilippo	Autosomal recessive	• progressive infarction
Maroteaux–Lamy (VI)	Autosomal recessive	• progressive demyelination • dural thickening
Sly (VII)	Autosomal recessive	High signal abnormalities may regress after bone marrow transplant

(a)

(b)

(c)

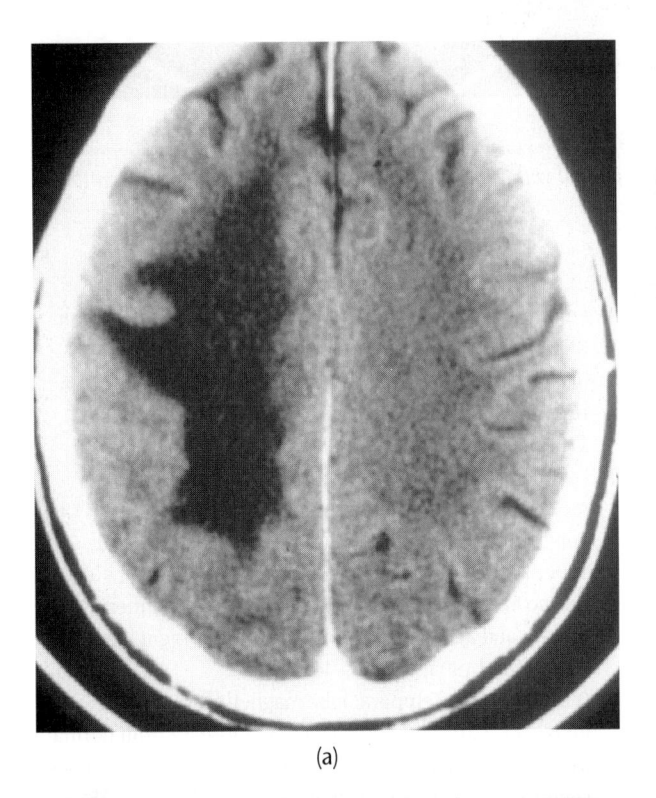

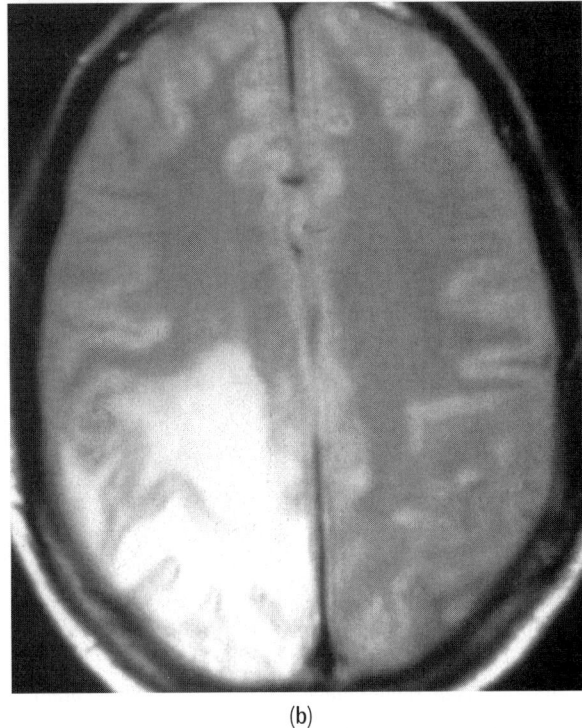

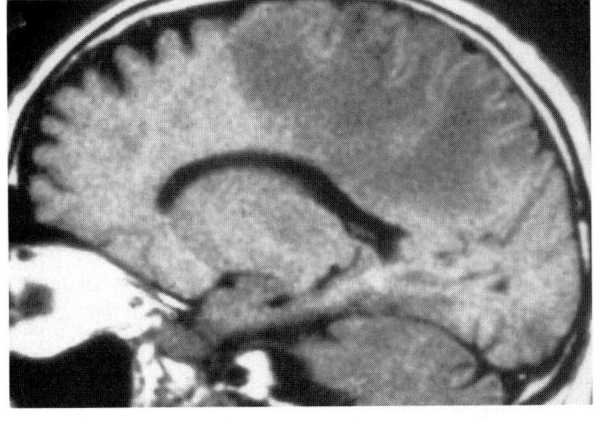

Figure 8.31 *Radiation-induced oedema following localized radiotherapy for cerebral lymphoma. CT images (a) demonstrate extensive areas of low attenuation within the centrum semi ovale. T2-weighted MRI (b) shows high signal involving both the grey and white matter. T1-Weighted parasagittal MR (c) shows the focal nature of the low signal abnormality which extends into the white matter of the gyri within the radiation fields.*

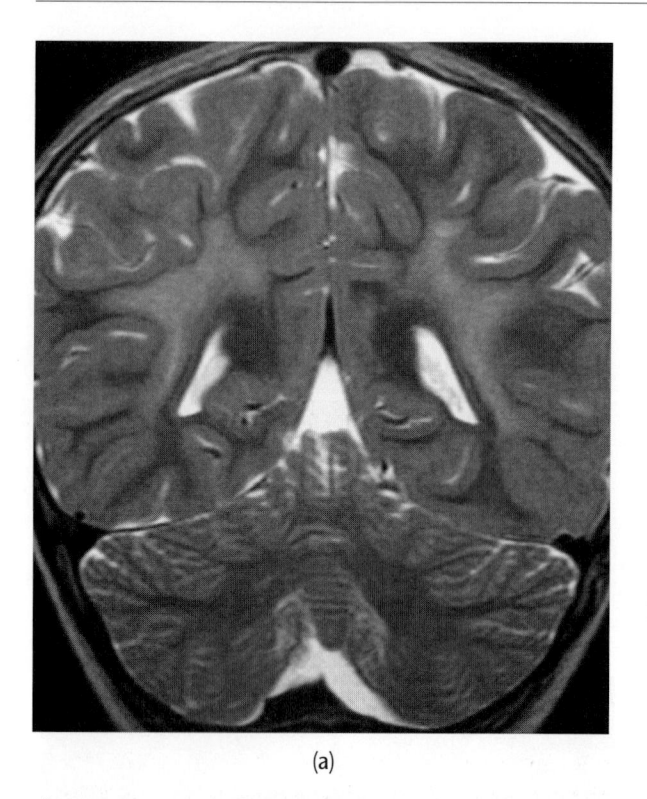

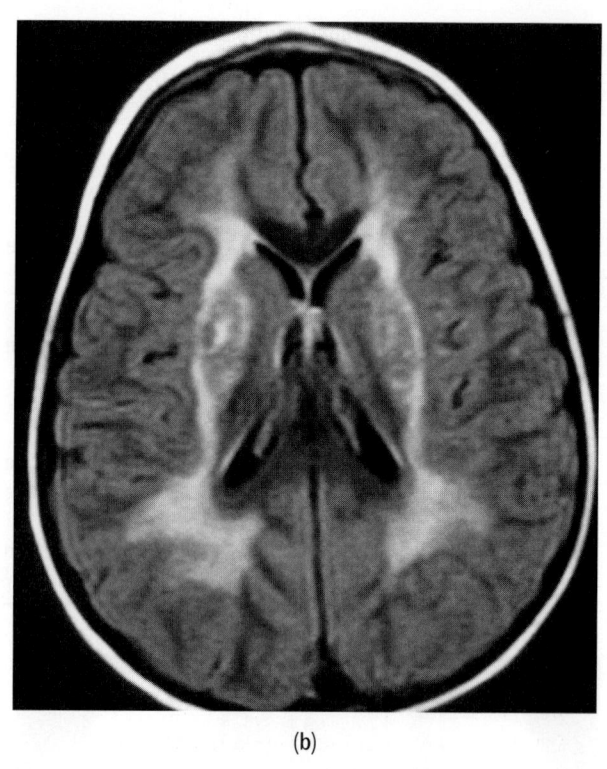

Figure 8.32 Coronal T2-weighted (a) and axial (b) FLAIR images in a patient with subacute leukoencephalopathy following intrathecal methotrexate. (Images courtesy of Dr S Sheppard.)

T2WI (Fig. 8.32). L-Asparaginase used in childhood leukaemia is associated with dural venous sinus thrombosis in up to 2% of cases.

References

1. Davis PC, Mirra SS, Alazraki N. The brain in older persons with and without dementia: findings on MR, PET, and SPECT images. *Am J Roentgenol* 1994; **162**: 1267–78.
2. Golomb J et al. Nonspecific leukoencephalopathy associated with aging. *Neuroimag Clin N Amer* 1995; **5**: 33–44.
3. Yetkin FZ et al. High-signal foci on MR images of the brain: observer variability in their quantification. *Am J Roentgenol* 1992; **159**: 185–8.
4. Almkvist O, Wahlund LO, Andersson-Lundman G, Basun H, Backman L. White-matter hyperintensity and neuropsychological functions in dementia and healthy aging. *Arch Neurol* 1992; **49**: 626–32.
5. George AE et al. Leukoencephalopathy in normal and pathologic aging: 1. CT of brain lucencies. *Am J Neuroradiol* 1986; **7**: 561–6.
6. Kobari M, Meyer JS, Ichijo M, Oravez WT. Leukoaraiosis: correlation of MR and CT findings with blood flow, atrophy, and cognition. *Am J Neuroradiol* 1990; **11**: 273–81.
7. George A, deLeon M, Golomb J, Kluger A, Convit A. Imaging the brain in dementia: expensive and futile? *Am J Neuroradiol* 1997; **18**: 1847–51.
8. Foundas AL, Leonard CM, Mahoney SM, Agee OF, Heilman KM. Atrophy of the hippocampus, parietal cortex, and insula in Alzheimer's disease: a volumetric magnetic resonance imaging study. *Neuropsychiat Neuropsychol Behav Neurol* 1997; **10**: 81–9.
9. Fox NC, Freeborough PA. Brain atrophy progression measured from registered serial MRI: validation and application to Alzheimer's disease. *J Magn Reson Imag* 1997; **7**: 1069–75.
10. Laakso M et al. The interuncal distance in Alzheimer disease and age-associated memory impairment. *Am J Neuroradiol* 1995; **16**: 727–34.
11. O'Brien JT et al. Temporal lobe magnetic resonance imaging can differentiate Alzheimer's disease from normal ageing, depression, vascular dementia and other causes of cognitive impairment. *Psychol Med* 1997; **27**: 1267–75.
12. Frackowiak RS. Imaging and Alzheimer disease: current issues [Editorial]. *Alzheimer Dis Assoc Disord* 1995; **9**: 5.
13. Neary D. Non Alzheimer's disease forms of cerebral atrophy. *J Neurol Neurosurg Psychiat* 1990; **53**: 929–31.
14. Julin P et al. Clinical diagnosis of frontal lobe dementia and Alzheimer's disease: relation to cerebral perfusion, brain atrophy and electroencephalography. *Dementia* 1995; **6**: 142–7.
15. Maeda A et al. Computer-assisted three-dimensional image analysis of cerebral amyloid angiopathy. *Stroke* 1993; **24**: 1857–64.
16. Caplan LR. Binswanger's disease – revisited. *Neurology* 1995; **45**: 626–33.

17 Awad IA, Johnson PC, Spetzler RF, Hodak JA. Incidental subcortical lesions identified on magnetic resonance imaging in the elderly. II. Postmortem pathological correlations. *Stroke* 1986; **17**: 1090–7.

18 Osborn A, Tong K. *Handbook of Neuroradiology: Brain and Skull*. 1996; St Louis: Mosby.

19 Atlas S. *Magnetic Resonance Imaging of the Brain and Spine*. 1996; Philadelphia: Lippincott–Raven.

20 Savoiardo M, Girotti F, Strada L, Ciceri E. Magnetic resonance imaging in progressive supranuclear palsy and other parkinsonian disorders. *J Neural Transm Suppl* 1994; **42**: 93–110.

21 Fukutani Y *et al*. Striatonigral degeneration combined with olivopontocerebellar atrophy with subcortical dementia and hallucinatory state. *Dementia* 1995; **6**: 235–40.

22 Mascalchi M, Dal Pozzo G. Magnetic resonance imaging of degenerative diseases of the central nervous system. *Ital J Neurol Sci* 1992; **13**: 105–11.

23 Bronnen R. MR of temporal mesial sclerosis: how much is enough? *Am J Neuroradiol* 1998; **19**: 15–18.

24 Mamourian A, Cho C, Saykin A, Poppito N. Association between size of the lateral ventricle and assymetry of the fornix in patients with temporal lobe epilepsy. *Am J Neuroradiol* 1998; **19**: 9–13.

25 Kato Y *et al*. Detection of pyramidal tract lesions in amyotrophic lateral sclerosis with magnetization transfer measurements. *Am J Neuroradiol* 1997; **18**: 1541–7.

26 van Walderveen MA *et al*. Correlating MRI and clinical disease activity in multiple sclerosis: relevance of hypointense lesions on short-TR/short-TE (T1-weighted) spin-echo images. *Neurology* 1995; **45**: 1684–90.

27 Boggild MD, Williams R, Haq N, Hawkins CP. Cortical plaques visualised by fluid-attenuated inversion recovery imaging in relapsing multiple sclerosis. *Neuroradiology* 1996; **38** (Suppl) **1**: S10–3.

28 Filippi M *et al*. Quantitative assessment of MRI lesion load in multiple sclerosis. A comparison of conventional spin-echo with fast fluid-attenuated inversion recovery. *Brain* 1996; **119**: 1349–55.

29 Gean-Marton AD *et al*. Abnormal corpus callosum: a sensitive and specific indicator of multiple sclerosis. *Radiology* 1991; **180**: 215–21.

30 Brainin M, Reisner T, Neuhold A, Omasits M, Wicke L. Topological characteristics of brainstem lesions in clinically definite and clinically probable cases of multiple sclerosis: an MRI-study. *Neuroradiology* 1987; **29**: 530–4.

31 Horowitz AL, Kaplan RD, Grewe G, White RT, Salberg LM. The ovoid lesion: a new MR observation in patients with multiple sclerosis. *Am J Neuroradiol* 1989; **10**: 303–5.

32 Baum K, Nehrig C, Schorner W, Girke W. Periventricular plaques in multiple sclerosis: irreversible? An MRI follow-up study. *Eur Neurol* 1992; **32**: 219–21.

33 Chakrabortty S *et al*. Intracerebral ring-enhancing lesions in a patient with multiple sclerosis: a case report. *Surg Neurol* 1995; **43**: 591–4.

34 DeLara F, Tartaglino L, Friedman D. Spinal cord multiple sclerosis and devic neuromyelitis optica in children. *Am J Neuroradiol* 1995; **16**: 1557–8.

35 Berger JR *et al*. Relapsing and remitting human immunodeficiency virus-associated leukoencephalomyelopathy. *Ann Neurol* 1992; **31**: 34–8.

36 Orrell RW. Grand rounds – Hammersmith Hospitals. Distinguishing acute disseminated encephalomyelitis from multiple sclerosis. *Br Med J* 1996; **313**: 802–4.

37 Baum PA, Barkovich AJ, Koch TK, Berg BO. Deep gray matter involvement in children with acute disseminated encephalomyelitis. *Am J Neuroradiol* 1994; **15**: 1275–83.

38 Kesselring J *et al*. Acute disseminated encephalomyelitis. MRI findings and the distinction from multiple sclerosis. *Brain* 1990; **113**: 291–320.

39 Schipper HI, Seidel D. Computed tomography in late-onset metachromatic leucodystrophy. *Neuroradiology* 1984; **26**: 39–44.

40 Wende S, Ludwig B, Kishikawa T, Rochel M, Gehler J. The value of CT in diagnosis and prognosis of different inborn neurodegenerative disorders in childhood. *J Neurol* 1984; **231**: 57–70.

41 Castellote A *et al*. MR in adrenoleukodystrophy: atypical presentation as bilateral frontal demyelination. *Am J Neuroradiol* 1995; **16**(Suppl): 814–5.

42 Masdeu JC *et al*. The open ring. A new imaging sign in demyelinating disease. *J Neuroimaging* 1996; **6**: 104–7.

43 Zwetsloot CP, Padberg GW, van Seters AP, Maaswinkel-Mooy PD, Onkenhout W. Adult adrenoleukodystrophy: the clinical spectrum in a large Dutch family. *J Neurol* 1992; **239**: 107–11.

9

Hydrocephalus

ROGER D LAITT, DAVID G HUGHES

Introduction	266	Hydrocephalus secondary to cerebrospinal fluid overproduction	275
Normal cerebrospinal fluid physiology	266	Treated hydrocephalus	275
Diagnosis of hydrocephalus	267	References	278
Non-communicating hydrocephalus	269		
Communicating hydrocephalus	272		

INTRODUCTION

Hydrocephalus can be defined as an excess accumulation of cerebrospinal fluid (CSF) in the normal CSF pathways of the brain due to an imbalance between CSF production and absorption. In practice this is almost always due to obstruction of CSF flow producing an increased volume of CSF within the brain. This results in an increase in intracranial pressure that may fluctuate. The effect on brain parenchyma depends on the extent and rapidity of increase of intracranial pressure, the cause of the hydrocephalus and the age of the patient. Ventriculomegaly secondary to poor brain development or to cerebral atrophy should not be considered to represent hydrocephalus and is excluded by definition.

Classification schemes are usually based on the observed level of CSF obstruction.[1] This is relevant to patient management with most schemes separating hydrocephalus into two main types. These are non-communicating or internal hydrocephalus and communicating or external hydrocephalus.[2] The terms obstructive and non-obstructive hydrocephalus are used less frequently in view of the fact that virtually all cases of hydrocephalus are obstructive. In non-communicating type hydrocephalus the obstruction to CSF flow is ventricular whereas in communicating type hydrocephalus the obstruction is extraventricular. The obstruction may be at multiple levels giving a combined type of hydrocephalus.

The clinical presentation of hydrocephalus depends on patient age at time of onset and the rapidity and duration of increased intracranial pressure. In children the presence of associated structural brain abnormalities is also a factor. In infants hydrocephalus usually results in enlargement of head circumference with splaying of sutures, bulging fontanelles and thinning of the vault. Mass effect produces ocular abnormalities including VIth nerve palsy and Parinaud's syndrome. The infant may be irritable and restless and there may be spasticity of lower limbs. In older children and adults the symptoms are those of raised intracranial pressure with early morning headache, nausea and vomiting. Ocular signs and lower limb spasticity are again common findings. Hypothalamic-pituitary dysfunction may be the presenting complaint in younger patients. Rapidly developing hydrocephalus usually presents early but slowly enlarging ventricles may initially remain asymptomatic.

NORMAL CEREBROSPINAL FLUID PHYSIOLOGY

Cerebrospinal fluid is produced by mesenchymal tissue that invaginates into the lateral, third and fourth ventricles. This tissue is known as the choroid plexus. It can be variable in size filling approximately 75% of the ventricular lumen *in utero* with this proportion falling as the brain and ventricular system develop. In life the choroid plexus calcifies with age as a normal finding. This is commonly seen in adults usually in the posterior third ventricle and in the body and temporal horns of the lateral ventricles. This calcification rarely exceeds 10mm in greatest dimension.

In the newborn the total CSF volume is approximately 50ml. This volume increases with brain development to approximately 150ml in the adult with about 25% of this being within the ventricular system. The choroid plexus produces approximately 80–90% of the total CSF with the remainder formed by brain and spine parenchyma.[3] The daily production of CSF from the choroid is in the order of 500ml or approximately 0.4ml per minute.

The CSF follows a defined pathway from the ventricular system into the subarachnoid space via the fourth ventricular exit foramina of Magendie and Luschka. From here CSF either enters the cisternal system or passes into the spinal subarachnoid spaces. The bulk of the CSF takes the cisternal route before flowing over the cerebral convexities; draining into the venous system via arachnoid granulations. These consist of multiple microscopic villi that protrude into the superior sagittal sinus and into other sinuses and large veins. Conventional theory is that these villi act as one-way valves allowing CSF to pass down a hydrostatic pressure gradient driven by a normal mean CSF pressure of 70–150mm of water into low pressure veins. It is also postulated that CSF drains into lymphatics and capillaries within the brain parenchyma. These alternate pathways may become important when there is obstruction to CSF flow with increased intracranial pressure allowing a new equilibrium between production and absorption of CSF to be reached. This is known as compensated or arrested hydrocephalus.[4]

The mechanism driving CSF from its site of production through the ventricular system to sites of CSF absorption has been debated. Phase contrast cine magnetic resonance imaging (MRI) has demonstrated that CSF flow is related to cardiac pulsation.[5] Systolic pressure waves produce expansion of cerebral arteries and then of the capillary bed. As the brain is in a confined space outflow of CSF and venous blood and also deformation of brain tissue vent this pressure increase. As a result the CSF has its own systolic and diastolic flow patterns which occur at different times in different anatomical locations producing a net flow of CSF from choroid plexus to arachnoid granulations.

DIAGNOSIS OF HYDROCEPHALUS

Whilst the referring clinician maybe suspicious for the presence of hydrocephalus the diagnosis is made by imaging with ventricular enlargement in the absence of poor brain development or atrophy. Ultrasound, if a suitable acoustic window is available, computed tomography (CT) and MRI are all sensitive modalities for assessing ventricular size. Ultrasound is limited by the availability of an acoustic window, usually the anterior fontanelle. This also results in reduced resolution of posterior structures due to distance-related attenuation of the ultrasound beam. The advantages of MRI over CT and ultrasound are that it more clearly demonstrates posterior fossa structures which may be important in assessing obstructive hydrocephalus. It has improved contrast resolution that allows examination of the ventricular system and subarachnoid spaces for the presence of webs, inflammatory membranes and subtle mass lesions. It can also be used to look at CSF flow, which is important in differentiating atrophic ventriculomegaly from communicating hydrocephalus, particularly normal pressure hydrocephalus.[6] Once the diagnosis has been made CT and ultrasound are adequate in assessing changes in ventricular size.

The differentiation of hydrocephalus from ventriculomegaly secondary to reduced brain volume is important in patient management. It can be difficult, particularly with communicating hydrocephalus, and a number of imaging parameters have been suggested to discriminate between these two entities. These are outlined in Table 9.1. These signs may be of limited value when viewed in isolation but in combination may allow discrimination between these two entities. Our ability to diagnose hydrocephalus has been improved by MRI and some of these signs are only seen with this modality.

The two most reliable discriminators between hydrocephalus and atrophy are the size of the temporal horns in relation to the size of the ventricular bodies[7] and enlargement of the third ventricular recesses.[8] The reasons why the temporal horns are of relatively small size in an

Table 9.1 Radiological features of hydrocephalus and atrophic ventriculomegaly

	Hydrocephalus	Ventriculomegaly
Temporal horns	Commensurate dilatation with lateral ventricular body	Less than body of lateral ventricle
Third ventricle	Enlargement of the anterior or posterior recesses Convex walls	Recesses not prominent Parallel walls
Mamillopontine distance	Reduced < 4mm	Normal
Cortical sulci	Effaced	Widened
Periventricular areas	Interstitial oedema	Normal/vascular disease
CSF flow voids on MRI	Prominent in third ventricle	Not prominent

268 Hydrocephalus

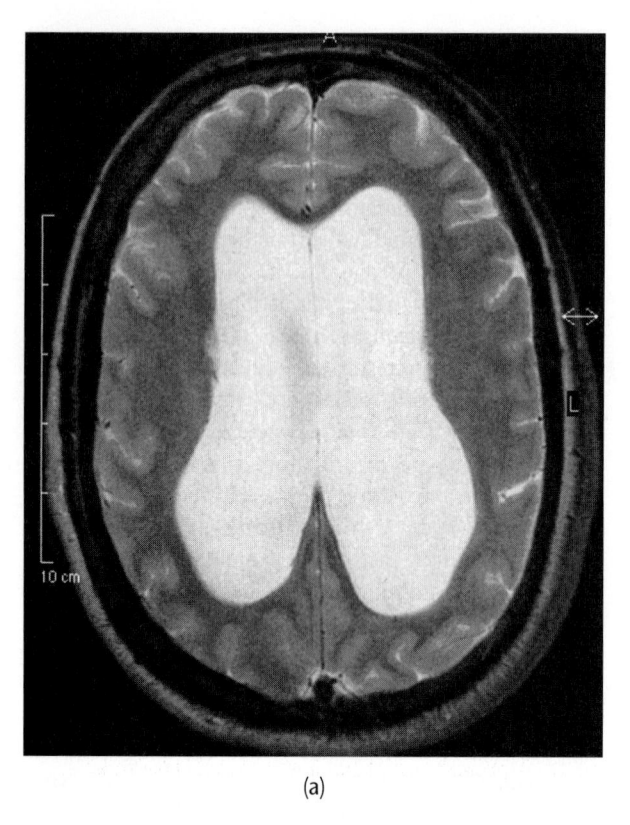

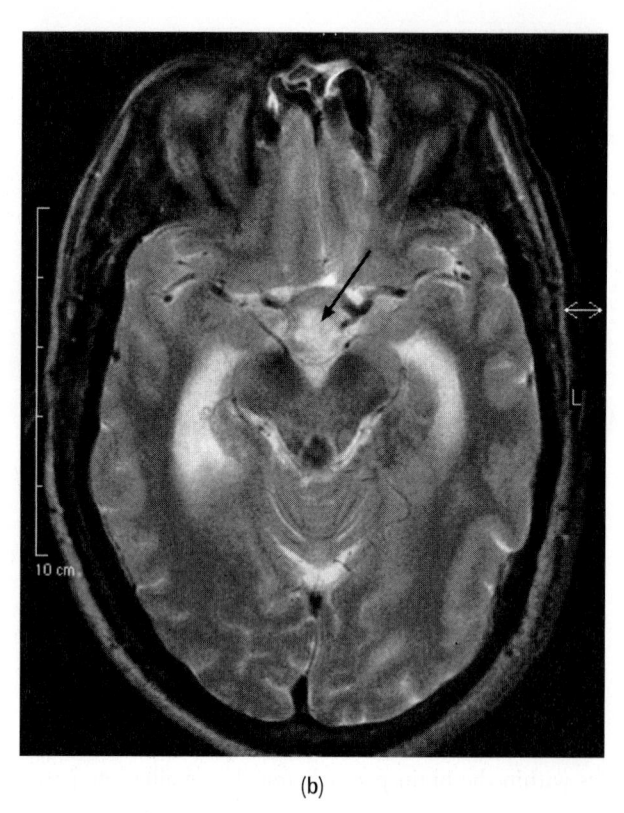

Figure 9.1 Communicating hydrocephalus in a 62-year-old male. (a) Axial T2-image with dilatation of the lateral ventricles. (b) Axial T2-image through the temporal horns showing commensurate dilatation of the temporal horns and the anterior recesses of the third ventricle (arrow).

atrophic brain is not entirely clear but may relate to the reduced volume of white matter tracts in this region compared with other brain areas. Attention should also be paid to the sylvian fissures when assessing temporal lobe atrophy. In hydrocephalus the temporal horns often show proportionate dilatation when compared with the ventricular body (Fig. 9.1). Enlargement of the third ventricular recesses is also a useful sign of hydrocephalus and can be clearly seen on sagittal MRI (Fig. 9.2). The mamillopontine distance is also assessed in this plane (Fig. 9.2). This is decreased in hydrocephalus due to inferior displacement of the third ventricular floor. Increased intraventricular pressure may result in transudation of CSF into the brain parenchyma causing periventricular interstitial oedema (Fig. 9.3). In older patients it is important to discriminate this from periventricular changes secondary to small vessel vascular disease. In hydrocephalus CSF flow can become hyperdynamic which can result in signal loss due to flow voids. This is best seen in the third ventricle and cerebral aqueduct (Fig. 9.4).

A disproportionate increase in ventricular size when compared with enlargement of cortical sulci is an important indicator of hydrocephalus. This is less reliable in infants and younger children with communicating hydrocephalus and is complicated by the fact that there is a normal variation in size of the subarachnoid spaces

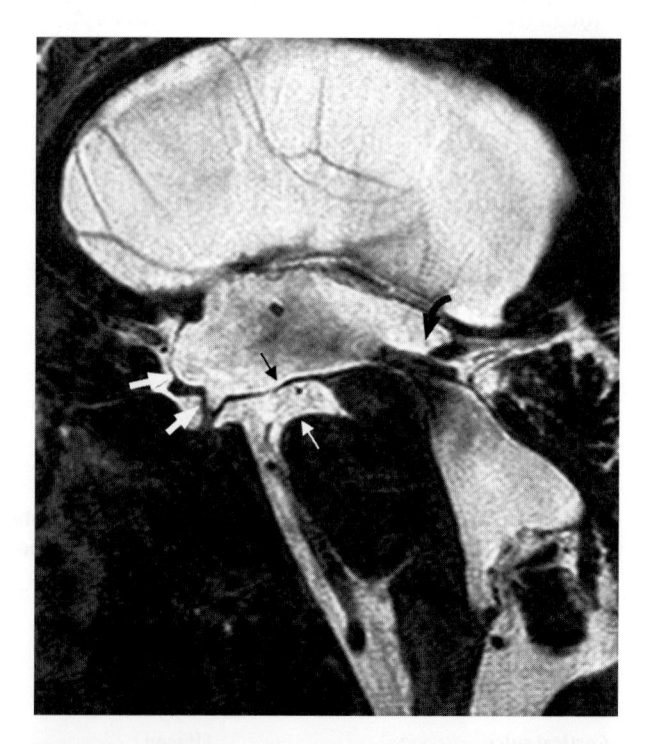

Figure 9.2 Sagittal T2-volume image demonstrating dilated chiasmatic and infundibular recesses of the third ventricle. The suprapineal recess is also dilated (curved arrow). The mamillopontine distance is assessed in this plane (short arrows).

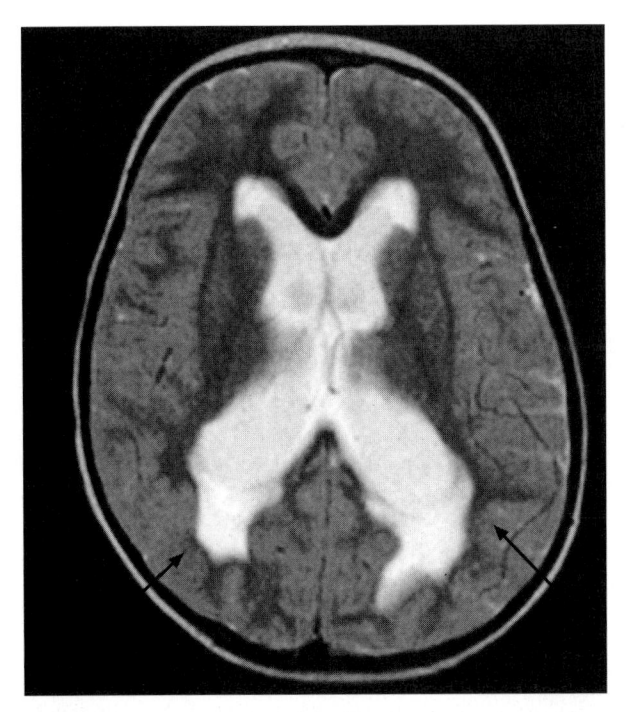

Figure 9.3 Non-communicating hydrocephalus in a 4-year-old girl due to fourth ventricular primitive neuroectodermal tumour. Axial T2-image demonstrating periventricular interstitial oedema (arrows).

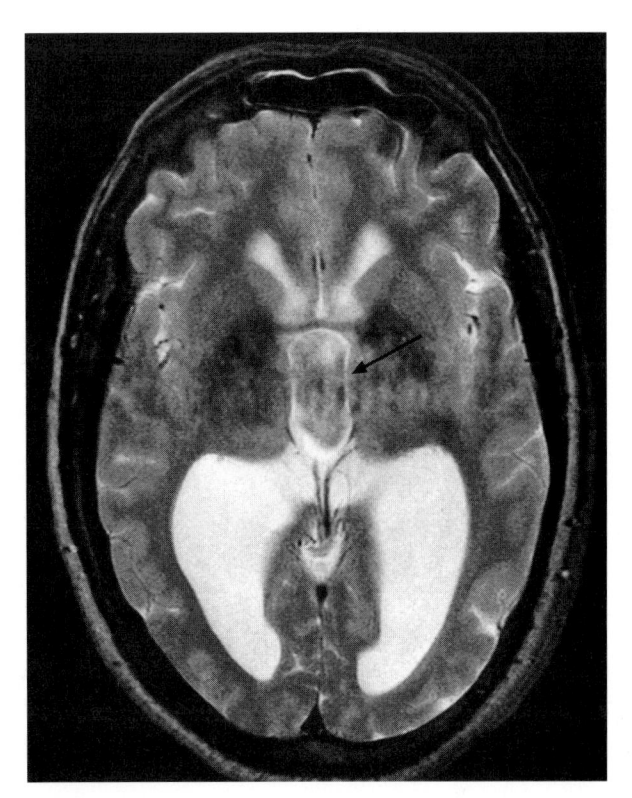

Figure 9.4 Normal pressure hydrocephalus. Axial T2-image at the level of the third ventricle with hyperdynamic CSF flow producing signal loss (arrow).

and ventricles in this age group.[9] Knowledge of head circumference is important here as a large head suggests hydrocephalus whereas a small head suggests atrophy. In adults similar difficulty maybe encountered in discrimination of atrophy and communicating hydrocephalus. Diagnostic errors can be minimized with detailed knowledge of clinical information and close collaboration with the referring clinician.

NON-COMMUNICATING HYDROCEPHALUS

This type of hydrocephalus, also known as internal hydrocephalus, is due to intraventricular obstruction of CSF flow. This can occur anywhere from the site of production of CSF by the choroid plexus to the fourth ventricular exit foramina. In reality obstruction is most commonly seen at sites where the CSF pathway is of small calibre, at the foramen of Monro, in the posterior third ventricle, in the cerebral aqueduct and in the fourth ventricle. Obstruction is most commonly secondary to tumours and the differential diagnosis largely depends on patient age and lesion location.

Lateral ventricular

Tumours causing obstruction in this region may be intraventricular or parenchymal. Intraventricular tumours in adults include meningiomas (Fig. 9.5), which are most commonly seen in the atrium, oligodendroglioma, subependymomas and central neurocytomas. In children tumours include primitive neuroectodermal tumours and choroid plexus papillomas. Extraventricular tumours can compress the ventricles trapping various parts. This usually occurs at the body or atrium with trapping of the temporal or occipital horns secondary to aggressive lesions such as anaplastic astrocytomas or metastatic disease. In both age-groups obstruction can be due to haemorrhage or infection with the production of fibrous webs. Choroid plexus cysts are non-neoplastic epithelial lined cysts, which are usually bilateral and incidental. A persistent cavum septum pellucium is a common developmental anomaly with persistence of normal fetal CSF space between the two septal leaves. It should not be confused with a mass lesion.

Foramen of Monro/anterior third ventricle

The classic cause of obstruction at this location is the colloid cyst of the third ventricle. This epithelial lined cyst is benign and arises from the anterosuperior aspect of the third ventricle between the columns of the fornix. These lesions are common in adults but rare in children. The hydrocephalus maybe intermittent and positional

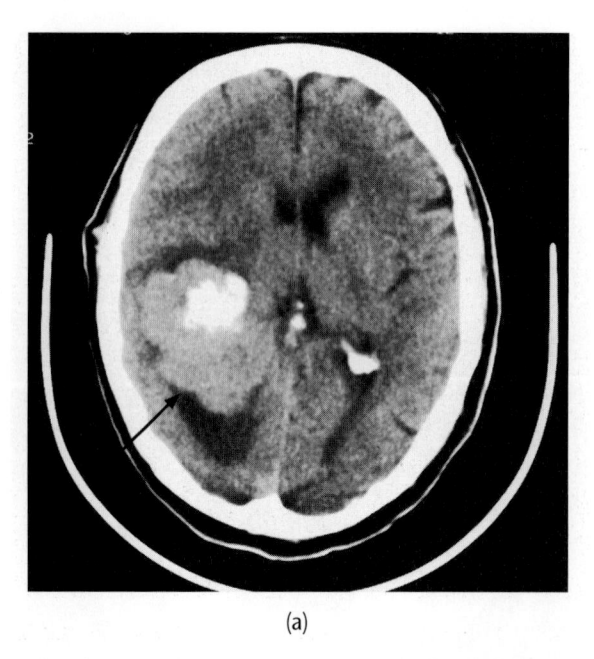

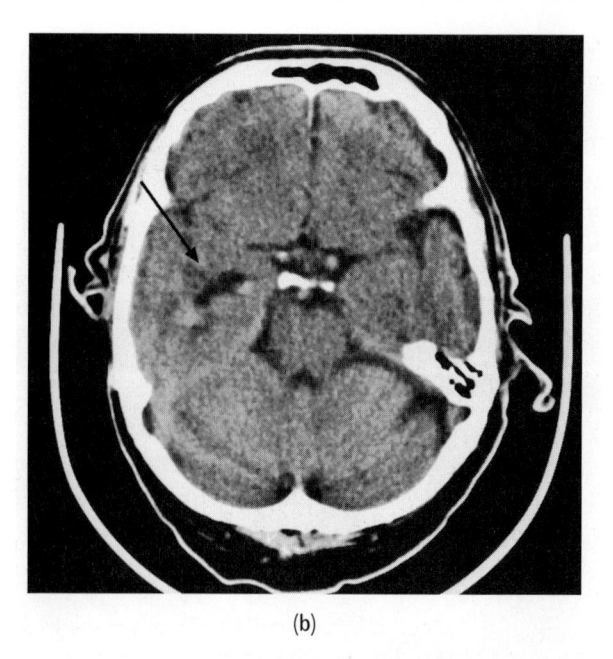

Figure 9.5 *A 77-year-old female with an intraventricular meningioma. (a) CT demonstrating a large partly calcified intraventricular tumour (arrow). (b) CT lower cut demonstrating a partly trapped temporal horn (arrow).*

and usually affects both ventricles. On CT the lesion is high density on unenhanced scans (Fig. 9.6). On MRI the signal intensity is variable due to cyst contents which include proteinaceous material and blood degradation products. Location is the clue to diagnosis. Other lesions can occur in this midline location such as astrocytomas, meningiomas, central neurocytomas and choroid plexus tumours.[10] Rarely, suprasellar tumours such as craniopharyngioma in children or pituitary macroadenoma and meningioma in adults can grow superiorly to obstruct the ventricles in this region. Giant aneurysms from the circle of Willis can also project superiorly. Lateral ventricular enlargement maybe symmetrical or predominantly one-sided. Lesions slightly off the midline may cause unilateral hydrocephalus such as a giant cell astrocytoma seen in association with tuberose sclerosis (Fig. 9.7).

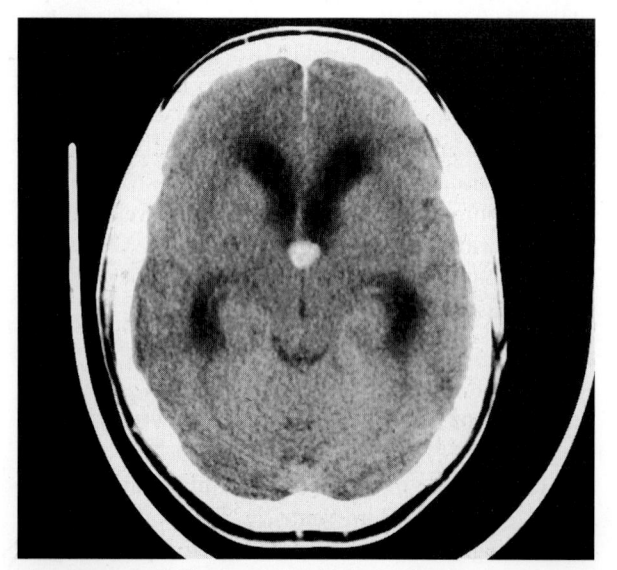

Figure 9.6 *Colloid cyst of the third ventricle in a 42-year-old man. CT scan demonstrates high density mass in the region of the forame of Monro.*

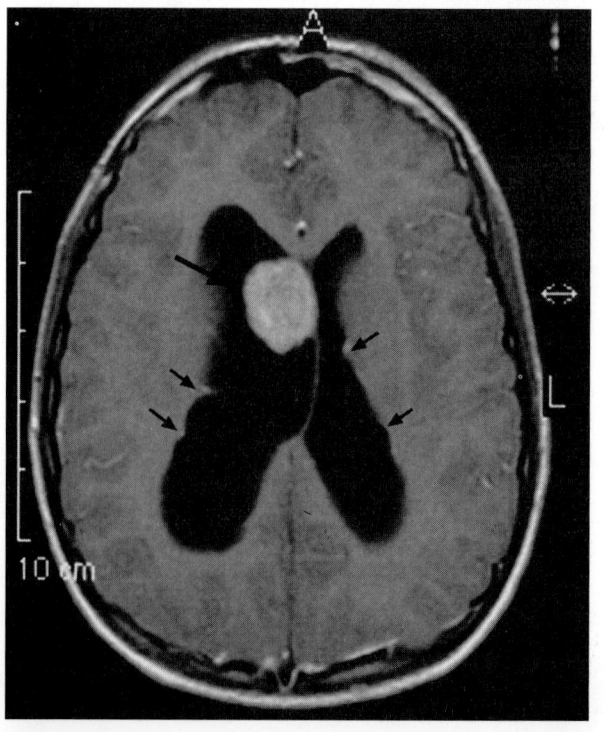

Figure 9.7 *Tuberose sclerosis in a 13-year-old boy. Axial post-contrast T1-image demonstrating an enhancing giant cell astrocytoma (long arrow) and subependymal nodules (short arrows).*

Posterior third ventricle and cerebral aqueduct

Tumours causing obstruction in this location are usually extraventricular. Pineal gland masses may be asymptomatic until they reach a size sufficient to obstruct the third ventricle and proximal aqueduct. In children this is a common site for germ cell tumours (Fig. 9.8). These lesions can metastasize throughout CSF spaces and cause obstruction to flow in other locations. In adults pineal cell tumours, such as pineocytomas, and pineal cysts predominate. Astrocytomas and metastases also occur here. Intrinsic cerebral tumours occur in the tectal plate posterior to the aqueduct and anteriorly in the brainstem. These lesions are usually astrocytomas. An enlarged vein of Galen in neonates is a rare cause of obstruction to the posterior third ventricle but this diagnosis is usually clinically evident.

Aqueduct stenosis can be developmental or acquired. The developmental form is often sporadic but can be familial with various forms of inheritance.[11] Clinical presentation can occur at any time from birth to adulthood. At CT there is dilatation of the lateral and third ventricles with a normal fourth ventricle. Care should be taken here, however, as the fourth ventricle is often of normal size in communicating hydrocephalus. In addition tectal plate tumours can be easily overlooked on CT. In this patient group MRI scanning is therefore strongly recommended to differentiate between benign and neoplastic aqueduct stenosis. The most common intrinsic lesion of the tectal plate is a glioma.

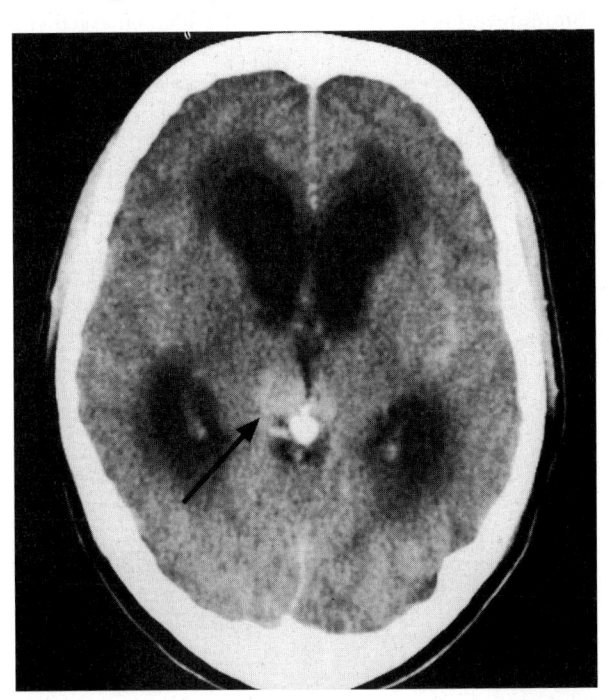

Figure 9.8 *Germinoma in a 24-year-old male causing compression of the posterior third ventricle (arrow). Post-contrast CT image demonstrates acute hydrocephalus with periventricular oedema.*

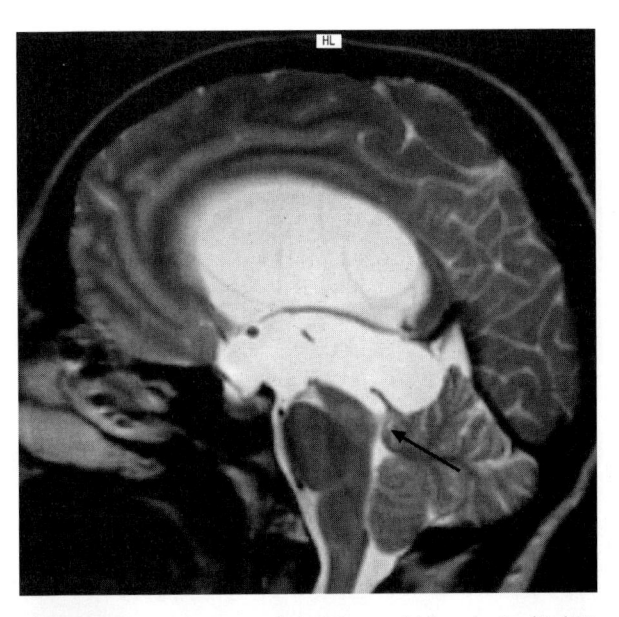

Figure 9.9 *Aqueduct stenosis in 18-year-old female. Sagittal T2-image demonstrating a benign web obstructing the cerebral aqueduct (arrow). There is prominent enlargement of the aqueduct proximal to the web. The suprapineal recess is also extremely prominent and has mass effect.*

Benign aqueduct stenosis can be secondary to acquired occlusion of the aqueduct with fibrous webs following haemorrhage or infection. These webs can also be developmental. They can be clearly defined using high resolution T2-weighted MRI scans,[12] which can also be of value in assessing suitability for endoscopic third ventriculostomy (Fig. 9.9). Acute hydrocephalus can also occur due to obstruction of the aqueduct following intraventricular or subarachnoid haemorrhage.[13]

Fourth ventricle

Primary fourth ventricular mass lesions are common in children but rare in adults. True intraventricular tumours include medulloblastomas, which are a type of primitive neuroectodermal tumour, ependymomas and choroid plexus tumours. In adults metastases are the most common tumour in this location.[14] Intrinsic mass lesions that may compress and obstruct the fourth ventricle include astrocytomas in both age groups, with haemangioblastomas and metastatic disease being more common in adults. Extraxial tumours such as acoustic neuroma can also obstruct the fourth ventricle (Fig. 9.10). Non-neoplastic lesions such as inflammatory masses or benign cysts are occasionally seen in this region. Acute hydrocephalus secondary to posterior fossa haemorrhage is an emergency situation and angiography maybe indicated prior to evacuation of the clot. Infarction can also produce brain swelling with obstruction to CSF flow. Obstruction of the fourth ventricular outflow foramina can be seen in subarachnoid or intraventricular haemorrhage and also in infection. In certain

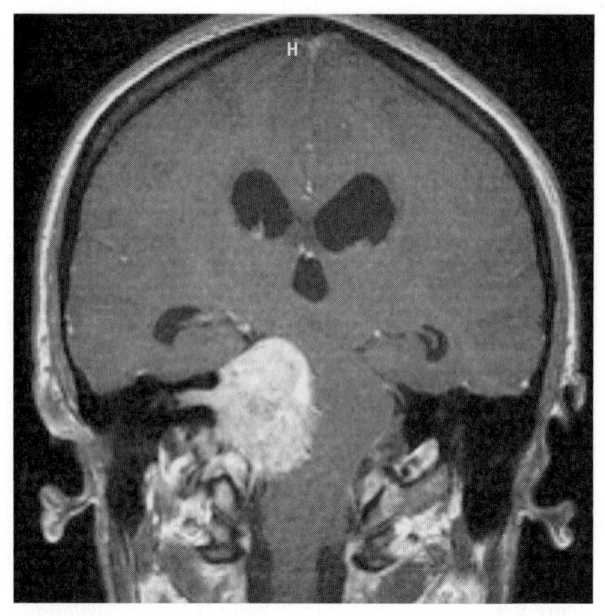

Figure 9.10 *Acoustic neuroma 45-year-old female. Coronal post-contrast T1-image demonstrating a large posterior fossa tumour with supratentorial hydrocephalus.*

circumstances the cerebral aqueduct and the fourth ventricular outflow foramina may become obstructed. This isolates the fourth ventricle which enlarges due to continued CSF production from contained choroid plexus. This is known as a trapped fourth ventricle, which can behave like a mass lesion. It is usually seen following shunting of the lateral ventricles but can occur *de novo* usually following infection (Fig. 9.11) or intraventricular haemorrhage.

Congenital malformations

There are two common anomalies involving the posterior fossa that are associated with hydrocephalus. These are the Chiari malformations and the Dandy–Walker malformations. The Chiari I malformation with cerebellar tonsillar ectopia may be associated with hydrocephalus. In the more complex Chiari II malformation hydrocephalus is almost a constant finding thought to be secondary to obstruction to the outflow of CSF from the fourth ventricle.[4]

The Dandy–Walker malformation is associated with hydrocephalus in 70–80% but the development may be delayed beyond infancy. This is usually a communicating type hydrocephalus with patent fourth ventricular exit foramina.

COMMUNICATING HYDROCPHALUS

In this type of hydrocephalus, also known as external hydrocephalus, there is free flow of CSF out of the fourth ventricle into the posterior fossa subarachnoid space. However, obstruction to CSF flow occurs between the basal cisterns and the arachnoid villi, between the arachnoid villi and the venous sinuses or most commonly due to a combination of both mechanisms. It is not usually possible to define the level of obstruction on imaging grounds. The pattern of ventricular enlargement may be similar in communicating and non-communicating types; however, depending on the site of CSF obstruction, cerebral sulci are usually more prominent in the communicating type and the ventricular enlargement

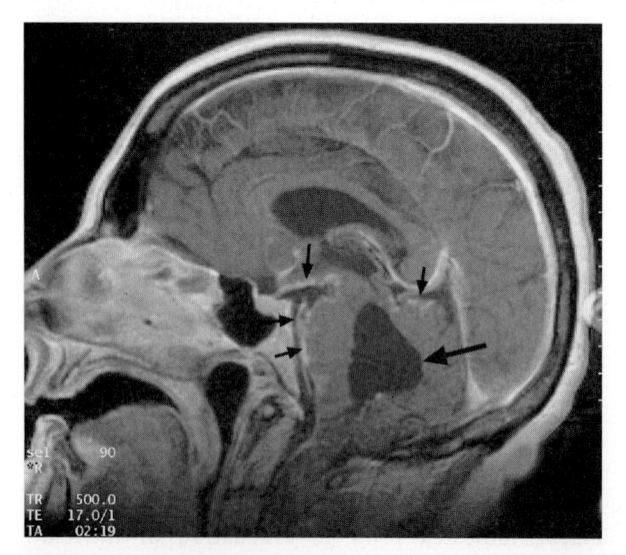

Figure 9.11 *Tuberculous meningitis in a 52-year-old female. Sagittal post-contrast T1-image demonstrates abnormal leptomeningeal (short arrows) enhancement with a dilated, trapped fourth ventricle (long arrow).*

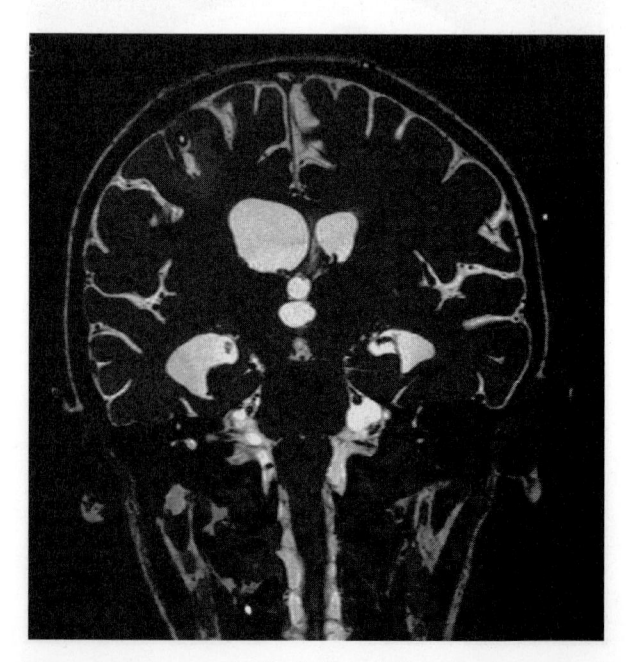

Figure 9.12 *Communicating hydrocephalus secondary to previous bacterial meningitis in an 11-year-old girl. Coronal CISS 3-D image demonstrating multiple inflammatory membranes in the basal cisterns and spinal subarachnoid spaces.*

less pronounced, particularly in the third ventricle. Periventricular oedema may also be less prominent.

This type of hydrocephalus is often secondary to diffuse disease involving the subarachnoid spaces. In children and adults this maybe due to meningeal infection with secondary scarring and membrane formation[12] (Fig. 9.12). Subarachnoid haemorrhage can result in a similar process impairing flow of CSF over the cerebral hemispheres. Both infection and haemorrhage may also have direct effects on the arachnoid villi with possible obstruction of CSF flow into the sinuses;[15] MRI may reveal haemosiderin staining of the pia-arachnoid following haemorrhage. This is seen as low signal on the surface of the brain on long TR sequences. Diffuse meningeal metastases, infection or inflammatory disease can also produce this type of hydrocephalus with enhancement of the pia-arachnoid on post-contrast scans (Fig. 9.13). Radiological differentiation of these three disorders maybe difficult.

As passage of CSF from the arachnoid villi to the venous sinuses is partly pressure-dependent an increase in venous sinus pressure may impair this process. This is seen with venous sinus thrombosis and arteriovenous shunting into the sinuses. Interestingly this increase in venous pressure is transmitted to the CSF but rarely produces ventricular enlargement in patients over about 3 years of age.[16] A similar situation is seen in benign intracranial hypertension (pseudotumour cerebri) which is also thought to be secondary to raised venous outflow pressure. The ventricles in this disorder are not enlarged by definition, as there is limited space for ventricular expansion and possibly alternative mechanisms for CSF outflow when venous pressures are raised. Raised venous pressures in patients under 2 years of age may produce a different picture with ventricular enlargement. This is thought to result from the increased compliance of the skull vault and parenchyma in these patients, which does not restrict ventricular dilatation.[4] A number of disorders with associated skull base hypoplasia, including achondroplasia, have ventricular enlargement as part of the syndrome[4] (Fig. 9.14). It is postulated that this enlargement is secondary to decreased cerebral venous outflow through small jugular foramina. This results in elevated venous pressure in the sagittal sinus reducing the pressure gradient across the arachnoid villi and thus impairing CSF outflow.

There are two types of communicating hydrocephalus that deserve more detailed comment. These are benign enlargement of the subarachnoid spaces in infancy and normal pressure hydrocephalus.

Benign enlargement of the subarachnoid spaces

There are a group of children who present with macrocephaly, usually in the first year of life. These children are

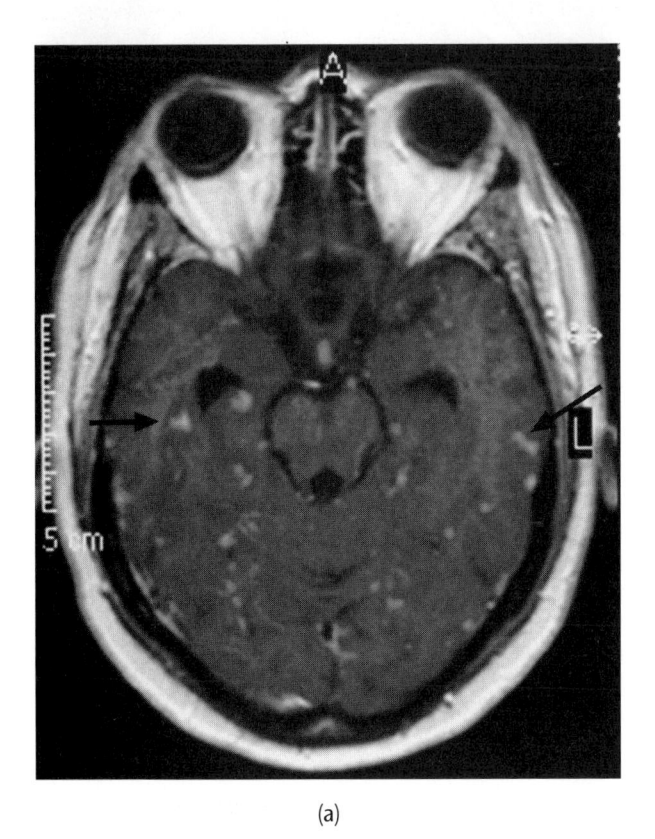

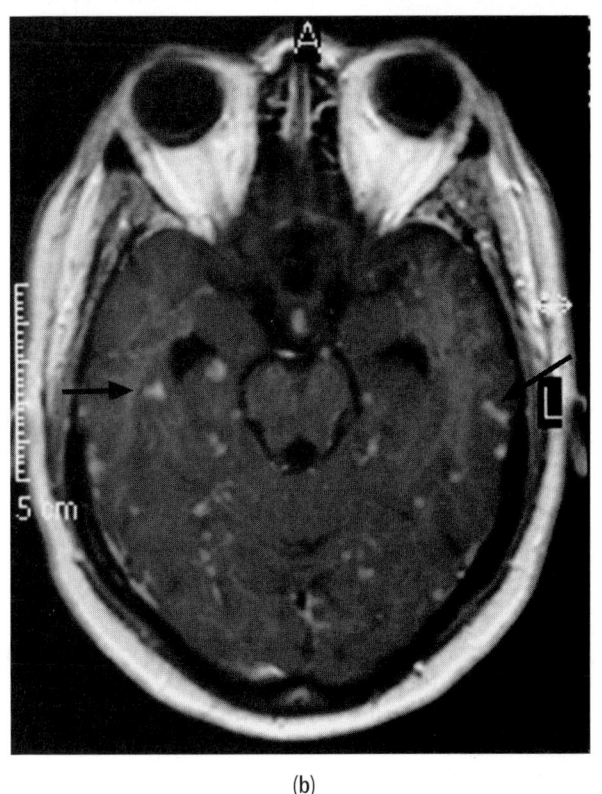

Figure 9.13 *(a),(b) Sarcoidosis in a 41-year-old man producing a communicating hydrocephalus. Post-contrast T1 images demonstrate multiple nodular areas of leptomeningeal enhancement with mild ventricular dilatation.*

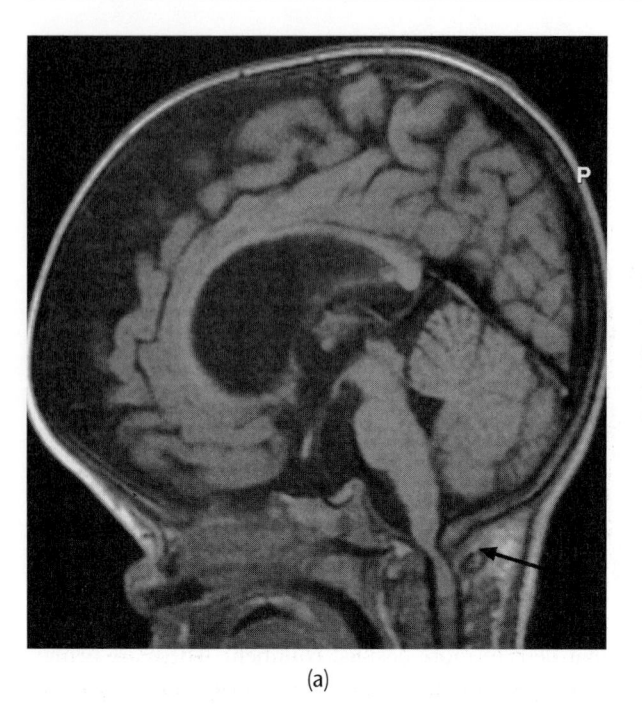

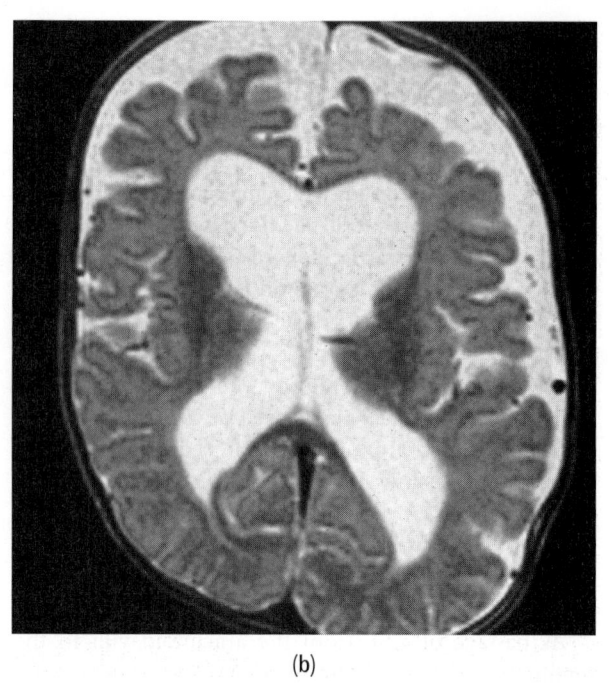

Figure 9.14 *Achondroplasia in a 1-year-old boy. (a) Sagittal T1-image demonstrating hypoplasia of the skull base with compression of the upper cervical cord at the foramen magnum (arrow). (b) Axial T2-image demonstrating a communicating hydrocephalus with prominence of the CSF spaces over the frontal lobes and ventricular enlargement.*

either neurologically normal or have mild developmental delay. Imaging demonstrates mild-to-moderate enlargement of the lateral and third ventricles with enlarged frontal subarachnoid spaces[17] (Fig. 9.15). The cause is unknown but may be secondary to defective CSF absorption due to delayed maturation of arachnoid villi. The natural history is usually good with normal development although a small minority of patients may develop progressive communicating hydrocephalus that requires treatment. Patients may also be at risk for subdural haematoma formation. Recognition of this syndrome is important for prognostic reasons. The findings should not be confused with cerebral atrophy, where head circumference is small, or subdural collections where the gyral pattern is effaced and not accentuated.

Normal pressure hydrocephalus

Normal pressure hydrocephalus is a disorder defined by a clinical triad of dementia, gait disturbance and urinary incontinence that is reversible with ventricular shunting.[18] It may be secondary to previous subarachnoid haemorrhage, trauma, infection or previous surgery. In the absence of these risk factors this syndrome is known as idiopathic normal pressure hydrocephalus. Imaging demonstrates ventriculomegaly and enlargement of the subarachnoid spaces in a pattern consistent with a communicating type hydrocephalus (Fig. 9.16). By definition the CSF opening pressure should be close to normal limits (< 180 mm of water).

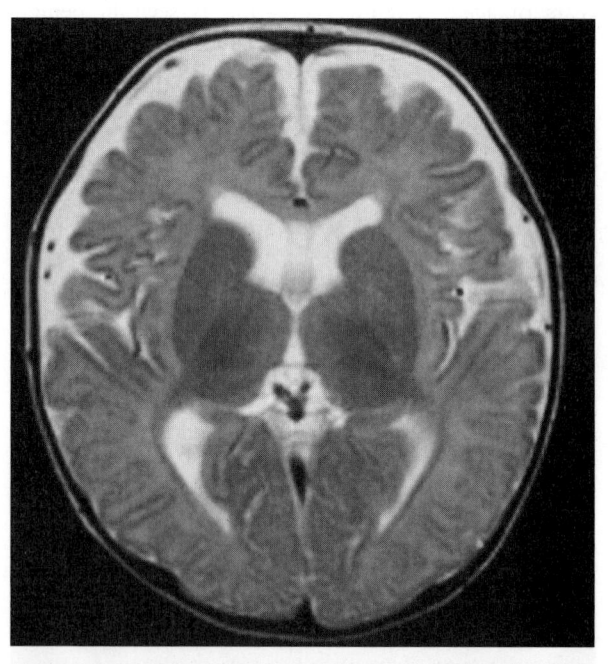

Figure 9.15 *Benign enlargement of the subarachnoid spaces in a 7-month-old infant with macrocephaly. Axial T2-image demonstrates prominence of the frontal subarachnoid spaces with mild ventricular enlargement.*

The problem lies in identifying which patients will respond to a shunting procedure. This is difficult as degenerative and vascular dementias can have similar clinical presentation and imaging findings particularly

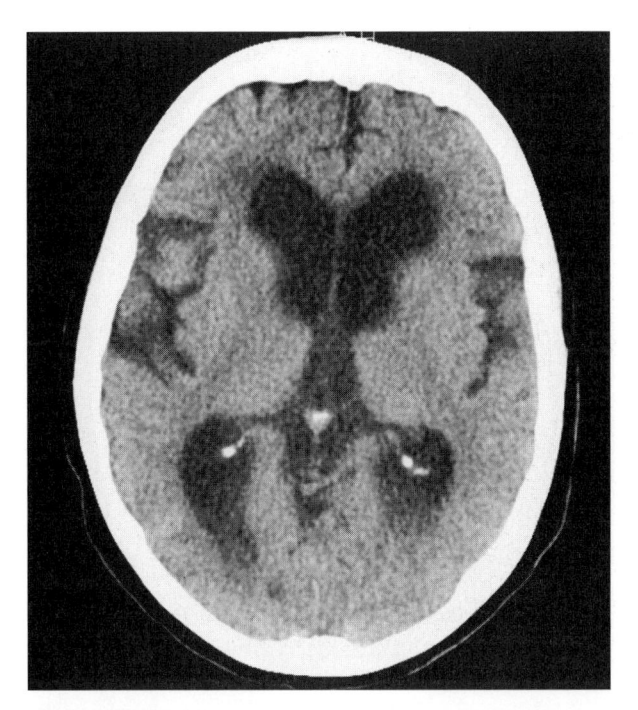

Figure 9.16 Normal pressure hydrocephalus in a 78-year-old man: CT scan demonstrates ventricular enlargement with prominent sylvian fissures in the absence of vascular disease.

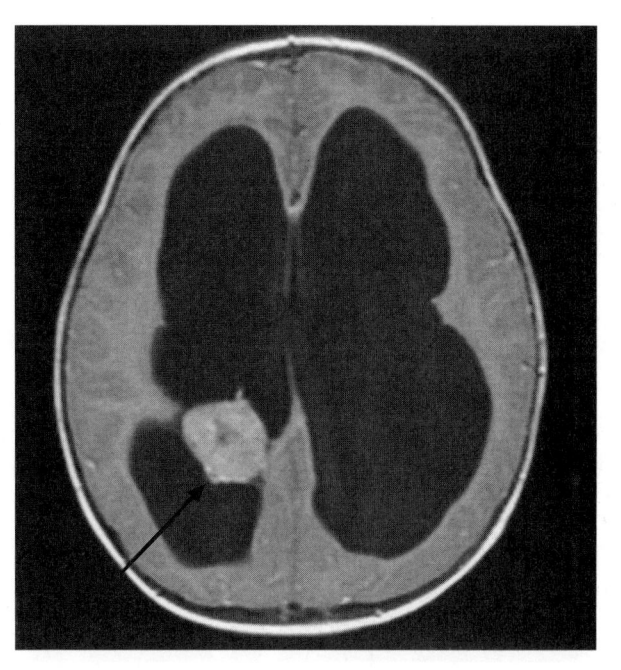

Figure 9.17 A 5-year-old male with a choroid plexus papilloma. Post-contrast T1-image demonstrates an enhancing intraventricular tumour (arrow) with hydrocephalus.

on CT. This is where the discriminators between hydrocephalus and atrophy described in Table 9.1 may be important. In reality, however, it is often still difficult to make a diagnosis on imaging grounds. There has been considerable interest in changes in CSF flow in normal pressure hydrocephalus with evidence that this flow becomes hyperdynamic. This is most noticeable in the cerebral aqueduct and posterior third ventricle where flow voids are seen on appropriate MRI sequences (Fig. 9.4). This flow void is thought to represent a decreased capacity for brain expansion in normal pressure hydrocephalus during cardiac systole resulting in increased pressure transmission to the ventricular system. This produces a secondary increase in intraventricular CSF flow. This increased flow can be quantified using cardiac gated phase contrast MRI[19] and does appear to help in predicting a successful outcome following shunting procedures.

This diagnosis should be made with caution in the absence of the clinical triad. In reality, patients often undergo a trial of lumbar puncture with drainage of CSF. If this produces a clinical improvement then shunting becomes a serious consideration.

HYDROCEPHALUS SECONDARY TO CEREBROSPINAL FLUID OVERPRODUCTION

Production of CSF by the choroid plexus can increase in the presence of a choroid plexus papilloma or in diffuse villous hyperplasia. These conditions usually affect infants and young children and can be detected *in utero*. Choroid plexus papilloma is a discrete mass that occurs most commonly in the lateral ventricles in children (Fig. 9.17) and the fourth ventricle in adults. There is a marked male predominance.[4] Villous hyperplasia of the choroid plexus is usually diffuse with enlargement of the choroid bilaterally.[20] The mechanism producing hydrocephalus in these conditions is complex. The popular theory is that production exceeds the ability of the arachnoid villi to drain CSF into the venous sinuses with a net increase in CSF volume and the development of hydrocephalus. This is almost certainly an oversimplification as the CSF produced has a high protein content that gives rise to a low grade leptomeningitis. This results in impairment of absorption of CSF at the arachnoid villi producing an obstructive hydrocephalus at this level. In reality it is likely that both overproduction and decreased absorption have a combined role in producing hydrocephalus in these conditions.

TREATED HYDROCEPHALUS

Medical therapy has a limited role in the control of hydrocephalus with CSF diversion with surgical shunts providing the pillar of treatment. The most common shunt employs external drainage of CSF controlled by an external valve. An occipital burr hole is most commonly used for shunt insertion with some surgeons preferring a frontal approach. The CSF can be diverted to a number

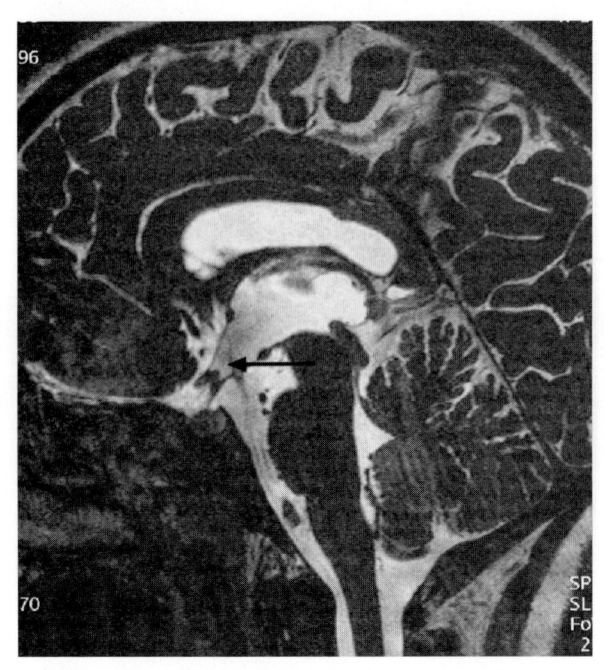

Figure 9.18 A 10-year-old girl after third ventriculostomy for aqueduct stenosis. Sagittal CISS 3-D image demonstrating a small defect in the floor of the third ventricle. A jet of CSF flow from the third ventricle to the basal cisterns can be clearly seen (arrow).

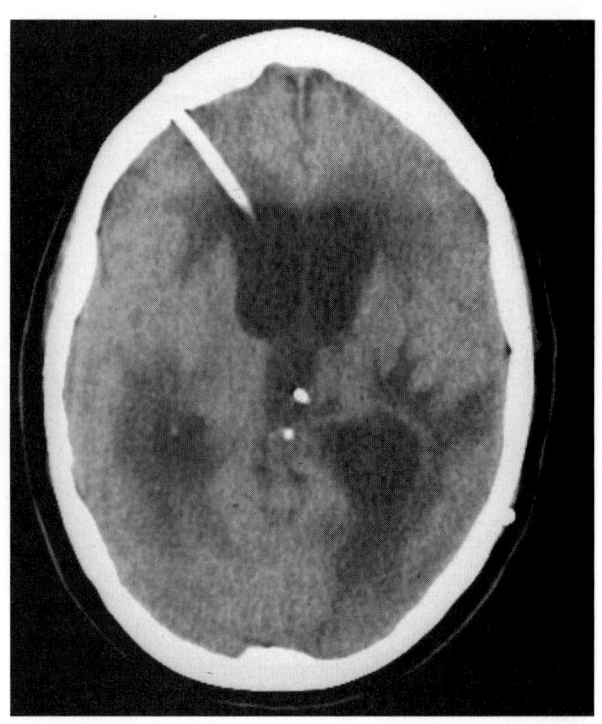

Figure 9.19 A 52-year-old female previously shunted for a posterior fossa tumour presents with symptoms of raised intracranial pressure. A CT brain scan demonstrates a right frontal shunt with acute hydrocephalus secondary to shunt obstruction.

of sites with the most common reservoir being the peritoneal cavity. Shunt malfunction occurs in up to 80% of patients with over half these complications being secondary to shunt obstruction.[21] To overcome some of the complications associated with long-term external ventricular shunting, internal CSF diversion with third ventriculostomy is being increasingly used in selected patients. This technique is of particular value for obstructive hydrocephalus distal to the third ventricle and can be performed endoscopically.[12] It requires careful planning with preoperative MRI in the sagittal plane to outline the anatomy of the third ventricular floor. The defect created in the third ventricular floor allows passage of CSF from the third ventricle to the basal cisterns bypassing the aqueduct and the fourth ventricle. Interestingly this procedure may also have some benefit in the long-term management of communicating hydrocephalus; MRI is of value in the follow-up of these patients and can demonstrate patency of the stoma (Fig. 9.18).

Shunt obstruction

Symptoms of shunt failure may be similar to the presenting symptoms of hydrocephalus including headache, vomiting, irritability, memory changes or change in seizure activity; CT brain allows comparison with previous scans in the assessment of ventricular size and may indicate a need for shunt revision (Fig. 9.19). The most common site of obstruction is the ventricular catheter,[21] commonly due to choroid plexus blocking drainage holes. Shunt obstruction may be confirmed with radioisotope examination or with fluroscopically guided injection of iodinated contrast media into the shunt reservoir.[22] Disconnections or breaks in shunt tubing are usually investigated with plain radiographs. MRI is of increasing value in the investigation of shunt malfunction. We have found the fluid attenuation inversion recovery sequence (FLAIR) to be of value in identifying shunt position; T2-sequences are also very sensitive for the detection of perishunt oedema, which is one of the earliest sign of shunt obstruction (Fig. 9.20). This occurs secondary to increased intraventricular pressure with CSF being forced into the brain parenchyma along the shunt path.

Shunt infection

This is the most serious complication and occurs on average in 7% of cases.[23] Infection can occur early after shunt insertion or late (> 3 months). Higher infection rates are seen with hydrocephalus secondary to previous intraventricular haemorrhage and in young infants; CT is of limited value in diagnosing infection, which requires direct CSF examination, although ependymal enhancement is seen with ventriculitis (Fig. 9.21). It is, however, useful to monitor possible associated changes in ventricular size.

Overdrainage

With drainage there is reduction in cerebral volume resulting in craniocerebral disproportion. Cortical draining veins can stretch and even minor trauma can result in subdural haematoma formation (Fig. 9.22). This usually occurs within 1–2 years of shunting. Post-shunt pachymeningeal fibrosis is a well recognized finding following shunting and can be diffuse (Fig. 9.23). This is possibly a reaction to chronic subdural fluid collections.[4] It is important to recognize this as a benign condition particularly in patients who have been shunted for tumours that may spread to the meninges.

Secondary sagittal craniosynostosis may occur following excessive drainage in children under 6 months old. Slit ventricle syndrome may occur up to 10 years following shunting. This is usually a high-pressure syndrome in patients with reduced intracranial volume due to early sutural closure. Patients usually present with intermittent symptoms of shunt failure. Imaging demonstrates small slit-like ventricles and loss of extra-ventricular CSF space. A trapped fourth ventricle can also be a consequence of overdrainage in the paediatric population with failure of CSF outflow due to obstruction of the aqueduct and the fourth ventricular exit foramina.

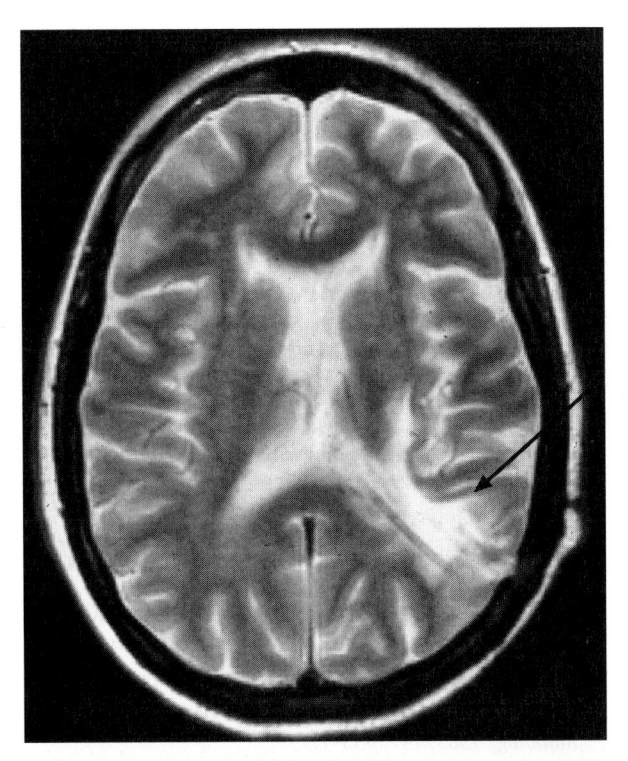

Figure 9.20 A 40-year-old female with symptoms of possible shunt malfunction. Axial T2-image demonstrates high signal around the shunt tubing consistent with oedema secondary to shunt obstruction.

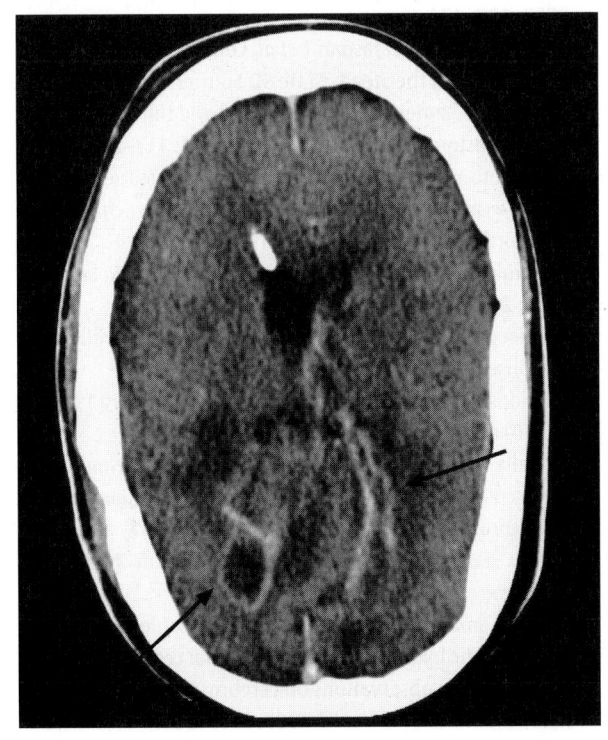

Figure 9.21 A 33-year-old female with Chiari II malformation and chronic hydrocephalus requiring long-term shunting. Axial post-contrast CT demonstrates ependymal enhancement (arrows) secondary to infective ventriculitis. Vault thickening is also seen as a feature of chronic shunting.

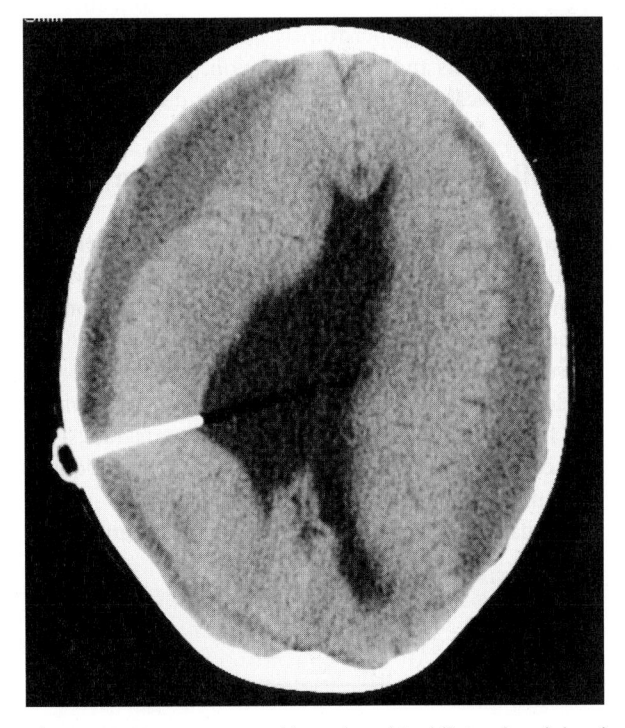

Figure 9.22 A 41-year-old male with bilateral subdural haematomas as a complication of overvigorous drainage of previously enlarged ventricles.

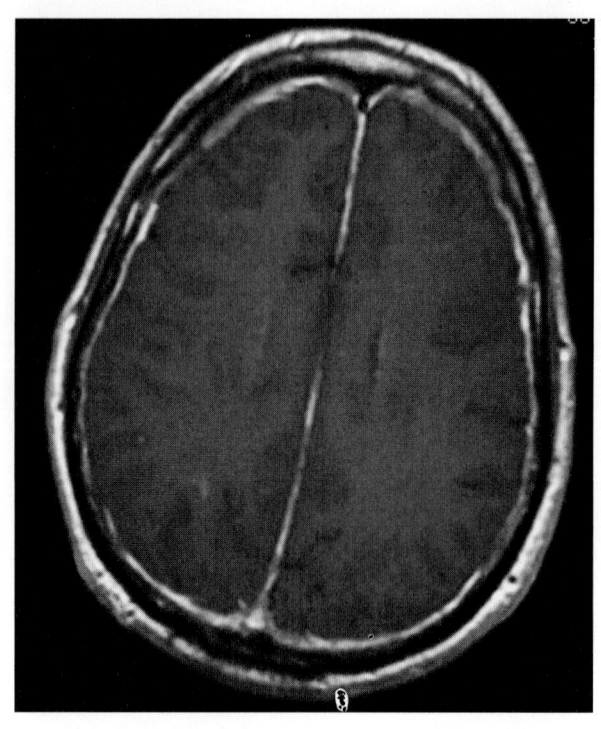

Figure 9.23 *Post-contrast T1-image in a 53-year-old man demonstrating diffuse meningeal enhancement secondary to previous ventricular shunting.*

Abdominal complications of ventriculoperitoneal shunts

These include ascites, small bowel obstruction, abdominal wall abscess, peritonitis, visceral perforation, abdominal cysts and hernia formation. These complications are investigated with plain films and CT.[21]

Complications of third ventriculostomy

The procedure may fail due to an inadequate opening of the third ventricular floor. In addition there are other membranes in the subarachnoid space, most notably Liliquists' membrane, which may also need to be divided for successful shunting.[12] A patent ventriculostomy can be demonstrated with high resolution T2-MRI where CSF flow produces phase dispersion and signal loss. This flow can be quantified using phase-contrast techniques.

Damage to normal structures can also occur such as the basilar artery with haemorrhage or aneurysm formation.

REFERENCES

1. Aronyk KE. The history and classification of hydrocephalus. *Neurosurg Clin N Amer* 1993; **4**: 606–7.
2. Naidich TF, McLone DG. Radiographic classification and gross morphological features of hydrocephalus. In: *Disorders of the Developing Nervous System: Diagnosis and Treatment* pp. 505–39. (Hoffman H, Epstein F (Eds), Oxford: Blackwell Scientific Publications, 1986.
3. McComb JG. Cerebrospinal fluid physiology of the developing foetus. *Am J Neuroradiol* 1992; **13**: 595–9.
4. Barkovich AJ. *Pediatric Neuroimaging*. Philadelphia: Lippincott-Raven, 1995.
5. Greitz D, Wirestam R, Franck A *et al*. Pulsatile brain movement and associated haemodynamics studied by magnetic resonance phase imaging. The Monro-Kellie doctrine revisited. *Neuroradiology* 1992; **34**: 370–80.
6. Bradley WG. MR prediction of shunt response in NPH: CSF morphology versus physiology. *Am J Neuroradiol* 1998; **19**: 1285–6.
7. Heinz ER, Ward A, Drayer BP *et al*. Distinction between obstructive and atrophic dilatation of the ventricles in children. *J Comput Assist Tomogr* 1980; **4**: 320–5.
8. Barkovich AJ, Edwards MSB. Applications of neuroimaging in hydrocephalus. *Pediat Neurosurg* 1992; **18**: 65–83.
9. Kleinman PK, Zito JL, Davidson RI, Raptopoulos V. The subarachnoid spaces in children: normal variations in size. *Radiology* 1983; **147**: 455–7.
10. Waggenspck GA, Guinto FC. MRI and CT of masses of the anterosuperior third ventricle. *Am J Neuroradiol* 1989; **10**: 105–10.
11. Haverkamp F, Wolfle J, Artez M *et al*. Congenital hydrocephalus internus and aqueduct stenosis: aeitiology and implications for genetic councelling. *Eur J Pediatr* 1999; **158**: 474–8.
12. Laitt RD, Mallucci C, Jaspan T *et al*. Constructive Interference in the Steady State 3D Fourier-transform MRI in the management of hydrocephalus and third ventriculostomy. *Neuroradiology* 1999; **41**: 117–23.
13. Yoshimoto Y, Ochiai C, Kawamata K *et al*. Aqueductal blood clot as a cause of acute hydrocephalus in subarachnoid haemorrhage. *Am J Neuroradiol* 1996; **17**: 1183–6.
14. Bilaniuk LT. Adult infratentorial tumours. *Semin Roentgenol* 1990; **25**: 155–73.
15. Massiecotte EM, Del Bigio MR. Human arachnoid villi response to subarachnoid haemorrhage: possible relationship to chronic hydrocephalus. *J Neurosurg* 1999; **91**: 80–4.
16. D'Avella D, Greenberg RP, Mingrino S *et al*. Alterations in ventricular size and intracranial pressure caused by sagittal sinus thrombosis. *J Neurosurg* 1980; **53**: 656–61.
17. Boaz JC, Edwards-Brown MK. Hydrocephalus in children. *Neuroimag Clin N Amer* 1999; **9**: 73–91.
18. Hakim S, Adams RD. The special clinical problem of symptomatic hydrocephalus with normal cerebrospinal fluid pressure: observations on cerebrospinal fluid hydrodynamics. *J Neurol Sci* 1965; **2**: 307–27.
19. Bradley WG, Scalzo D, Queralt J *et al*. Normal pressure hydrocephalus: evaluation with cerebrospinal fluid measurements at MR imaging. *Radiology* 1996; **198**: 523–9.
20. Britz GW, Kim DK, Loeser JD. Hydrocephalus secondary to diffuse villous hyperplasia of the choroid plexus. Case

report and review of the literature. *J Neurosurg* 1996; **85**: 689–91.
21 Naidich TP. Assessment of shunted hydrocephalus and complications of shunt therapy. *AARS Categorical Course Syllabus* 1992; 207–13.
22 Goeser CD, McLeary MS, Young LW. Diagnostic imaging of ventriculoperitoneal shunt malfunctions and complications. *Radiographics* 1998; **18**: 635–51.
23 Quigley M, Reigel D, Kortyna R. Cerebrospinal fluid shunt infections. Report of 41 cases and a critical review of the literature. *Pediatr Neurosci* 1989; **15**: 111–20.

10

Advanced techniques in neuroradiology

ALAN JACKSON, STEVE WILLIAMS

Introduction	280	Magnetization transfer and diffusion weighted imaging	285
Perfusion imaging	280	Magnetic resonance spectroscopy	287
Quantification of contrast-enhancement	284	References	291
Functional imaging	284		

INTRODUCTION

Improvements in computed tomography (CT) and magnetic resonance imaging (MRI) hardware, MR sequences and image processing are continuously extending the repertoire of the diagnostic neuroradiologist. Although the majority of the data presented in this book refer to standard CT and MRI techniques it is clear that the clinical role of these newer methods will progressively increase. In many cases the exact clinical benefits and role of new imaging methodologies is not yet entirely clear. The purpose of this chapter is to provide an introductory overview of some of these methods. Since it is not appropriate in a book of this type to attempt to be comprehensive we will focus on a range of techniques which already have some direct clinical role or which seem likely to become increasingly important in the near future. Many of these new methods are aimed at the identification of microstructural changes, beyond the true spatial resolution of MRI or at the production of physiological measurements.

PERFUSION IMAGING

The measurement of cerebral perfusion is a vital component of clinical diagnosis and management in a wide range of brain diseases. Despite this there is no ideal method for the imaging of cerebral perfusion in clinical cases. Single photon emission computed tomography (SPECT) using the radio-labelled blood-flow tracer technetium-99m hexamethyl propylene amime oxime (^{99}Tc HMPAO) provides the most clinically acceptable method at the present time. ^{99m}Tc HMPAO crosses the blood–brain barrier and is taken up by brain cells at a rate proportional to the local cerebral blood flow. The isotope is trapped and fixed within cells, providing a memory of perfusion at the time of injection. The isotope is a short-lived (6h half-life), high energy-emitter which can be detected by SPECT for up to a few hours after injection. In patients with reduced regional perfusion, deficits in ^{99m}Tc HMPAO uptake are clearly identified and can be quantified to some extent. However, there are several significant disadvantages with this technique. First SPECT images reflect the distribution of ^{99m}Tc HMPAO within brain tissue following an initial uptake phase. This distribution will be affected not only by pathological variations in perfusion but will also reflect regional atrophy and, to a lesser extent physiological activation. In addition the technique requires a prolonged period of data collection and produces relatively low spatial resolution.

Xenon-enhanced computed tomography

Xenon is a highly soluble inert gas that can be safely used as an X-ray contrast medium. Inhalation of xenon produces a progressive increase of xenon partial pressure in the plasma and extracellular fluid with a consequent reduction in CT attenuation. At steady-state, the concentration of xenon in the tissues reflects regional perfusion allowing calculation of absolute blood flow. This technique has remained unpopular due to the general anaesthetic properties of xenon, which can cause confusion and somnolence in some patients. However, the increased acquisition speed of spiral CT allows measurements of cerebral perfusion through the whole brain to be made in under 1 minute.[1] This acquisition speed is combined with improvements in post-processing technology which allow the images to be acquired without a lengthy equilibration phase, so that the subject's exposure to the gas is minimized. Despite the simplicity and accuracy of this technique its popularity remains limited.

Magnetic resonance imaging of cerebral perfusion

The measurement of cerebral perfusion with MRI has been the subject of extensive research. Two generic approaches to determining cerebral blood flow (CBF) have been described. The first of these is to quantify the amount of blood flowing into a slice of brain by magnetically tagging protons in the blood flowing into it. The second technique is to use rapid MRI to trace the passage of a bolus of contrast media through the brain using the resulting signal intensity change to calculate cerebral perfusion. This second technique, known as dynamic contrast-enhanced MR perfusion imaging, is the simpler of the two methods and is becoming widely used in clinical practice.

DYNAMIC CONTRAST-ENHANCED MR PERFUSION IMAGING

The production of cerebral blood flow maps by dynamic contrast-enhanced MRI requires the accurate measurement of the transient changes in gadolinium concentration which occur as a contrast bolus passes through the brain.[2,3] The technique requires a rapid intravenous injection of contrast media over a period of 2–3 seconds, which is chased by an injection of normal saline given at the same rate. This technique is designed to deliver a tight bolus of contrast into the superior vena cava in order to minimize bolus dispersion between intravenous injection and its arrival at the carotid arteries. The signal change in the brain produced by the passage of this bolus can be recorded by measuring relaxivity (T1-weighted images [T1WI]) or susceptibility (T2*-weighted images [T2*WI]) effects; T1WI require small quantities of contrast but are highly susceptible to tissue enhancement and produce relatively poor signal-to-noise ratios in the brain parenchyma while T2*WI produce a more profound signal change in the brain parenchyma since the susceptibility effects of contrast occur not only in the blood vessels but also in the normal tissue surrounding them. Most perfusion imaging is therefore conducted with T2*-weighted sequences.

Whatever imaging sequence is chosen it must accurately record the transient signal change occurring during bolus passage. Since the bolus will, on average have an overall width of no more than 20 seconds high-speed imaging is essential. Several studies have shown that the time resolution of these images should be in the region of 2 seconds or less since lower temporal resolutions give rise to significant errors in the calculation of cerebral blood volume (CBV) and CBF.[4] This requirement for high temporal resolution has led to the widespread use of echo planar imaging methods. Many workers have employed single shot echo planar sequences although the use of multishot, multislice echo planar methods is also common.

Introduction of T2*-sensitive volume imaging techniques has also been described. The PRESTO technique (principles of echo shifting with a train of observations)[5] combines an echo planar volume acquisition with echo shifting to increase T2* sensitivity. This method may be combined with navigator echo correction to reduce image blurring produced by patient movement. The development of fast echo planar-based volume imaging techniques like PRESTO allows imaging of the whole brain volume in the 2 seconds available. Nonetheless the number of voxels that can be sampled is severely limited by the temporal resolution required and this is, in turn, directly related to the gradient performance of the MRI scanner. A typical PRESTO perfusion sequence would have a matrix of $64 \times 64 \times 40$. In many cases higher spatial in-plane resolution is required in which case the number of slices acquired must be reduced.

The images produced by all these techniques demonstrate a short-lived drop in signal intensity corresponding with the passage of the contrast bolus through the brain's vascular bed. This signal change must be analysed to produce the required measurements of CBV, CBF and mean transit time (MTT). Fortunately this analysis can be performed using simple models of tracer kinetics. The first step in the analysis is to translate the change in signal intensity to a contrast concentration time curve. In T1WI a simple linear dependency between signal intensity and contrast concentration can be assumed over quite a wide range. In T2*WI the concentration of contrast is approximately directly proportional to the rate of change of T2*, commonly referred to as $\Delta R2$. Examination of the $\Delta R2$ time curve from an area of grey matter demonstrates the transient increase in contrast concentration during bolus passage (Fig. 10.1). According to standard tracer kinetics

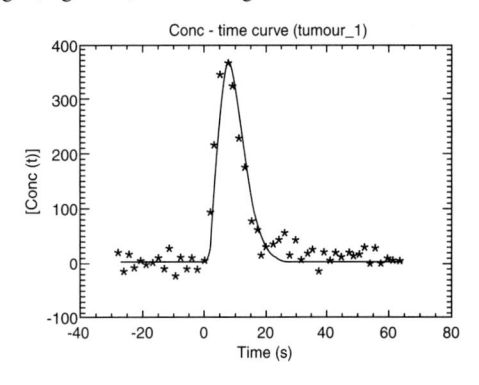

Figure 10.1 *The change in contrast concentration against time in a single voxel from a malignant brain tumour. Data points are fitted to a gamma variat curve shown as a line which is then used to calculate haemodynamic variables.*

the area under this curve is proportional to the CBV and the width of the curve is proportional to the MTT. The central volume theorem states that CBF is equal to CBV divided by MTT. Using these relationships all three parameters can be simply calculated on a voxel by voxel basis. This allows the production of parametric maps of CBV, MTT and CBF. In addition the time taken for the bolus to arrive in the voxel (T0) and the time taken to reach peak concentration (TTP) can easily be derived and are also commonly used to produce parametric maps (Colour plate 3).

Dynamic contrast-enhanced perfusion MR techniques are now available on most commercial imaging systems. These sequences combined with the matched image analysis software produce maps of CBV, CBF, MTT, T0 and TTP. There are, however, a number of potential drawbacks with this approach to the measurement of cerebral perfusion. The bolus of contrast must be rapidly administered and must remain coherent in its first passage through the brain. In patients with cardiac arrhythmias or poor cardiac function this may not occur giving rise to poor quality parametric images. This technique assumes that the bolus of contrast media remains entirely within the intravascular compartment throughout its first pass through the brain, which is clearly untrue in the presence of enhancement and particularly in malignant cerebral tumours. This is of particular importance since the measurement of CBV appears to be a useful prognostic indicator in a wide range of cerebral malignancies (Colour plate 4). More important, the technique does not produce absolute measurements of CBV or CBF. This means that no reference to normal values can be confidently made and assessment of the images relies on the presence of asymmetry or focal regional change. Because of this shortcoming images produced by dynamic contrast-enhanced imaging are better referred to as relative CBV and CBF (rCBV and rCBF).

Several approaches to this problem have been described, each attempting to produce CBF maps with true quantitative values. The most commonly used technique is to measure the width of the bolus that enters the brain in the carotid artery and to use this to improve the measurements of mean transit time obtained in the individual brain voxels.[2] This technique, known as deconvolution, is a simple approach to the production of CBF values which appears to produce an approximate correction factor that allows values of CBF to be compared between patients. Nonetheless the deconvolution technique is far from ideal and may have problems in specific diseases, particularly where arterial stenoses and occlusions are present.[6]

DYNAMIC CONTRAST-ENHANCED CT PERFUSION IMAGING

First-pass bolus analysis techniques can also be used with CT data. The use of fast spiral CT acquisitions have produced first-pass bolus data with standard X-ray contrast media which has sufficient time resolution to allow calculation of CBF and CBV.[7] However, on most systems this will allow the acquisition of only one or two slices with the appropriate dynamic resolution. The introduction of multislice CT systems will, however, make this methodology far more attractive since it adds no additional imaging time or contrast dose to a standard CT contrast-examination.

MEASUREMENT OF CEREBRAL PERFUSION BY SPIN TAGGING

Several MR perfusion imaging techniques which avoid the need for intravenous contrast injection have been described. These techniques use pulsed labelling of arterial spins by radiofrequency inversion pulses and use images acquired with and without labelling to measure regional perfusion. Most of these techniques use inversion pulses to label blood which will enter the sampling slice. This results in a reduction of signal in the slice when the 'spin label' is applied. The technique is complicated by loss of the spin label due to the relatively short T1 of the inflowing blood compared with the rate of passage of the blood through the brain. Thus, although arterial tagging in the neck is theoretically optimal from a biological standpoint and works well in small animals, it is extremely difficult to implement in humans.

Alternative approaches of labelling spins immediately adjacent to the imaging plane has its own problems regarding direction of inflow, selection of the optimal inflow times and inadvertent labelling of venous inflow. This has given rise to a number of alternative approaches to spin labelling which include echo planar MRI with alternating radio-frequency (EPISTAR), flow sensitive alternating inversion recovery (FAIR), uninverted FAIR (UNFAIR), and quantitative imaging of perfusion using single subtraction (QUIPPS). Review of these techniques and their specific problems has been published by Patel et al.[8] In general these techniques are complex to implement and produce very small (<2%) signal changes. This places significant demands on sequence design and means that some of these techniques perform poorly in patients with reduced cerebral perfusion. Despite this these techniques appear extremely promising as a method of quantitative perfusion imaging and further development of spin-tagging methodologies can be expected.

Clinical applications of perfusion imaging

Despite its potential shortcomings dynamic contrast enhanced susceptibility MRI has been used in a wide range of clinical applications. In patients with carotid and vertebral artery disease the maintenance of regional

CBF depends on the dilation of pial arterials with a consequent increase in the volume of blood vessels within the brain. This will produce an increase in the CBV map which may be seen particularly in the watershed areas of the forebrain. In fact, the dilatation of cerebral vessels has a more marked effect on the speed of contrast passage so that larger changes are seen in maps of T0 and TTP (Colour plate 4).[9] As the brain's autoregulatory mechanisms fail to compensate adequately for the reduced cerebral perfusion pressure, then the CBF maps will eventually show regional decreases in perfusion. This pattern of blood flow changes allows identification of the areas of brain most severely affected, the efficiency with which the Circle of Willis is supplying collateral flow and the extent in which the autoregulatory mechanism has been expended.

In patients with established stroke, perfusion imaging will clearly demonstrate the extent of the area which has been subject to reduction in CBF.[10] This is potentially of considerable clinical importance since some of the tissue within this area of reduced perfusion may well be capable of salvage, either by reperfusion or the use of cerebral protective agents. The identification of areas of established stroke by the use of diffusion imaging can be combined with perfusion mapping to identify areas of perfusion/diffusion mismatch. The presence of these areas of viable but hypoperfused brain tissue forms the basis for many proposed strategies of stroke treatment.

Dynamic contrast-enhanced imaging also has a significant role in the assessment of patients with cerebral tumours.[11] One of the principle features of a wide range of tumours is abnormality of the blood supply and of the microvascular structure within the tumour itself. Increases in local CBV enable the identification of areas of increased malignancy within low-grade gliomas. In addition the detection of regional changes in CBV provides an indicator of dedifferentiation which can be used in planning tumour therapy. The simplest and most effective method for the detection of these abnormalities is MR perfusion imaging. The use of MR perfusion imaging in tumours is complicated by the presence of increased endothelial permeability which occurs in areas of malignant dedifferentiation. This increased permeability allows extravasation of contrast into the extracellular space to produce the familiar contrast-enhancement effects.

In areas of high capillary permeability, leakage of contrast during the passage of the bolus leads to an increase in signal within enhancing voxels due to the relaxivity effects of the contrast within the extracellular space. When imaging sequences with mixed T1- and T2*-sensitivity are used, these relaxivity effects reduce the magnitude of the susceptibility induced signal drop induced by passage of the contrast bolus (Fig. 10.2). This can result in severe underestimation of CBV and CBF values. This relaxivity effect can be minimized by the use of low flip angle acquisitions although the signal-to-noise ratio

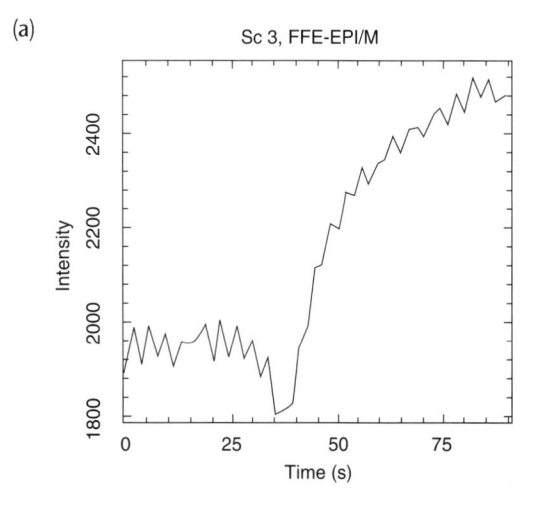

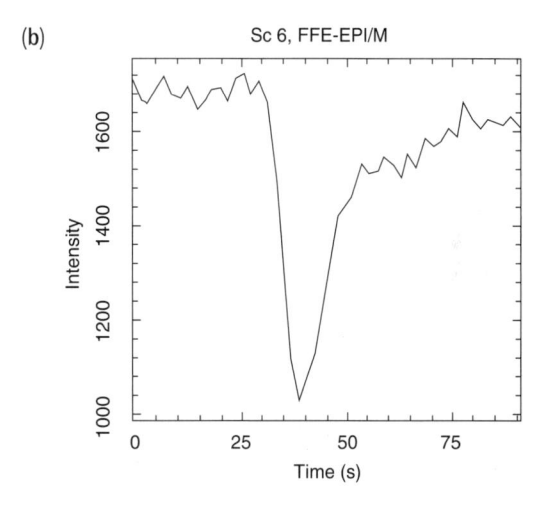

Figure 10.2 *(a) Signal intensity changes with time in a large acoustic neuroma using a 2-D FFE sequence with a 35° flip angle and no pre-enhancement (mixed T1- and T2-weighting). Note the immediate signal rise above baseline due to relaxivity effects. (b) Signal intensity changes with time in the same patient following a pre-enhancement dose of contrast. Note the normal signal drop and recovery phase.*

of the contrast time curve will be adversely affected. More effectively pre-administration of a contrast dose 10–15 minutes prior to the perfusion examination will pre-saturate tissues so that any T1 changes caused by contrast bolus passage will be markedly reduced. These simple techniques allow rapid routine imaging of rCBV and rCBF even in very vascular tumours and provide methods for the clinical demonstration of regional increases in CBV (Colour plate 5). In gliomas these areas of increased CBV represent the most malignant area of the tumour and should form the target for diagnostic biopsy.

Dynamic contrast-enhanced MR perfusion imaging can also be used in a wide range of other cerebrovascular diseases. Colour plates 6–8 demonstrate abnormalities of MR perfusion imaging in a number of disorders including Alzheimer's disease. Despite this the technique remains developmental and will continue to evolve as it passes into clinical practice. In particular we should expect to see the production of quantitative maps of cerebral blood flow to replace the relative blood flow maps currently produced by most commercial systems.

QUANTIFICATION OF CONTRAST-ENHANCEMENT

The time course of tissue-enhancement has been of interest in many disease states, particularly in the diagnosis and classification of tumours. In recent years it has been increasingly appreciated that tumour growth is dependent on the development of new blood vessels, known as angiogenesis, which is stimulated by the release of growth factors from tumour cells. These growth factors directly increase the permeability of capillary membranes allowing easier passage of metabolites into and out of the tumour as well as stimulating the proliferation of blood vessel lining cells and the growth of new cells.[12]

The development of new therapeutic approaches to cancer targeting these growth factors has led to an increased interest in the measurement of the permeability of the capillary endothelium. The presence of high endothelial permeability in tumours has been implicated in the formation of peritumoural oedema and tumour cysts and it has also been suggested that high permeability supports the generation and viability of haematogenous metastases.[13,14] Imaging studies to measure endothelial permeability rely on the accurate measurement of marker concentrations in the blood stream and in the tumour over time. By application of an appropriate pharmacokinetic model the effective permeability between the blood stream and tumour can be calculated.

Several appropriate pharmacokinetic models have been described. The most commonly used model described by Brix[15] calculates a transfer constant (K12) which relates to the passage of contrast between the blood stream and the tumour interstitium and which is related to vascular permeability. More comprehensive models described by Tofts et al.[16] and by Larsson et al.[17] attempt to calculate true absolute values for endothelial permeability surface area product (k). The rationale for these, more complex and methodologically demanding, approaches is to produce a measurement which is independent of variables such as instrument gain, contrast dose, patient cardiovascular status etc. This makes these models attractive for monitoring changes in tumour vasculature during treatment and in determining the surrogate endpoints for treatment in longitudinal comparison and multicentre trials. The Tofts model produces two independent variables: the surface area endothelial permeability product (k) and the contrast distribution volume (vl) which corresponds to the size of the extracellular space (Colour plate 9). Values of k and vl are highly reproducible and are independent of the scanner type. They show a close correlation with the aggressive behaviour of tumours across many tumour types (Fig. 10.3).

FUNCTIONAL IMAGING

Identification of regional neuronal activity using MRI techniques is now well established. Neuronal activation produces an increase in capillary blood flow within the region of activation. This increase in flow is greater than would be required to simply meet the increased neuronal oxygen demand. Consequently there is a regional reduction in the overall concentration in deoxyhaemoglobin due to haemodilution. Since deoxyhaemaglobin is a paramagnetic compound, producing focal changes in magnetic field intensity, this produces a small but detectable increase in MR signal on T2*WI. This signal change is referred to as blood oxygen level dependent (BOLD) contrast and forms the basis of most functional MRI techniques. Although the signal changes caused by BOLD seldom exceed 10%, they can be separated from background image noise by the use of multiple image repetitions combined with statistical techniques to analyse the significance of any variation in signal which is observed. Most functional imaging experiments have

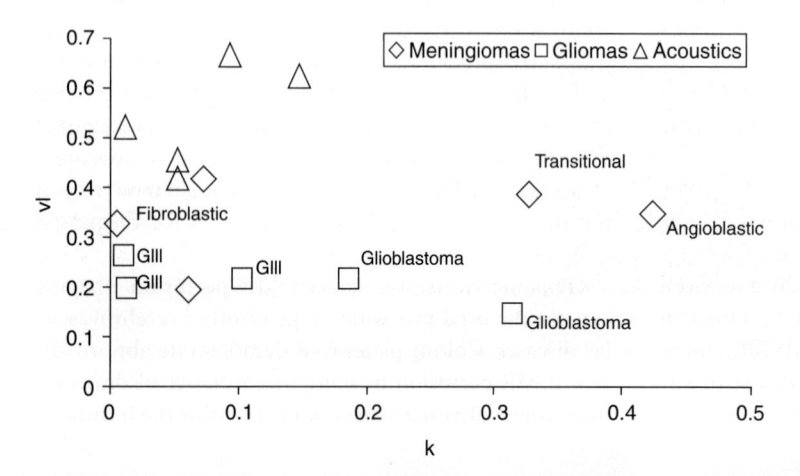

Figure 10.3 A plot of endothelial surface area permeability product (k) against contrast distribution space (vl) in 15 patients with cerebral tumours. Patients with acoustic neuroma show high values of vl in keeping with the known histological characteristics of the tumour. High values of k (>0.15) as seen only in patients with glioblastoma and aggressive meningiomas.

been conducted using a block paradigm. A typical example of this is identification of the motor cortex using a motor task. The subject lies in the MR scanner and performs a simple motor activity such as apposition of the thumb and fingers. A series of MR images is obtained over a period of time during which the subject is asked to perform a task and then to rest. This is repeated to produce several blocks of images during which the task was performed and several blocks in which it was not.

The use of simple statistical measures such as *t*-tests or non-parametric probability tests to compare images 'with task' to images 'without task' allows the construction of probability maps, which show the location of the cortex involved (Fig. 10.4, Colour plate 10). This technique has been widely used in the cognitive neurosciences and is increasingly used in neuroradiological practice to identify eloquent areas of cortex. This can be of considerable use prior to surgery, helping the surgeon to avoid injury to sensitive areas of cortex (Colour plate 11a,b). Combinations of these functional tests are also being examined as potential alternatives to the Wada tests in the assessment of surgery for focal epilepsy.

More recently the BOLD technique has been further developed to allow the use of single stimuli combined with stimulus locked responses. In this technique a series of short-lived stimuli are applied during a period of continuous image acquisition. Signal averaging allows the identification of typical short-lived BOLD responses in the affected areas of the brain without the need for continuous block activity. This has simplified paradigm design to some extent although this technique has not as yet been used in clinical practice.

MAGNETIZATION TRANSFER AND DIFFUSION WEIGHTED IMAGING

Magnetization transfer imaging (MTI) and diffusion weighted imaging (DWI) provide new MR contrast mechanisms of potential use in clinical neuroradiology. Both techniques can be used to detect abnormalities beyond the resolution of conventional MRI and provide additional information about changes in cellular and molecular composition of tissue.

Magnetization transfer imaging

Magnetization transfer contrast results from the presence of two separate pools of protons within tissue: 1) bound immobile protons associated with macromolecules such as myelin and 2) mobile protons associated with free water. Pulsed MTI is achieved by application of an off-resonance radiofrequency before the pulse sequence in order to preferentially saturate protons in the bound pool. These bound protons then transfer magnetization to mobile protons in free water producing a drop in signal intensity. The change in net signal intensity depends on the strength of the saturation pulse and on the structure of the macromolecular matrix. The amount of magnetization transferred can be represented as the magnetization transfer ratio (MTR). Decreases in MTR are seen in areas of demyelination, inflammation, Wallerian degeneration and in human and experimental brain tumours. The measurement of MTR appears to be unaffected by tissue anisotropy and is increasingly used as a method of quantifying abnormalities in isotropic white matter tracts affected by inflammatory and ischaemic disease. Despite this, the exact clinical benefits of MTI remain unclear, while MTR is thought to reflect the structural integrity of tissues with an important contribution from myelin and axons. In multiple sclerosis decreases in MTR appear maximal during the acute enhancing phase, slowly recovering as lesions mature.[18] This suggests that MTI may provide a tool for elucidating pathophysiology and for monitoring treatment in multiple sclerosis. It has also been shown that MTR can improve the accuracy of tumour classification. Kurki *et al.*[19] found MTR to be superior to other MR techniques in the classification of intra-axial tumours allowing accurate differentiation between low-grade astrocytomas, haemangioblastomas and craniopharyngiomas. Taylor-Robinson *et al.*[20] demonstrated a correlation between globus pallidus MT contrast and blood ammonia levels which also correlated to the severity of hepatic encephalopathy in patients with liver dysfunction. These observations suggest that MTR images may become an increasingly important feature of diagnostic imaging strategies in a number of brain diseases.

DIFFUSION WEIGHTED IMAGING

Diffusion weighted imaging sequences have been available for many years but it is only recently that the technique has become widely clinically available. The diffusion technique depends on motion-related signal loss induced by the use of large matched dephasing gradients. These gradients will have no effect on the MR signal unless motion is present within the sample volume.

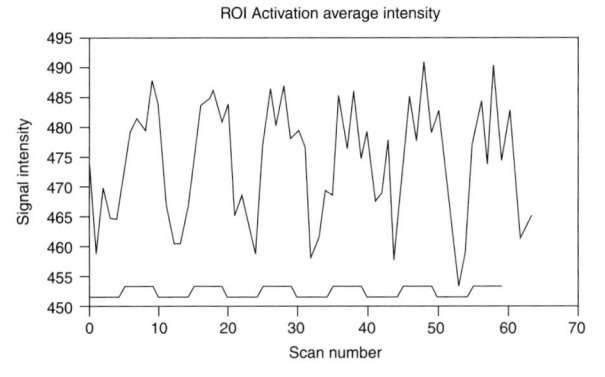

Figure 10.4 *Time course of signal changes in the visual cortex during visual stimulation. The subject was shown a flashing checkerboard with intermittent periods of rest. The visual stimulus causes periodic elevation of the signal.*

The presence of Brownian diffusion of water within the sample will, however, produce signal loss proportional to the strength of the dephasing gradients and the degree of diffusion, which occurs in the interval between the application of the two gradients. Acquisition of several images using increasing diffusion gradient strengths allows calculation of the apparent diffusion coefficient (ADC) for each pixel. The value of the ADC is dependent on the gradient strengths, duration and spacing and is thus not a true diffusion coefficient, and comparison of absolute values between sites must be made with caution. Water diffusion itself in the brain is affected by the viscosity and tortuosity of the intracellular and extracellular spaces, and by the presence of barriers to diffusion, such as cell membranes and myelin sheaths. Although the biophysical basis of pathological changes in water diffusion is not well understood, changes in cell volume leading to expansion or shrinkage of the extracellular space appear to play an important role. Diffusion has inherently directional properties and is properly represented as a tensor.

Traditionally ADC measurements have been acquired along a single axis of the main magnet bore, but the measurements then become highly sensitive to the precise alignment of the gradient axis with anisotropic structures such as white matter. By acquiring three images, sensitized along all three principle axes, the effects of anisotropy can be removed by constructing the trace of the diffusion tensor. However, three measurements are insufficient to characterize anisotropy, and as interest in diffusional anisotropy has increased more workers are now measuring the full tensor. This requires measurement in six directions,[21] but the clinical value of a full tensor description is as yet unclear.

The clinical use of DWI depends on the ability of the imaging sequence to correct for small physiological patient movements that occur during image acquisition. Patient movements can be minimized by rapid imaging and most diffusional sequences are now based on single shot echo planar imaging (EPI), fast spin echo (FSE), gradient and spin echo (GRASE) or multi-shot EPI techniques. Because of the long scan times DWI images are also sensitive to phase shifts, which vary from view to view. To correct for this many DWI sequences use a double echo technique in which the fast echo carries spatial information and the second 'navigator echo' has no spatial encoding. Variations in the phase of the navigator induced by motion are then used to correct phase errors occurring in the fast imaging echo. These navigator echo corrected images show significant reduction in movement-related phase echo and make clinical DWI realistically achievable.

CLINICAL USES OF DIFFUSION WEIGHTED IMAGING

The clinical role of DWI is already well defined in some areas and continues to grow, as more stable imaging techniques become widely available. The largest application of DWI is likely to be in the investigation of cerebral ischaemia. In both clinical studies and animal models DWI demonstrates a rapid fall in ADC with a gradual return to normal followed by an increase over baseline values.[22] In acute stroke, demonstrations of decreased ADC may be the only imaging abnormality, whilst T2 images remain normal.[23] In the late phase of stroke, areas of increased ADC allow confident identification of lesions which are at least several days old and correspond to cellular breakdown with loss of diffusional barriers.[24] The identification of an area of T2 abnormality with ADC values around normal may indicate either cellular recovery or progressive cellular necrosis. In these cases DWI alone is not sufficient to predict outcome and evidence of the perfusional status of the tissue must be sought. This combination of DWI and perfusion imaging often known as the 'brain-attack' protocol offers considerable promise for the assessment of acute stroke, for treatment planning and for the assessment of new therapeutic strategies.[10,25,26]

Other clinical uses for DWI are less well defined. The ability to measure regional anisotropy has led several groups to examine the potential utility of DWI in white matter development and white matter disease. In the newborn the ADC of white matter is considerably greater than in adults and there is a close correlation to the gestational age with ADC dropping as gestational age increases. Measurements of diffusional anisotropy do not show a similar correlation and it has been suggested that ADC measures reflect brain water content whilst diffusional anisotropy gives information concerning brain microstructure.[27] This conclusion is supported by observations in multiple sclerosis where diffusion imaging identifies significantly abnormal water diffusion properties in otherwise normal appearing white matter.

Use of DWI can also allow one to distinguish between lesion types with the highest diffusion seen in destructive (T1 hypointense) lesions and the greatest changes in anisotropy found in inflammatory (gadolinium enhancing) lesions.[28] In addition, DWI has been used to visualize the degree and distribution of white matter tract lesions in a variety of disease states including tumours, trauma and stroke. It also has potential applications in the investigation of cerebral tumours.

In patients with epidermoid tumours of the posterior fossa DWI allows confident demonstration of the tumour which can be isointense to CSF on all conventional MR sequences. The DWI characteristics of cerebral abscess are also suggested to be of diagnostic use with abscesses showing high signal on DWI images compared with benign cystic brain tumours which appear hypointense.[29] More excitingly changes in ADC observed after tumour therapy in both human and animal models appear to correlate closely with histological changes taking place within the tumour. Chenevert et al.[30] used diffusion measurements in an animal tumour model undergoing treatment and showed a strong increase in ADC prior to tumour regression. The use of DWI may therefore provide a useful adjunct to monitoring radio and chemotherapy in cerebral malignancy.

MAGNETIC RESONANCE SPECTROSCOPY

Introduction and historical perspective

The frequency of the MR signal is used in imaging to encode *spatial* information via the application of magnetic field gradients, but in magnetic resonance spectroscopy (MRS), it is used to encode *chemical* information. This use stems from the fact that atomic nuclei in different chemical environments resonate at slightly different frequencies, such that, for example, the hydrogen nuclei (protons) in water resonate at a different frequency from those in fat. Protons in different parts of the same molecule also resonate at different frequencies, for example the CH_3 and CH protons in molecules such as lactate and alanine. This chemical specificity of MRS has led to its ubiquitous application in chemistry laboratories – no chemical compound is synthesized or natural product isolated without an MR spectrum being recorded.

Applications in chemistry and biochemistry have been developing continually since the mid-1960s, with the first studies of intact biological systems taking place in the early 1970s. The first human spectra were published in 1981 a few years after the first human images (1976–1977), but at about the same time as clinical evaluation of MRI started. Since then the growth in the use of MRI has far outpaced that of spectroscopy, and the penetration of MRS into routine clinical practice has been minimal. This situation may be about to change as a result of technical improvements and software development within the industry.

Initially human MRS was the preserve of a few well-funded research centres, dedicated to performing spectroscopy with specialized instruments. MRS required high field magnets (1.5 Tesla or greater), with excellent field homogeneity and well controlled eddy currents; requirements which were neither met nor necessary for diagnostic imaging in the 1980s and early 1990s. However, these requirements are needed for the fast imaging techniques, such as EPI which are finding increasing use in neuroradiology. As a result, virtually all modern 1.5T scanners are, at least in principle, technically capable of performing spectroscopy. At the same time, the major manufacturers have made carrying out spectroscopy examinations both easier and quicker. Many of the set-up procedures, such as homogeneity

(a)

(b)

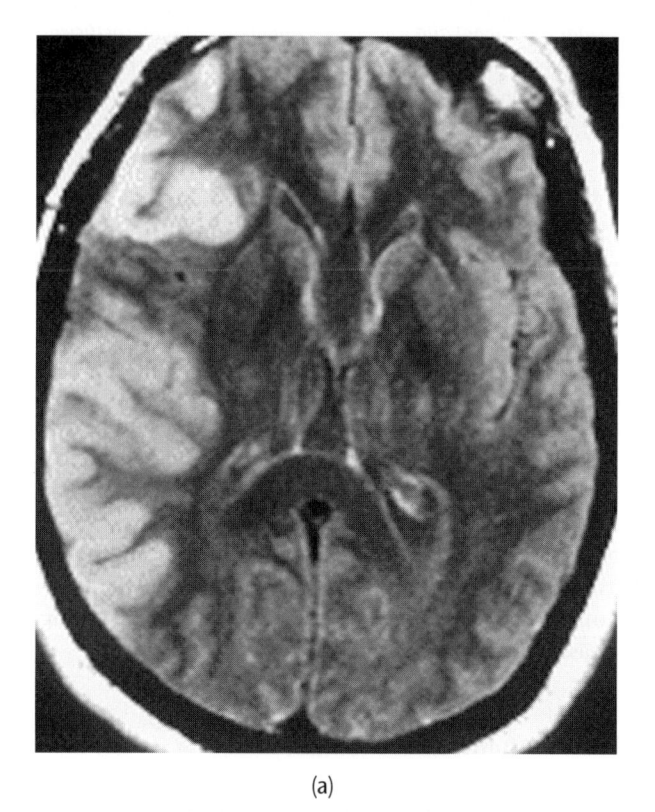

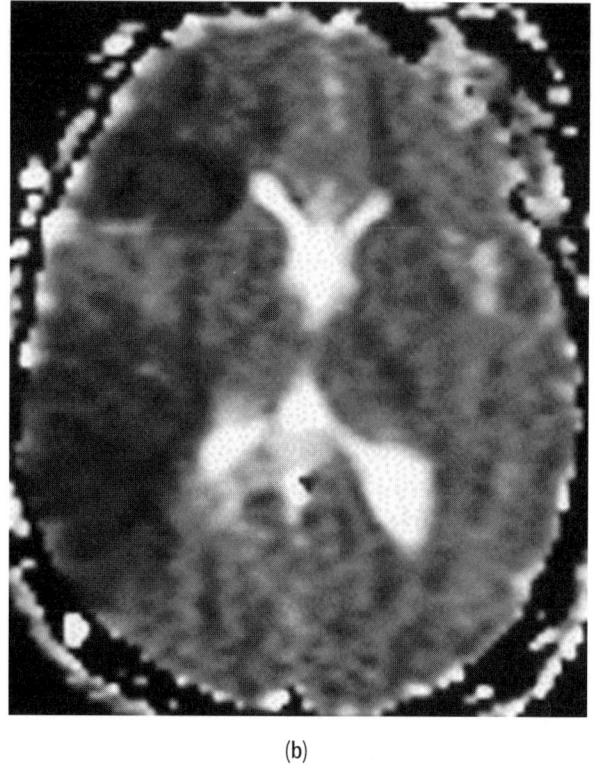

Figure 10.5 *Right-sided middle cerebral artery stroke imaged 3 hours after onset. (a) Fast FLAIR image demonstrates extensive signal abnormality in the distribution of the middle cerebral artery. (b) Apparent diffusion coefficient (ADC) image shows extensive areas of decreased ADC in the distribution of the stroke.*

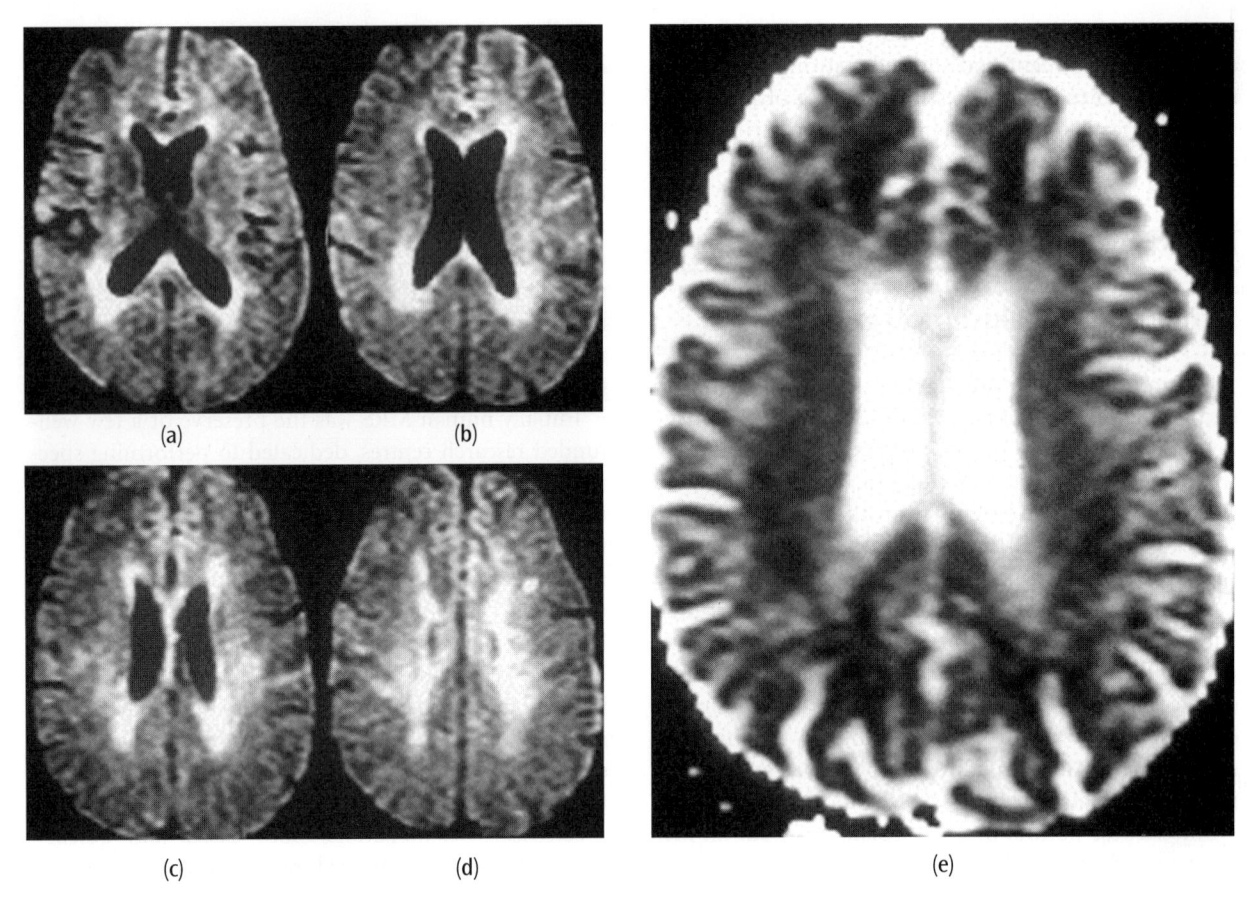

Figure 10.6 *Diffusion weighted images in a patient with multiple sclerosis. Images (a)–(d) show the primary images acquired with a combination of diffusion and T2-weighting. Note the extensive periventricular high signal abnormality. (e) Apparent diffusion coefficient image calculated using the data in image (b) together with two other diffusion weighted images at the same level. Note the high diffusion coefficient in CSF and the areas of high diffusion coefficient lesions in the immediate periventricular region. Comparing the image with Colour plate 12 it is clear that the extent of abnormality demonstrated by diffusion weighted imaging is less extensive than that seen on the primary images from which the ADC is calculated.*

adjustment (*shimming*), coil tuning, water suppression and gradient trimming, which used to be performed manually, requiring both skill and experience and taking several minutes, are now carried out automatically. Improvements in acquisition techniques enable either good quality single voxel spectra from relatively small volumes (<10 ml) to be acquired in a few minutes, or spectroscopic images of brain slabs to be acquired in 10–20 minutes (providing better spatial resolution with wider brain coverage). As a result a spectroscopy examination need not always be a dedicated study, but can be performed after an imaging protocol. The processing, quantification and display of spectroscopic data has also become more accessible in the late 1990s, and the application of sophisticated computational methods is reducing the amount of manual input required for reliable data processing.

As a result, at the turn of the century the opportunities for MRS to have a clinical impact are greater than before, and the purpose of this section is to give an overview of the information available from spectroscopy and give specific examples of its clinical utility. Our intention is not to crystal-ball gaze and predict what MRS may do in 2005 or 2010, but rather to look at applications in the late 1990s and give a practising neuroradiologist sufficient knowledge to determine whether MRS may be useful in clinical practice now or in the near future. We only discuss proton (^{1}H) spectroscopy, since the use of other nuclei (carbon, phosphorus, nitrogen) is likely to remain a research activity, both for reasons of lower MR sensitivity and the additional hardware requirements for performing measurements on these nuclei.

What can MRS measure?

In comparison to most other techniques of chemical or biochemical analysis, such as infrared or ultraviolet spectroscopy, chromatography, mass spectrometry, microelectrodes etc, MRS is relatively insensitive: in living tissue it can only detect compounds at concentrations of about 1 mmol/litre or greater, compared with micro- nano- or pico-mol/litre for other methods. However, its ability to see well-defined regions deep within tissue and its specificity in identifying separate biochemical compounds means it is the only technique able to measure important brain metabolites completely non-invasively. Figure 10.7 a,b as shows an example of a human brain ¹H spectrum, illustrating the compounds which can be detected. In the remainder of this section their significance to brain function and medicine is considered.

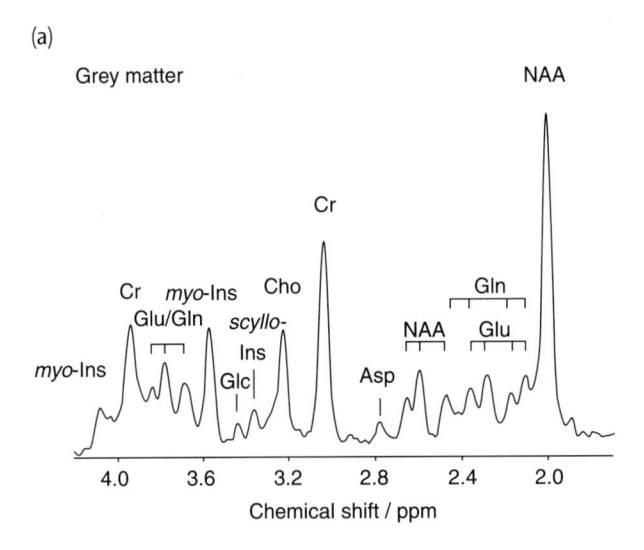

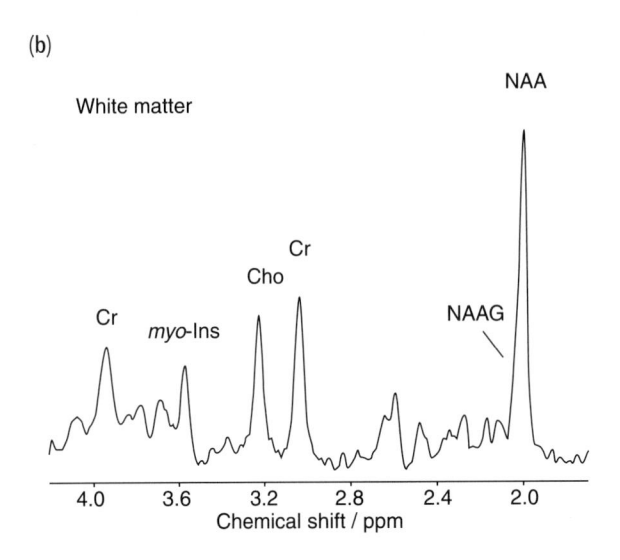

Figure 10.7 *Short echo time STEAM spectra from human brain. ¹H spectra are shown from the grey matter (18 ml volume) and white matter (12 ml) of a young healthy adult. Each acquisition took 6.4 min (TR/TE/Nex 6000/20/64). Metabolites are assigned as – NAA: N-acetylaspartate; NAAG: N-acetylaspartylglutamate; Glu: glutamate; Gln: glutamine; Asp: aspartate; Cr: creatine plus phosphocreatine; Cho: choline containing compounds; Ins: inositol; Glc: glucose. (Reproduced with permission from Ref. 38.)*

N-ACETYLASPARTATE, CREATINE AND CHOLINE-CONTAINI]NG COMPOPUNDS

These three resonances are the most intense signals in a normal brain spectrum, and the only ones usually detected in long echo time (TE>120 ms) spectra. N-Acetylaspartate (NAA) is present predominantly in neurons, and has assumed considerable importance as a marker of neuronal loss or dysfunction. It is, for example, reduced or absent in most brain tumours, in multiple sclerosis lesions and in stroke infarcts. Initially, loss of NAA was assumed to be irreversible and therefore to be associated with loss of neuronal cells. However, there is now good evidence from studies of multiple sclerosis and mitochondrial disorders (MELAS), that decreases in NAA can be reversed.[31] Taken together with biochemical evidence that NAA is synthesized in mitochondria, and that its synthesis is disrupted in damaged mitochondria, a loss of NAA can be considered as evidence of disturbed energy metabolism in neurons.

An example of the clinical utility of NAA measurements is provided by its use in several centres worldwide in aiding planning for epilepsy surgery. In patients with refractory temporal lobe epilepsy selected for partial resection, accurate lateralization of the seizure focus is essential. For example, in the epilepsy surgery programme carried out at Great Ormond Street Hospital for Children in London, bilateral measurements of NAA are routinely used as part of surgical planning.[32] The MRS measurements are taken from an 8ml volume in the temporal lobe which includes the hippocampus, but is considerably larger than it. Nevertheless in the majority of cases NAA is reduced ipsilateral to the seizure focus, suggesting that there is diffuse damage to tissue surrounding the focus, and that biochemical abnormalities are present in tissue which appears normal on imaging. In other cases there is evidence of a bilateral reduction in NAA, providing evidence for neurochemical dysfunction contralateral to the seizure focus. In those cases in which all the non-invasive assessments of seizure lateralization are concordant (surface EEG, volumetric and relaxometric MRI, MRS), the surgeon will not usually require invasive measurements to confirm the side of the focus. An example of the spectra recorded in such studies is given in Fig. 10.8a,b,c.

The creatine signal is the sum of signals from both creatine and phosphocreatine. Although these are important energy metabolites, involved in maintaining ATP during acute hypoxic/ischaemic events and in facilitating transport of ATP equivalents within the cytosol, the ¹H resonance does not change acutely during disruptions to energy metabolism, since total creatine remains unaltered. The creatine signal is most often used as a reference to calculate metabolite ratios such as NAA/creatine or choline/creatine. These ratios have been shown to change in a number of diseases, but the use of ratios, although valuable in certain circumstances can be misleading.

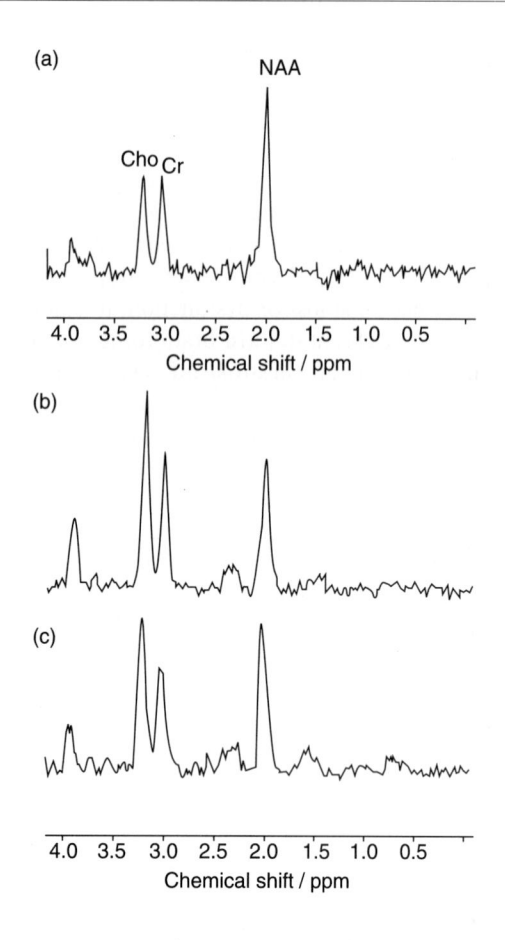

Figure 10.8 ¹H Spectra in temporal lobe epilepsy in children. (a) A long echo time (TR/TE/Nex 1660/135/128) PRESS spectrum from an 8 ml volume in the temporal lobe of a normal control. N-acetylaspartate (NAA), creatine/phosphocreatine (Cr) and choline containing compounds (Cho) are the only metabolites detected under these conditions. The ratio NAA/(Cr + Cho) is 0.91. In (b) and (c) spectra from the right (b) and left (c) temporal lobes of an age-matched child with a clinical right temporal epilepsy focus are shown. The ratio NAA/(Cr + Cho) is 0.44 on the right (focus) and 0.52 on the left. This case is an example of bilateral biochemical abnormality, though the severity of the abnormality provides confirmation of lateralization. (Reproduced with permission from Ref. 32.)

The signal assigned to choline-containing compounds (Cho) consists mainly of resonances from glycerophosphocholine and phosphocholine, which are metabolites involved in pathways of membrane synthesis and degradation. Minor contributions to the Cho resonance at 3.20–3.22 ppm come from choline itself and phosphoethanolamine, which are also membrane-related metabolites. The Cho signal is elevated in brain tumours, and has proved to be reliable marker of tumour mass. Spectroscopic imaging of brain tumour patients promises to be of particular value in identifying viable areas within tumours in order to guide biopsy. In a conventional tumour image it is difficult to distinguish peritumour oedema, from necrotic regions, and actively metabolizing regions. However, a metabolite map, constructed from a spectroscopic imaging data set allows this to be done. Oedema will be essentially free of metabolites, with the exception of low levels of lactate which may have diffused out of cells. Necrotic cells are also characterized by high lactate, whereas the viable cancer cells are distinguished by high Cho, and this is the area which should be biopsied (see Colour plate 12).

Another potentially important application of spectroscopy in cancer diagnosis, lies in the use of computer-based statistical methods to automatically interpret spectral patterns and assign the spectra to tumour type and grade. Following work from a number of groups worldwide on the application of pattern recognition, neural networks and discriminant analysis to cancer NMR spectra (both *in vitro* and *in vivo*, in animals and in man), the feasibility of this approach has been demonstrated.[33] Further developments to remove the need for an experienced spectroscopist in the data processing stage will be necessary if these methods are to achieve wider clinical utility.

LACTATE

As the end-product of anaerobic glycolysis, lactate is elevated acutely following hypoxia/ischaemia and has been used extensively in experimental studies as an early marker of acute stroke. However, this is less valuable in a clinical context, since stroke is rarely studied within 1–2 hours of onset, and in any event DWI can provide essentially the same information (regions of energy failure) with better temporal and spatial resolution. The value of metabolite measurements in acute stroke, particularly NAA and lactate, may lie in refining prognostic indicators of clinical outcome, but there is conflicting evidence on this issue.[34,35]

GLUTAMATE, GLUTAMINE, OTHER AMINO ACIDS

Glutamate is the most concentrated organic molecule in the brain (10–15 mmol/litre), but because of its complex NMR spectrum, it is not detectable at long echo times (TE>120 ms). The signal from glutamate is distributed amongst a large number of resonances effectively diluting its intensity, and in addition signal cancellation occurs as the echo time is prolonged. However, the use of short echo times (30 ms >TE) has allowed glutamate and glutamine to be studied in a number of diseases. For example, chronic hepatic encephalopathy has been shown by ¹H MRS to be associated with increased glutamine and decreased *myo*-inositol in the brain.[36] The spectroscopic measurements correlate well with clinical measures of severity, and may provide good markers of disease progression/treatment. Detection of other amino acids, such as γ-aminobutyrate (GABA), alanine or aspartate is less straightforward, by virtue of their low concentration and/or overlap with other more intense resonances. Nevertheless MRS has been used to measure GABA in the brains of epilepsy patients undergoing treatment with GABA-raising drugs.[36] These studies raise the possibility of using MRS measurements in pharmacology in a variety of ways including *in vivo* pharmacokinetics, dose ranging studies and dose targetting in individual patients.

GLUCOSE AND INOSITOL

Short echo time spectroscopy enables detection of signals from glucose, *myo*-inositol and *scyllo*-inositol. *Myo*-inositol is often considered as a glial marker, though the evidence to support this is less strong than that which suggests NAA is a neuronal marker. However, it does appear to be an important indicator of osmotic stress in brain cells, and its decrease in hepatic encephalopathy is thought to reflect an osmotic disturbance in glial cells. It has been proposed that measurements of *myo*-inositol by MRS may be useful in monitoring therapy in osmotically stressed patients, in which the treatment must be finely judged in order to be effective without being damaging. The importance of glucose to brain function needs no explanation, but whether the ability to measure brain glucose non-invasively will have any impact on patient management is less clear.

High field magnets

The development of MR in all research areas, from analytical chemistry, through biochemistry to MRI has always been to higher field magnets. At the beginning of the 1990s protein chemists aspired to 500 MHz magnets operating at 11.7 Tesla, now they are looking to 23 Tesla. In MRI 1.5 Tesla is considered 'high field', but there are a number of human imaging systems now at 3 and 4 Tesla. These very high field systems bring considerable benefits to spectroscopy in terms of increased signal-to-noise and spectroscopic resolution. These benefits are now being realized through an understanding of some of the particular problems associated with high field MR in humans.[37] However, it is not clear that the increased cost of these systems, when interfaced to a standard console from one of the major manufacturers, will bring sufficient benefits to normal diagnostic imaging to warrant their installation outside major research centres. As such, the impact of high field MRS on radiological practice will be limited.

Concluding remarks

In the early 1980s, MRI was sometimes considered a threat to the traditional role of radiologists – indeed it was joked that NMR was an acronym for 'No More Radiologists', and that the technical skills required to carry out and perform MR exams would remain the preserve of medical physicists. In fact, the converse is nearer to the truth, and the almost complete penetration of MRI into clinical practice has come about because each successive generation of instruments has integrated new MR methods into a readily accessible package, so that the latest research methods are available for the widest possible patient population. If spectroscopy is also to become more than a research tool, then similar developments must take place, so that a clinician can be confident of getting reliable, quantifiable information routinely from an MRS examination, without having to call on the help of experts to carry out every study. As a result of the advances described in this chapter, spectroscopy may now be in a position to be more routinely exploited in neuroradiology.

REFERENCES

1 Hagen T, Bertyla K, Piepgrass U. Correlation of regional cerebral blood flow measurements by stable Xenon CT and perfusion MRI. *J Comput Assist Tomogr* 1999; **23**: 257–64.
2 Rempp KA, Brix G, Wenz F, Becker CR, Guckel F, Lorenz WJ. Quantification of regional cerebral blood flow and volume with dynamic susceptibility contrast-enhanced MR imaging. *Radiology* 1994; **193**: 637–41.
3 Rosen BR, Belliveau JW, Vevea JM, Brady TJ. Perfusion imaging with NMR contrast agents. *Magn Reson Med* 1990; **14**: 249–65.
4 Boxerman JL, Rosen BR, Weisskoff RM. Signal-to-noise analysis of cerebral blood volume maps from dynamic NMR imaging studies. *J Magn Reson Imag* 1997; **7**: 528–37.
5 Lui G, Sobering G, Duyn J, Moonen C. A functional MRI technique combining principles of echo-shifting with a train of observations (PRESTO). *Magn Reson Med* 1993; **30**: 764–8.
6 Ostergaard L, Sorensen AG, Kwong KK, Weisskoff RM, Gyldensted C, Rosen BR. High resolution measurement of cerebral blood flow using intravascular tracer bolus passages. Part II: Experimental comparison and preliminary results. *Magn Reson Med* 1996; **36**: 726–36.
7 Hunter G, Hamberg L, Ponzo J, Huang-Hellinger R, Morris P *et al.* Assessment of cerebral perfusion and arterial anatomy in hyperacute stroke with three-dimensional functional CT: Early clinical results. *Am J Neuroradiol* 1998; **19**: 29–37.
8 Patel MR, Siewert B, Warach S, Edelman RR. Diffusion and perfusion imaging techniques. *Magn Reson Imag Clin N Amer* 1995; **3**: 425–38.
9 Kluytmans M, van der Grond J, Klijn CJM. Measurement of hemodynamic changes in patients with severe carotid lesions: A clinical perfusion weighted imaging study. In: *5th Scientific Meeting of the International Society for Magnetic Resonance in Medicine.* Vancouver, Canada, 1997.
10 Barber PA, Darby DG, Desmond PM, Yang Q, Gerraty RP *et al.* Prediction of stroke outcome with echoplanar perfusion- and diffusion-weighted MRI. *Neurology* 1998; **51**: 418–26.

11 Aronen HJ, Glass J, Pardo FS, Belliveau JW, Gruber ML et al. Echo-planar MR cerebral blood volume mapping of gliomas. Clinical utility. *Acta Radiol* 1995; **36**: 520–8.

12 Amoroso A, Del Porto F, Di Monaco C, Manfredini P, Afeltra A. Vascular endothelial growth factor: a key mediator of neoangiogenesis. A review. *Eur Rev Med Pharmacol Sci* 1997; **1**: 17–25.

13 Goldman GK, Bharara S, Palmer CA, Vitek J, Tsai JC et al. Brain edema in meningiomas is associated with increased vascular endothelial growth factor expression. *Neurosurgery* 1997; **40**: 1269–77.

14 Jensen RL. Growth factor-mediated angiogenesis in the malignant progression of glial tumors: a review. *Surg Neurol* 1998; **49**: 189–95.

15 Brix G, Semmler W, Port R, Schad L, Layer G, Lorentz W. Pharmacokinetic parameters in CNS Gd-DTPA enhanced MR imaging. *J Comput Assist Tomog* 1991; **15**: 621–8.

16 Tofts P, Berkowitz B, Schnall M. Quantitative analysis of dynamic Gd-DTPA enhancement in breast tumours using a permeability model. *Magn Reson Med* 1995; **33**: 564–8.

17 Larsson H, Stubgaard M, Frederiksen J, Jensen M, Henriksen O, Paulson O. Quantitation of blood-brain carrier defect by magnetic resonance imaging and gadolinium-DTPA in patients with multiple sclerosis and brain tumors. *Magn Reson Med* 1990; **16**: 7–13.

18 Hanyu H, Imor Y, Sakurai H, Iwamoto T, Takasaki M, Shindo H, and K. Abe, Diffusion-weighted magnetic resonance and magnetization transfer imaging in the assessment of ischemic human stroke. *Intern Med* 1998; **37**: 360–5.

19 Kurki T, Lundbom N, Valtonen S. Tissue characterisation of intracranial tumours: the value of magnetisation transfer and conventional MRI. *Neuroradiology* 1995; **37**: 515–21.

20 Taylor-Robinson SD, Oatridge A, Hajnal JV, Burroughs AK, McIntyre N, deSouza NM. MR imaging of the basal ganglia in chronic liver disease: correlation of T1-weighted and magnetisation transfer contrast measurements with liver dysfunction and neuropsychiatric status. *Metab Brain Dis* 1995; **10**: 175–88.

21 Werring DJ, Clark CA, Parker GJ, Miller DH, Thompson AJ, Barker GJ. A direct demonstration of both structure and function in the visual system: combining diffusion tensor imaging with functional magnetic resonance imaging. *Neuroimage* 1999; **9**: 352–61.

22 Schlaug G, Siewert B, Benfield A, Edelman RR, Warach S. Time course of the apparent diffusion coefficient (ADC) abnormality in human stroke. *Neurology* 1997; **49**: 113–9.

23 Geijer B, Brockstedt S, Lindgren A, Stahlberg F, Norrving B, Holtas S. Radiological diagnosis of acute stroke. Comparison of conventional MR imaging, echo-planar diffusion-weighted imaging, and spin-echo diffusion-weighted imaging. *Acta Radiol* 1999; **40**: 255–62.

24 Fitzek C, Tintera J, Muller-Forell W, Urban P, Thomke F et al. Differentiation of a recent and old cerebral infarcts by diffusion-weighted MRI. *Neuroradiology* 1998; **40**: 778–82.

25 Lovblad KO, Baird AE, Schlaug G, Benfield A, Siewert B et al. Ischemic lesion volumes in acute stroke by diffusion-weighted magnetic resonance imaging correlate with clinical outcome. *Ann Neurol* 1997; **42**: 164–70.

26 Berry I, Ranjeva JP, Duthil P, Manelfe C. Diffusion and perfusion MRI, measurements of acute stroke events and outcome: present practice and future hope. *Cerebrovasc Dis* 1998; **8** (Suppl 2): 8–16.

27 Neil JJ, Shiran SI, McKinstry RC, Schefft GL, Snyder AZ et al. Normal brain in human newborns: apparent diffusion coefficient and diffusion anisotropy measured by using diffusion tensor MR imaging. *Radiology* 1998; **209**: 57–66.

28 Werring DJ, Clark CA, Barker GJ, Thompson AJ, Miller DH. Diffusion tensor imaging of lesions and normal-appearing white matter in multiple sclerosis. *Neurology* 1999; **52**: 1626–32.

29 Kim YJ, Chang KH, Song IC, Kim HD, Seong SO et al. Brian abscess and necrotic or cystic brain tumor: discrimination with signal intensity on diffusion-weighted MR imaging. *Am J Roentgenol* 1998; **171**: 1487–90.

30 Chenevert TL, McKeever PE, Ross BD. Monitoring early response of experimental brain tumors to therapy using diffusion magnetic resonance imaging. *Clin Cancer Res* 1997; **3**: 1457–66.

31 De Stefano N, Matthews PM, Arnold DL. Reversible decreases in N acetylaspartate after acute brain injury. *Magn Reson Med* 1995; **34**: 721–7.

32 Cross JH, Connelly A, Jackson GD, Johnson CL, Neville BR, Gadian DG. Proton magnetic resonance spectroscopy in children with temporal lobe epilepsy. *Ann Neurol* 1996; **39**: 107–13.

33 Various Authors. Reviews of applications of pattern recognition methods in the analysis and classification of tumour NMR spectra. *NMR Biomed* 1998; **11**: 148–234.

34 Wardlaw JM, Marshall I, Wild J, Dennis MS, Cannon J, Lewis SC. Studies of acute ischemic stroke with proton magnetic resonance spectroscopy: relation between time from onset, neurological deficit, metabolite abnormalities in the infarct, blood flow, and clinical outcome. *Stroke* 1998; **29**: 1618–24.

35 Gillard JH, Barker PB, van Zijl PC, Bryan RN, Oppenheimer SM. Proton MR spectroscopy in acute middle cerebral artery stroke. *Am J Neuroradiol* 1996; **17**: 873–86.

36 Williams SR. Cerebral amino acids studied by nuclear magnetic resonance spectroscopy *in vivo*. *Prog Nuclear Mag Res Spectrosc* 1999; **34**: 301–26.

37 Hetherington HP, Pan JW, Chu WJ, Mason GF, Newcomer BR. Biological and clinical MRS at ultra-high field. *NMR Biomed* 1997; **10**: 360–71.

38 Frahm J, Hanefeld F. Localized proton magnetic resonance spectroscopy of cerebral metabolites. *Neuropaediatrics* 1996; **27**: 64–9.

Colour plates

Plates 1 and 2
also appear in Chapter 2 in black and white as Figures 2.5 and 2.32

Plates 3–12
are discussed in Chapter 10

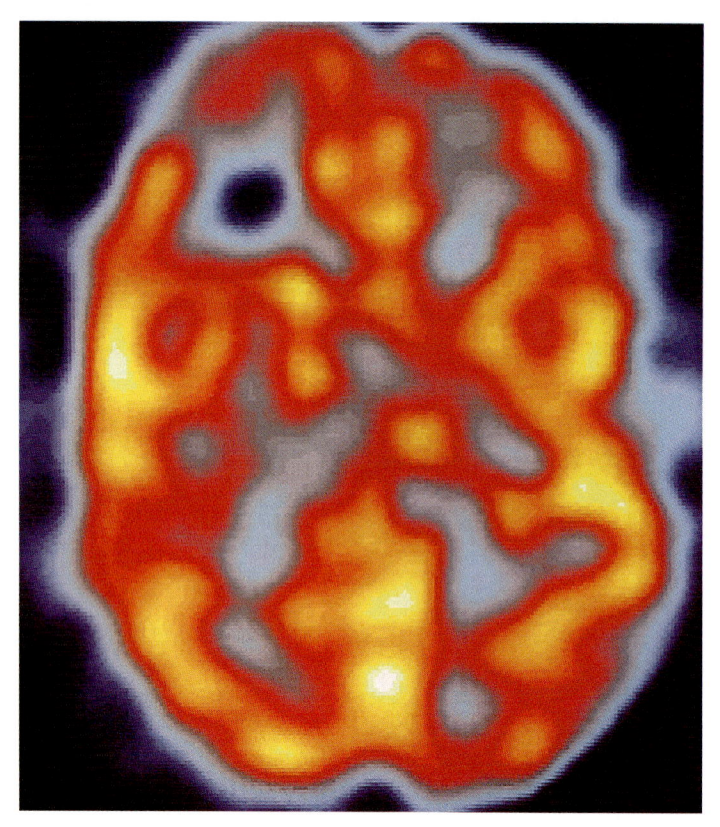

Plate 1 (Figure 2.5) *SPECT in the early subacute stage of a head-injured 35-year-old man shows hypoperfusion adjacent to a right frontal contusion but also shows unexpected hypoperfusion of the left frontal lobe where there was no evidence of injury on CT.*

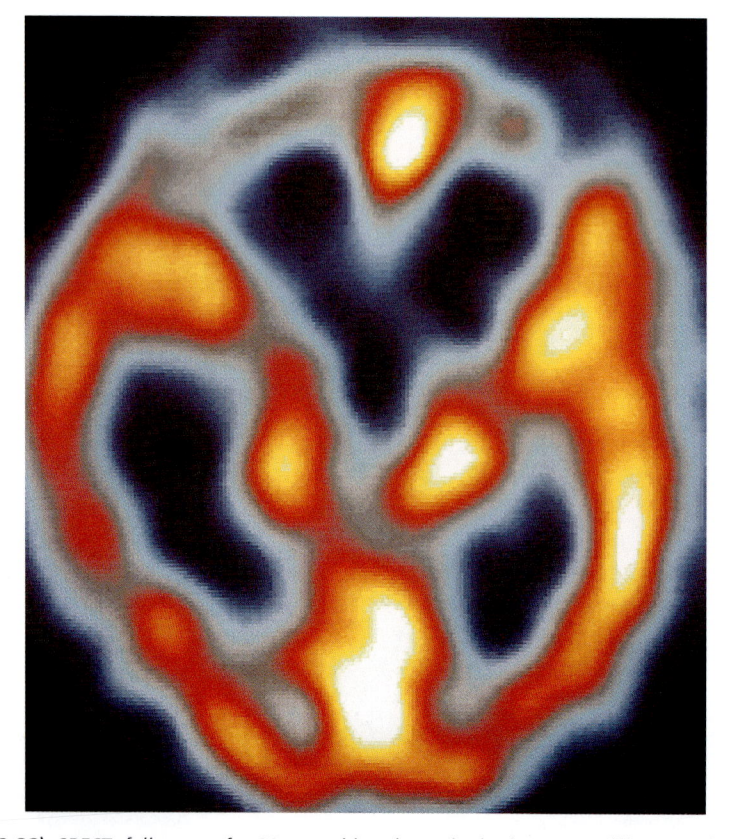

Plate 2 (Figure 2.32) *SPECT: follow-up of a 28-year-old patient who had a severe diffuse axonial injury. Perfusion pattern shows markedly reduced functioning cortex with a pattern consistent with diffuse atrophy.*

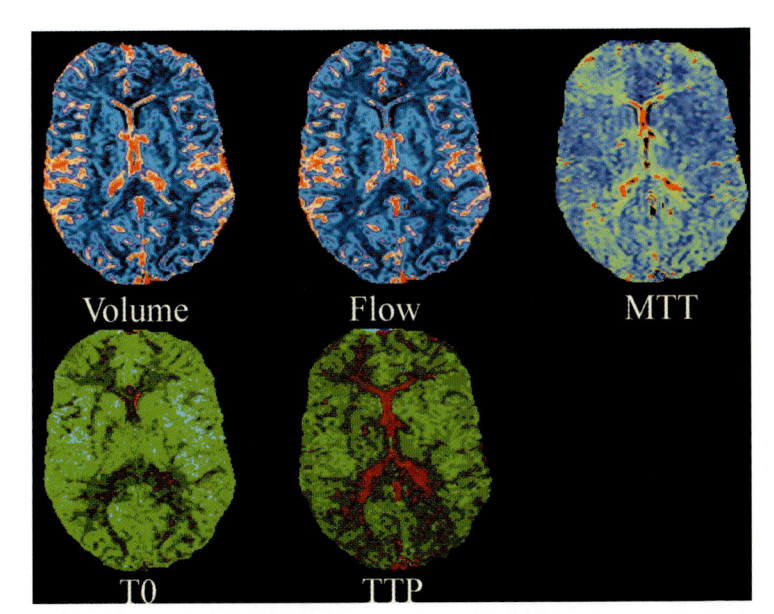

Plate 3 *Parametric imaging of perfusion-related haemodynamic variables calculated from dynamic susceptibility contrast-enhanced MRI. Images show relative cerebral blood volume (Volume); relative cerebral blood flow (Flow); mean transit time (MTT); time to contrast arrival (T0); and time to peak concentration (TTP). The distribution of cerebral blood volume and cerebral blood flow shows clear anatomical demarcations. MTT, T0 and TTP maps all show slight prolongation in the anterior and posterior cerebral watersheds.*

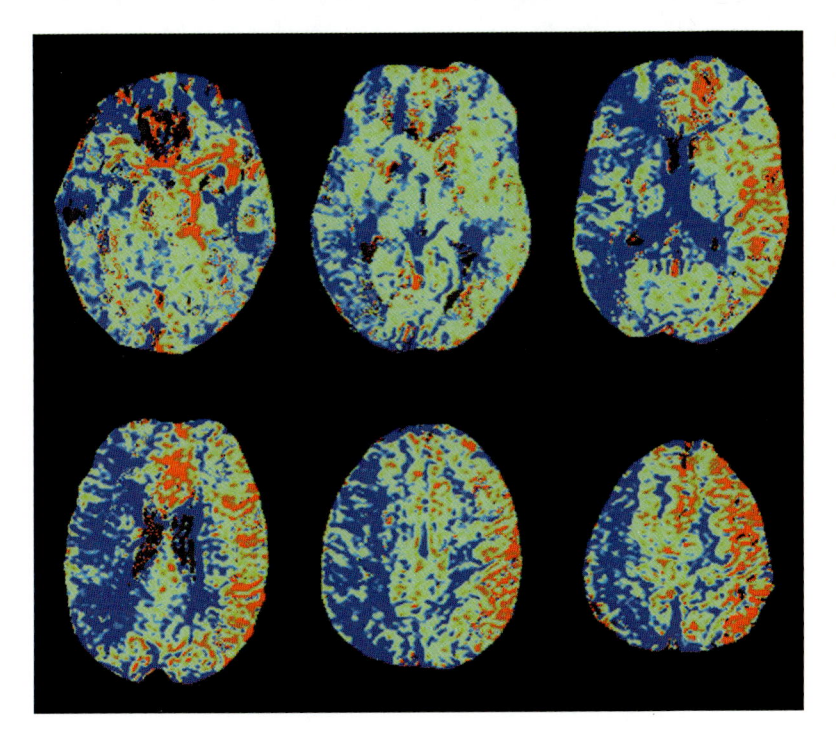

Plate 4 *Time to peak concentration (TTP) maps from dynamic susceptibility contrast-enhanced imaging in a patient with severe right-sided carotid stenosis. The images show marked asymmetry with prolongation of TTP in the distribution of the right middle cerebral artery and its watershed zones. The changes are most marked in the areas of the watershed and deep white matter.*

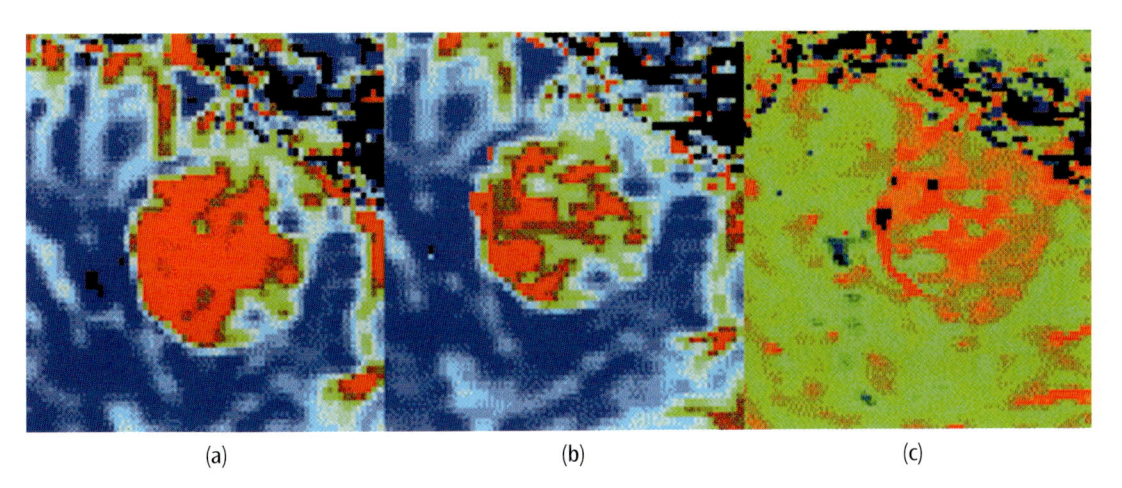

Plate 5 *Parametric image of (a) relative cerebral blood volume, (b) relative cerebral blood flow, and (c) mean transit time in an acoustic neuroma showing the high vascularity and uneven distribution and speed flow.*

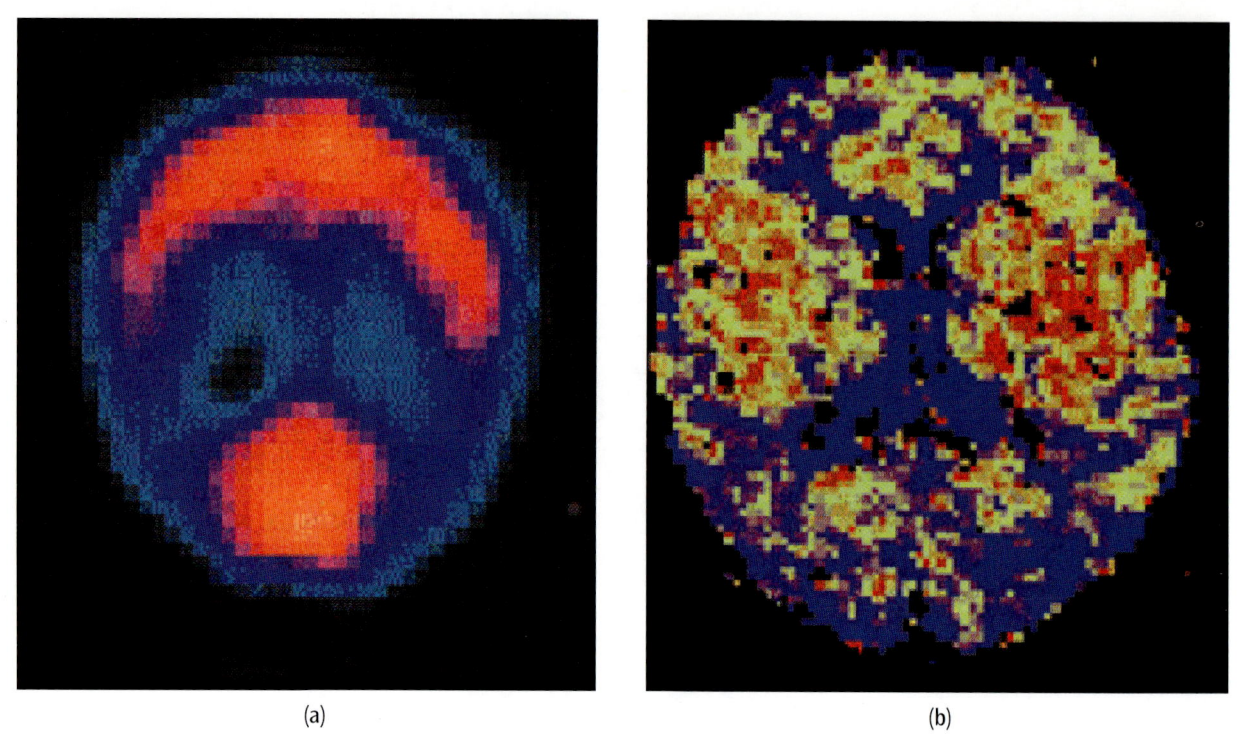

Plate 6 Images from a patient with Alzheimer's disease. (a) ^{99m}Tc HMPAO SPECT image in the axial plane demonstrates bilateral parietal areas of underperfusion. (b) Time to peak concentration (TTP) map from dynamic susceptibility contrast-enhanced imaging sequence shows corresponding areas of prolonged TTP in the posterior parietal and occipital cortices.

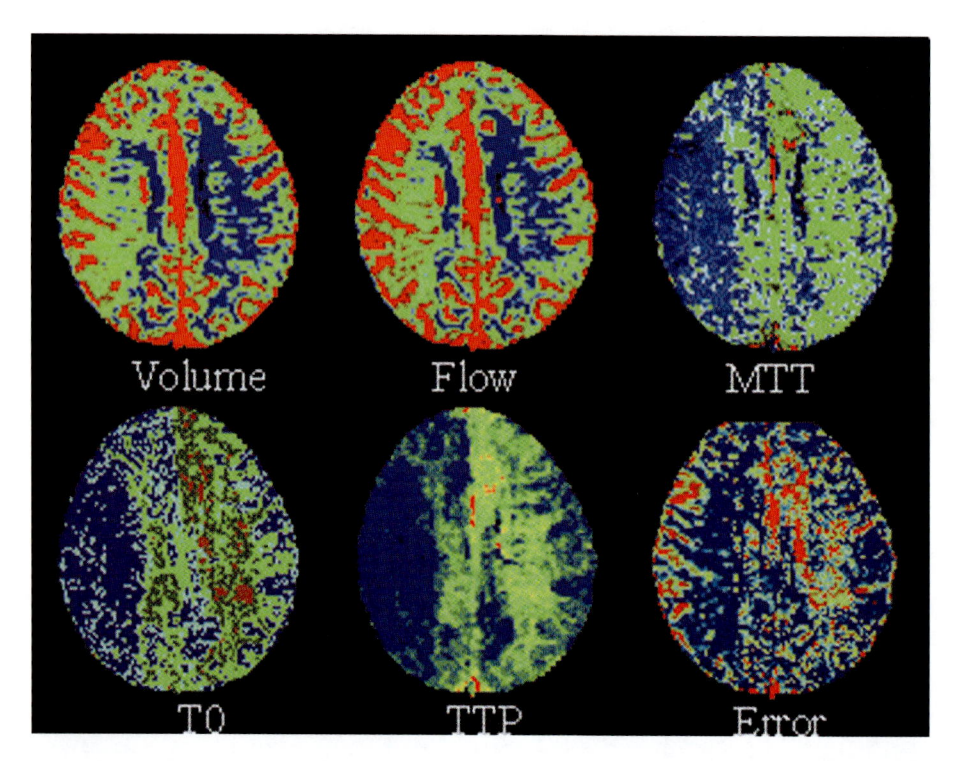

Plate 7 Perfusion images from a patient with right-sided hyperperfusion syndrome, 24 hours after carotid endarterectomy. Note the increase in relative cerebral blood volume (Volume), relative cerebral blood flow (Flow) and the decrease in mean transit time (MTT), time to contrast arrival (T0) and time to peak concentration (TTP) associated with rapid passage of increased volumes of blood through the middle and anterior cerebral artery territories.

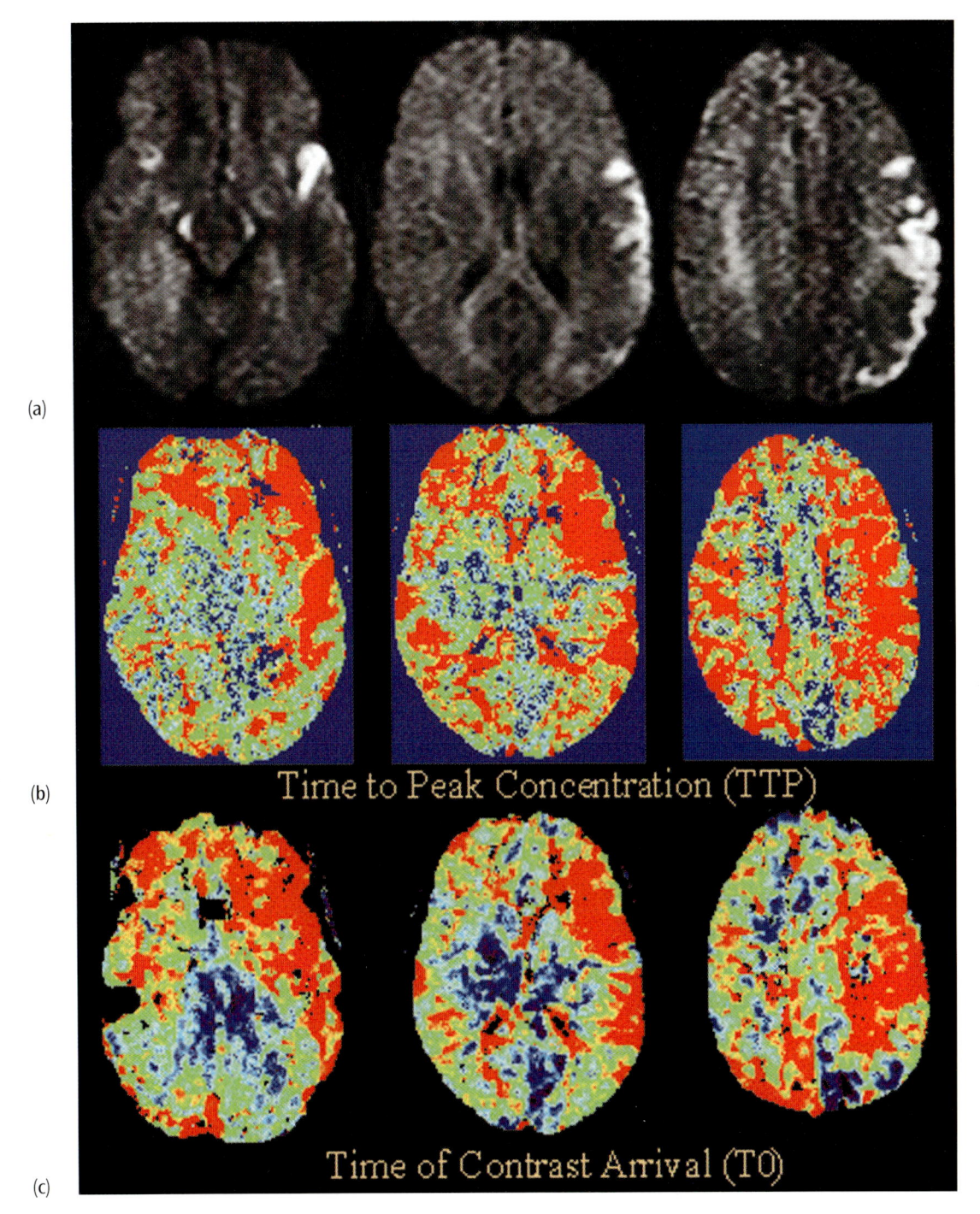

Plate 8 *(a) Diffusion weighted images in a patient with moyamoya syndrome showing extensive left-sided cortical infarction (high signal). (b) Parametric image of TTP. (c) Parametric image of T0. Red areas in these images represent abnormally delayed contrast arrival. The images show widespread disturbance of cerebral flow affecting both hemispheres.*

(a) (b) (c)

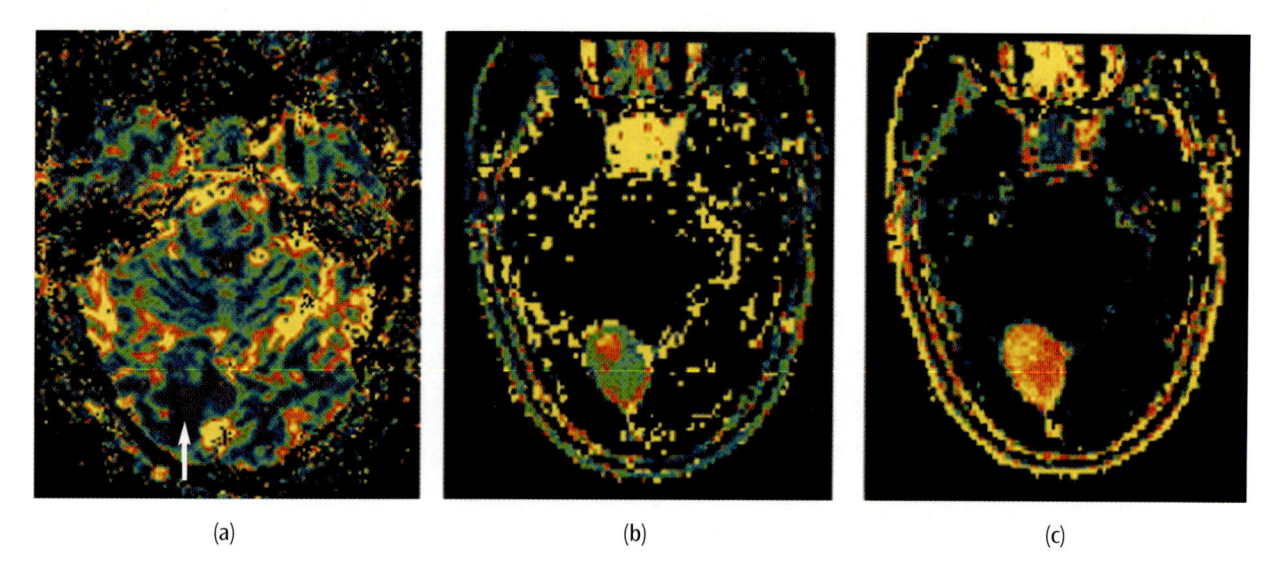

Plate 9 *Parametric images in a patient with a low-grade tentorial meningioma. (a) Cerebral blood volume map calculated from T2-weighted dynamic susceptibility contrast-enhanced imaging shows a very low cerebral blood volume within the tumour itself (arrow). (b) Map of endothelial surface area permeability product shows an area of moderately high permeability (red) in the centre of a tumour which has intermediate permeability (green). (c) Contrast distribution space shows high contrast distribution space suggesting a large extracellular fraction within the tumour.*

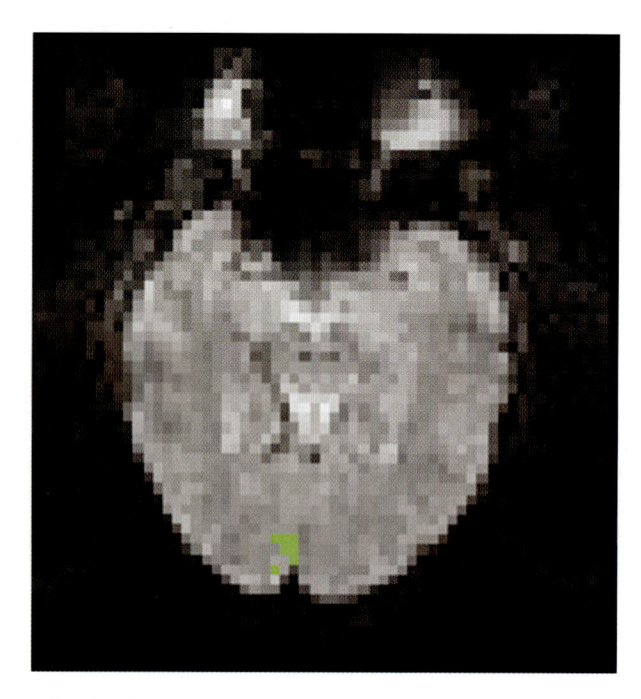

Plate 10 *Parametric map of the visual cortex response. Green areas represent voxels which show a signal change with the same time variation as the stimulus ($p<0.01$).*

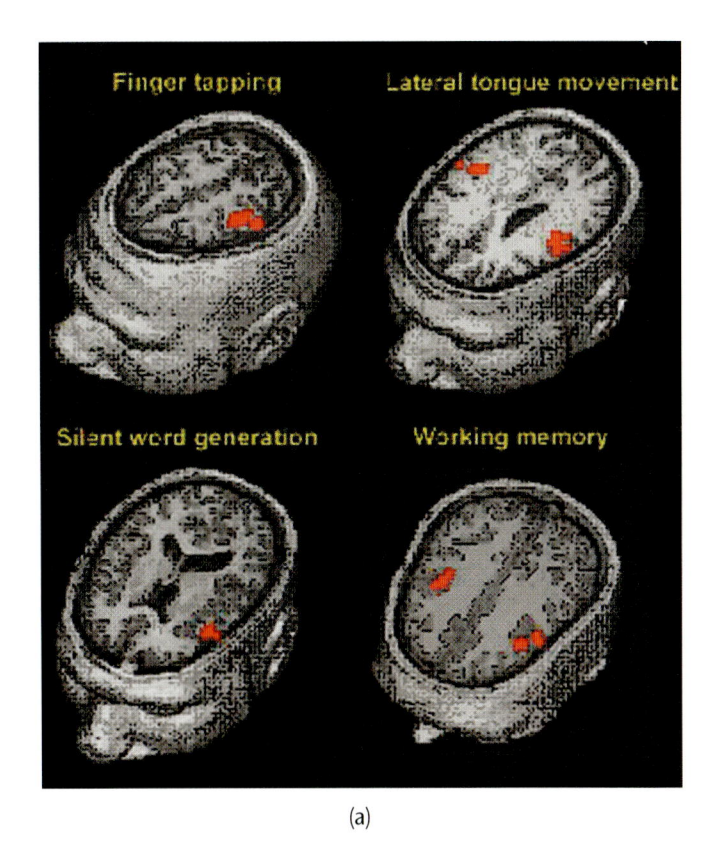

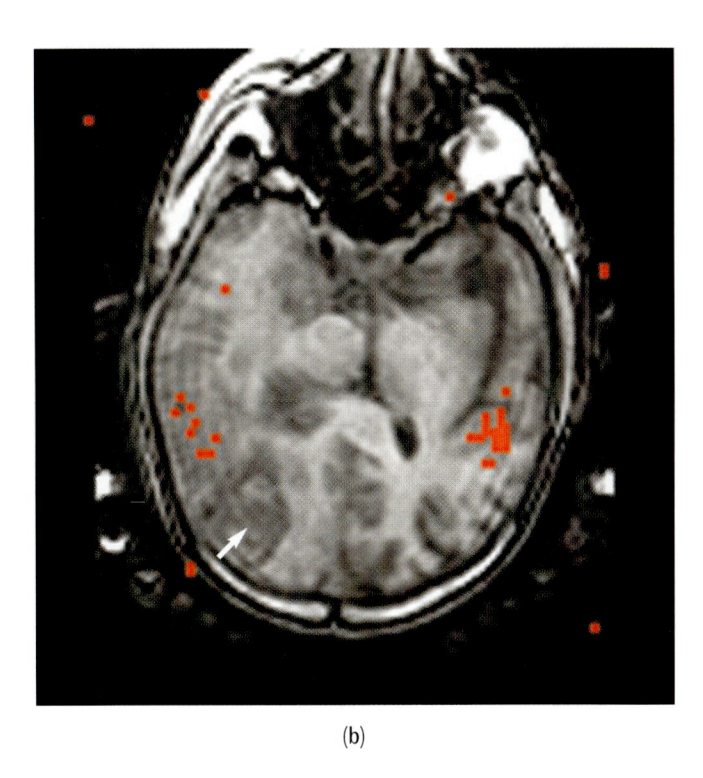

Plate 11 *(a) Three-dimensional renderings of functional imaging using the BOLD (blood oxygen level dependent) technique in a normal volunteer to demonstrate areas of eloquent cortex. (Courtesy Dr P Folkers, Philips Medical Systems.) (b) Identification of auditory cortex in a patient with a right-sided astrocytoma (arrow) prior to surgery.*

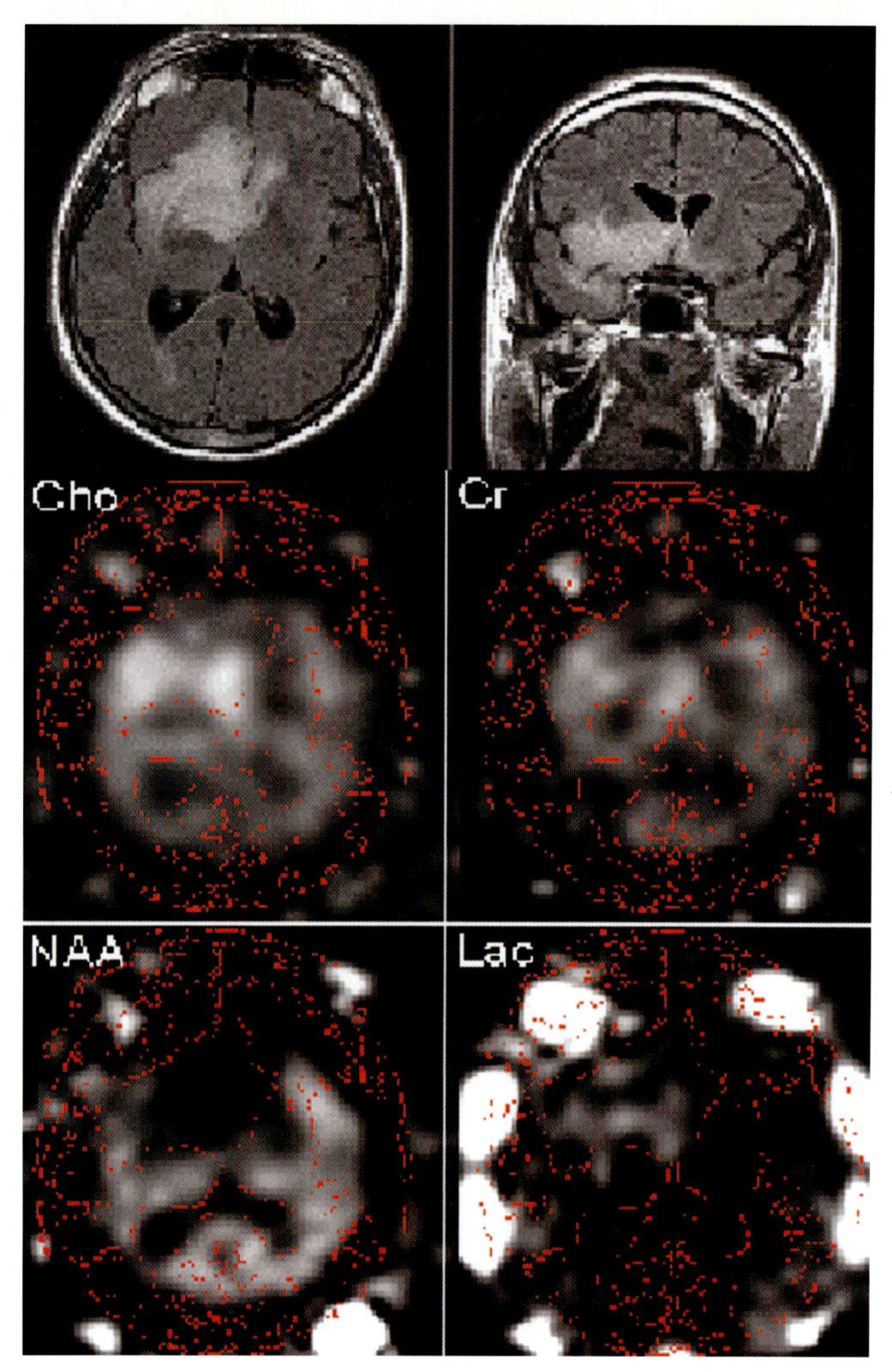

Plate 12 Spectroscopic imaging of a patient with a primary cerebral glioma. The anatomical, T1-weighted, contrast-enhanced images show the location of the tumour mass. The outline of the axial image is overlayed on the Cho (choline containing compounds), Cr (creatine plus phosphocreatine), NAA (N-acetylaspartate) and Lac (lactate) spectroscopic images. Although the tumour appears relatively homogenous on the anatomical scan, it can be seen that Cho and Cr are high within a small region towards the edge of the tumour mass. Lactate is elevated over a larger region, though the lactate image is probably contaminated by lipid, which can be seen in other peripheral regions of the brain. The elevated Cr and Cho regions correspond to active tumour mass. (Image courtesy of Philips Medical Systems UK.)

Index

Note: page numbers in **bold** refer to figures, those in *italics* refer to tables and those prefixed by CP refer to colour plate numbers. Abbreviations used in subheadings are: ADEM = acute disseminated encephalomyelitis; CT = computed tomography; MR = magnetic resonance; PML = progressive multifocal leukoencephalopathy.

abscesses **23**, 230–2, **231**, **232**
 differential diagnoses 103, 113
 diffusion weighted imaging 287
 pituitary 131, **133**
 after traumatic injury 95
N-acetylaspartate (NAA) signals CP12, 289–90, **289**, **290**
achondroplasia 273, **274**
acoustic schwannomas 33, **34**
 and hydrocephalus 271, **272**
 MR perfusion imaging CP5, **283**
 in neurofibromatosis 55, 57, **57**, 154
 perfusion imaging **284**
acquired immunodeficiency syndrome (AIDS) 108, 110, 215–22, **223**
acrocephaly 52, **54**
acute disseminated encephalomyelitis (ADEM) 113, 235–6, **235**, 258, **259**
adenomas, pituitary 32, 126–31, **129–30**, **131**, **132**
adrenoleukodystrophy *260*, 261, **262**
aesthesioneuroblastomas 110
ageing brain 26, 241–5, **242–4**
 dementia 245–8, **246–9**, *248*, 274–5
agyric lissencephaly 62, **64**
AIDS (acquired immunodeficiency syndrome) 108, 110, 212, 215–22, **223**
alanine 291
alcohol-associated degeneration 252, *252*
Alexander's disease *260*
Alzheimer's disease CP6, 245–6, **246**
aminobutyrate 291
amphetamines *164*, 177–8, **178**
amyloid angiopathy 179, **180**, 247
amyotrophic lateral sclerosis 254
anaesthesia, children 45
anatomy of brain
 axial images **7–11**
 cerebellopontine angle **19**
 cerebral artery territories **20–1**
 computed tomography **12–16**
 coronal images **3–6**
 parasellar region **16–17**
 pineal region **18**
 sagittal images **1–2**
 suprasellar cistern **16–17**
aneurysms 33, *165*, 170–2
 catheter angiography 166, **168**, 170, 171, 175
 extra-axial haemorrhage 163, *164*

haemorrhage in children 182, **184**
 and hydrocephalus 270
 interventional neuroradiology 182–3, **185**
 intraparenchymal haemorrhage *165*, 171, 172–3
 mycotic 231–2
 or pituitary adenomas 130, **132**
 subarachnoid haemorrhage 163, **164**, **167**, **169**, 170–2
 subdural haemorrhage 171
angiographically occult vascular malformations 174, **175**, **176**, 182
angiomas
 cavernous 174, **175**, 182
 venous 174
angiopathies *187*, 204–5
 amyloid 179, **180**, 247
 moyamoya disease CP8, 204
apparent diffusion coefficient (ADC) 286–7, **287**, **288**
aqueduct stenosis 271, **271**, **276**
arachnoid cysts **36**, 126, **128**, 160, **161**
Arnold–Chiari (Chiari II) malformation 47, **47**, **277**
arterial dissection
 craniocervical 203
 extra-axial haemorrhage *164*
arterial stenoses, perfusion imaging CP4, **282**
arteriovenous fistulae 95
arteriovenous malformations (AVM)
 calcification 39
 haemorrhage *165*, 172–3, **173**, 174–5
  children 182, **183**
  extra-axial 163, *164*
  hypertensive patients 176, **177**
 interventional neuroradiology 183–4, **185**
 intraventricular 119, **121**
 Osler–Weber–Rendu syndrome 182, **183**
aspartate signals **289**, **290**, 291
aspergillosis 236–7
astrocytomas
 calcification 38, 99
 children 24, 140–2, **143**, 145
 ependymal seeding 30
 giant cell **29**, 104, **105**, 115, 270, **270**
 and hydrocephalus 270, **270**, 271
 intraventricular **28**, **29**, 115
 magnetization transfer imaging 286
 and neurofibromatosis 55–6, 58
 perfusion imaging **284**

supratentorial intra-axial 99–103, **100–3**, 104, **105**, 106
 tuberous sclerosis 29, 59, **60**
autism 252
axial images **7–11**
axial region
 parasellar lesions 33
 suprasellar lesions 32, 33

bacterial endocarditis 231, **232**
basal ganglia diseases 249–51, **251**, *252*
basilar tip aneurysms 171
Behçet's disease 103, 113
benign enlargement of subarachnoid spaces 273–4, **274**
benign intracranial hypertension 273
Binswanger disease 199, **201**
birth trauma 179–80
block paradigm, functional imaging CP10, 285
BOLD (blood oxygen level dependent) imaging CP11, 285
bone infections 96
bovine spongiform encephalopathy (BSE) 235
brain anatomy *see* anatomy of brain
brain injuries *see* traumatic injuries
brainstem gliomas 24, *141*, 145, **146**
brainstem haematomas 84, **86**
brainstem infarction 196, **196**
Brix model, endothelial permeability 284
'butterfly' gliomas 99, **100**

calcification **38–9**
 choroid plexus 38, 116, 151, 266
 craniopharyngiomas 38, 131, **133**
 cytomegalovirus 39, 213, **213**
 giant cell astrocytomas 29, 104, **105**
 gliomas 38, 99, 103, 104, **105**
 HIV 215, **215**
 pineal region tumours 120, 121
 Sturge–Weber syndrome 39, 62
 toxoplasmosis 39, 214, **214**
 tuberous sclerosis **30**, 59, **60**
Canavan's disease 259, *260*
capillary telangiectasias 174, 182
carotid endarterectomy 202
carotid stenosis CP4
catheter angiography
 cerebral ischaemia 202
 haemorrhage 166, 168, **168**, 170, 171, 175

cavernous angiomas 174, **175**, 182
central neurocytomas
    and hydrocephalus 270
    intraventricular 28, 114, 115, **115**, 116
central neurofibromatosis
    (neurofibromatosis type 2) 55, 57–8,
    57, **58**
central pontine myelinosis 258, **260**
cephaloceles 45–6, **46**
cerebellar lobes, anatomy **20–1**
cerebellar tonsils 46–7, 272
cerebello-olivary degeneration *252*
cerebellopontine angle (CPA) anatomy **19**
cerebellopontine angle (CPA) tumours 34,
    152–5, *153*, 158–9
cerebral abscesses *see* abscesses
cerebral amyloid angiopathy 179, **180**, 247
cerebral arterial ectasia 203–4, **204**
cerebral artery territory anatomy **20–1**
cerebral atrophy
    ageing brain 241
    dementias 245, 246–7, **246**, **247**
    after traumatic injury 96
cerebral cortex, functional imaging
    CPs10–11, 285, **285**
cerebral infarction *see* infarction
cerebral ischaemia 187
    angiopathies 204–5
    cerebral arterial ectasia 203–4, **204**
    craniocervical arterial dissection 203
    diffusion weighted imaging 286
    imaging strategies 202–3
    traumatic injury 92–3, **93**
    see also infarction
cerebral lobes, anatomy **20–1**
cerebral neuroblastomas *see* primitive
    neuroectodermal tumours
cerebral perfusion imaging CPs3–9, 280–4
cerebritis 227, 230–1
cerebromalacia 81, 94, **94**
cerebrospinal fluid
    in hydrocephalus *see* hydrocephalus
    physiology 266–7
cerebrospinal fluid fistulae 94
cervical spine injuries 75–6
chemodectomas *see* paragangliomas
chemotherapy-induced disease 262, 264,
    264
chest, traumatic injuries 76
Chiari malformations 46–7, **46**, **47**, 272, **277**
children
    cerebral abscesses 230
    cerebral infarction 207–10, **208–10**
    cerebral venous infarction 205–6, 227
    choroid plexus papillomas 28
    congenital abnormalities *see* congenital
        abnormalities
    congenital infections 212–15
    craniopharyngiomas **32**, 131, **133**
    diffusion weighted imaging 286–7
    dysembryoplastic neuroepithelial
        tumours 106, **106**
    ependymomas **25**, 114, 145–6, **147–8**
    epilepsy surgery 289–90, **290**
    gangliogliomas 108
    gliomas 23, 24
        astrocytomas **24**, 140–2, *141*, **142**, **143**,
        145

xanthoastrocytomas 103–4
haemorrhage **163**, 179–82, *180*, **181**, **183**,
    184
hamartomas 30
head injuries 77, **78**, **85**
hydrocephalus 266, 268–9
    communicating 273–4
    non-communicating **269**, 271, 272
    treatment **276**, 277
leukodystrophies 258–62
meningiomas 123
meningitis 222, 225, 226–7, **228–9**, 229
    hydrocephalus **272**, 273
pineal cell tumours 121
pineal germ cell tumours 120
primitive neuroectodermal tumours 108
    medulloblastomas **24**, 142–5, **143**, **144**
sedation 45
tuberculosis 229, 236
choline-containing compound signals CP12,
    289, 290, **290**
chordomas 156–7, **157**
choroidal cysts 118, **120**
choroid plexus
    calcification **38**, 116, 151, 266
    CSF physiology 266, 267, 275
    villous hyperplasia 275
choroid plexus carcinomas 116
choroid plexus cysts 28, 269
choroid plexus papillomas
    and hydrocephalus 116, 269, 275, **275**
    infratentorial intra-axial *141*, 151, **151**,
    152
    intraventricular **28**, 116, **117**
    or schwannomas 154
clivus meningioma 32
clover leaf skull deformity 52
coagulopathies *164*, 173
cocaine *164*, 177–8, 205
coccidioidomycosis 237
Cockayne's syndrome 259, *260*
colloid cysts **28**, 117–18, **118**, **119**
    and hydrocephalus 28, 269–70, **270**
colpocephaly **66**, 69
communicating artery aneurysms **170**, 171
congenital abnormalities 44
    cephaloceles 45–6, **46**
    Chiari malformations 46–7, **46**, **47**, 272,
    277
    in corpus callosum **66**, **67**, 69
    cortical dysplasia **65**, 67, 213
    craniosynostosis 51–2, **53**, **54**
    CT techniques 44–5, 52, 59, 62
    Dandy-Walker complex 50–1, **51**, 272
    dorsal induction disorders 45–7, 272, **277**
    grey matter diseases 249–51, 254
    grey matter heterotopia **64**, 65–7
    holoprosencephaly 47–9, **48**, **49**
    infections 212–15
    Joubert syndrome 51, **52**
    lissencephaly 62, **64**
    megalencephaly 52, 54–5, **54**
    MR techniques 44
        craniosynostosis 52
        myelination 70–1, *70*
        neurofibromatosis 57, 58, *58*
        Sturge-Weber syndrome 62
        tuberous sclerosis 59

Von Hippel-Lindau disease 62
myelination **68–9**, 70–1, **70**
neuronal migration disorders 62–9, 213
phakomatoses 44, 55
    melanocytic 62
    neurofibromatosis 55–8, **55–8**
    Sturge-Weber syndrome 39, 62, **63**
    tuberous sclerosis 29, **30**, 58–9, **59**, **60**,
    270
    vascular 62, 182
    Von Hippel-Lindau disease **25**, 59–62,
    61, 147, 149
pial arteriovenous malformations **173**,
    174, 182
polymicrogyria **65**, 67, 213
rhombencephalosynapsis 51
schizencephaly **65**, 67
septo-optic dysplasia 49, **49–50**
ventral induction disorders 47–52, 272
white matter diseases 258–62, *263*
congenital cysts
    arachnoid **36**, 126, **128**, 160, **161**
    dermoids 158, 159
    epidermoids **34**, 126, 128, 152, *153*,
    158–9
contrast-enhanced CT, perfusion imaging 282
contrast-enhanced MRI
    cerebral infarction 190–1, **191**, 192–3
    cerebral venous infarction 207
    congenital abnormalities 44, 57, 58, 62
    haemorrhagic infarction 194, **195**
    perfusion imaging CPs3–9, 281–4, **281**
    supratentorial tumours 98, 99
        astrocytomas 100, 102–3
        metastases 110, 112, **112**, 113
        pituitary 126–7, **129–30**, 130
contusions 80, 81, **81–3**, 84, 87, 90
coronal images
    brain anatomy **3–6**
    supratentorial tumours 99
corpus callosum
    congenital anomalies **66**, **67**, 69
    and lacunar infarcts 199
cortex, functional imaging CPs10–11, 285,
    285
cortical dysplasia (polymicrogyria) **65**, 67,
    213
cortical tubers, tuberous sclerosis 59, **59**
cranial nerve, scan protocols *138*, *139*
cranial nerve schwannomas
    acoustic *see* acoustic schwannomas
    in neurofibromatosis **55**, 57–8, 154
craniocervical arterial dissection 203, **204**
craniopharyngiomas **32**
    calcification **38**, 131, **133**
    and hydrocephalus 270
    intraventricular 131, **134**
    magnetization transfer imaging 286
    supratentorial 131–6, **133–4**
craniosynostosis 51–2, **53**, **54**, 277
creatine signals CP12, **289**, 290, **290**
Creutzfeldt-Jakob disease 235
cryptococcal infections 110, 118, 220, **224**,
    236
CT perfusion imaging 281–2
cysticercosis 118
cytomegalovirus (CMV) infection **39**, 212–13,
    213, 222

Dandy–Walker complex 50–1, **51**, 272
deconvolution technique 282
deep (diffuse) white matter hyperintensities
(DWMH) **26**, 243–4, 246, 248
dementia 245–8, **246–9**, *248*
  Alzheimer's disease CP6, 245–6, **246**
  normal pressure hydrocephalus 248, **249**,
    268, **269**, 274–5
demyelinating diseases
  central pontine myelinosis 258, **260**
  infective 257–8
    ADEM 113, 235–6, **235**, 258, **259**
    PML 215, 218, **224**, 258, **258**
  or lacunar infarcts 199
  multiple sclerosis **27**, **31**, 103, 113, 254–7,
    288
  periventricular hyperintensities 243
dermoids 158, *159*
Devic's disease 256
diffuse axonal injury CP2, 77–80, **77**, **78–80**,
  85
diffuse (deep) white matter hyperintensities
  (DWMH) **26**, 243–4, 246, 248
diffusion weighted imaging (DWI) 285,
  285–7, **287**, **288**
digital subtraction angiography 202–3
dolichocephaly 51
dorsal induction disorders 45–7, 272, **277**
drug abuse
  cerebral infarction 204–5
  and haemorrhage *164*, 176–8, **178**
  neurodegenerative disorders *252*
  septic emboli 231, **232**
Duplex carotid ultrasound 202
dural arteriovenous malformations 174–5
Duret haematomas 84, **86**
dynamic contrast-enhanced CT perfusion
  imaging 282
dynamic contrast-enhanced MR perfusion
  imaging CPs3–9, 281–4, **281**
dysembryoplastic neuroepithelial tumours
  (DNTs) 23, 103, 106, **106**, 108
dysplastic gangliocytoma of the cerebellum
  151

eccentric target sign 217–18, **218**
echinococcosis 238–9
echo planar imaging methods 281, 282
ecstasy 177–8
ectasia
  cerebral arterial 203–4, **204**
  in neurofibromatosis *55*
emboli, septic 231, **232**
empty triangle (delta) sign 206, **206**
empyemas
  extradural 37
  subdural **37**, 227, **228**
encephalitis 214, 232–6
endocarditis, bacterial 231, **232**
endothelial permeability, perfusion imaging
  CP9, 283–4
ependymal cysts 118
ependymal tumour seedlings 30
ependymomas
  children **25**, 114, 145–6, **147–8**
  and hydrocephalus 271
  infratentorial intra-axial **25**, 145–6, **147–8**
  intraventricular 114, **114**, 115

  in neurofibromatosis *55*, 58
  or schwannomas 154
epidermoid cysts
  infratentorial extra-axial **34**, 152, *153*,
    158–9, **159**, **160**
  supratentorial extra-axial 126, **128**
epilepsy
  scan protocols *137*, *138*
  spectroscopic imaging 289–90, **290**, 291
  after traumatic injury 96
EPISTAR 282
Epstein–Barr virus 234–5
état lacunaire (criblé) 247
extra-axial haemorrhage *see* haemorrhage,
  extra-axial
extra-axial lesions *see* infratentorial lesions,
  extra-axial; supratentorial lesions,
  extra-axial
extradural empyemas 37
extradural haemorrhage *see* haemorrhage,
  extradural

Fabry's disease *263*
facial fractures **74**, 75, **75**, 94
FAIR 282
fistulae, after trauma 94, *95*
flow sensitive alternating inversion recovery
  (FAIR) 282
foramen of Monro, hydrocephalus 269–70,
  270
Fragile X syndrome 252
Friedreich's ataxia *252*, 254
frontotemporal dementia 246–7, **247**
functional imaging CPs10–11, 284–5
fungal infections 236–7
  cryptococcus 110, 118, 220, **224**, 236

GABA 291
gangliocytomas 108
gangliogliomas **107**, 108
Gaucher's disease *263*
germ cell tumours 120, **122**, **123**, 271
germinal matrix haemorrhage 181–2
germinomas 120, **122**, **271**
giant cell astrocytomas
  and hydrocephalus 270, **270**
  intraventricular **29**, 115
  supratentorial intra-axial 104, **105**
  tuberous sclerosis 29, 59, **60**
glioblastomas 99, **284**
gliomas
  'butterfly' 99, **100**
  calcification 38, 99, 103, 104, **105**
  ependymal seeding 30
  gliomatosis cerebri 104, 106
  and hydrocephalus 270, **270**, 271
  infratentorial intra-axial 24
    children **24**, 140–2, **143**, 145, **146**
    oligodendrogliomas 151
  intraventricular **28**, **29**, 114, 115, 116–17,
    118
  magnetization transfer imaging 286
  in neurofibromatosis 55–6, **55**, 58
  perfusion imaging 283, 284, **284**
  pineal region 121–2, **125**
  spectroscopic imaging CP12
  supratentorial intra-axial **22**, 99–103, 104,
    105, 106, 108, 113

  supratentorial intraventricular 114, 115,
    116–17, **118**
  tectal plate 271
  and tuberous sclerosis 29, 59, **60**
gliomatosis cerebri 104, 106
glomus tumours *see* paragangliomas
glucose signals **289**, 290
glutamate signals **289**, 290
glutamine signals **289**, 290
grey matter diseases 245
  of basal ganglia 249–51, **251**, *252*
  dementia CP6, 245–8, **246–9**, *248*, 274–5
  mitochondrial encephalomyelopathies
    252–4, *252*
  temporal mesial sclerosis 251–2, **253**
  Wernicke's encephalopathy 252
grey matter heterotopias **31**, **64**, 65–7

haemangioblastomas
  and hydrocephalus 271
  infratentorial intra-axial **25**, *141*, 142, 147,
    149, **149**, **150**
  magnetization transfer imaging 286
  in Von Hippel–Lindau disease **25**, 60–2,
    61, 147, 149
haemangiopericytomas 155–6
haematomas 23
  or haemorrhagic tumours 173–4
  indications for CT in traumatic brain
    injury 76–7
  parenchymal 40–1, 43
  or haemorrhagic infarction 179, *179*
  see also haemorrhage, intraparenchymal
  subdural *see* haemorrhage, subdural
haemorrhage
  aneurysms *165*, 171–2
  catheter angiography 166, **168**, 170,
    170, 171, 175
  children 182, **184**
  interventional neuroradiology 182–3,
    185
  intraparenchymal haemorrhage *165*,
    171, 172–3
  subarachnoid haemorrhage 163, **164**,
    167, 170–2, **170**
  children 163, 179–82, *180*, **181**, **183**, **184**
  extra-axial 37, **37**, 162–4
  extradural 162
    extra-axial 162, **163**
    supratentorial extra-axial 37
    traumatic **82**, 84, **85**, **89**, 90
  and hydrocephalus 271, 272
  imaging pathophysiology 165–7, *169*
  imaging protocols 167–70
  infratentorial 165, *165*
  interventional neuroradiology 182–4, **185**
  intraparenchymal 162, 165, **166**, **167**, 171,
    172–4
    cerebral amyloid angiopathy 179, **180**,
      247
    haematoma or haemorrhagic tumour
      173–4, **173**
    hypertensive 173, 175–6, **177**
    infarction 178–9, **178**, *179*, **179**
    substance abuse 176–8, **178**
    vascular malformations 172–3, 174–5,
      176, **177**, 182, 183–4

haemorrhage – *continued*
    intraventricular 162, 171
        extra-axial 164, **165**
        traumatic 84–5
    maturation on imaging 84, *86*, 169
    and metastases 113, *164*, 173–4, **173**
    subarachnoid 162, 163, *164*, *169*, 170–1
        CT pathophysiology 166
        CT protocols 168–70, **169**, *170*
        extra-axial 163, **164**
        herniations 167
        neonates 180–1
        traumatic 86–7, **87**
    subdural **42**, 43, 162
        CT pathophysiology 166
        extra-axial **37**, 162–3, **163**
        non-traumatic causes *164*, 171
        with shunted hydrocephalus 277, **277**
        traumatic **83**, 87–90, **87–9**, 91
    supratentorial 37, **37**, 165, *165*
        into pituitary adenomas 128, 130, **130**
    in toxoplasmosis lesions 216, **221**
    traumatic intracerebral haematomas 81, **83**, 84, **84**, **85**, 86
haemorrhagic infarction 178–9, **178**, **179**, 194–5, **195**
Hallervorden–Spatz disease 249
hamartomas
    differential diagnoses 102, 115
    in tuberous sclerosis 29, **30**, 59, **59**
harlequin eye deformity 51
headaches, scan protocols *137*, *138*
head injuries *see* traumatic injuries
hepatic encephalopathy, spectroscopic imaging 291
herniations
    and intracranial haemorrhage **167**, 172
    after traumatic injury **86**, **89**, 90–2
herpes simplex (HSV) infections 39, 212, 214, 222, 232–4
heterotopias **31**, **64**, 65–7
high field magnets 291
hippocampal sclerosis 251–2, **253**
histiocytosis 103, **104**
HIV (human immunodeficiency virus) infection 215–16, **216–21**, **223**, **225**
    congenital 212, 215, **215**
holoprosencephaly 47–9, **48**, **49**
human immunodeficiency virus *see* HIV
Hunter's disease *263*
Huntington's disease 249
Hurler's disease *263*
hydatid cysts 238–9
hydrocephalus 266
    Chiari malformations 47, 272, **277**
    choroid plexus papillomas 116, 269, 275, **275**
    communicating type 266, 272–5
    with CSF overproduction 275
    Dandy–Walker complex 51, 272
    diagnosis 267–9, *267*, **268–9**
    meningitis 226, 229, **272**, 273
    non-communicating type 266, 269–72
    normal CSF physiology 266–7
    normal pressure 248, **249**, 268, **269**, 274–5
    shunt therapy 274, 275–8, **276**, **277**, **278**
    after traumatic injury 85, 92, 95

hyperperfusion syndrome CP7
hypertensive intraparenchymal haemorrhage 173, 175–6, **177**
hypoxia, profound neonatal **209**, 210
hypoxic–ischaemic syndrome 196, 198

infarction **22**, **27**, 187, 188–9
    absent flow void 190, **190**
    AIDS patients 222
    cerebral venous **22**, 205–7, **206**, **207**, 227
    children 207–10, **208–10**
    craniocervical arterial dissection 203, **204**
    cytotoxic oedema **189**, 190, 191
    drug abuse 204–5
    evolution 189–94, **189–94**
    fogging effect 193–4, **193**
    gadolinium enhancement 190–1, **191**, 193
    gliosis 194, **194**
    gyral hyperintensity 194, **194**
    haemorrhagic 178–9, **178**, **179**, 194–5, **195**
    hyperdense middle cerebral artery 190, **191**
    iodinated contrast medium 192–3
    lacunar 198–9, **200**, **201**
    magnetic resonance angiography 200–2, 207, **207**
    moya moya disease CP8, 204
    parenchymal change **189**, 190, 191–2, **192**
    posterior circulation 196, **196**, **197**, 198
    and strokes 187
    systemic lupus erythematosus 204
    after traumatic injury 92, **92**, 93, **93**
    vascular dementia 247
    vasogenic oedema 191
    Wallerian degeneration **190**, 194
    watershed 196, 198, **199**
infections 212
    in AIDS patients 110, 215–22
    cerebral abscesses 230–2, **231**, **232**
    congenital 212–15
    cytomegalovirus 39, 212–13, **213**, 222
    demyelinating 215, 218, **224**, 235–6, 258
    encephalitis 214, 232–6
    fungal 236–7
        cryptococcus 110, 118, 220, **224**, 236
    herpes simplex 39, 212, 214, 222, 232–4
    HIV 212, 215–16, **216–21**, **223**, **225**
    and hydrocephalus 226, 229, 272, 273, 276, **277**
    or lymphomas 110, 216–18, **222**, **223**
    meningitis *see* meningitis
    parasitic 237–9, **237**
    PML 215, 218, **224**, 258, **258**
    rubella 39, 214–15
    sarcoidosis **238**, 239, **239**, 273
    syphilis 110, 220
    toxoplasmosis 39, 212, 213–14, 215, 216–18, **217–21**
    after traumatic injury 95–6
    tuberculosis 220, 222, **225**, 229, **230**, 236, **272**
infective demyelination 257–8
    ADEM 113, 235–6, **235**, 258, **259**
    PML 215, 218, **224**, 258, **258**
inflammatory parasellar masses **135**, 136
infratentorial haemorrhage 165, *165*

infratentorial lesions 140
    extra-axial 152
        chordomas 156–7, **157**
        congenital cysts **34**, 152, *153*, 158–60, **161**
        haemangiopericytomas 155–6
        lipomas 158
        meningiomas **34**, *153*, 154–5, **156**
        metastases *153*, 154
        normal structure 35
        paragangliomas **35**, *153*, 154, 158, **158**, **159**
        schwannomas **34**, 152–4, *153*, **155**, **156**
    intra-axial
        in adults 142, 146–9
        astrocytomas **24**, 140–2, *141*, **142**, **143**, 145
        brainstem gliomas **24**, *141*, 145, **146**
        in children 140–6, 151
        choroid plexus papillomas *141*, 151, **151**, **152**
        dysplastic gangliocytoma of cerebellum 151
        ependymomas **25**, *141*, 145–6, **147–8**
        haemangioblastomas **25**, *141*, 142, 147, 149, **149**, **150**
        medulloblastomas **24**, *141*, 142–5, **143**, **144**
        metastases *141*, 146–7, 149, 150
        oligodendrogliomas 151
        subependymomas 150
inositol signals **289**, 291
internal auditory meatus (IAM) 34, **35**, 154, **154**, **155**
internal carotid artery bifurcation aneurysms 171
interventional neuroradiology 182–4, **185**
intra-axial lesions *see* infratentorial lesions, intra-axial; supratentorial lesions, intra-axial
intracranial haemorrhage *see* haemorrhage
intracranial pressure
    hydrocephalus 266
    meningitis 226, **226**
    scan protocols *137*
    after traumatic injury 90, 91, 92
intraparenchymal haemorrhage *see* haemorrhage, intraparenchymal
intraventricular haemorrhage *see* haemorrhage, intraventricular
intraventricular lesions
    arteriovenous malformations 119, **121**
    astrocytomas **28**, **29**, 115
    central neurocytomas 28, 114, 115, **115**, 116
    choroid plexus papillomas **28**, 116, **117**, 269
    craniopharyngiomas 131, **134**
    cysts **28**, 117–18, **118**, **119**, **120**
    ependymomas 114, **114**, 115
    gliomas **28**, 116–17, **118**
    and hydrocephalus 116, 269, 271
    meningiomas **29**, 114, 115–16, **116**
    metastases 119
    subependymomas 114–15
iron deposition 244–5, **245**
ischaemia 187
    angiopathies 204–5

cerebral arterial ectasia 203–4, **204**
deep white matter hyperintensities 244
diffusion weighted imaging 286
imaging strategies 202–3
traumatic injury 92–3, **93**
see also infarction

Joubert syndrome 51, **52**

kleeblattschadel deformity 52
Krabbe's disease 259, *260*, 261, **261**

labyrinthine schwannomas 57–8
lacerating injuries 80–1, 84, **84**, 87
lactate signals CP12, 290–1
Langerhan's histiocytosis 103, **104**
Larsson model, endothelial permeability 284
Leigh's syndrome 251
leukoaraiosis 244
leukodystrophies 258–62
leukoencephalopathy 262, **264**
leukomalacia, periventricular **209**, 210
Lhermitte–Duclos disease 151
lipid metabolism disorders *263*
lipomas
    corpus callosum anomalies **67**, 69
    infratentorial extra-axial 158
    pineal region 120
lissencephaly 62, **64**
lumbar punctures 226
Lyme disease 236
lymphocytic adenohypophysitis 131
lymphomas 30, 108–10
    in AIDS patients 108, 110, 215, 216–18, **222**, **223**
    differential diagnoses
        astrocytomas 103
        meningiomas 110, 116, 125
        metastases 147, 149
        toxoplasmosis 110, 216–18, **222**
    metastatic 110, **111**

macrocephaly, benign enlargement of subarachnoid spaces 273–4, **274**
magnetic resonance spectroscopy (MRS) CP12, 287–91
magnetization transfer (MT) imaging 285–6
Marburg type multiple sclerosis 256
Maroteaux–Lamy syndrome *263*
measles infection 235, 258
medulloblastomas **24**, 108, *141*, 142
    children 142–5, **143**, **144**
    and hydrocephalus 271
megalencephaly 52, 54–5, **54**
melanocytic phakomatoses 62
melanomas, malignant **36**
MELAS syndrome 252–3, **253**
meningeal disease, diffuse **36**
meningiomas
    causing hydrocephalus 269, 270, **270**
    differential diagnoses 110, 114, 116, 125, 155
        pituitary adenomas 131, **132**
    infratentorial extra-axial **34**, *153*, 154–5, **156**
    intraventricular **29**, 114, 115–16, **116**
    in neurofibromatosis 55, **57**, 58
    parasellar **134**, 136

perfusion imaging **284**
suprasellar **32**, 131, **132**
supratentorial extra-axial **36**, 122–5, **126**, **127**, **128**
supratentorial intraventricular 114, 115–16, **116**
meningitis 222, 225–6, **226**, **227**
    acute lymphacytic 229
    chronic 229, **230**
    complications 226–7, **228**, **229**
    cryptococcal 220
    differential diagnoses 110, 226
    and hydrocephalus 226, 229, **272**, 273
    lumbar punctures 226
    after traumatic injury 95
    tuberculous 220, 222, **225**, 229, **230**, 272
MERRF syndrome 253
metabolic disease, calcification **38**
metachromatic leukodystrophy *260*, 261, **261**
metastases
    AIDS patients 222
    and haemorrhage 113, *164*, 173–4, **173**
    and hydrocephalus 271
    infratentorial extra-axial *153*, 154
    infratentorial intra-axial *141*, 146–7, 149, 150
    supratentorial extra-axial **36**, 125
    supratentorial intra-axial **22**, 103, 110, **111**, 112–13, **112**, **113**
    supratentorial intraventricular 119
metastatic lymphomas 110, **111**
methylene dioxymethylamphetamine 177–8
microcephaly, congenital infections 213, 214
middle cerebral artery aneurysms **167**, 171
middle cerebral artery hyperdensity 190, **191**
mitochondrial encephalomyelopathies 252–4, *252*
motor neuron disease 254
moyamoya disease CP8, 204
MR perfusion imaging CPs3–9, 281–4, **281**
mucopolysaccharidoses *263*
mucormycosis 236–7
multiple sclerosis **27**, 254–7, **255**, **256**, **257**
    or astrocytomas 103
    diffusion weighted imaging **288**
    or metastases 113
    periventricular lesions **31**, 255, **257**
multisystem atrophy (Parkinson plus syndromes) 250–1, **251**, *252*
mycotic aneurysms 231–2
myelination
    ageing brain 241
    congenital disorders **68–9**, 70–1, **70**

neonates
    cerebral abscesses 230
    cerebral infarction 207, **209**, 210
    cerebral venous infarction 205–6
    congenital infections 212–15
    diffusion weighted imaging 286–7
    haemorrhage 179–82, *180*, 182
    hamartomas 30
    hydrocephalus 271
    leukodystrophies 259
    meningitis 222, 225, 226–7
    sedation 45

nerve lesions, scan protocols *139*
nerve palsies, scan protocols *138*
nerve sheath tumours *see* neurofibromas; schwannomas
neurinomas *see* schwannomas
neurocutaneous melanosis 110
neurocutaneous syndromes *see* phakomatoses
neurocysticercosis 237–8, **237**
neurocytomas 28, 114, 115, **115**, 116, 270
neurodegenerative diseases 241, 245
    of basal ganglia 249–51, **251**, *252*
    dementia CP6, 245–8, **246–9**, *248*, 274–5
    mitochondrial encephalomyelopathies 252–4, *252*
    temporal mesial sclerosis 251–2, **253**
    Wernicke's encephalopathy 252
    see also white matter diseases
neurofibromas 33, *55*, 56
neurofibromatosis 55–8, **55–8**
    schwannomas in 33, *55*, 57–8, **57**, **58**, 154
neuromyelitis optica 256
neurosarcoidosis 238, 239, **239**, 273
neurosyphilis 220
neurulation disorders, primary 45–7
    Chiari malformations 46–7, **46**, **47**, 272, **277**
normal pressure hydrocephalus 248, **249**, 268, **269**, 274–5

olfactory groove meningiomas **32**
oligodendrogliomas
    calcification 38, 99, 103, **105**
    infratentorial intra-axial 151
    supratentorial intra-axial 99, 103, **105**
    ventricular 28, 114, 116, **118**
olivopontocerebellar degeneration 250, **251**, *252*
optic nerve gliomas 55–6, **55**
Osler–Weber–Rendu syndrome 182, **183**

pachygyric lissencephaly 62
pachymeningeal fibrosis 277, **278**
paediatric imaging *see* children
palsies, scan protocols *138*
paragangliomas (glomus tumours)
    infratentorial extra-axial **35**, *153*, 154, 158, **158**, **159**
    or schwannomas 154
parasellar region
    anatomy **16–17**
    axial lesions **33**
    supratentorial lesions **134**, **135**, 136
parasitic infections 237–9, **237**
parenchymal haematomas *see* haematomas, parenchymal
Parkinson plus syndromes 250–1, **251**, *252*
Parkinson's disease 249–50
Pelizaeus–Merzbacher syndrome 259, *260*
perfusion imaging CPs3–9, 280–4
pericallosal artery aneurysms 171–2, **172**
periventricular hyperintensities (PVH) **26**, 243, **244**, 246, 248
phakomatoses 44, 55
    melanocytic 62
    neurofibromatosis 55–8, **55–8**
    Sturge–Weber syndrome 39, 62, **63**

phakomatoses – *continued*
   tuberous sclerosis 29, **30**, 58–9, **59**, **60**, **270**
   vascular 62, 182
   Von Hippel–Lindau disease **25**, 59–62, **61**, 147, 149
pial arteriovenous malformations **173**, 174, 182
pinealoblastomas 121
pinealocytomas 121, **124**, 271
pineal region 119–20
   anatomy **18**
   cysts 122, 271
   germ cell tumours 120, **122**, **123**
   gliomas 121–2, **125**
   pineal cell tumours 121, **124**, 271
   tumours causing hydrocephalus 271
pituitary masses **32**
   abscesses 131, **133**
   adenomas **32**, 126–31, **132**, 270
plagiocephaly 51, **53**
pneumocephalus 90, **91**
polymicrogyria **65**, 67, 213
pontine myelinosis 258, **260**
post-concussion syndrome 96
posterior fossa
   common neoplasms **24**, **25**, **34**
   congenital anomalies 50–1, **50**, 51, **52**, 272
   normal structures **35**
   see also infratentorial lesions
posterior inferior cerebellar artery aneurysms (PICAs) 171
PRESTO technique 281
primitive neuroectodermal tumours (PNETs) 108
   differential diagnoses 103, 108, **108**, 114
   and hydrocephalus 269, 271
   medulloblastomas **24**, 142–5, **143**, **144**
progressive multifocal leukoencephalopathy (PML) 215, 218, **224**, 258, **258**
progressive supranuclear palsy 250
proton spectroscopy CP12, 287–91
pseudoaneurysms 95, **95**
pseudotumour cerebri 273

quantification of contrast enhancement 284, **284**
quantitative imaging of perfusion using single subtraction (QUIPPS) 282

radiotherapy-induced disease 113, 262, **263**
raised intracranial pressure *see* intracranial pressure
Rathke pouch cysts 136
relaxivity effects, perfusion imaging 283–4, **283**
rhombencephalosynapsis 51
rubella 39, 214–15

sagittal images **1–2**
Sanfilippo's syndrome *263*
sarcoidosis **238**, 239, **239**, 273
scaphocephaly 51, **53**
Schilder type multiple sclerosis 256–7
schizencephaly **65**, 67
schwannomas **33**, **135**, 136
   and hydrocephalus 271, **272**

infratentorial extra-axial **34**, 152–4, *153*, **155**, **156**
   in neurofibromatosis **33**, **55**, 57–8, **57**, **58**, 154
   perfusion imaging CP5, **283**, **284**
sedation, children 45
seizures, scan protocols *138*
sellar lesions
   axial region **32**
   craniopharyngiomas 131–6, **133–4**
   pituitary adenomas 126–31, **129–30**, **131**, **132**
septic emboli 231, **232**
septo-optic dysplasia 49, **49–50**
shunt therapy, hydrocephalus 274, 275–8, **276**, **277**, **278**
Shy–Drager syndrome 250
sickle cell disease 204, **205**
single photon emission CT (SPECT) 280
   Alzheimer's disease CP6
   head injuries CP1, 77, **78**, 96
      contusions 81
      perfusion changes CP2, 93–4, **93**
      subdural haemorrhage 88, **91**
sinovenous occlusion, cerebral 205–7
skull fractures 74–5
slit ventricle syndrome 277
Sly syndrome *263*
spectroscopy CP12, 287–91
spinal injuries 75–6
spin tagging 282
spongiform encephalopathy 235
striatonigral degeneration 250
strokes 187–8
   cerebral imaging strategies 202
   diffusion weighted imaging 286, **287**
   haemorrhagic infarction 178–9, **178**, *179*, **179**
   perfusion imaging 283
   spectroscopic imaging 290–1
   vascular dementia 247
Sturge–Weber syndrome 39, 62, **63**
subacute leukoencephalopathy 262, **264**
subacute necrotizing encephalomyelopathy 251
subacute sclerosing panencephalitis 235
subarachnoid haemorrhage *see* haemorrhage, subarachnoid
subarachnoid spaces, benign enlargement 273–4, **274**
subcortical ischaemic encephalopathy (Binswanger disease) 199, **201**
subdural effusions, meningitis 227
subdural empyema **37**, 227, **228**
subdural haematomas *see* haemorrhage, subdural
subependymal giant cell astrocytomas (SGCAs) 29, 59, **60**
subependymal nodules (SENs) 29, **30**, 59, **60**, **270**
subependymomas 114–15, 150
substance abuse
   cerebral infarction 204–5
   and haemorrhage *164*, 176–8, **178**
   neurodegenerative disorders 252, *252*
   septic emboli 231, **232**
sudanophilic leukodystrophies 259, *260*
suprasellar cistern **16–17**

suprasellar lesions, axial region **32**, **33**
   see also craniopharyngiomas
supratentorial haemorrhage 37, **37**, 165, *165*
   into pituitary adenomas 128, 130, **130**
supratentorial lesions 98
   CT principles 98–9
   CT scan protocols *137–9*
   extra-axial **36–7**, 122
      congenital cysts **36**, 126, **128**
      meningiomas **36**, 122–5, **126**, **127**, **128**
   intra-axial **22–3**, 122
      abscesses **23**, 103, 113
      aesthesioneuroblastomas 110
      dysembryoplastic neuroepithelial tumours 103, 106, 108
      ganglioglioma **107**, 108
      gliomas **22**, 99–104, **105**, 106, 108, 113
      infarcts **22**, 103
      lymphomas 103, 108–10, **111**
      metastases **22**, 103, 110, **111**, 112–13
      primitive neuroectodermal tumours 103, 108, **108**
   intraventricular 114
      arteriovenous malformations 119, **121**
      central neurocytomas 114, 115, **115**, 116
      choroid plexus papillomas 116, **117**
      cysts 117–18, **118**, **119**, **120**
      ependymomas 114, **114**, 115
      gliomas 116–17, **118**
      meningiomas 114, 115–16, **116**
      metastases 119
      subependymomas 114–15
   MRI principles 99
   MRI scan protocols *137–9*
   parasellar **33**, **134**, **135**, 136
   pineal region 119–22, **123**, **124**, **125**
   pituitary abscesses 131, **133**
   sellar region
      craniopharyngiomas 131–6, **133–4**
      pituitary adenomas 126–31, **129–30**, **131**, **132**
syphilis 110, 220
systemic lupus erythematosus (SLE) 113, 204

tapeworm infection 237–8, **237**
^{99m}Tc HMPAO 280
tectal plate tumours 271
temporal mesial sclerosis 251–2, **253**
teratomas, pineal 120, **123**
thalamo-ventricular haemorrhage 181
third ventriculostomy 276, **276**, 278
Tofts model, endothelial permeability 284, **284**
TORCH 39, 212–15
toxoplasmosis 39, 212, 213–14, 215, 216–18, **217–21**
tracer kinetic models 281–2, **281**
transient ischaemic attack (TIA) 187
traumatic injuries 73
   abscesses after 95
   arteriovenous fistulae after 95
   brain displacement after **86**, **88**, 90
   cerebral atrophy after 96
   cerebromalacia after 81, 94, **94**
   cerebrospinal fluid fistulae 94
   cervical spine assessment 75–6
   chest assessment 76

classification 73–4, *74*
contusions 80, 81, **81–3**, 84, 87, 90
diffuse axonal injury CP2, 77–80, 85
epilepsy after 96
extradural haemorrhage **82**, **85**, **89**, 90
facial skeleton **74**, 75, **75**, 94
generalized hemisphere swelling 92
haemorrhage
    extradural **82**, 84, **85**, **89**, 90
    intracerebral haematomas 81, **83**, 84, **84**, **85**, **86**
    intraventricular 84–5
    maturation on imaging 84, *86*
    subarachnoid 86–7, **87**
    subdural **83**, 87–90, **87**, **88–9**, **91**
herniation **86**, **89**, 90–2
hydrocephalus 85, 92, 95
indications for CT 76–7, 96
indications for MRI 77, 96
infarcts 92, **92**, 93, **93**
infections 95–6
ischaemic damage 92–3, **93**
lacerations 80–1, 84, **84**, 87
perfusion changes CP2, 93–4, **93**
plain radiography 74–5
pneumocephalus 90, **91**
post-concussion syndrome 96
pseudoaneurysms 95, **95**
raised intracranial pressure 90, 91, 92
skull 74–5, 95
SPECT CP1, 77, **78**, 96
    contusions 81
    perfusion changes CP2, 93–4, **93**
    subdural haemorrhage 88, **91**
subdural haemorrhage **87**, 88, **88**, 90
vascular damage 92–4, 95, **95**
trigeminal nerve
    scan protocols *139*
    schwannomas **135**, 154, **156**
    in neurofibromatosis **33**, 57, **57**
trigonocephaly 51, **53**

tuberculosis 220, 222, **225**, 236
    differential diagnoses 110, 113
    multiple tuberculomas **236**
    tuberculous meningitis 220, 222, **225**, 229, **230**, **272**
tuberculum sella meningioma **32**
tuberous sclerosis 29, **30**, 58–9, **59**, **60**
    and hydrocephalus **270**
tubers
    or astrocytomas 102
    tuberous sclerosis 59, **59**

unilateral megalencephaly 52, 54–5, **54**
uninverted FAIR (UNFAIR) 282

varicela zoster virus 222
vascular damage, traumatic injury 92–4, 95, **95**
vascular dementia 247–8, *248*, **248**
vascular malformations
    calcification **39**
    congenital 62, 182
    haemorrhage *165*, 172–3, **173–6**, 174–5
        children 182, **183**
        extra-axial 163, *164*
        hypertensive patients 176, **177**
        interventional neuroradiology 183–4, **185**
        intraventricular 119, **121**
vasculitis *164*, 204–5
venous angiomas 174
venous infarction **22**, 205–7, **206**, **207**, 227
ventricular shunts 274, 275–8, **276**, **277**, **278**
ventriculitis
    meningitis 226–7
    shunt infection 276, **277**
ventriculomegaly 267–9, *267*
ventriculostomy 276, **276**, 278
Virchow–Robin spaces (VRS) **26**, 198–9, **201**
    ageing brain 242–3, *242–3*, **244**
visual cortex, functional imaging CP10, 285, **285**

Von Hippel–Lindau (VHL) disease **25**, 59–62, **61**, 147, 149
Von Recklinghausen disease (neurofibromatosis type 1) 55–7, **55**, **56**

water, diffusion weighted imaging 286–7
Wernicke's encephalopathy 252
Whipple's disease 103, 113
white matter
    diffuse (deep) hyperintensities **26**, 243–4, 246, 248
    diffusion weighted imaging 286–7
    periventricular hyperintensities **26**, 243, **244**, 246, 248
    unidentified neurofibromatosis objects **55**, 56
white matter diseases 241, 254
    central pontine myelinosis 258, **260**
    chemotherapy-induced 262, 264, **264**
    diffusion weighted imaging 287
    infective demyelination 257–8
        ADEM 235–6, 258, **259**
        PML 215, 218, **224**, 258, **258**
    leukodystrophies 258–62
    multiple sclerosis **27**, **31**, 103, 113, 254–7, **288**
    radiotherapy-induced 262, **263**
    tuberous sclerosis 59
Wilson's disease 249, **250**

xanthoastrocytomas 103–4, **105**
xenon enhanced CT 280–1